S0-DIS-498

Basic Issues in Hearing

The **8th International Symposium on Hearing** has been sponsored by the *Rijksuniversiteit Groningen*, the *Royal Netherlands Academy of Arts and Sciences*, the *Heinsius-Houbolt Fund*, the Foundation *Steun het Gehoorgestoorde Kind*, the Foundation *Keel-, Neus- en Oorheelkunde*, the Foundation *Groninger Universiteitsfonds*, and the companies *Tracor Europa* and *Bernafon Nederland B.V.*

Colophon:
Text layout by Alja Mensink.
All authors used word processors to develop their papers, and submitted the manuscripts either on diskette or through international computer net using the EARN-link in Groningen. The text files, produced with a dozen different word processors, were translated using R-DOC/X™ (Advanced Computer Innovations) or, in a few cases, 'manually', to PC-Write™ (Quicksoft). PC-Write version 2.71 was tailored to optimize printout on a Hewlett-Packard LaserJet™ II printer, using HP's K-(Times Roman™ and mathematical) and U-(Helvetica™)-fontcartridges. hd.

Previous symposia:

1. 1969: Driebergen, Netherlands. *Frequency Analysis and Periodicity Detection in Hearing*. Edited by R.Plomp and G.F.Smoorenburg (Sijthoff, Leiden) 1970.
2. 1972: Eindhoven, Netherlands. *Hearing Theory*. Edited by B.L.Cardozo (I.P.O., Eindhoven).
3. 1974: Tutzing, F.R.Germany. *Facts and Models in Hearing*. Edited by E.Zwicker and E.Terhardt (Springer Verlag, Berlin).
4. 1977: Keele, Great Britain. *Psychophysics and Physiology of Hearing*. Edited by E.F.Evans and J.P.Wilson (Academic Press, London).
5. 1980: Noordwijkerhout, Netherlands. *Psychophysical, Physiological and Behavioural Studies in Hearing*. Edited by G.van den Brink and F.A.Bilsen (Delft University Press, Delft).
6. 1983: Bad Nauheim, F.R.Germany. *Hearing- Physiological Bases and Psychophysics*. Edited by R.Klinke and R.Hartmann (Springer Verlag, Berlin).
7. 1986: Cambridge, Great Britain. *Auditory Frequency Selectivity*. Edited by B.C.J.Moore and R.D.Patterson (Plenum Press, New York).

RF290
I58
1988

Basic Issues in Hearing

Proceedings of the 8th International Symposium on Hearing

Paterswolde, Netherlands, April 5–9, 1988

Edited by

H. Duifhuis
Biophysics Department
University of Groningen
The Netherlands

J. W. Horst and H. P. Wit
Institute of Audiology
University Hospital Groningen
The Netherlands

NO LONGER THE PROPERTY
OF THE
UNIVERSITY OF R.I. LIBRARY
18787416

1988

Academic Press
Harcourt Brace Jovanovich, Publishers
London San Diego New York Berkeley Boston
Sydney Tokyo Toronto

ACADEMIC PRESS LIMITED
24/28 Oval Road, London NW1 7DX

United States. Edition published by
ACADEMIC PRESS INC.
San Diego, CA 92101

Copyright © 1988 by
ACADEMIC PRESS LIMITED
All rights reserved. No part of this book may be reproduced
in any form by photostat, microfilm, or any other means,
without written permission from the publishers

ISBN: 0-12-223346-8

Printed in Great Britain by St Edmundsbury Press Limited
Bury St Edmunds, Suffolk

Preface

The 8th International Symposium on Hearing continues the European tradition, started in 1969, of organizing interdisciplinary symposia which focus on current issues in hearing. A comparison of the proceedings of the successive symposia (cf. p.*ii*) shows strong developments in this research field, which is emphasized by M.R. Schroeder on the following pages. The contributed papers, which were intermingled in the actual program in order to stimulate the interdisciplinary interaction, are presented in a more traditional order in this book: After the invited paper section (R. Plomp and E. Zwicker) the sections are arranged from peripheral to central issues in hearing.

At the previous meeting in Cambridge (1986) it was decided to organize the present one in Groningen in 1988 rather than in 1989, in order to get out of synchrony with the I.U.P.S. satellite symposia. From now on, it is the intention to go back to a three year cycle. The next symposium is planned near Bordeaux in 1992.

A successful symposium is impossible without the splendid cooperation of all participants, but also without esssential sponsoring (p.*ii*). We gratefully acknowledge that we had both. We also thank the section chairmen B. Scharf, I. Pollack, G.F. Smoorenburg, E.F. Evans and F.A. Bilsen for their cooperation. We acknowledge particularly the essential role of our organizing crew: ms. F. Slichter, ms. W. Kanis, P. van Dijk, P.J. Kuipers, J. van Maarseveen and H.M. Segenhout. Finally we appreciate the smooth and pleasant cooperation with Academic Press, which we contacted at an untimely late stage.

H. Duifhuis
J.W. Horst
H.P. Wit

Groningen, 10 May 1988.

Nineteen years and still growing - and growing younger*

Manfred R. Schroeder

Drittes Physikalisches Institut, University of Göttingen, F.R. Germany

Ladies and Gentlemen,
Dear Friends in HEARING!

Well, the Dutch have done it again!

Diek Duifhuis, Wiebe Horst and Hero Wit and their teams from Groningen have put together a most interesting and wide ranging scientific program and the social side, too, excels in every respect - as witness tonight's engaging concert and dinner.

The hotel is truly delightful, with most comfortable rooms, bikes for hire to circle the lake and an exotic swimming pool cum sauna. Our hearty thanks to our Dutch colleagues who made it all possible. And, of course, it is a great pleasure to see so many of our old friends again, friends from the Netherlands and from (almost) around the world.

This is the 8th Symposium on Hearing and the 4th held in "Holland" (if you forgive me for placing Eindhoven and Groningen in Holland). And as we pause to give thanks, we should remember particularly Reinier Plomp, who started it all in Driebergen in 1969 and Guido Smoorenburg the guiding hand behind Reinier.

Appropriately, the Driebergen meeting started off with three basic contributions from the two fields that underly our joint effects: physiology and psychophysics: Spoendlin and Keidel talked about the cochlea and the unforgettable Jan Schouten revisited the (perhaps I should say *his*) residue.

The influence that Jan has had on our field, and its strength in the Netherlands, through these symposia and through the creation of the Instituut voor Percerptie Onderzoek (IPO) at Eindhoven and through his many students is inestimable. I remember with particular pleasure Willem van Bergeijk (commonly mispronounced Vanbergic in the States) who was working with - hold your breath - *animals* at Bell Labs. (His killyfish seemed to be influenced by the phases of the *moon*, until it was revealed that the water in Willem's tank was changed precisely every four weeks. And I remember his and Capranica's bull frog cage labelled "Rana rana" on the outside and, on the inside, for the frogs to see, "Homo sapiens".)

Looking back over the last nineteen years, we can see that we have come a *long* way. The *residue*, which still occupied the first symposium, is laid to rest thanks to the combined efforts of De Boer, Cardozo and Ritsma, in particular.

* *After dinner speech at the 8th International Symposium on Hearing*

And *pitch perception* in general is now well understood with few if any mysteries left. In fact, even such astounding pitch paradoxes in which the pitch of a tone complex goes *down* when all frequencies are doubled [1] are satisfactory explained by the theories of Goldstein, Terhardt and Wightman. Monaural phase perception, too, is better understood now, although the great variety of different timbres engendered by monaural phase changes remain a goldmine for further research [2].

Since the Driebergen meeting, the emergence of new experimental techniques has benefitted our field in a variety of ways. *On-line signal processing* has given a great boost both to psychophysical and neurophysiological "data acquisition" (called simply *measurement* in the dark ages). Capacitive probes, laser interferometry and the Mössbauer method have sharpened our understanding of basilar membrane (BM) motion. Intracellular recording has given us our first inside view of hair cell potentials.

The *nonlinearity* of the BM, which first looked like a nonlinear compliance and then like a nonlinear *resistance*, stands now revealed, by otoacoustic emissions, as a saturating *active* mechanism. And at this meeting we have learned, from studies using the patch clamp method, that the active mechanism may be mediated by *outer hair cell (OHC) motility*. Thus, the OHCs have finally found their proper function, and so have the long puzzling efferent fibres.

We, the hearing people, used to be criticized as *poor cousins* of the visual community. But over the last twenty years, hearing *has* caught up with vision in its understanding of basic mechanisms. But where will the *future* lead us - or *we* it? Looking back, we recognize that much of our progress came from the judicious applications of new methods foreign to our field: on-line computing, laser interferometry, the Mössbauer method, intracellular recording, the patch clamp method and other supremely sensitive techniques. In the future we make further progress by drawing more heavily on the emergent understanding of *neural networks* and other new theoretical and instrumental capabilities, such as the superconducting SQUID for measuring minute currents and the tunneling microscope for observing molecular structures.

I also hope the future wil see a further expansion of our work on monaural and binaural hearing of impaired listeners and on speech perception - the ultimate goal of our *sense* of hearing.

Let me conclude with a quote from Jan Schouten at the Driebergen meeting. As you know, Jan put great store in the "eternal triangle" of *Perception*, *Physiology* and *Theory* and he said:

"Finally, with respect to the three sides of our triangle, the importance of cooperation and mutual inspiration cannot be sufficiently stressed."

Amen!

[1] Schroeder, M.R. (1986). "Auditory paradox based on fractal waveform," J.Acoust.Soc.Am. 79, 186-189.
[2] Schroeder, M.R. (1986). "Flat-spectrum speech," J.Acoust.Soc.Am. 79, 1580-1583.

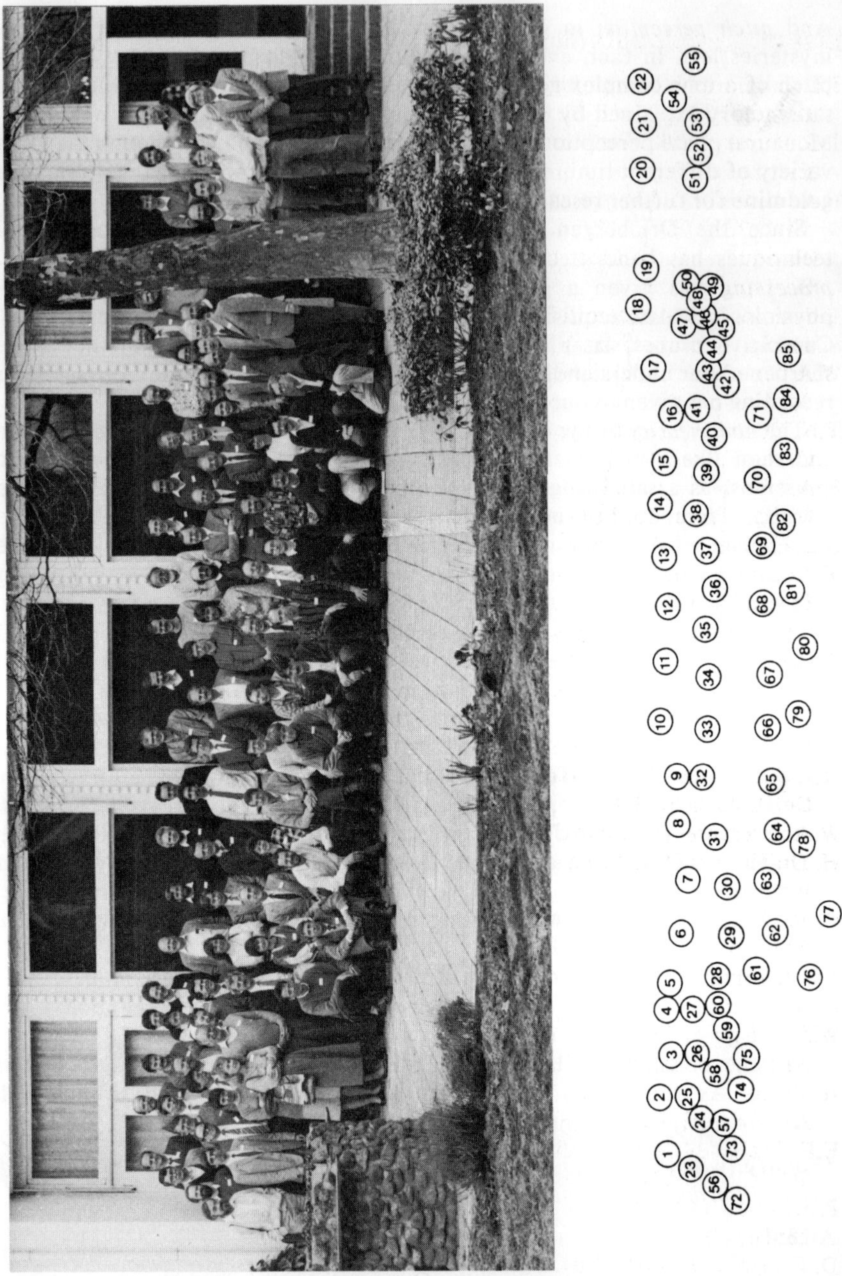

List of participants (numbers refer to photo)

J.J. Ashmore (44), Dept.Physiology, Medical School, University Walk, Bristol, BS8 1TD, U.K.
J.G. Beerends (20), Inst.for Perception Research, Postbus 513, 5600 MB Eindhoven, NL
F.A. Bilsen (43), Lab. voor Technische Natuurkunde, T.U.Delft, Postbus 5046, 2600 GA Delft, NL
J. Blauert, L.allgem.Electrotechn.& Akustik, Ruhr-Universität, D-4630 Bochum 1, BDR
E.de Boer (54), Academisch Medisch Centrum, Rm D2-210, Meibergdreef 9, 1105 AZ Amsterdam, NL
W.A.C.v.d.Brink (79), TNO Institute for Perception, Postbus 23, 3769 ZG Soesterberg, NL
T.N. Buell (21), Dept. Psychology, University of California, Berkeley, CA 94720, USA
R.A.J.Buwalda, Lab. Medische Fysica, AMC, Universiteit van Amsterdam, Meibergdreef 15, 1105 AZ Amsterdam, NL
B.L. Cardozo (40), Ankermonde 39, 3434 GB Nieuwegein, NL
Y. Cazals (65), Lab.d'Audiology Expérimental, Université Bordeaux II, Inserm unité 229,Hôpit Pellegrin, Bordeaux, 33076, France
J.A. Costalupes (51), Box 14992, Minneapolis, MN 55414, USA
A.C. Crawford (69), Physiological Laboratory, University of Cambridge, Cambridge, BC2 3EG, UK
B. Delgutte (22), RLE MIT & Eaton Peabody Lab, Mass. Eye and Ear Infirmary, 243 Charles Street, Boston, MA 02114, USA
R.J. Diependaal, Fac.Wiskunde en Informatica, T.U.Delft, Postbus 356, Delft, 2600 AJ, NL
W.A. Dreschler (33), AMC Klinische Audiologie, 1105 AZ Amsterdam, NL
H. Duifhuis (68), Biophysics Department, Rijksuniversiteit Groningen, Westersingel 34, 9718 CM Groningen, NL
P. van Dijk (10), Institute of Audiology, University Hospital Groningen, P.O.Box 30.001, 9700 RB Groningen, NL
J.J. Eggermont (24), Dept.of Psychology, The University of Calgary, Calgary, Alberta, T2N 1N4, Canada
W.J.M. Epping (67), Dept. Medical Physics & Bioph., K.Universiteit Nijmegen, Postbus 9101, 6500 HB Nijmegen, NL
A. Erell, Dept.E.Comm., Cntrl & Comp.Syst., Tell Aviv University, Ramat Aviv, 69978, Israel
E.F. Evans (30), Communication & Neuroscience, University of Keele, Keele Staffs, ST5 5BG, England
P.F. Fahey (85), Dept of Physics/EE, University of Scranton, Scranton, PA 18510, USA
D. Fantini (49), MRC Inst.of Hearing Research, University Park, Nottingham, NG7 2RD, England

H. Fastl (57), Institute of Electroacoustics, Technical University München, Arcisstr.21, D-8000 München 2, BRD
R.R. Fay (26), Parmly Hearing Institute, Loyola University of Chicago, 6525 N. Sheridan Rd., Chicago, IL 60626, USA
J.M. Festen (31), Experimentele Audiologie, KNO, Acad.Ziekenh. Vrije Universiteit, de Boelelaan 1117, 1081 HV Amsterdam, NL
M. Florentine (42), CommResLab/DeptSp.LngPath.Audiol, Northeastern University, Dept.Electr.& Computer Eng., Boston, MA 02115, USA
W. Gaik (36), L.allgem.Electrotechn.& Akustik, Ruhr-Universität, D-4630 Bochum 1, BRD
A.H. Gitter (82), Dept. Otolaryngology, University of Würzburg, Josef-Schneider-Str. 11, D-8700 Würzburg, BRD
D.M. Green (6), Dept. Psychology, University of Florida, Gainesville, FL 32611, USA
J.H. Grose (7), Dept. of Surgery, Univ. North Carolina Med.School, Div. of Otolaryngology, Chapel Hill, NC 27514, USA
E.R. Hafter (15), Dept. Psychology, University of California, Berkeley, CA 94720, USA
J.W. Hall (53), Dept. of Surgery, Univ. North Carolina Med.School, Div. of Otolaryngology, Chapel Hill, NC 27514, USA
G.B. Henning (16), Dept. Experimental Psychology, Oxford University, South Parks Rd., Oxford, OX1 3UD, England
A. Hoekstra (73), Audiologisch Centrum Prof.J.J.Groen Stichting, Zangvogelweg 150, 3815 DP Amersfoort, NL
K. Horner (64), Lab.d'Audiology Expérimental, Université Bordeaux II, Inserm unité 229,Hôpit Pellegrin, Bordeaux, 33076, France
J.W. Horst, Institute of Audiology, University Hospital Groningen, P.O.Box 30.001, 9700 RB Groningen, NL
T. Houtgast (58), TNO Institute for Perception, Postbus 23, 3769 ZG Soesterberg, NL
A.J.M.Houtsma (39), Inst.for Perception Research, Postbus 513, 5600 MB Eindhoven, NL
E. Javel (23), Boys Town National Institute, 555 North 30th Street, Omaha, NE 68131, USA
D.T. Kemp, Inst. Laryngology and Otology, Gray's Inn Road, London, WC1X 8EE, England
D.O. Kim (55), Div. of Otolaryngology, Univ. of Connecticut Health Ctr, Farmington, CT 06032, USA
R. Klinke, Zentrum der Physiologie, J.W.Goethe Universität, Theodor-Stern-Kai 7, D-6000 Frankfurt 70, BRD
A. Kohlrausch (19), Drittes Physikalisches Institut, Universität Göttingen, Bürgerstrasse 42-44, D-3400 Göttingen, BRD
B. Kollmeier (2), Drittes Physikalisches Institut, Universität Göttingen, Bürgerstrasse 42-44, D-3400 Göttingen, BRD
P. Kolston (50), Wiskunde en Informatica, T.U.D., Julianalaan 132, 2628 BL Delft, NL

C. Köppl (74), Institut für Zoologie, Lichtenbergstr. 4, D-8046 Garching, BRD
P. Kraft, Audiologisch Centrum, Stationsweg 26, 8911 AJ Leeuwarden, NL
C.J. Kros (81), Physiological Laboratory, University of Cambridge, Cambridge, BC2 3EG, UK
J.A.P.de Laat (28), KNO, Academisch Ziekenhuis Leiden, Postbus 9600, 2300 RC Leiden, NL
E.R. Lewis (25), Electr.Research Lab., University of California, Berkeley, CA 94720, USA
G.R. Long (29), Dept.Audiol.& Speech Sciences, Purdue University, West Lafayette, IN 47907, USA
M.E. Lutman (52), MRC Inst.of Hearing Research, University Park, Nottingham, NG7 2RD, England
G.A. Manley (72), Institut für Zoologie, Lichtenbergstr. 4, D-8046 Garching, BRD
S. McAdams (5), Inst.Rech.&Coord.Acoust./Musique, 31 rue Saint-Merri, Paris, F-75004, France
R. Meddis (8), Dept Human Sciences, University of Technology, Loughborough LE, LE11 3TU, U.K.
W.J. Melssen (80), Dept. Medical Physics & Bioph., K.Universiteit Nijmegen, Postbus 9101, 6500 HB Nijmegen, NL
M.I. Miller (32), Dept EE etc & Inst.Biomed.Comp., Washington University, 700 South Euclid Avenue, St. Louis, MO 63110, USA
B.C.J.Moore (78), Dept.of Experimental Psychology, University of Cambridge, Downing Street, Cambridge, CB2 3EB, England
P.M. Narins (34), Dept of Biology, University of California at LA, Los Angeles, CA 90024, USA
S.T. Neely (84), Boys Town National Institute, 555 North 30th Street, Omaha, NE 68131, USA
S.J. Norton (75), Dept.Hearing and Speech, University of Kansas Med.Center, 320 H.C.Miller Building, Kansas City, KS 66103, USA
A.R. Palmer (3), MRC Inst.of Hearing Research, University Park, Nottingham, NG7 2RD, England
R.D. Patterson (9), MRC Applied Psychology Unit, 15 Chaucer Road, Cambridge, CB2 2EF, England
J.O. Pickles (17), Dept of Physiology, Med.School, University of Birmingham, Birmingham, B15 2TJ, England
R. Plomp (38), TNO Institute for Perception, Postbus 23, 3769 ZG Soesterberg, NL
I. Pollack (13), Mental Health Res. Institute, University of Michigan, 205 Washtenaw Place, Ann Arbor, MI 48109-0720, USA
V.F. Prijs (62), KNO, Academisch Ziekenhuis Leiden, Postbus 9600, 2300 RC Leiden, NL
A. Rees (4), MRC Inst.of Hearing Research, University Park, Nottingham, NG7 2RD, England
G. Reuter (74), Dept. Otolaryngology, University of Würzburg, Josef-

Schneider-Str. 11, D-8700 Würzburg, BRD
V.M. Richards (27), Dept. Psychology, University of Florida, Gainesville, FL 32611, USA
R.J. Ritsma (60), Rijksstraatweg 20a, 9752 AD Haren, NL
M. Rodenburg (45), Afd. Biomed.Natuurk.en Technologie en afd.KNO, Erasmus Universiteit, Dr Molewaterplein 50, 3015 GE Rotterdam, NL
S. Rosen (70), Dept Phonetics & Linguistics, University College London, 4 Stephenson Way, London, NW1 2HE, England
B. Scharf (63), Auditory Perception Lab., Northeastern University, Boston, MA 02115, USA
N.A.M.Schellart, Lab. Medische Fysica, AMC, Universiteit van Amsterdam, Meibergdreef 15, 1105 AZ Amsterdam, NL
R. Schoonhoven (76), KNO, Academisch Ziekenhuis Leiden, Postbus 9600, 2300 RC Leiden, NL
M.R. Schroeder (59), Drittes Physikalisches Institut, Universität Göttingen, Bürgerstrasse 42-44, D-3400 Göttingen, BRD
S.A. Shamma (83), Dept.EE & Systems Res. Center, University of Maryland, College Park, MD 20742, USA
N. Slepecky (71), Institute for Sensory Research, Syracuse University, Syracuse, NY 13244-5290, USA
D.W. Smith (1), Dept. of Otolaryngology, 7308 Medical Sciences Bldg., University of Toronto, Toronto, Ontario M5S 1A8, Canada
J. Smolders (56), Zentrum der Physiologie, J.W.Goethe Universität, Theodor-Stern-Kai 7, D-6000 Frankfurt 70, BRD
G.F. Smoorenburg (61), Instituut voor Zintuigfysiologie, Postbus 23, 3769 ZG Soesterberg, NL
J. Smurzynski (18), Inst.for Perception Research, Postbus 513, 5600 MB Eindhoven, NL
M. Souter (46), Inst. Laryngology and Otology, Gray's Inn Road, London, WC1X 8EE, England
I.H.M. van Stokkum (35), Dept. Medical Physics & Bioph., K.Universiteit Nijmegen, Postbus 9101, 6500 HB Nijmegen, NL
R.S. Tyler, Dept. Otol. Head & Neck Surgery, University of Iowa, Iowa City, IA 52242, USA
H. Versnel (66), KNO, Academisch Ziekenhuis Leiden, Postbus 9600, 2300 RC Leiden, NL
J.P. Wilson (48), Communication & Neuroscience, University of Keele, Keele Staffs, ST5 5BG, England
H.P. Wit (77), Institute of Audiology, University Hospital Groningen, P.O.Box 30.001, 9700 RB Groningen, NL
S. Wolf (37), L.allgem.Electrotechn.& Akustik, Ruhr-Universität, Bochum 1, D-4630, BDR
R.J. Wubbels (12), Biophysics Dept., LAN, Rijksuniversiteit Groningen, Westersingel 34, 9718 CM Groningen, NL
E. Zwicker (41), Institute of Electroacoustics, Technical University München, Arcisstr.21, D-8000 München 2, BRD

Contents

Section 4: Neurophysiology and neural information 154

Section 5: Psychophysics of pure and complex tones 294

First author (**n**) and comments index (*n*)

Section 1

Invited review papers

Two distinguished colleagues who played a major role in the initiation of the European "*International Symposium on Hearing*" *series, present a personal view on two decades of developments in hearing research.*

A personal view on tone perception research

Reinier Plomp

TNO Institute for Perception, Soesterberg, and
Department of Otolaryngology, Free University Hospital, Amsterdam
The Netherlands

This paper was written by invitation of the organizers of this symposium to present, on the basis of an involvement in tone perception research during more than 30 years, my view on its past and future. This challenge is so personal that I can only answer it by telling about my own way in the past together with an outlook on research I would like to do if I had another 30 years to go.

Inspired by von Helmholtz

When I started in 1953 as a physicist trained in acoustics, there was no tradition in psychoacoustical research in the Netherlands apart from the clinically oriented work by H.C. Huizing in Groningen and J.J. Groen in Utrecht. My task was to set up research in audition and speech perception within a group involved in vision. M.A. Bouman, the head of this group, was a strong adherent of the view that applied and basic research should go hand in hand. It is understandable that the subject matter of my first experiments was the auditory analogue of temporal integration in vision (Plomp and Bouman, 1959; Plomp, 1961) followed by a study on forward masking (Plomp, 1964a).

In the mean time I had made a discovery that fully determined the direction of my interests and the course of my future studies. I read von Helmholtz's (1863) "Die Lehre von den Tonempfindungen als physiologische Grundlage fur die Theorie der Musik" and became (inevitably) highly impressed by the author's extraordinary capability in listening to everyday sounds, describing their sensations, and explaining them in a comprehensive hearing theory. At the same time I studied Stevens and Davis' book "Hearing - Its Psychology and Physiology", dating from 1938 but in the fifties still one of the main sources in the field. In the "Perspective" added to the text, E.G. Boring compared this book with the one by von Helmholtz, concluding: "Certainly we are ready now for a new *Lehre von den Tonempfindungen* to orient us among the complexities of the new physiological acoustics which is now so successfully answering questions which Helmholtz posed." My main reaction was: is this statement true? Can we say that Stevens and Davis presented the solutions to questions to be considered central in von Helmholtz's approach? My answer was no.

Von Helmholtz's starting point was the complex tone such as produced by musical instruments and the human voice. He explained that, owing to the ear's frequency-analyzing power, we are able to hear out the lower harmonics individually. Although he treated quite extensively the interference of sinusoidal components, manifesting itself in combination tones, beats and dissonance, the author never forgot that the tones in everyday life are *not* sinusoidal but compositions so that he had to deal with questions such as the single pitch of complex tones, the possible role of phase relations, and the origin of timbre. In every respect von Helmholtz's treatment was practical in the sense that he had in mind the sounds we hear in everyday life.

When we compare this treatment with the approach of Stevens and Davis, the difference is striking. In their book we are as it were in another world, the world of the sinusoidal tone of the laboratory rather than the complex sound of the outer world. This difference in attention had immense consequences for the choice of the questions discussed. The properties of 'pure' tones (hearing threshold, difference limen for frequency and intensity, pitch, loudness) and the interactions of two tones (beats, combination tones) are treated but many of the questions considered by von Helmholtz as being of central significance (e.g. timbre, limit of frequency resolution, pitch of complex tones) get almost no attention. Therefore, the book by Stevens and Davis is *not* an "update" of von Helmholtz's comprehensive approach but a reduction to the perception of sinusoidal stimuli. Of course, this holds not only for their book; it is a general characteristic of the literature a quarter of a century ago. This might have been a necessary stage in the development of hearing theory, but it is a rather restricted, not to say even misleading, approach.

So, the question I asked myself was: now, 100 years after von Helmholtz, can we say that the problems discussed by him in a more qualitative way are in the meantime investigated more quantitatively? I concluded that this was not the case. This conclusion was the starting point of a series of experiments for which I had only to reread *Die Lehre von den Tonempfindungen* and to formulate its main points of interest. The result was a series of articles on subjects all inspired by von Helmholtz. Since the greater part of the early literature on these topics was in the German language and not easily accessible for the modern student, I provided most of the articles with historical reviews. Let me present a short overview of these experiments.

(1) *Hearing out the partials.* In Part 1 of his treatise, von Helmholtz deals with the ear's capacity to analyze, up to a certain limit, a periodic sound wave into its sinusoidal components. This capacity is known as Ohm's acoustical law. As no systematic study on the limits of hearing out these components had been done, my first experiments were devoted to this question (Plomp, 1964b). In

one of the experiments the listener was provided with a three-way switch; in the middle position he heard a complex tone comprising 12 harmonics. In the other two positions simple tones were presented, one coinciding in frequency with a harmonic and the other with a frequency half-way between this and the next higher or lower harmonic. The listener had to decide which of these simple tones was also a part of the complex sound. I found that, even under the most favourable conditions, not more than the first 5 to 7 harmonics could be distinguished individually, in agreement with the critical-bandwidth concept.

(2) *Combination tones*. After having considered the ear's frequency-analyzing power, von Helmholtz begins Part 2 with an exposition on combination tones as a second restriction on Ohm's acoustical law. Thanks to the enigmatic nature of these tones in a pre-electronic age, they got much more attention in the 19th century than after the introduction of electronic amplifiers around 1920. As almost no data were available on the sensation level of primary tones at which combination tones become audible, this became my next topic (Plomp, 1965). In retrospect, these experiments were most important for the notion that the detectability threshold of the combination tone $2f_1$-f_2 depends so strongly on the frequency difference f_2-f_1 that it must be related to the ear's frequency resolution and, by implication, must have its origin in the inner ear. No wonder that this cubic difference tone received so much attention in later studies on the inner ear's nonlinearity.

(3) *Roughness and dissonance*. Subsequently, von Helmholtz discusses in Part 2 the interference of tones and its underlying role in the perceptual difference between dissonant and consonant chords. Experiments on this role were started by considering the effect of the frequency separation of two simple tones on the degree of roughness/dissonance. It appeared that a chord sounds most dissonant for a frequency difference of about one quarter of the critical bandwidth and sounds consonant for frequency differences beyond the critical bandwidth (Plomp and Levelt, 1965). In the same paper, this knowledge was used to explain the perceptual singularity of musical intervals consisting of two complex tones with simple frequency ratio ("tonal consonance") in a more quantitative (but essentially identical) way than von Helmholtz could do in his time. Statistical analyses of chords in musical compositions confirmed the important role of the critical bandwidth in music. Right at the time that Levelt and I were performing these experiments, Kruskal published his well-known papers on nonmetric multidimensional scaling (Kruskal, 1964a, 1964b). This made it attractive to verify the role of harmonics in the perception of musical intervals by means of a nonverbal technique (triadic comparisons). We received the program on cards from the author and Levelt had to go to Dusseldorf (West Germany) to find a computer on which the program could be run (Levelt, van de Geer and Plomp, 1966). I guess that this was the first time that multidimensional scaling was applied in this country.

(4) *Beats*. Still one question was left: can the beats of mistuned consonances, a main topic of interest in the 19th century, be explained fully by the occurrence of combination tones and the interference of nearly coinciding

partials? From my experiments with pairs of simple tones, I concluded that beats may also have their origin in periodic waveform variations as such, possibly converted into timing variations in nerve discharges (Plomp, 1967a).
(5) *Pitch of complex tones*. In treating the audibility of harmonics in Part 1 of his book, von Helmholtz was quite aware that we perceive complex tones as having a single pitch coinciding with the pitch of the fundamental. He followed Ohm as a promotor of the essential role of the fundamental versus Seebeck who denied this role in favor of the periodicity of the complex waveform. This generally accepted view could no longer be maintained after Schouten's pioneering experiments in 1938-1940 in which he demonstrated that the fundamental can be removed without any effect on the pitch (cf. Schouten, 1940). But, if the fundamental is not essential, which harmonics do determine pitch? I studied this question by means of complex sounds of which the frequencies of the first *m* harmonics were shifted 10% downwards and the higher harmonics 10% upwards. The subjects were requested to decide whether the pitch of this signal was higher or lower than the original complex tone (Plomp, 1967b). The results showed that the dominant region shifts from the fourth to fifth harmonics for tones with fundamental frequencies below 200 Hz down to the fundamental itself above 2000 Hz. Below I will return to the interpretation of these results.
(6) *Timbre*. Another subject of von Helmholtz's Part 1 still left unexplored was the perception of timbre. Multidimensional scaling, referred to under (3), was just the tool required to study the multidimensionality of timbre. By means of triadic comparisons, we could verify that the effect of phase on the timbre of complex tones is relatively small compared with the effect of spectral shape (Plomp and Steeneken, 1969). In exploring the relation between timbre and spectral shape, we adopted principal-components analysis to find the main dimensions of spectral differences (Plomp, Pols and van de Geer, 1967). Now having techniques for investigating the main dimensions for timbre differences as well as for spectral differences, the two approaches could be combined; a very good agreement was observed (Pols, van der Kamp and Plomp, 1969; Plomp, 1970). This result encouraged us to study the spectral differences between vowels pronounced by large groups of speakers more extensively, showing how well this perception-oriented approach could be used for automatic recognition of vowels (Klein, Plomp and Pols, 1970; Pols, Tromp and Plomp, 1973; van Nierop, Pols and Plomp, 1973). This led to an early system of automatic word recognition (Pols, 1971).

This condensed review may be sufficient to demonstrate the highly stimulating role of von Helmholtz' *Die Lehre von den Tonempfindungen* for my research. I would not like to suggest, however, that no other important studies were done in this field at the same time. From my own group I may refer to G.F. Smoorenburg's experiments on the pitch of two-tone complexes and the role of cubic combination tones, to T. Houtgast's psychophysical exploration of the role of lateral suppression which stimulated so many experiments, and to the more recent work by J. Vos on the perception of pure and tempered musical intervals. I cannot mention all others contributing in the same years to a better understanding of tone perception. I am happy that most of them are participants in this symposium.

As a result, our knowledge of tone perception, particularly frequency resolution, nonlinearity, interference phenomena and pitch of complex tones, increased considerably within the period 1955-1975. In order to confront this progress in psychoacoustics with the electrophysiological state of the art, an international conference was organized in Driebergen, the Netherlands, in 1969. The title of that meeting: "Frequency analysis and periodicity detection" reflects what was considered to be the hot issue of that time. This successful conference was the beginning of a series of which the present is the eighth.

Intermezzo: Pitch theory

I come back to the experiments on the pitch of complex tones because they illustrate so well how difficult it is for a researcher to look in an unbiased way at his data. As I mentioned, Schouten had investigated in 1938-1940 that the fundamental is not essential for perceiving the low pitch of complex tones resulting in his "residue pitch", based on the periodicity of the higher harmonics unresolved by the ear. Since J.C.R. Licklider's demonstration that the low pitch of a group of higher harmonics remains undisturbed when low-frequency noise is introduced to mask a fundamental possibly created by nonlinear distortion in the ear, the problem seemed to be settled in favor of the periodicity theory. Along these lines I concluded in my pitch study: "The experimental results strongly suggest that the pitch of complex tones is based on periodicity rather than on frequency." (Plomp, 1967b).

However, I should have realized that, actually, the data did not support this suggestion at all. I overlooked a third possibility, already referred to by de Boer (1956) in his dissertation: the low pitch of complex tones may be derived from spectral cues of harmonics resolved by the ear rather than from the fundamental or from temporal cues of unresolved higher harmonics. The finding that the third to fifth harmonics are most dominant in pitch perception should have kept me from drawing the wrong conclusion from the data. I consider this as a very instructive (and shocking) illustration of how vigilant we have to be in keeping our mind open and trying alternative explanations instead of going the easy way of following the fashion of the moment.

End of a period

As I decided after my part-time appointment at the Free University in 1972 to focus my attention on the effects of hearing impairment on speech intelligibility and the role of possible underlying psychoacoustical parameters, I thought it worthwhile to conclude the previous period by preparing a book on the state of the art. The title: *Aspects of Tone Sensation* (Plomp, 1976) explicitly refers to von Helmholtz' book on which it depends so strongly for its topics. This monograph gives a much more honest balance of the contributions of many investigators than I presented above.

I think that my main reason for publishing this book was the feeling that in the midseventies an important period in the development of tone perception research was coming to an end. At that time the scene was radically different from the one twenty years before. An international community of researchers had studied various aspects of hearing theory that were very tightly related. Frequency resolution, phase sensitivity, pitch perception, lateral suppression, nonlinear effects, all these phenomena appeared to be connected and had to be integrated. Looking backwards, it is remarkable to see how many young investigators became so fascinated by what was going on in tone perception research that, without any formal steering, they joined this movement and contributed to its progress. This was particularly so in this country but also abroad many were inspired by the main issues in this field of research.

It seems to me that this period was an important stage in the development of hearing theory. Simplifying the situation, we may say that in the beginning most attention was paid to how the ear perceives sinusoidal vibrations, as we saw above in the reference to the book by Stevens and Davis. This led inevitably to a rather restricted picture of tone perception in which several cardinal aspects were overlooked. The perception of complex tones cannot be fully understood by studying only simple tones. Also here, the total is more than the sum of the parts. We needed to study complex sounds in order to find out about pitch and timbre.

Spectro-temporal pattern analysis

We are now more than a decade after the research covered by *Aspects of Tone Sensation*. Further progress has been made. This is not the place to give a survey of extensions and modifications of earlier views. I will restrict myself to three recent developments.

(1) *Profile analysis*. About five years ago, Green introduced this term into audition to denote the phenomenon that the ear is very sensitive to differences between tone complexes of which only the intensity of a single component is varied (for a recent review, see Green and Bernstein, 1987). The use of the intensity difference limen as a criterion was made impossible by introducing random differences in the presentation levels of the two complexes to be compared. Apparently the ear is able to use spectrally global rather than local information in comparing spectral shapes. This interesting phenomenon may be highly relevant for understanding why speech perception is so invariant to intensity differences.

(2) *Co-modulation masking release*. Hall, Haggard, and Fernandes (1984) were the first to publish an effect that may be considered as an extension of the one just discussed. They found that the detection of a simple tone in a narrow band of noise is strongly improved by adding a second narrow band of noise with exactly the same temporal envelope as the first. This intriguing phenomenon, usually referred to as co-modulation masking release (CMR),

was confirmed by several other investigators. As in profile analysis, random differences in presentation level appeared to be of minor importance (Hall, 1986).

(3) *Perceptual grouping*. Although the work in this area started earlier than the studies just discussed, it is mentioned last because it has the widest scope. In 1975, van Noorden published his important dissertation on what he called: temporal coherence in the perception of tone sequences (main results in van Noorden, 1977). Together with the investigations by Bregman and coworkers on auditory streaming (for a review, see McAdams and Bregman, 1979), they represent important new developments on the perception of sequences of sound as we have in speech and music.

Whereas in profile analysis steady-state stimuli are used, this is no longer the case with co-modulation masking release and perceptual grouping. In the latter two topics not only spectral information, but also temporal information is involved. This illustrates that tone-perception research has entered a new era in which the stimuli are characterized by spectro-temporal patterns. We saw above that experiments with simple tones are not suited to explain pitch and timbre as properties of complex tones. Similarly, we may state that experiments in which either the spectral or the temporal properties are the variables - however important they may be - will not be sufficient to explain the perception of sounds spectrally varying in time. In other words: in order to understand how the complex sounds of everyday life are perceived, we cannot skip the stage in which stimuli with all typical properties of everyday sounds are our objects of study.

How further?

We should not conclude, however, that studying the perception of stimuli with spectra varying in time is the end of the long road of tone perception research. Even if we could investigate all aspects involved, we would still be far behind knowing the real capacity of our hearing. Usually in daily life we do not have the simple case of a single sound source in quiet but the much more complicated condition of different simultaneous sound sources. In speech perception, the other sources may be considered as disturbances; in music the ability to hear different tones at the same time belongs to its essence. With our present knowledge, it is possible to design an equipment recording the variations in pitch, loudness and spectrum of a dynamic sound. But this equipment would fail completely if presented with more than one simultaneous sound streams. The analysis of sound of the peripheral ear in terms of frequency components - although an essential condition - is totally inadequate to explain how sound streams are separated from each other as individual percepts.

Again I may refer to von Helmholtz who was quite aware of this problem: "Now there are many circumstances which assist us first in separating the musical tones arising from different sources, and secondly, in keeping together the partial tones of each separate source. Thus when one musical tone is heard for some time before being joined by the second, and then the second continues after the first has ceased, the separation in sound is facilitated by the succession of time. We have already heard the first musical tone by itself, and hence know immediately what we have to deduct from the compound effect for the effect of this first tone. Even when several parts proceed in the same rhythm in polyphonic music, the mode in which the tones of different instruments and voices commence, the nature of their increase in force, the certainty with which they are held, and the manner in which they die off, are generally slightly different for each." (von Helmholtz, 1863; English translation, p. 59).

The discrimination of simultaneous sounds, or more generally: of sound streams, may be considered as the highest task in auditory processing. It may be instructive to try to order the most striking capacities of the hearing organ in a scheme, with the more basic ones at the bottom and the more complex ones at the top, see next page. Of course, the significance of this ordering may be locally rather low, but this does not touch the general idea. Partly these capacities are typically peripheral, partly of central origin (with a vague transitional range).

The distinction between a peripheral level and a central level in tone perception is closely related to the type of physiological processes involved. The core of the peripheral level is a rather extensively studied acoustico-hydrodynamic system, with clear "special purpose" properties. On the other hand, we have centrally almost unexplored neuronal structures which seem to be much less specific for hearing. Von Helmholtz's brilliant idea of comparing the cochlea with a system of strings tuned to different freqencies from high to low was a milestone in the development of peripheral hearing theory. We still wait for a comparable breakthrough in modelling central auditory processing.

Let us return to the psychophysical aspect. We should realize that the kind of phenomenon under study determines the best experimental approach to be applied. Psychoacousticians have been very successful with forced-choice procedures in exploring phenomena considered to be of peripheral origin. In most cases the listener's task was to detect a change in some parameter. The phenomenon was "hard" and the condition could be repeated again and again without any problem.

As is visualized in the last column of the scheme, we get more and more into trouble if we try to maintain the detection approach with repeated presentations in studying phenomena of a more central nature. The audibility of a sound is a condition for its perception but hearing is much more than that. The challenge in everyday life is recognition rather than detection. This is most clear in the separation of simultaneous sound streams, according to the scheme the most complex task of the auditory system. Recognition implies that previous experience, training and expectation play essential roles. This is radically different from the situation in, for example, masking experiments; therefore, the experimental approach should be radically different.

level	phenomenon	method
	TOP	
central	separation of sound streams perceptual grouping continuity in time co-modulation masking release pitch of complex tones profile analysis timbre perception	recognition, single presentations
peripheral	lateral inhibition forward masking frequency discrimination amplitude discrimination phase effects combination tones masking patterns	detection, repeated presentations
	BOTTOM	

I have the impression that psychoacousticians are still rather reluctant to adapt their experimental methods to the requirements of studying central aspects of tone perception. This is reflected in the literature on perceptual grouping in which qualitatative demonstration of effects plays a much larger role than quantitative determination of the role of the various variables. In my opinion, the only way to overcome this impasse is to adapt the procedure to the problem by eliminating the effects of training and bias as much as possible. Instead of presenting the same (or almost the same) condition again and again, we should change over to single presentations as we do in speech perception experiments. The same stimulus may be used again but only after so many others in between that every presentation may be considered as a fresh one. Along this line, our experimental approach will become more and more representative of everyday experience, just what we need to find the ultimate laws of how sounds are perceived by the auditory system. This is the kind of research I would like to do if I had another 30 years to go.

References

de Boer, E. (1956). *On the 'Residue' in Hearing* (Doctoral Dissertation, University of Amsterdam).

Green, D.M., and Bernstein, L.R. (1987). "Profile analysis and speech perception," in: *The Psychophysics of Speech Perception*, edited by M.E.H.

Schouten (Nijhoff, Dordrecht), pp. 314-327.
Hall, J.W. (**1986**). "The effect of across-frequency differences in masking level on spectro-temporal pattern analysis," J.Acoust.Soc.Am. **79**, 781-787.
Hall, J.W., Haggard, M.P., and Fernandes, M.A. (**1984**). "Detection in noise by spectro-temporal pattern analysis," J.Acoust.Soc.Am. **76**, 50-56.
Klein, W., Plomp, R., and Pols, L.C.W. (**1970**). "Vowel spectra, vowel spaces, and vowel identification," J.Acoust.Soc.Am. **48**, 999-1009.
Kruskal, J.B. (**1964a**). "Multidimensional scaling by optimizing goodness of fit to a nonmetric hypothesis," Psychometrika **29**, 1-27.
Kruskal, J.B. (**1964b**). "Nonmetric multidimensional scaling: a numerical method," Psychometrika **29**, 115-129.
Levelt, W.J.M., van de Geer, J.P., and Plomp, R. (**1966**). "Triadic comparisons of musical intervals," Brit.J.Mathemat.Statist.Psychol. **19**, 163-179.
McAdams, S., and Bregman, A. (**1979**). "Hearing musical streams," Comp. Music J. **3**, No. 4, 26-43.
Plomp, R. (**1961**). "Hearing threshold for periodic tone pulses," J.Acoust. Soc.Am. **33**, 1561-1569.
Plomp, R. (**1964a**). "Rate of decay of auditory sensation," J.Acoust.Soc.Am. **36**, 277-282.
Plomp, R. (**1964b**). "The ear as a frequency analyzer," J.Acoust.Soc.Am. **36**, 1628-1636.
Plomp, R. (**1965**). "Detectability threshold for combination tones," J.Acoust. Soc.Am. **37**, 1110-1123.
Plomp, R. (**1967a**). "Beats of mistuned consonances," J.Acoust.Soc.Am. **42**, 462-474.
Plomp, R. (**1967b**). "Pitch of complex tones," J.Acoust.Soc.Am. **41**, 1526-1533.
Plomp, R. (**1970**). "Timbre as a multidimensinal attribute of complex tones," in *Frequency Analysis and Periodicity Detection in Hearing*, edited by R. Plomp and G.F. Smoorenburg (Sijthoff, Leiden), pp. 397-411.
Plomp, R. (**1976**). *Aspects of Tone Sensation - A Psychophysical Study* (Academic Press, London).
Plomp, R., and Bouman, M.A. (**1959**). "Relation between hearing threshold and duration for tone pulses," J.Acoust.Soc.Am. **31**, 749-758.
Plomp, R., and Levelt, W.J.M. (**1965**). "Tonal consonance and critical bandwidth," J.Acoust.Soc.Am. **38**, 548-560.
Plomp, R., Pols, L.C.W., and van de Geer, J.P. (**1967**). "Dimensional analysis of vowel spectra," J.Acoust.Soc.Am. **41**, 707-712.
Plomp, R., and Steeneken, H.J.M. (**1969**). "Effect of phase on the timbre of complex tones," J.Acoust.Soc.Am. **46**, 409-421.
Pols, L.C.W. (**1971**). "Real-time recognition of spoken words," IEEE Trans. Comp. **C-20**, 972-978.
Pols, L.C.W., van der Kamp, L.J.T., and Plomp, R. (**1969**). "Perceptual and physical space of vowel sounds," J.Acoust.Soc.Am. **46**, 458-467.
Pols, L.C.W., Tromp, H.R.C., and Plomp, R. (**1973**). "Frequency analysis of Dutch vowels from 50 male speakers," J.Acoust.Soc.Am. **53**, 1093-1101.

Schouten, J.F. (**1940**). "The residue and the mechanism of hearing," Proc. Kon.Ned.Acad.Wetensch. **43**, 991-999.
Stevens, S.S., and Davis, H. (**1938**). *Hearing - Its Psychology and Physiology* (Wiley, New York).
van Nierop, D.J.P.J., Pols, L.C.W., and Plomp, R. (**1973**). "Frequency analysis of Dutch vowels from 25 female speakers," Acustica **29**, 110-118.
van Noorden, L.P.A.S. (**1975**). *Temporal Coherence in the Perception of Tone Sequences* (Doctoral Dissertation, Eindhoven Technological University).
van Noorden, L.P.A.S. (**1977**). "Minimum differences of level and frequency for perceptual fission of tone sequences ABAB," J.Acoust.Soc.Am. **61**, 1041-1045.
von Helmholtz, H. (**1863**). *Die Lehre von den Tonempfindungen als physiologische Grundlage fur die theorie der Musik.* (Vieweg & Sohn, Braunschweig). English translation by A.J. Ellis, *On the Sensations of Tone as a Physiological Basis for the Theory of Music* (reprinted by Dover, New York, 1954).

Comments

Tyler:

I wonder about the interpretation of tasks that require very long periods of training, for example 30 or 40 weeks. It is certainly important to determine the limits of auditory perception. However it may be that in these tasks the subjects are being trained to use cues that they do not normally utilize in typical conversation. Therefore, tasks that do not require very long periods of training are probably more appropriate for understanding speech perception.

Green:

I certainly agree that listener training is a very important aspect of research on the perception of complex tones. Many of these experiments require a large amount of training and the degree of training must be monitored very carefully in any study. I must disagree with your suggestion on the use of "naive" subjects. In my experience "naive" subjects come with various degrees of training. Certainly their initial level of performance is very different. Trying to find an "unsophisticated" observer may be just as difficult as training to subject to asymptotic performance.

Reply by Plomp:

These comments refer to the spoken version of my paper in which I spent more attention to the last paragraph of the written version: the need to adapt our experimental methods to the requirements of studying central aspects of tone perception. I discussed some experiments in which the results strongly depend on (1) the acoustic context of the stimulus, (2) naive listening, and (3) the effect of long training. As the two comments show, different positions on the role of training are hold. In my opinion, the need for a long training period should warn the experimenter that he may be studying the plasticity of the brain rather than "hard" properties of the auditory process.

Psychophysics and physiology of peripheral processing in hearing

Eberhard Zwicker

Institute of Electroacoustics
Technical University München, F.R. Germany

Introduction

Presenting this paper, I feel somewhat uncomfortable. I am used to report on psychoacoustical results, on physiologically measured facts, or on models which describe both. Now, I am asked to give a review of the tendencies about what happened during the last seven symposia of this kind, which cover a period of almost 20 years. There is no physical measurement I can do on that, there is not more than one subject to be asked, namely myself. There are very few real facts about tendencies, but mostly opinions and - unfortunately - only my own opinion. Therefore, I have to apologize for not mentioning all the very important contributions to these meetings, but just to recall some most important tendencies seen from my point of view.

The most important basic goal of all the seven meetings always was to bring researchers working in the scientific field of hearing together and to combine their views. They stem from the field of psychophysics and behavioral studies on the one hand, and from the field of neurophysiology, physiology and anatomy on the other hand. Using this subdivision and abbreviating it by PB and NP, but for a combination of both just using P+P, the papers held at the different symposia can be categorized as follows:

	PB	NP	P+P	Σ
Driebergen (1969)	19	14	1	34
Eindhoven (1972)	13	9	1	23
Tutzing (1974)	12	19	-	31
Keele (1977)	23	20	-	43
Noordwijkerhout (1980)	39	26	2	67
Bad Nauheim (1983)	26	29	3	58
Cambridge (1986)	14	31	2	47
Σ =	146	148	9	303

The last meeting seems to be an exception. In all other meetings, the two fields have been very well balanced - within a tolerance of less than ± 3 dB! The combination of the two fields of science introduces a problem since in psychoacoustics mostly humans are subjects, while in physiology mostly animals are searched on. Knowing this, it is not always advisable to compare the corresponding data directly. The basic structure of the hearing system, however, especially around the cochlea, seems to be relatively similar so that quite often comparisons may be allowed, at least for mammals.

The content of this paper will be subdivided into two sections. A review of the seven symposia will be given from the point of view what happened in the past. This can only be a comprehensive summary pointing towards appeared new ideas, important results and new facts. The second part will contribute to the questions "where are we today" and "what shall we do in future?". Again, I have to apologize that this is my own personal view and not a median value of the several hundred participants of the seven former meetings. I know that in the last part, I undertake the very dangerous step to view towards future. I am sure, there are many other opinions with regard to this question. However, since I have recognized through my life that my own voice is not always of influence, I feel not too uncomfortable, because everybody will do anyhow what he/she wants to do and not what I am proposing!

Since I have been asked by the organizers to concentrate on peripheral effects, I try to do so. Additionally, I will focus on monaural hearing. In order to save space, I will mention the seven symposia just by the years they have taken place and will not use references in the following part.

Review of seven symposia

The first meeting in 1969 on "Frequency analysis and periodicity detection in hearing" was the base line for all consecutive symposia. I am sure that all the participants of that meeting as well as of the following meetings join me in making the statement that the efforts of Prof. Reinier Plomp in combining the psychoacousticians and the physiologists in hearing are very worthy of merit. We all thank him very much for this stimulating idea, which he realized in such a superb form.

One of the very important contributions of the first meeting was to find expressions and items, which have been useful and understandable to both categories of scientists. It really needed almost the whole meeting, before the members of the different groups were able to understand the other group up to 95%. This process which was very strong at the first symposium, is still in progress, and is an important contribution of each of the following meetings. There is not only a difference in expressions which have to be discussed, but quite often the same expression is used, however, the meaning is different or at least the method leading to the result is quite different. This has been a source of several misunderstandings which could be cleared up in the meetings. The first meeting was also an update of the results available at that time. Although the meeting was concentrated on frequency analysis and periodicity detection, the basic contributions in the review papers have been of great importance for mutual introduction into the fields. Many facts outlined at that time are still guidelines and are referred now-a-days as classic data.

In 1972, "Hearing Theory" was the title, and the theory concentrated mostly on pitch. It was interesting for me to realize, how much the pitch theory of Terhardt, developed basically for already in 69, as well as the pitch theories of Whiteman and Goldstein are based on what is existent already after peripheral preprocessing, namely the frequency selectivity of the peripheral hearing system. However, at that time we still were very uncertain about the fact, where this frequency selectivity occurs. The title of Evans' paper "Does frequency sharpening occur in the cochlea?" was typical for that situation.

At the 1974-meeting in Tutzing we all appreciated very much the introductions into the neuro-anatomy of the cochlea by Engström as well as by Spöndlin and by Flock. Nevertheless, the discussion on cochlear mechanics has opened many questions. Not only the discrepancy between neurophysiologically measured data from the eighth nerve, and physiologically measured data from the basilar membrane displacement showed strong differences, but also the ideas of a "second filter" remained doubtful. On the other hand, the "marriage" between psychoacousticians and physiologists started to produce small "seedlings" like for example the psychoacoustical equivalent of tuning curves, proposed by Zwicker and by Vogten. In addition, it was found as a common result that nonlinear effects play an important rule not only in one, but in both of the fields as expressed by Rhode, Dallos, Pfeiffer, and Smoorenburg and Bilsen. The general discussion also made clear that there must be something in the peripheral hearing system, which enables the ear to transform the large dynamic range of about 80 to 100 dB into a much smaller range of only 40 or 50 dB transferred towards the brain.

At the 1977-meeting in Keele, the discussion on this subject was continued. It became already clear that a compression must take place within the mechanics of the cochlea. This means that nonlinear effects seem to influence very strongly peripheral preprocessing. The question, where the sharp frequency selectivity is installed, was further discussed by Zwislocki, assuming an interaction between inner and outer hair cells. Duifhuis as well as Houtgast further discussed the nonlinear effects, which were introduced by Scharf as slightly level-dependent critical bandwidth. The contributions to pitch theory by de Boer, Moore and van den Brink added to the understanding of most of the effects. Although there was a new "seedling" born, called masking-period pattern as an equivalent to period histograms, the contributions by Viemeister and by others made clear that the psychoacoustically measured facts in temporal resolution can not be understood without equivalent further investigations in neurophysiology.

The 1980-meeting in Noordwijkerhout already gained by the discovery of otoacoustic emissions by Kemp. Wilson as well as Wit and Ritsma, besides others, contributed more data to this phenomenon. Triggered by this effect,

Kim *et al.* proposed active cochlea models, while Allen offered a cochlear micromechanic model, similar to Zwislocki's ideas. Additional contributions were made at that meeting which partly added to the understanding of peripheral processing, partly seem to complicate this understanding. It became clear at that time that some kind of nonlinear active feedback within the cochlea is needed and that the compression of the dynamic range may partly be installed through the phase locking in the nerve fibers.

The 1983-meeting in Bad Nauheim contributed important parts to the peripheral signal processing. Most impressive was the comparison of basilar membrane-, hair cell-, and neural responses by Johnstone, Partuzzi and Sellick. The paper made clear that the sharp frequency selectivity is not only available in the neural response of the fiber but also in the hair cell and even in basilar membrane displacement. Their date also made clear that the equivalent of low-frequency masking-period patterns and corresponding period histograms can be seen already in the displacement of the basilar membrane. This and other papers pointed to the fact that very careful preparation is needed in order to get results which correspond with normal life. It also became clear that many of the former data have been misleading because of imperfect preparation techniques. On the other hand it was shown at this meeting that the otoacoustic emissions are a good tool in order to investigate peripheral processing within the cochlea of humans without injury. It was shown psychoacoustically by Fastl that modulation plays an important role in hearing and that fluctuation strength as well as pitch strength are interesting psychoacoustical values to be measured in order to quantify these perceptions. These responses to temporal variations together with other results have led to the question whether nonsimultaneous masking as well as simultaneous masking are produced within the cochlea by the same sources. Using otoacoustic emissions, this question could be answered by the relatively general statement that simultaneous masking is due to processing within the cochlea, i.e. peripheral, while nonsimultaneous masking is due to processes within or behind the first synapses.

At the 1986-meeting in Cambridge, Klinke as well as Crawford and Fettiplace contributed data from non-mamals. Together with the additional views on the evolution of mechanisms of frequency selectivity in vertebrates by Manley, these contributions give impressions about the possibilities of nature, to use different ways in order to come to the same solution, namely frequency selectivity in the hearing system. Evidence for a proposed active mechanical process in the outer hair cells was shown by Hudspeth, by Zenner, by Ashmore, and by Brownell. The discussions at this meeting also made clear that even after seven of these meetings we still may have to be very careful in using such common phrases as "just noticeable difference" or "difference limen". It seems that there are still 2% of expressions left which may have different meanings in different areas, in different laboratories, and in different heads.

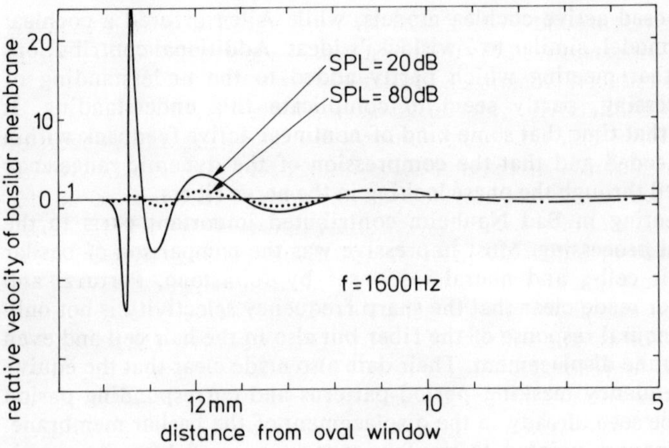

Figure 1: Relative velocities of the basilar membrane's travelling wave produced by a 1600-Hz tone of low level (20 dB, solid) and of high level (80 dB, dotted). The two waves are equalized at the right, i.e. towards oval window. Note the gain at low levels and the shift of the maximum. Data adopted from (Zwicker, 1986) and plotted on linear scale.

Present knowledge and open questions

Up to about 6 kHz, it is generally accepted that the sound pressure at the eardrum is the value responsible for the produced sensation. Since the transmission in the **middle ear** from the eardrum to the oval window is also mostly known and assumed to behave linearly up to about 80 dB, it seems reasonable to state that the peripheral part of the sound processing system up to the oval window is successfully investigated. Only at very high frequencies, some leakage remains.

Signal processing within the **inner ear** got strongly lightened during the last 10 years: It became clear that active processes are involved and that extreme nonlinear characteristics take place. The combination of psychoacoustical research and of the appropriate use of otoacoustic emissions in human subjects has led to these results. We have some idea about the functional behaviour of the hydromechanics of the inner ear together with the activity of outer hair cells and the organ of Corti (see for example Zwicker 1986). It seems reasonable that the traveling waves assumed so far are existent only at high levels (see the dotted line in Fig. 1), while the activity of the outer hair cells becomes dominant at low levels and sharpens the envelope of the traveling wave drastically towards a more strongly peaked form (see solid line in Fig. 1). The peak reached at low levels is shifted towards the helicotrema in relation to that reached at high levels. The example outlined in Fig. 1 also indicates the strong nonlinearity which may either be expressed as a reduction of the gain by 26 dB when enlarging the level from 20 dB to 80 dB, or by the phrase that low levels around 20 dB are 26 dB more amplified than high levels near 80 dB. The important result is the reduction of the dynamic range which in our example is reduced from 60 dB to 34 dB.

How this additional **activity** at lower levels is achieved is still a mystery - at least to me. The outer hair cells are commonly the favourites as producers of this activity. The mobility of these cells, however, seems to be a fact which may become effective at very high levels, but not at low levels of 20 dB. There, the displacement of the basilar membrane is near 10^{-6} mm without and about 10^{-5} mm with an additional gain of 20 dB. Such small values seem not to be able to elicit currents efficient enough to produce the necessary motion. The effect should also show the compression-like nonlinearity as measured using otoacoustic emissions and $(2f_1\text{-}f_2)$-distortion products. Therefore, my own thoughts go more in the direction of electro-mechanical transducers installed within the membranes of the cells, which are very thin and therefore produce relatively large capacity and large field strength. Such transducers often follow strong nonlinear behaviour and, therefore, seem to be predestinated for the active sources in question.

The travelling wave in the human inner ear can not be measured and analyzed directly. Therefore, the otoacoustic emissions represent an important tool for indirect measurements. The **frequency selectivity** can be measured by suppression tuning curves, which show the level of a suppressor tone as a function of its frequency which is just needed to reduce the amplitude of spontaneous, simultaneously evoked, or of delayed evoked emissions for a certain amount, for example 3 or 6 dB. Such suppression tuning curves are indicated in Fig. 2 and are compared with psychoacoustically measured tuning curves. All of these curves show the same behaviour which corresponds very well with that of the neurophysiological tuning curves of single fibers measured in animals. There is, however, a small but distinct difference: the four kinds of tuning curves plotted in Fig. 2 all show a marked difference between the frequency of the probe tone or of the emission and that frequency which corresponds to the lowest point of the tuning curve or to the center frequency of the U-shaped valley. This effect is not or at least not as clearly seen in neurophysiological tuning curves. The source or the reason of this difference remains hidden and may be discussed in future meetings.

Another very interesting feature of all kinds of human otoacoustic emissions is the most probable critical band rate distance between neighouring frequencies of emissions. This distance was found to be a **constant value of 0.4 Bark** (Dallmayr, 1985, 1987), which corresponds to a distance along the basilar membrane of 0.5 mm. We assume that this distance is closely correlated with the traveling wave in the human inner ear. There, the phase difference of the traveling wave corresponding to the place distance of a half millimeter amounts near the characteristic frequency to ±180°, values which create most likely other emissions. However, this is an assumption only, which has to be proven. Nevertheless, there seems to be a possibility to obtain information about the characteristics of traveling waves in human inner ears through data of otoacoustic emissions.

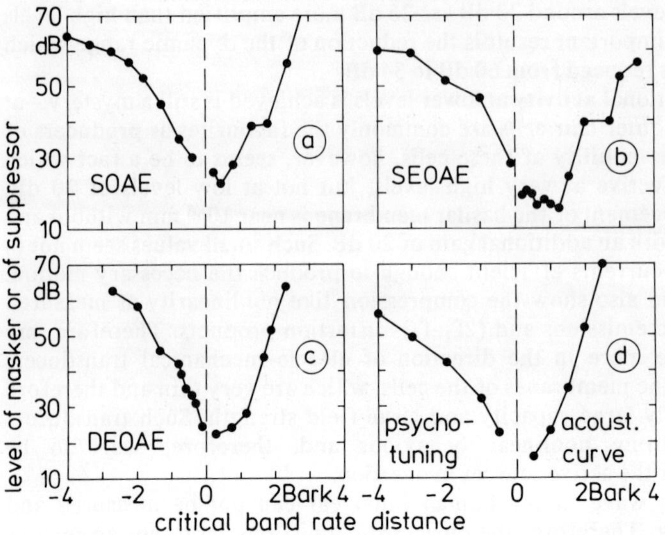

Figure 2: Suppression-tuning curves, i.e. level of a suppressor tone necessary to reduce an otoacoustic emission for 3 dB as a function of the suppressors frequency which is expressed in the the frequency of the emission in belong to spontaneous, simultaneously evoked, and delayed evodata are adopted from Dallmayr (1985, 1987), and Wilson (1983), respectively. Panel (d) shows corresponding data of psychoacoustical tuning curves (Zwicker & Schorn 1978).

Another interesting result on the **source of masking** was also revealed through emissions. It could be demonstrated that all simultaneous masking - at least for smaller levels of the test tone - is achieved within the cochlea and the nonlinearity of its signal processing. Simultaneous masking covers not only classical masking patterns but also tuning curves as well as masking-period patterns produced by low-frequency maskers with all their temporal characteristics (Scherer, 1988). Non-simultaneous masking, on the other hand, is not produced within the cochlea, but in or behind the first synapses within the neural pathway. Although there are a few data of post-stimulus effects available measured in single fibers of mammals, we are still confronted with a lack of neurophysiological data which simulate as much as possible the paradigm used in psychoacoustical post-stimulus masking measurements.

The **critical bandwidth** was also discussed somewhat during the last ten years. There are two kinds of questions to be asked. One is connected with the size of the critical band width, the other with the source of it. Most of the discussion was about the size, while the question about the source was mostly ignored. Summarizing all the data available on this subject, it seems that most of the early data from the 50ies have been verified, if either free-field condition of sound presentation or earphones with equalizers which take care

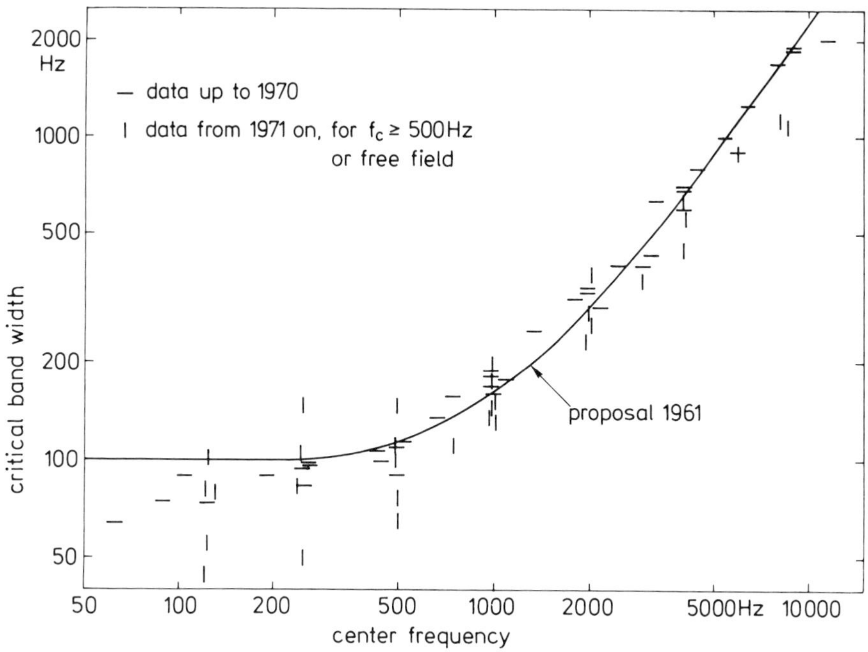

Figure 3: Collection of data indicating the critical bandwidth as a function of the center frequency. Horizontal bars belong to data from up to 1970; vertical bars steam from data published later than 1970. Below a center frequency of 500 Hz, only data produced in free-field or equivalent free-field condition using equalized earphones are plotted. The solid line indicates the proposal agreed on by an international commission.

of simulating free-field conditions are used. It may be pointed out again - as we from our Institute have done very often - that normal earphones (including 95% of the ones used in psychoacoustical laboratories) show a frequency response with a shape of a band pass with slopes near 300 Hz and 3 kHz. With all the cheap electronics available, it does not make sense to spend many expensive hours of listening through earphones without equalizers and produce very questionable data this way. Much more efficient is the direct use of equalizers in front of the earphone if one is not able - and this is mostly the case - to use free-field conditions. All the data available on critical bandwidth using reasonable acoustical presentation are shown in Fig. 3 in comparison with the dependence of critical bandwidth on frequency as proposed by a commission of ISO. Taking into account the interindividual variation and the influences of the methods used to determine indirectly the width of the critical band, I am surprised how close the published data agree to each other and also to the internationally proposed frequency dependence.

The only open question, which can not be answered scientifically but only by practical reasons, is the width at very low frequencies. The actual data - from the 50ies as well as the new ones - point towards a critical bandwidth near 80 Hz at the low frequency end. Since this is the end not only of the frequency scale (0 Hz) but also of the audible frequency range (20 Hz) we suggested 25 years ago to assume the lowest critical band width to be 100 Hz from 0 Hz to 100 Hz or 80 Hz, if counted from 20 Hz to 100 Hz. Often, I use the phrase "until the contrary is proven, the former opinion is held". Therefore, I wait until someone offers real hard data on the critical band width at a center frequency of 50 Hz! Instead of discussing too far this almost unsolvable question, we rather should search towards the source of the critical bandwidth. In general, it seems reasonable to assume that it is created within the inner ear. However, there are still a few unsolved problems: why is critical band width at low levels and even at threshold in quiet almost the same (within 40%) as at medium levels, and why is it still about the same at high levels, where we would expect much larger band width in relation to that near threshold, where the feedback creates much stronger frequency selectivity?

Very often we hear and read of a comparison between data produced using **simultaneous** masking and data produced through **nonsimultaneous**, preferable post-stimulus **masking**, but also pulsation threshold. I like to point out, that such two data sets can rarely be compared directly. We know since many years that post-stimulus masking does not behave linearly, does not decay exponentially, but depends on masker duration (see Fig. 4a). Therefore, it is possible only in very rare cases, or only as a very first approximation to use such non-simultaneous paradigms for the determination of auditory frequency selectivity. No question that simultaneous masking behaves nonlinearly, too. However, this nonlinearity is concentrated on the slopes of masking and not at the center. The bandwidth of a filter is indicated by the frequency distance of the 3 dB-points which are close to what is meant by "center". The steepness of the slopes of a filter and of masking does not influence band width very much. Post-stimulus masking, on the other hand, shows a strong change of the masking pattern at the center if plotted for different delay times as shown in Fig. 4b. This means that the still acceptable approximation for simultaneous masking of assuming a linear system is not possible for post-stimulus masking data used to describe frequency selectivity. The human hearing system, as many other sensory systems, extensively uses nonlinear effects. Our physical and electrotechnical thinking is influenced very strongly by mathematics in such a way that we preferably think in linear systems for which the frequency and the time-domain are exchangeable. This is **not** so, if nonlinearities are involved as is for sure the case in our hearing system, even in its peripheral part. The mixture of linear and nonlinear systems leads to effects and characteristics which are much less easy to predict and need thoughts which - unfortunately - can not be so simply be modeled via computers as it is possible for linear systems. However, nature can not exist without nonlinearity, so we better adapt to this situation in our future scientific activity.

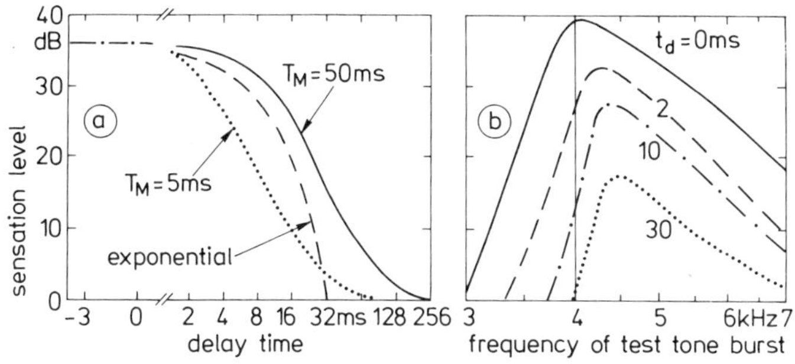

Figure 4: Part (a) shows the decay of post-stimulus masking for masker durations of 5 and 50 ms. (Adopted from Zwicker and Fastl, 1972; and Scherer, 1988). The broken line corresponds to an exponential decay with a time constant of 8 ms. Part (b) indicates schematically the shift of the masking pattern (test tone burst level as a function of its frequency) with increasing delay time in post-stimulus masking towards higher frequencies. Masker frequency is 4 kHz. Adopted from (Fastl, 1979).

To summarize my views on **peripheral signal processing** of our hearing system, my impression today is that the hydrodynamical linear system of the inner ear is superimposed by a highly nonlinear system which uses feedback in order to produce the frequency selectivity as well as the temporal resolution as well as dynamic compression needed to create that ingenious part of signal processing, which is preceding the neural processing. The saturating nonlinearity within the feedback loop seems to produce the outstanding characteristics. For very faint sounds, the feedback acts near the point of oscillation, and therefore the ear is not only very sensitive, but also very sharply tuned, a fact very useful for just audible sounds. For loud sounds, on the other hand, the feedback loop's gain is automatically strongly reduced through the compressive nonlinearity so that not only the large sensitivity is reduced which is not needed for high levels - but also the tuning widened so that temporal resolution is strongly enlarged, an important fact in order to verify speech communication. The nonlinearity installed in the feedback loop plays, therefore, an important role, it is the stabilizing factor in the system. In technical systems - analog or digital! - stabilization occurs at the highest possible "power" available, as for example in the formerly used feedback-radio-receivers, or in the well known system of - unwanted! - acoustical feedback through microphone-amplifier-loudspeaker in a room, or - also very well known because of its large power resource - the feedback system of an atomic power plant. In extreme contrast to that - and therefore much more save! -, the hearing system uses a nonlinearity at very low amplitudes, so low that oscillation - if it occurs - remains stabilized at inaudibly low levels. This way, a situation, which in any case should be avoided in technical systems because of strong danger, becomes very useful and handy. The inaudible oscillations measured as spontaneous otoacoustic emission are a by-product of a normally functioning hearing system with its admirable features. An other by-product is also well known: the unexpected large ($2f_2$ - f_2)-distortion products. These distortion products appear especially for narrow frequency distance of the two primaries. This indicates that the nonlinearity appears only within single channels as characterized by the frequency selectivity. This kind of nonlinearity only within channels is the basis of the astonishing fact that we are sensitive to a nonlinearity of only 1% of our audio system, although the nonlinearities installed in our inner ear are so large that an expression in percent is not possible. Much research activity is needed to solve all the open questions which concentrate mostly on the detailed functions of all the parts within scala media!

A few more **comments** on the strategy of **further research** as well as of **further symposia** may lead to, and may be the conclusion. During the last 10 years it appeared the tendency to offer a model for the results of sometimes only one experiment. Most often, such models are not useful to describe results of other experiments and are, therefore, not very helpful. The more experimental results can be described by one and the same model, the more interesting is the model. Therefore, it may proposed to be more restrictive in offering very selective or specialized models, while more general but still quantitative models are always very welcome for further discussion.

The basic goal of all the symposia, namely to superimpose and to combine psychoacoustics and neurophysiology was and is **the** important base of most of the success created so far. This goal has not lost one bit of its importance. On the contrary, it seems more important now-a-days because of the tendency for more and more specialization. Hearing researchers of the last century - to mention for example von Helmholtz as one of the outstanding - have been thinking very widely not only in the field of hearing, but in very many other disciplines. Today, we are much more specialized and therefore have to cooperate with other specialists or, at least, have to communicate with each other. All what enhances this strategy is very welcome and should be accepted. From this point of view, I like to propose that at the end of the symposia open questions may be formulated, possible ways towards solutions indicated, and researchers willing to contribute to the question named, which may report at the next symposium on the subject. Most important is again the view from different directions towards the same subject. I like to close this paper by expressing many thanks, especially to all the organizers of former symposia and of this symposium as well as to the many contributors from inside and from outside Europe, and by wishing all of you very effective further symposia.

References

Dallmayr, C. (**1985**). "Spontane oto-akustische Emissionen, Statistik und Reaktion auf akustische Störtöne," Acustica **59**, 67-75.

Dallmayr, C. (**1987**). "Stationary and dynamic properties of simultaneous evoked otoacoustic emissions (SEOAE)," Acustica **63**, 243-255.
Fastl, H. (**1979**). "Temporal masking effects: III. Pure tone masker," Acustica **43**, 282-294.
Scherer, A. (**1988**). "Erklärung der spektralen Verdeckung mit Hilfe von Mithörschwellen- und Suppressionsmustern." Submitted to Acustica.
Wilson, J.P. (**1980**). "Evidence for a cochlear origin for acoustic re-emissions, threshold fine-structure and tonal tinnitus," Hearing Res. **2**, 233-252.
Zwicker, E. (**1986**). "A hardware cochlear nonlinear preprocessing model with active feedback," J.Acoust.Soc.Am. **80**, 146-153.
Zwicker, E. and Fastl, H. (**1972**). "Zur Abhängigkeit der Nachverdeckung von der Störimpulsdauer," Acustica **26**, 78-82.
Zwicker, E. and Schorn, K. (**1978**). "Psychoacoustical tuning curves in audiology," Audiology **17**, 120-140.

Section 2

Sensory cell physiology

The sensory transducer, the hair cell, is an essential element in the auditory (and related) system(s). Progress is made in analyzing isolated inner and outer hair cell properties using refined optical, electrophysiological and biochemical techniques. The first five papers focus on mammalian cochlear hair cells, the sixth compares hair cell structures in birds and mammals.

Non-linear electrical properties of guinea-pig inner hair cells: a patch-clamp study

C.J. Kros and A.C. Crawford

The Physiological Laboratory, Downing Street, Cambridge CB2 3EG, United Kingdom.

Introduction and methods

Intracellular recordings in lower vertebrate hair cells strongly suggested the presence of time- and voltage-dependent conductances modifying the receptor potential so that it is not linearly dependent on the transducer current, resulting in an electrical resonance (Crawford and Fettiplace, 1981). The main conductances involved have subsequently been shown to be a calcium-dependent potassium conductance and a calcium conductance (Lewis and Hudspeth, 1983; Art and Fettiplace, 1987).

Recent current injection experiments in inner hair cells *in vivo* showed evidence for some outward rectification of the cell's membrane (Nuttall, 1985; Dallos, 1986; Russell, Cody and Richardson, 1986).

Here we describe a preparation of isolated inner hair cells developed in order to study the membrane properties of these cells using the patch-clamp technique (Hamill *et al.*, 1981). A similar approach has been taken for guinea-pig outer hair cells by Ashmore and Meech (1986).

Inner hair cells were isolated mechanically from the apical region of cochleas of pigmented guinea-pigs, killed by cervical dislocation. The isolation procedure resembled that reported by Lim and Flock (1985), but no enzymatic treatment was used. The cells were mostly grouped in clusters; occasionally truly isolated cells were found. The extracellular solution used was bicarbonate-free Hanks' MEM (Gibco), modified by the addition of 10 mM HEPES-NaOH, pH 7.3 at 38°C. The composition of the salts (in mM) was: 137 NaCl, 0.3 Na_2HPO_4, 5.4 KCl, 0.4 KH_2PO_4, 1.3 $CaCl_2$, 0.5 $MgCl_2$, 0.4 $MgSO_4$. In some experiments 1 mM $CdCl_2$ was added.

Cells were maintained during the experiments on a heated compound microscope stage at 35-38°C and viewed using differential interference contrast optics with a ×40 water immersion objective. They were superfused with tissue-culture medium at a flow sufficient to change the bath volume every 5 minutes. The medium was not oxygenated.

The patch-clamp electrometer included a facility for partly compensating the series resistance of the pipettes. Both voltage clamp and current injection experiments could be performed on the same cells. Pipettes were filled (in mM) with: 140 KCl, 5 EGTA-KOH, 0.3 $CaCl_2$, 5 $MgCl_2$, 2.5 Na_2ATP and 5 HEPES-KOH, pH 7.2. In some experiments CsCl replaced KCl and the Na-salts of EGTA and HEPES were used. The series resistance after compensation ranged from 2.5 to 6 MΩ. The inner hair cell's capacitance was 9 ± 2 pF (mean ± S.D., n = 8). The time constant of the voltage clamp in all experiments presented here was faster than 100 μs.

Results and discussion

The cells had resting potentials of -68 ± 3 mV (mean ± S.D., n = 15) and developed large time- and voltage-dependent outward currents when clamped to potentials more positive than this. To examine these currents cells were held at -74 mV (a potential at which all time- and voltage-dependent conductances were turned off). An example is shown in Fig. 1. The upper part shows the membrane currents that developed when the potential was stepped through the range of voltages indicated by each trace. Currents developed over the first 10 ms of the step, the onset becoming faster as the cell was

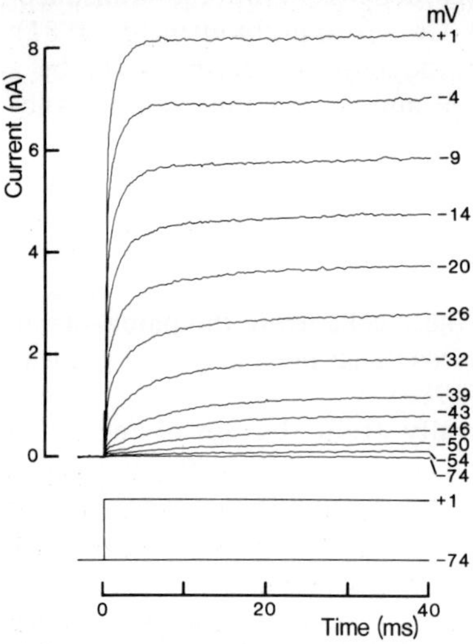

Figure 1. Membrane currents (upper part) of an inner hair cell under voltage clamp. Lower part: voltage step protocol; absolute membrane potentials (corrected for MΩ series resistance) shown by each current trace (averaged from 4 repetitions). Leakage and capacity current subtracted.

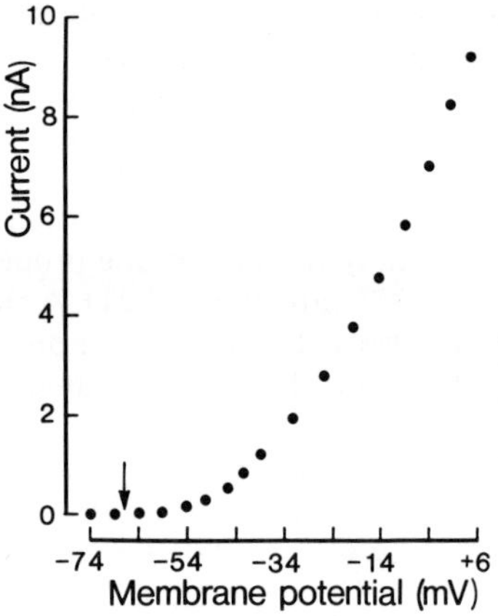

Figure 2. Steady state current-voltage relationship for the cell of Fig. 1. Mean values of the currents are plotted against the absolute potentials to which the cell was 4.3 stepped. Outward current is plotted upwards. Arrow indicates resting potential (-67 mV).

depolarized further. Hyperpolarizing steps (not shown) showed only a small instantaneous current consistent with an ohmic leakage conductance of 1-2.5 nS. The onset showed no appreciable initial delay but its rise could not be described by a single exponential process. The steady state values of the membrane current at different potentials are illustrated in Fig. 2. Similar curves were obtained in 17 other experiments. For large depolarizations the slope conductance increased to about 266 nS, from a value of about 1.9 nS negative to the resting potential. Note that the potential range over which the conductances were activated is quite small: most of the conductance turned on in the range -50 to -30 mV.

To investigate further this strong outward rectification the membrane was depolarized to -19 mV for a period sufficient for the current to reach a steady level, and then returned to a more hyperpolarized potential. This voltage protocol is illustrated schematically in the lower part of Fig. 3. A proportion of the ionic channels opened on depolarization close following the step. The resulting tail current is determined by the time course of closure of the channels and the electromotive force driving current flow. Such tail currents will reverse at a potential where the electromotive force is zero (Hodgkin and Huxley, 1952). It can be seen in the example of Fig. 3 that this coincides with a value of -74 mV. In 10 cells the reversal potential was -76 ± 2 mV (mean ± S.D.), close to the expected potassium equilibrium potential of -86 mV. This indicates that the potassium ion is the main charge carrier, but there is a small contribution from other ionic species as well (Hodgkin, 1958).

In experiments in which caesium replaced potassium in the patch pipette all outward currents were suppressed. Since caesium blocks potassium channels (Yellen, 1984), this observation also indicates that the outward

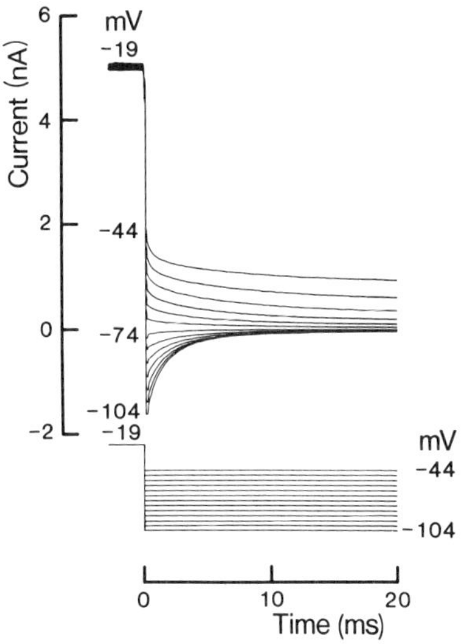

Figure 3. Reversal of membrane tail currents when the membrane potential is returned from a value of -19 mV to one of 13 levels between -104 and -44 mV in 5 mV increments. Upper part: tail currents. Lower part: schematic representation of the voltage protocol. Zero time corresponds to the instant of repolarization; the current during the preceding 40 ms when the cell was held at -19 mV is also shown. The uncompensated series resistance was 3.0 MΩ. Each trace averaged from 23 repetitions. Leakage and capacity current subtracted.

current is carried by potassium ions. Caesium-filled cells showed a much smaller inward current when depolarized to potentials as positive as 0 mV, which was probably partly carried by calcium ions.

To determine whether the potassium currents were calcium-dependent, as in other hair cells (Lewis and Hudspeth, 1983; Ashmore and Meech, 1986; Art and Fettiplace, 1987) 1 mM cadmium ion was added to the superfusion medium and suppressed reversibly all currents evoked by depolarizing steps. Since cadmium ions block the calcium channel (Hagiwara and Byerly, 1981) it seems that the outward potassium currents are indeed calcium-dependent, and that part of the inward current seen in caesium-filled cells is carried by calcium ions. These findings suggest that inner hair cells contain a calcium-activated potassium conductance and a calcium conductance, similar in magnitude to those reported previously in the hair cells of lower vertebrates (Lewis and Hudspeth, 1983; Art and Fettiplace, 1987). The presence of the calcium conductance is not surprising since these cells presumably use it to control release of synaptic transmitter. It remains to be seen whether the calcium-activated potassium conductance can shape the receptor potentials in a way as important as its role in lower vertebrate hair cells. It is certainly the case that the operating range of this conductance coincides with the membrane potential range of the receptor potentials (Cody and Russell, 1987), unlike the observations of Ashmore and Meech (1986), who found considerably smaller calcium-dependent potassium currents in guinea-pig outer hair cells activated only at potentials far depolarized from the resting potential.

Acknowledgements

This work was supported by the M.R.C. and Trinity College Cambridge. We would like to thank Professor H.B. Barlow for the loan of equipment and Dr. R. Fettiplace for helpful discussions throughout the course of this work.

References

Art, J.J., and Fettiplace, R. (**1987**). "Variation of membrane properties in hair cells isolated from the turtle cochlea," J.Physiol. **385**, 207-242.

Ashmore, J.F., and Meech, R.W. (**1986**). "Ionic basis of membrane potential in outer hair cells of guinea pig cochlea," Nature **322**, 368-371.

Cody, A.R., and Russell, I.J. (**1987**). "The responses of hair cells in the basal turn of the guinea-pig cochlea to tones," J.Physiol. **383**, 551-569.

Crawford, A.C., and Fettiplace, R. (**1981**). "An electrical tuning mechanism in turtle cochlear hair cells," J.Physiol. **312**, 377-412.

Dallos, P. (**1986**). "Neurobiology of cochlear inner and outer hair cells: intracellular recordings," Hearing Res. **22**, 185-198.

Hagiwara, S., and Byerly, L. (**1981**). "Calcium channel," Ann.Rev.Neurosci. **4**, 69-125.

Hamill, O.P., Marty, A., Neher, E., Sakmann, B., and Sigworth, F.J. (**1981**). "Improved patch-clamp techniques for high-resolution current recording from cells and cell-free membrane patches," Pflügers Archiv. **391**, 85-100.

Hodgkin, A.L. (**1958**). "The Croonian Lecture: Ionic movements and electrical activity in giant nerve fibres," Proc.Roy.Soc. B. **148**, 1-37.

Hodgkin, A.L., and Huxley, A.F. (**1952**). "The components of membrane conductance in the giant axon of Loligo," J.Physiol. **116**, 473-496.

Lewis, R.S., and Hudspeth, J. (**1983**). "Voltage- and ion-dependent conductances in solitary vertebrate hair cells," Nature **304**, 538-541.

Lim, D.J., and Flock, Å. (**1985**). "Ultrastructural morphology of enzyme-dissociated cochlear sensory cells," Acta Otolaryngol. **99**, 478-492.

Nuttall, A.L. (**1985**). "Influence of direct current on dc receptor potentials from cochlear inner hair cells in the guinea pig," J.Acoust.Soc.Am. **77**, 165-175.

Russell, I.J., Cody, A.R., and Richardson, G.P. (**1986**). "The responses of inner and outer hair cells in the basal turn of the guinea-pig cochlea and in the mouse cochlea grown in vitro," Hearing Res. **22**, 199-216.

Yellen, G. (**1984**). "Ionic permeation and blockade in Ca^{2+}-activated K^+-channels of bovine chromaffin cells," J.Gen.Physiol. **84**, 157-186.

Auditory transduction steps in single inner and outer hair cells

Alfred H. Gitter and Hans-Peter Zenner

Department of Otolaryngology,
University of Würzburg, D-8700 Würzburg, West Germany

Introduction

Inner and outer hair cells are the site of transduction of the mechanical sound stimulus into an electrical signal in the mammalian cochlea. It was postulated, that this mechano-electrical process is based upon K^+ fluxes through hair cell membranes. Appropriate ion channels have been identified in cell membranes of outer hair cells (Gitter, 1984; Gitter *et al.*, 1986; Ashmore and Meech, 1986). In addition, however, the mechanical stimulus is modulated by an active, possibly electro-mechanical, transduction process which is located in the outer hair cells. Techniques for preparation of single outer hair cells and short time culture of viable single hair cells (Brownell *et al.*, 1985; Zenner *et al.*, 1985; Flock *et al.*, 1986) have allowed the investigation of some characteristic features of mammalian auditory receptor cells, although an experimental approach to isolate inner hair cells was still lacking. Here we present single inner and outer hair cells, which can be isolated from guinea pig cochleae, as cellular model for the investigation of auditory transduction processes.

Microsurgical isolation of inner and outer hair cells

Guinea pigs of both sex with positive Preyer's reflex were decapitated. The temporal bone was removed and cooled to 4 °C. Then the lateral wall of the cochlea was opened with forceps. The membraneous labyrinth of each turn was transferred into droplets of cell culture medium in a standard cell culture dish mounted on an inverted microscope. Here, and in all subsequent steps, the hair cells were bathed in Hank's medium, which was adjusted to 300 mOsm/l by the addition of NaCl. Addition of collagenase (final concentration 1 mg/ml) eased the subsequent isolation of single cells, but was not essential. Fine needles of non-corrosive steel with a tip diameter of 10 - 100 μm allowed the manual dissection of the surface preparation. Single cells were separated from surface preparations by a short impact with the needle thus producing a jet stream in the vicinity of the cells. The yield of isolated hair

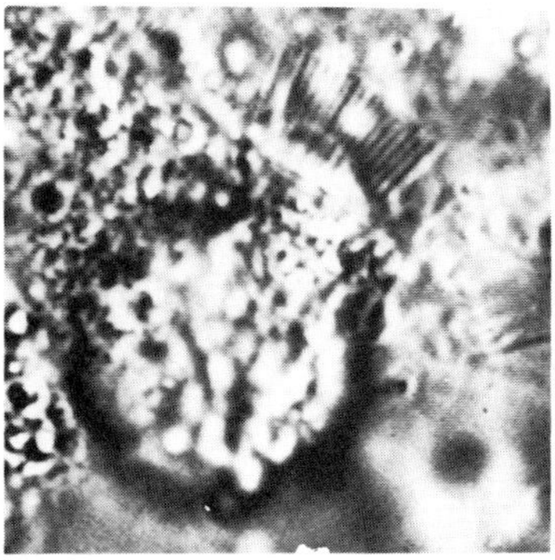

Figure 1. Micrograph of an inner hair cell isolated from guinea pig cochlea. Note the stereocilia.

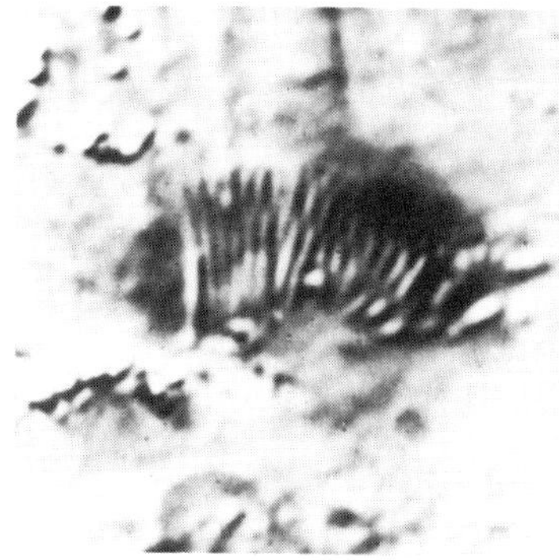

Figure 2. Cuticular region of an inner hair cell imaged by light microscopy with contrast enhancement.

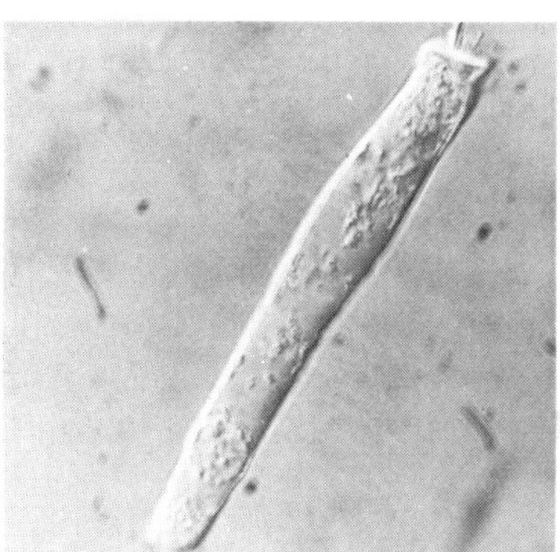

Figure 3. Single outer hair cell with the characteristic cylindrical cell body and cuticular plate.

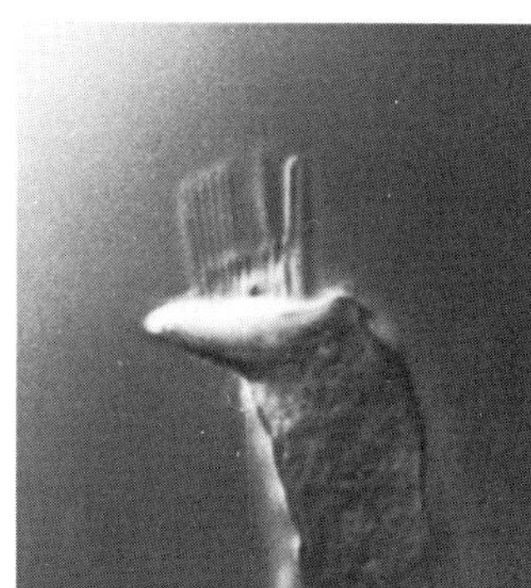

Figure 4. Cuticular region of a single outer hair cell. Note the different length of stereociliary rows.

cells consisted predominantly (≥ 95%) of outer hair cells. The single hair cells were often free of visible morphological defects and the characteristic configuration of stereocilia was preserved (see light microscopy images, figures 1-4).

Cell membrane integrity of isolated hair cells

Hair cells without morphological defects (changes in shape, cloddy structures or Brownian motion in the cytoplasm) usually excluded Trypan Blue. Moreover, iontophoretic application of Lucifer Yellow through impaled microelectrodes labelled the whole cell. This suggested integrity of the cell membrane. Partial staining of the cytoplasm was never observed. Nucleus and cuticular plate appeared brighter than the cytoplasm. Furthermore, the dye-coupling indicated electrical coupling of the cytoplasmic space.

Cell potential of isolated outer hair cells

The cell membrane potential difference of isolated outer hair cells had been measured using patch-clamp techniques to proof their viability (Zenner *et al.*, 1985a). Stable negative cell potentials (± 2 mV) of -45 ± 16 mV (mean ± SD, n = 17) with a minimum value of -69 mV had been registered for at least 5 min (Gitter *et al.*, 1986). Additional experiments with microelectrode

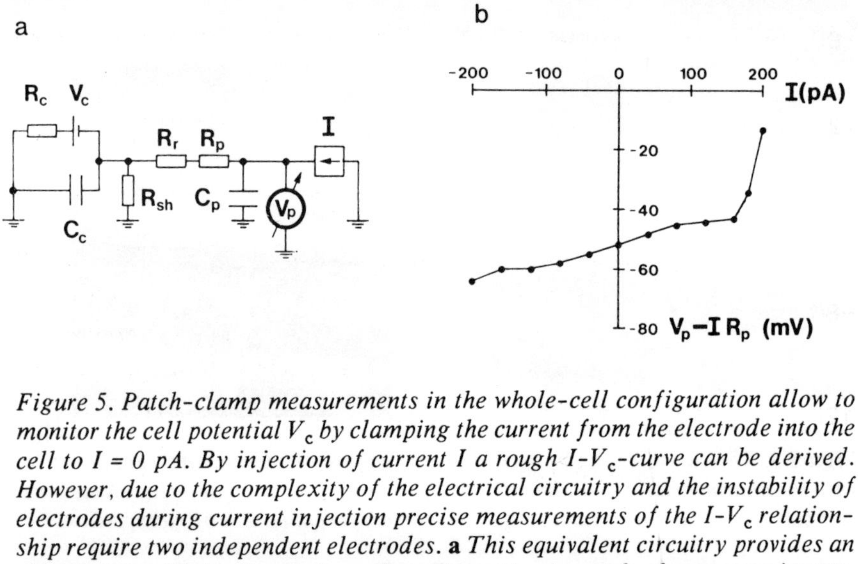

Figure 5. Patch-clamp measurements in the whole-cell configuration allow to monitor the cell potential V_c by clamping the current from the electrode into the cell to $I = 0$ pA. By injection of current I a rough I-V_c-curve can be derived. However, due to the complexity of the electrical circuitry and the instability of electrodes during current injection precise measurements of the I-V_c relationship require two independent electrodes. **a** *This equivalent circuitry provides an electrical model for the whole-cell configuration in patch-clamp experiments. The patch-clamp amplifier delivers a current I and measures the pipette voltage V_p.* **b** *I-V_c curve of an one-electrode patch-clamp experiment in the whole-cell configuration with an outer hair cell. V_p-$I{\cdot}R_p$, which approximates the cell potential V_c, was plotted as function of the injected current I, which was varied over a range of ± 200 pA. Here was the pipette input resistance R_p = 10 MΩ. The resting membrane potential was $V_c = V_p (I = 0) = -52 \pm 1$ mV before and after the depicted curve was registered.*

impalements usually showed an immediate decay of measured cell membrane potentials accompanied by morphological changes indicating cell death. However, in some experiments negative cell potentials of -42 ± 17 mV (mean ± SD, n = 22) could be registered. In one experiment a potential of -70 mV was registered for 2 minutes. The registrations exhibited oscillations of the potential which had not been observed in the previous patch-clamp recordings. The scatter of measured potentials may in part be due to the more or less harsh experimental conditions. It may also reflect a physiological variance. However, these results contradict the hypothesis of a cell membrane

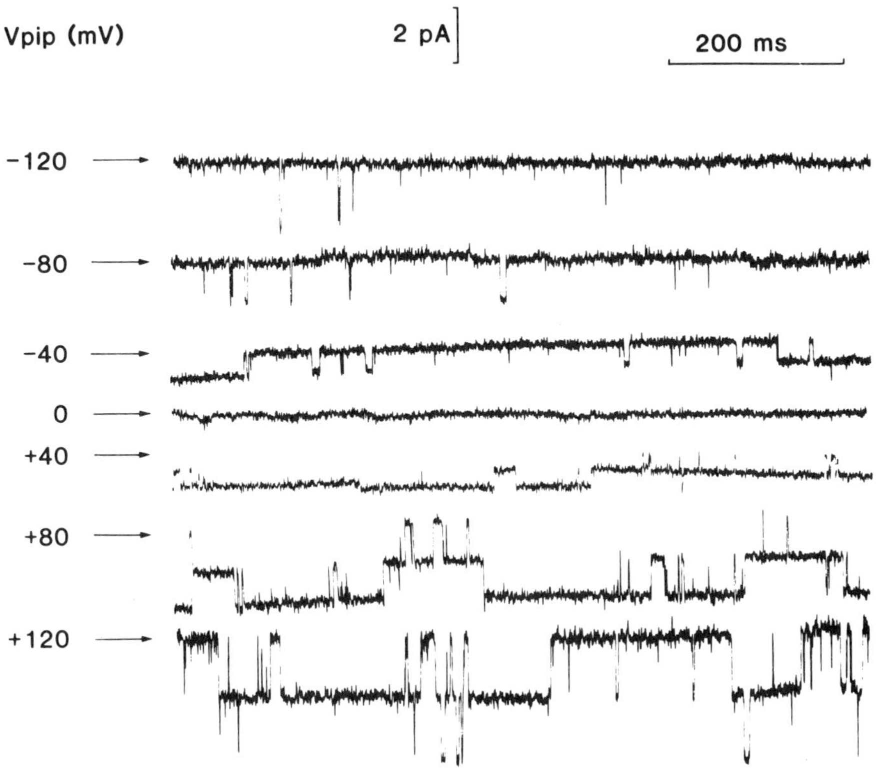

Figure 6. Current through the patch-clamp electrode as function of time. The recordings belong to an experiment with a cell-attached patch of the lateral cell membrane of an inner hair cell. The series of traces reflects different command voltages V_{pip} of the electrode. The transitions between different current levels correspond to the opening and closing of two similar ion channels. These channels exhibited a voltage-dependent kinetic and had a linear I-V_{pip} relationship with a slope conductance of 18 pS, each. The reversal potential $V_{rev} = V_{pip}(I = 0)$ was near 0 mV.

resting potential near 0 mV which would hyperpolarize following stimulation of the outer hair cells (Brownell *et al.*, 1985). Resting potentials up to -70 mV were also measured in vivo (Dallos *et al.*, 1982).

Ion channels in the lateral cell membrane of inner hair cells

The recent approvement of our dissection techniques allowed the investigation of ion channels in the lateral cell membrane of inner hair cells. The patch-clamp technique was applied to cell-attached and excised patch configurations. All experiments were performed at room temperature (24 °C). The patch pipette was filled with isotonic Ringer solution, containing in mmol/l: NaCl 95, KCl 50, $CaCl_2$ 1.5, $MgCl_2$ 1, HEPES 5, pH was adjusted to 7.4 with 2.5 mmol/l NaOH. So far three types of ion channels have been found. They exhibited in cell-attached patches conductivities of 9.9 ± 2.6 pS (mean ± SD, n = 7 experiments), 20.8 ± 2.8 pS (mean ± SD, n = 7), and 49.5 ± 1.8 pS (mean ± SD, n=3), respectively. Maxi-K^+-channels were not found, although they had frequently been observed in outer hair cells.

Slow outer hair cell motility

An increase of the K^+-concentration in the bath solution of isolated outer hair cells depolarized the cell membrane and led to slow

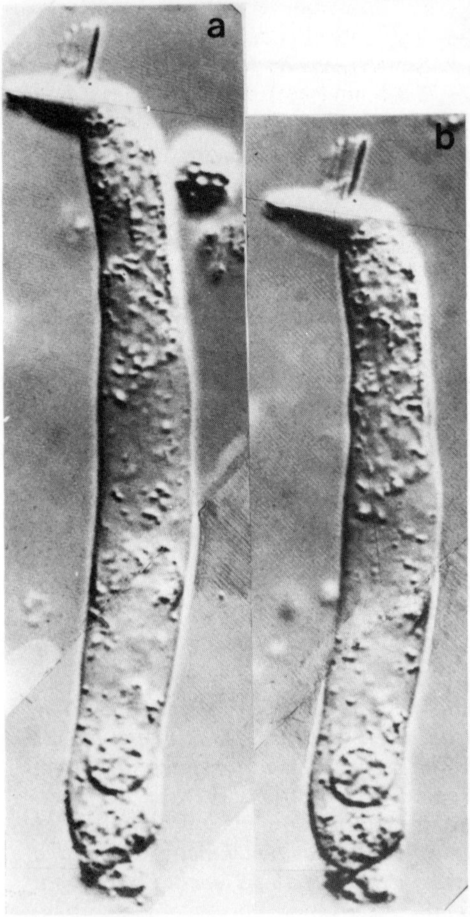

Figure 7. Micrographs showing an outer hair cell before (a) and after (b) exchange of the standard culture medium (containing 6 mmol/l potassium) to Ringer solution with increased (70 mmol/l) K^+ concentration. The cell length decreased ($\partial L/L$ = 0.15) and the angle between cuticular plate and the longitudinal axis of the cell body became 3.5° smaller. The angle between cuticular plate and stereocilia remained constant. Thereby the tilting movement of the cuticular plate induced a shear movement of the stereocilia.

motile responses (Zenner *et al.*, 1985b). The cell body contracted and the sterecilia were deflected by a tilting movement of the cuticular plate. Furthermore, following an increase in the intracellular Ca^{2+}-level isolated outer hair cells showed longitudinal contractions in the presence of ATP (Flock *et al.*, 1986, Zenner, 1986). Our experiments revealed, that outer hair cells possess actin-dependent motor properties, which are controlled by intracellular Ca^{2+} and calmodulin. Therefore they possibly adjust actively the mechanical properties of the basilar membrane during auditory stimulation (Zenner, 1986). The slow changes of the cell length (and thus the cytoskeleton) as well as the tilting movement of the cuticular plate could control the operation point of the stereocilia. Moreover, outer hair cells could modulate the mechanical characteristics of the cochlear partition during adaptation and TTS. They may contribute to the homeostasis of the basilar membrane location. Furthermore, the slow motile mechanisms may protect the vulnerable cochlear partition against high sound pressure levels. In additional experiments the relationship of outer hair cell elongation ∂L and applied force F could be detected by pulling cells mechanically in a glass pipette. For outer hair cells of 3rd turn, 1st row, $L = 72 \pm 5\ \mu m$ (mean ± SD, n=11) was here $\partial L/(L \cdot F) = 2.0 \cdot 10^6 \pm 9 \cdot 10^5\ N^{-1}$ (mean ± SD, n=21). The elongation was accompanied by an increase of cell volume and was for $\partial L/L \leq 0.04$ almost, but not completely, reversible. Irreversible destruction of the cells happened for $\partial L/L \geq 0.1$.

Fast outer hair cell motility

Electrically induced motile responses of isolated outer hair cells had first been described by Brownell *et al.* (1985). Recently we could demonstrate, that in an alternating electrical field outer hair cells are capable of fast cell length oscillations with frequencies up to the kHz range (Zenner *et al.*, 1987). With an improved technique we could measure motility for frequencies up to 30 kHz. Oscillations of outer hair cell length L were also detectable with intracellular injection of alternating current I through impaled microelectrodes. Ashmore (1987) presented an elaborate kinetic analysis for frequencies up to 10 kHz. In our experiments depolarizing current (-2 nA) led to contraction, hyperpolarizing current (+2 nA) to elongation of the cell body. For outer hair cells of the 3rd turn was $\partial L/\partial I = 0.3 \pm 0.1\ \mu m/nA$ (mean ± SD, n=12) and $\partial L/\partial t = 0.012 \pm 0.004\ \mu m/ms$ (mean ± SD, n=8). With intracellullar and extracellular stimulation the electrically induced motile response was not inhibited by dinitrophenol, cytochalasin B, and phalloidin. Thus, in contrast to ATP-dependent slow motile responses the electrically evoked motility does not require ATP nor is it driven by actin-myosin activity. The underlying mechanism remains obscure, but it represents a fast electro-mechanical transduction process. Rapid movements induced by this process may interfere cycle-by-cycle with the travelling wave. Thus, near hearing threshold they could amplify and tune the travelling wave.

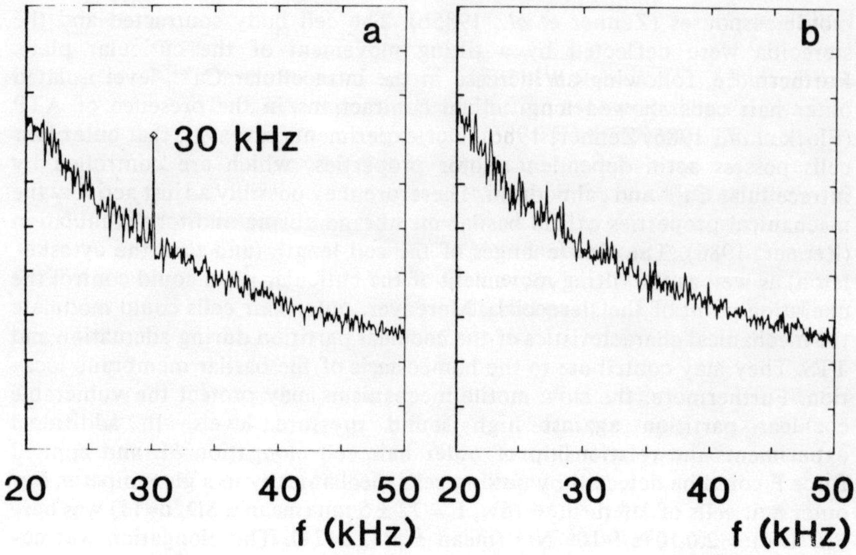

Figure 8. Length oscillation of an outer hair cell (3rd turn) exposed to an alternating electrical field (1 kV/m) of 30 kHz. Shown here are the power density spectra of (a) the experiment and (b) a control (stimulus without cell). The cell length oscillated following the stimulus cycle-by-cycle.

Mechano-electrical and electro-mechanical transduction in hair cells

Mechano-electrical transduction, sited in hair cells, is the basis for sound reception in the mammalian cochlea. Ion channels may play a key role in this process. They were found in apical (Gitter *et al.*, 1986) and basolateral (Gitter *et al.*, 1984; Gitter *et al.*, 1986; Ashmore and Meech, 1986) membranes of outer hair cells and in the lateral membrane of inner hair cells (see above). They contribute probably to de- and repolarization of the hair cells. In outer hair cells the changes of the cell potential (Dallos *et al.*, 1982) may lead to motile responses, thus establishing an electro-mechanical transduction process. In cochlear micromechanics slow and fast motile responses of outer hair cells may contribute to frequency selectivity, negative damping, TTS or adaptation processes.

Acknowledgments

The expert technical assistance of S. Brändler, E. Holzer, and U. Höfling is gratefully acknowledged. Cand. med. R. Zimmermann and M. Rudert collaborated in some experiments. The Deutsche Forschungsgemeinschaft supported this work with a Leibniz grant to H.P.Z.

References

Ashmore, J.F., Meech, R.W. (**1986**). "Ionic basis of membrane potential in outer hair cells of guinea pig cochlea", Nature **322**, 368-371.

Ashmore, J.F. (**1987**) "A fast motile response in guinea-pig outer hair cells: the cellular basis of the cochlear amplifier", J.Physiol. **388**, 323-347.

Brownell, W.E., Bader, C.R., de Ribeaupierre, Y. (**1985**). "Evoked mechanical responses of isolated cochlear outer hair cells" Science **227**, 194-196

Dallos, P., Santos-Sacchi, J., Flock, A. (1982). "Intracellular recordings from cochlear outer hair cells", Science **218**, 582-584.

Flock, Å., Flock, B., Ulfendahl, M. (**1986**). "Mechanisms of movement in outer hair cells and a possible structural basis", Arch.Otorhinolaryngol. **243**, 83-90.

Gitter, A.H., Zenner, H.P., Frömter, E. (**1984**). "Patch-clamp studies on mammalian inner ear hair cells", Workshop on noise analysis and related techniques, Leuven (Belgium).

Gitter, A.H., Zenner, H.P., Frömter, E. (**1986**). "Membrane Potential and Ion Channels in Isolated Outer Hair Cells of Guinea Pig Cochlea", ORL J. Otorhinolaryngol.Relat.Spec. **48**, 68-75.

Zenner, H.P., Gitter, A.H., Zimmermann, U., Schmitt, U., Frömter, E. (**1985a**). "Die isolierte, lebende Haarzelle - ein neues Modell zur Untersuchung der Hörfunktion", Laryngol.Rhinol.Otol. **64**, 642-648.

Zenner, H.P., Zimmermann, U., Schmitt, U. (**1985b**). "Reversible contraction of isolated mammalian cochlear hair cells", Hearing Res. **18**, 127-133.

Zenner, H.P. (**1986**) "Motile responses in outer hair cells" Hearing Res. **22**, 83-90.

Zenner, H.P., Zimmermann, U., Gitter, A.H. (**1987**). "Electrically induced fast motility of isolated mammalian auditory sensory cells", Biochem. Biophys.Res.Comm. **149**, 304-308.

Comments

Narins:

Burt Evans has clearly shown (ARO abstracts 1987, Clearwater Florida) a systematic gradient in the upper cut-off frequency along the longitudinal axis of the mammalian basilar membrane. That is, long OHC's at the apical end have relatively low cut-off frequencies for stimulus-induced contractibility, whereas short OHC's at the basal end are capable of much higher frequencies of movement - up to 8 kHz in his preparation.

Wilson:

Does the response at 30 kHz come from a hair cell from the 30-kHz region? Would you expect a hair cell from a specific region to respond mechanically more strongly to the appropriate frequency?

Reply by Gitter:

The depticted 30 kHz motility (Fig.8) stemmed from a 3rd turn outer hair cell. Burt Evans (Abstracts of the ARO Midwinter Meeting, 1987) reported a correlation between cell length and corner frequency of electrically induced length oscillations.

Kros and Crawford:

We would like to comment on your section on ionic channels in inner hair cells. You mentioned that you have so far only found rather small-conductance channels with preference for potassium ions but a low selectivity.

We have studied some cell-attached patches in the basolateral cell membrane of the inner hair cell at room temperature. The patch-pipettes were filled with (mM): 142 KCl, 0.9 $MgCl_2$, 1.3 $CaCl_2$, 10 HEPES-NaOH, pH 7.4.

We found among others channels with a large unit conductance of 120 ± 14 pS (mean ± S.D, n=4) in every patch, with a reversal potential about 45 to 65 mV depolarized from the holding potential of the pipette (0 mV). This suggests a selective potassium permeability, compatible with the whole-cell currents we reported in this meeting.

Is it possible that the lower conductances that you report arise from your use of higher sodium concentrations in the pipette filling solution and from the lower resting potentials of about 20 mV of your inner hair cells?

Reply by Gitter:

The mechanical dissection technique and short-time culture conditions of inner hair cells from guinea-pig cochlea were similar in your and our experiments. But there is a striking difference in the resting potentials of the isolated cells. This discrepancy may in part be explained by the different temperature of the preparations and by different recording techniques for the cell potentials (patch-clamp/conventional microelectrodes). It is, however, astonishing, that your measurements exhibit more negative resting potentials than are found *in vivo* (x - 40mV). I suppose, that although both preparations delivered viable cells, the physiological state of them may be different. It is therefore difficult to compare patch-clamp experiments performed in the on-cell configuration, since also different test solutions were used in the pipettes. In addition, the data base of single-channel recordings of inner hair cells is, even if we pool our observations, still to small as to allow a correlation between the level of whole-cell properties and the underlying molecular basis (ionic channels).

Ashmore

Figure 6 shows an outer hair cell undergoing a 15% shortening and a tilt of the cuticular plate. This is a difficult experiment because any differential adhesion of the cell to the bottom of the chamber could provide a twist as solutions are changed. However one explanation is that in lunate cells from the apical region, large shortenings might be expected to be accompanied by a straightening of the cell. In the intact cochlea, the cuticular plates of OHC are believed to be held rigidly by the reticular lamina by crosslinking filaments. This suggests that a coupling between longitudinal forces and the stereocilial torque would have to be strong before having any effect on the micromechanics. As a minimum requirement, it seems important to demonstrate that the tilt of the cuticular plate is reversible. If shorter OHCs from the cochlear basal region are used, then the cuticular plate and the long axis of the cell would initially be more nearly perpendicular, although the shorter optical lever provided by the stereocilia would make measurement difficult.

In cells undergoing a maximal reversible length change of 2% under patch pipette control, and which were held away from the chamber side, I find no evidence for a tilt of the cuticular plate.

Reply by Gitter:

The tilting movement of the cuticular plate of single outer hair cells is reversible and does not depend on adhesive interactions. We observed it also under conditions where a change of cell length was not observable (i.e., when the cells were exposed to an alternating electrical field perpendicular to the longitudinal cell axis). Furthermore, *in situ* experiments (perfusion of the perilymphatic space of the cochlea with medium of increased K^+-concentration) were performed by us and thin-sections of the organ of Corti exhibited a decrease of the outer hair cell length and a rotation of the longitudinal outer hair cell axis relative to the lamina reticularis.

What is the stimulus for outer hair cell motility?

J.F.Ashmore

Department of Physiology, Medical School
University Walk, Bristol BS8 1TD, U.K.

Introduction

The patch recording technique has revealed a variety of conductances, predominantly potassium conductances, in the hair cell membrane (Lewis and Hudspeth, 1983; Ashmore & Meech, 1986). A further extension of these techniques can be applied to the observation that isolated outer hair cells are motile (Brownell, Bader, Bertrand and de Ribaupierre, 1985). It can be shown that such outer hair cell length changes can be driven at acoustic frequencies (Ashmore, 1987a).

The outer hair cell system is clearly capable of responding to changes of potential applied as a command step from a patch pipette. It does so by generating forces along the axis cylinder, which although appearing as length changes in isolated cells, may be able to modify the mechanics of the cochlear partition. Although one proposal has been that the active hair cell mechanics involves a release of the basilar membrane from (negative) mechanical feedback (Mountain, 1985), linear modelling of the cochlear partition suggests that sharp basilar membrane tuning can be obtained if outer hair cells oppose fluid damping, i.e. by providing positive feedback (Neely and Kim, 1986; Geisler, 1986; Ashmore 1987a). In this view, the outer hair cell has to produce a force which opposes fluid damping, i.e. a force which lags the displacement.

This paper is concerned with how such motility might be linked to the primary input signal in hair cells, the transduction step coupling mechanical displacement to electrical events in hair cells.

Methods

Conventional patch clamp techniques were used to record whole cell currents. Outer hair cells were obtained from the guinea pig organ of Corti, by either enzymatic treatment (Trypsin 0.5 mg/ml) or by gentle mechanical trituration. They were maintained in tissue culture medium, (L15), which approximates the composition of perilymph. The mechanically sensitive component was studied using mechanically dissociated cells only. Tight seals were usually formed on the basal surface of the cell. Pipettes were filled with (in mM): K 140, Mg 2, HEPES 10, (pH 7.4), and BAPTA 10, to mimic a highly calcium buffered intracellular medium. Inclusion of such calcium buffers, although theoretically reducing Ca to below 10nM, did not inhibit cell motility (Holley and Ashmore, 1988).

Cells were mechanically stimulated by viscous coupling of a 3 μm diameter probe to the hair cell stereocilia. The probe was moved either as a step or by a 880 Hz pulse train 5 μm of the cell apical surface. The fluid flow could be measured by observing the particulate flow around the cell. Attempts at direct coupling of the probe with the stereocilia produced small currents (<15 pA). The most likely explanation is that a smaller fraction of the stereocilia were then deflected.

Results

Cell dialysis

Since the membrane is selectively permeable to potassium (Ashmore & Meech, 1986), whole cell currents could be reduced by replacing the K in the pipette with 140Na or 140Cs. In both cases the steady state magnitude of the length change were not affected (Figure 1), even though the cell input resistance was reduced from 15 nS (with K_i=140 mM) to 5 nS (with

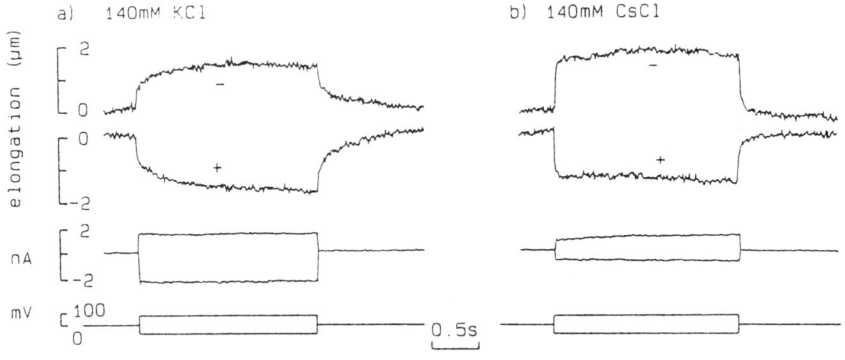

Figure 1: Effect of cell dialysis with different permeant ions. The pipette was filled with a) 140 mM KCl and b) 140 mM CsCl, both solutions buffered with EGTA (500µM) to 0.01Ca. Internal Cs blocks 0.7 of the presumed K conductance of the cell. Both cells recorded within 10 minutes from the same cochlea. Cell resting lengths, a) 77 µm, b) 69 µm. Photosensor responses (top), to hyperpolarizing/depolarizing commands (-/+) measured as in Ashmore (1987a). Command potentials delivered from holding potentials a) -33 mV, b) -20 mV.

Cs_i=140 mM), and the current flow through the cell membrane reduced accordingly. In the experiment shown, a slower component was apparent with K as the dialysing cation, but the initial rates of elongation were not significantly different. Thus in this type of experiment, where the energy for the motion is being provided by the command to the recording pipette, potential but not current appears to be the stimulus. This is consistent with a simple physico-chemical mechanism associated with the cell cortex or plasma membrane.

Transduction currents

To link the motion to the normal *in vivo* stimulus, the mechanically-sensitive transducer of the cell was studied in the whole cell configuration. The stereocilia were deflected by fluid coupling to a probe attached to a piezo-electric driver. Figure 2 shows that, under these conditions, a mechanically-evoked current can be recorded. The time course, both at onset and relaxation, was effectively determined by the pattern of solution flow around the sterocilia. The current was reversibly blocked by bath application of di-hydro-streptomycin (Ashmore, 1987b).

The slope conductance of the current was 0.7 nS at hyperpolarized potentials. This is consistent with inferred *in vivo* values (see Discussion). The nonlinearity of the I-V curve is likely to have arisen from a higher selectivity for Na over K of the transduction pathway. The selectivity correction is not made below.

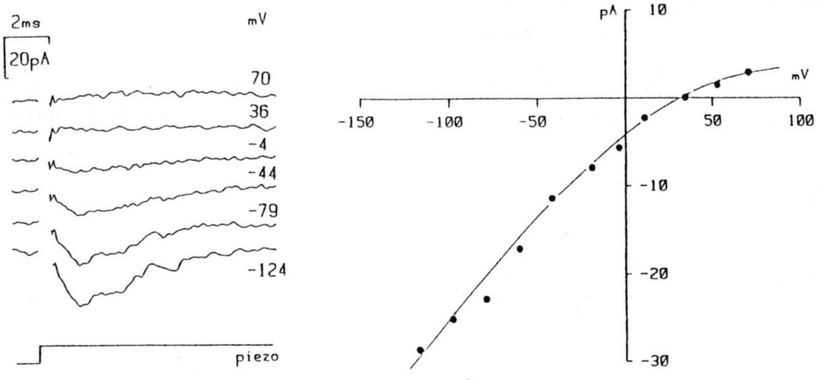

Figure 2: Mechanically-sensitive currents in outer hair cells. Left, responses to a step pulse applied to the driver of the probe. Only the mechanically-sensitive component is shown at different holding potentials (mV). The switching artifact has been removed. Signal averages (10x). Pipette contained K 140 mM, BAPTA, 10. Cell in perilymph solution (L15). Right, I-V curve for the responses, smooth curve drawn by eye. Non-linearity and positive reversal arise from higher selectivity to Na.

Discussion

Outer hair cells possess a mechanically-sensitive current which has characteristics of the transducer current. It is of the correct magnitude to generate the receptor potential seen in hair cells from *in vivo* recordings, (Russell *et al.*, 1986).

The available evidence supports the idea that the motile response in outer hair cells is potential-dependent. This is consistent with experiments in which agents designed to block a variety of known cell motile systems can be shown to be ineffective in blocking outer hair cell motility driven through a patch pipette (Holley and Ashmore, 1988). The simplest types of physico-chemical models, associated with a feature of the cell plasma-membrane and cortex thus appears to be responsible for the mechanism. The main objection to such a potential-sensing mechanism is however that the cell membrane capacitance would filter out any potential changes. The cochlear microphonic can certainly be measured above 10kHz, but the phasic outer hair cell receptor potential measured with a microelectrode at these frequencies, suggests that it is considerably attenuated (Cody and Russell, 1987; Dallos, 1985).

First consider the case where the cell is modelled as a finite cable, and current is injected at the apical end. At high frequencies, however, the cell will no longer be at equipotential, and a larger potential change will be generated near the cuticular plate. In the steady state, the space constant $\lambda = (G_b R_i)^{-1/2}$ is about 750 μm, i.e. about 10 times longer than the cell. Thus for steps >20 ms the cell would effectively be at isopotential. When the cell is driven at a frequency f, the magnitude $|\lambda|$ decreases by a factor $(1+4\pi^2\tau^2 f^2)^{-1/4}$ where τ is the membrane time constant. Taking τ=1.2 ms (Ashmore 1987a), the space constant would be reduced by 2.8× at 1 kHz, and 8.7× at 10 kHz assuming that the membrane conductance is uniformly distributed along the

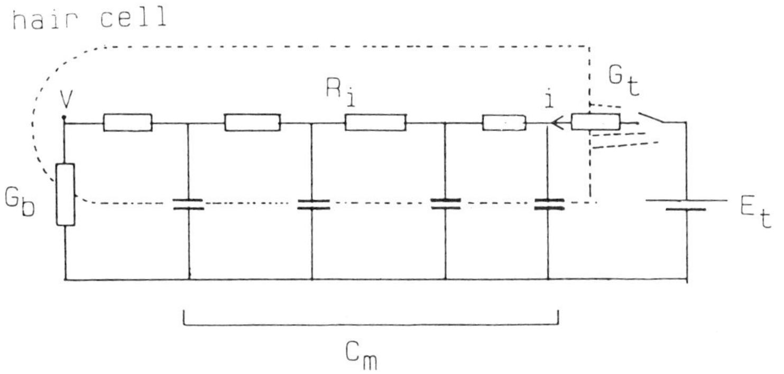

Figure 3. Equivalent circuit of the outer hair cell conductances. G_t=transducer conductance, with driving force E_t. G_b=conductance of cell base, which here may include shunt due to efferent action. C_m=capacitance of cell membrane, here shown distributed. R_i=100 ohm-cm, intracellular axis resistance.

cell. This suggests that outer hair cells, both from the apical and basal turns of the cochlea, are about 1 space constant long at acoustic frequencies. The cell is therefore effectively at isopotential over the range of frequencies of interest, but a small phase difference in membrane potential can exist along the cell. Under the latter conditions the resistance of the cytoplasmic axis cylinder limits the rate of spread of potential.

The results above show that the outer hair cell transducer conductance is less than 1 nS and is likely to account for less than a fraction 0.1 of the total cell input conductance (typically G_b=20 nS). There are several consequences of this electrical mismatch. It implies that outer hair cell I-V curves will be determined largely by the properties of the basolateral membrane, and so that the non-linearities observed in outer hair cell recordings *in vivo* will not reflect any properties of the transducer channel. Secondly, the receptor potential generated within the cell core is anticipated to be at most a fraction $G_t/(G_t+G_b)$ of the transducer driving force, E_t. Since E_t=160 mV approximately, the measured low frequency receptor potentials are close to the predicted 10 mV (Russell *et al*., 1986; Dallos, 1985). The inner hair cell transduction conductance is likely to represent a larger fraction of the cell input conductance since larger inner hair cell potentials are regularly observed. Thirdly, a phase shift in the outer hair cell membrane potential relative to the transducer current, would be expected at frequencies above $(G_t+G_b)/(2\pi C_m)$ on the basis of the simplest equivalent circuit (Figure 3). Inserting values, G_b=20 nS, G_t=0.8 nS and C_m=27 pF, this frequency would be about 120 Hz, so that at higher frequencies, the potential and hence the axial force would lag stereocilial displacement by 90°. Nevertheless if the hair cell membrane can be polarised by 10 mV, then the anticipated force would be sufficient to elongate the cell by 200 nm, which is observable. However, at 1 kHz, the receptor potential would be 0.7 mV in a lumped equivalent circuit model.

Larger potentials along the cell would only be obtained if outer hair cells are specialized with a low channel density along the apical portion of the basolateral cell membrane, and/ or the specific resistance of the axis cylinder is increased. Although the patch clamp is a poor sampling technique, reported K(Ca) channels are recorded exclusively from patches at the basal end of the cell (Ashmore and Meech, 1986), consistent with the former possibility. In this case the magnitude and phasing of potential in the OHC will be determined by the low pass filter characteristics of the transducer and capacitance of the apical cell membrane and would require that intracellular current flow be restricted, for example, to the space immediately between the cisternae and the plasmamembrane. There is currently no evidence supporting this possibility.

The arguments above suggest that opening of transducer channels may lead to axial force generation in outer hair cells by coupling via membrane potential. The mechanism has an intrinsic phase lag for the force of 90° required in simple models of outer hair cell function in which fluid damping of the basilar membrane is opposed. Nevertheless, a microelectrode inserted at or near the basal end of the cell would record an attenuated receptor potential at acoustic frequencies. If the efferent synapses causes a shunting of the membrane conductance, it should be effective to control the spread of current within the cell at frequencies above 1 kHz if the above estimates of the cell space constants are correct.

Acknowledgements
This work was supported by the Medical Research Council.

References

Ashmore, J.F. (**1987a**). "A fast motile response in guinea-pig outer hair cells: the cellular basis of the cochlear amplifier". J.Physiol. **388**, 323-347.

Ashmore, J.F. (**1987b**). "A mechanically-evoked current in outer hair cells isolated from the guinea-pig cochlea". J.Physiol. **372**, 37P.

Brownell, W.E., Bader, C., Bertrand, D. and De Ribaupierre, Y. (**1985**). "Evoked mechanical responses of isolated cochlear outer hair cells". Science **227**, 194-196.

Cody, A.R. and Russell, I.J. (**1987**). "The responses of hair cells in the basal turn of the guinea pig cochlea." J.Physiol. **383**, 551-569.

Dallos, P. (**1985**). "Response characteristics of mammalian cochlear hair cells" J.Neurosci. **5**, 1591-1608.

Geisler, C.D. (**1986**). "A model of the effect of outer hair cell motility on cochlear vibrations". Hearing Res. **24**, 125-132.

Holley, M.C. and Ashmore, J.F. (**1988**). "On the mechanism of a high-frequency force generator in outer hair cells isolated from the guinea pig cochlea". Proc.Roy.Soc. Lond.B. **232**, 413-429.

Holton, T. and Hudspeth, A.J. (**1986**). "The transduction channel of hair cells from the bullfrog characterized by noise analysis". J.Physiol. **375**, 195-227.

Lewis, R.S. and Hudspeth, A.J. (**1983**). "Voltage- and ion-dependent conductances in solitary vertebrate hair cells". Nature **304**, 538-541.

Mountain, D.C. (**1986**). "Active filtering by hair cells", in *Peripheral Auditory Mechanisms* edited by J.B.Allen, J.L.Hall, A.Hubbard, S.T.Neely and A.Tubis. (Springer, Berlin), pp ? .

Neely, S.T. and Kim, D.O. (**1986**). "A model for active elements in cochlear biomechanics". J.Acoust.Soc.Am. **79**, 1472-1480.

Russell, I.J, Cody, A.R. and Richardson, G.P. (**1986**). "The responses of inner and outer hair cells in the basal turn of the guinea-pig cochlea an in the mouse cochlea grown in vitro". Hearing Res. **22**, 199-216.

Comments

Gitter:

1. From your experiments you derive a Na^+ -selectivity of the transduction channels. Does that mean, the transduction currents were to be carried by

Na^+-ions *in vivo*?

2. According to your measurements depicted in Fig. 2 the whole-cell current which is induced by mechanical step pulses builds up rather slowly. Is that consistent with the idea of phase-locked cycle-by-cycle electro-mechanical transduction as source of the cochlear amplifier?

Replies by Ashmore:

1. No.

2. I have used viscous coupling between the probe and the OHC stereocilia because the V-shaped geometry of the stereociulia makes them difficult to deflect efficiently. Direct displacement of a section of two stereocilias away does produce, however, a small non-adapting tuward current suggesting that OHC transduction is sensitive to displacement, (cf.: Prog.Brain Res. 74, Ch. 1, 1988). The mechanically-sensitive current in Fig. 2 are transient because the array is responding to fluid flow around the cell apex and a reflects primarily details of the microscopic flow and not the kinetics of the transduction channel.

Outer hair cell motility - Calcium involvement in the pharmaco-mechanical response.

N. Slepecky, M. Ulfendahl & Å. Flock

Institute for Sensory Research, Syracuse University, Syracuse, NY, USA
Department of Physiology II, Karolinska Institute, Stockholm, Sweden

Introduction

Cells in the body are sensitive to their surroundings and respond to signals present in their external environment. These stimulus-induced responses occur normally and often serve as a mechanism by which a cell can effect change, and as a mechanism by which a cell can modulate its own sensitivity. Examples of such motile events include muscle contraction, mitosis, cell migration, neuron outgrowth, organelle transport, exocytosis and photoreceptor outer segment movement. *In vitro*, many of these forms of cell motility can be observed in specific cell types after depolarization (an electro-mechanical response) or after application of a chemical substance (a pharmaco-mechanical response), which mimic physiological stimulation. In almost all these forms of cell motility, cell shape changes are mediated by a rise in intra-cellular free calcium and calcium activation of an actin myosin interaction.

Intact isolated outer hair cells *in vitro* have recently been observed to change their shape in response to the application of chemical substances. Depolarization by high potassium or application of neurotransmitter substances such as acetylcholine causes isolated outer hair cells to shorten. This observed cell motility may represent the physiological response of outer hair cell to stimulation by these same substances *in vivo*. In the intact cochlea, outer hair cells could often be exposed to potassium since this ion would be expected to increase along the basolateral surface of the cell as a result of potassium flow through the cell during transduction, and especially after acoustic overstimulation. Acetylcholine, a neurotransmitter substance, is thought to be released from the efferent nerve terminals which synapse directly onto the base of the outer hair cells. Thus stimulus induced changes in outer hair cell shape in the intact cochlea could affect individual hair cell within the organ of Corti as well as affect the mechanics of the cochlear partition to alter frequency selectivity and sensitivity of the auditory system.

For these reasons we have further studied outer hair cell motility in order to determine the mechanism involved in shortening.

Outer hair cell response to stimulation

The potassium-induced outer hair cell response occurs after depolarization of the cell, immediately after the application of an isotonic solution containing potassium. We have recently shown that the shortening can be reversible (Slepecky *et al.*, 1988a); soon after the application of a solution containing potassium in the form of potassium gluconate or potassium methylsulfate, a potassium-shortened cell returns almost to its normal length, even in the continued presence of potassium.

Thus outer hair cell motility appears to be similar to the contraction - relaxation cycle seen in muscle after depolarization. In both striated and smooth muscle, cells respond immediately to the elevation of extracellular potassium. The depolarization causes a rise in the intracellular free calcium which activates actin and myosin interaction and contraction. After this stimulus-induced response, although the cell is no longer sensitive to the external potassium, it returns to its normal shape only when the intracellular calcium ion concentration is lowered (either by extrusion of calcium from the cell or by sequestration of the calcium in the internal membrane system of the sarcoplasmic reticulum).

Several results of ours suggest that the potassium-induced response seen in these hair cells is not caused by a decreased osmolarity of the solutions. The potassium-induced shortening can not be prevented by increasing the osmolarity of the medium with sucrose (Slepecky *et al.*, 1988b). The potassium-induced shortening can be blocked by pretreatment of the cell with tetracaine and N-ethylmaleimide. Moreover, a return to almost normal cell shape occurs even in the continued presence of the potassium solution.

Outer hair cells also respond to the application of other chemical substances. Outer hair cells observed during application of a solution containing the presumed efferent neurotransmitter acetylcholine shorten (Brownell *et al.*, 1985; Slepecky *et al.*, 1988a). In one instance, after the initial shortening, an outer hair cell returned to its original length. This response is also similar to the response seen in muscle after the application of acetylcholine, a known transmitter of the efferent "motor" nervous system.

In response to the application of the charged macromolecule cationized ferritin, isolated outer hair cells have been observed to shorten (Flock *et al.*, 1986; Slepecky *et al.*, 1988a). This suggests that hair cells could be sensitive to voltage changes and is again similar to results in muscle where excitation is thought to be coupled to contraction by intramembrane charge movement through channels connecting the cell membrane to the sarcoplasmic reticulum.

Outer hair cell structure

Although hair cell ultrastructure has been investigated for many years, it is only recently that the attention of the studies has focused on the differences between inner and outer hair cells. Outer hair cells have morphological similarities with muscle cells. It has long been known that actin and myosin are present at the apical surface of hair cells (Flock *et al.*, 1982; Drenckhahn *et al.*, 1982). In guinea pigs, actin is present in an infracuticular network of filaments (Zenner, 1986; Thorne *et al.*, 1987), as a cortical network lining the lateral wall (Flock *et al.*, 1986) and in the cytoplasm (Slepecky *et al.*, 1988b). Moreover hair cells have an elaborate system of membranous cisterns which line the lateral wall and which are connected to the hair cell plasma membrane by pillar structures, similar to the relationship of the sarcoplasmic reticulum with the T-tubule membrane in muscle cells. A rise in intracellular calcium is known to induce cell shape changes in muscle and non-muscle cells. Calcium influx or release from intracellular storage sites is the signal which regulates actin and myosin interaction. Experiments using permeabilized cells have suggested that calcium is involved with outer hair cell shortening (Flock *et al.*, 1986; Zenner, 1986; Schacht and Zenner, 1986).

Mechanisms involved in shortening

For all of the above reasons it was suggested that hair cell shortening is caused by a mechanism similar to that which causes muscle contraction. The actin containing systems in hair cells - the infracuticular network, the cortical filaments at the lateral wall, and the cytoplasmic system - have all been suggested to mediate cell shape changes in outer hair cells.

To further test the hypothesis that outer hair cell shape changes are similar to other forms of muscle and non-muscle forms of cell motility, more criteria have to be met. 1) Not only cytoskeletal and contractile proteins need to be present in hair cells, but regulatory proteins must be present as well. 2) The cytoskeleton of the hair cells must be arranged to allow interaction of these proteins, and a change in their distribution must correlate with a change in cell shape. 3) Calcium would be involved in the shortening event.

Contractile and regulatory proteins

Our recent results using immunocytochemistry have demonstrated the presence of cytoskeletal and regulatory proteins in outer hair cells which could affect cell shape. A spectrin-like protein has been found in the cuticular plate and along the lateral wall of outer hair cells. Spectrin is an actin binding protein which crosslinks actin filaments, attaches actin filaments to the cell membrane and affects rigidity of the cell membrane to influence cell shape. Calmodulin, an important calcium-binding regulatory protein in smooth muscle, is localized throughout the cytoplasm of outer hair cells. In muscle, calcium-calmodulin dependent enzyme activation regulates myosin phosphorylation and subsequent interaction of myosin with actin.

Cytoskeletal arrangement

Results of staining hair cells with antibodies to actin and with phalloidin demonstrate that actin is distributed throughout the outer hair cell body, but that some actin containing areas may not be essential for shortening. The infra-cuticular network contains actin, is present in guinea pig outer hair cells, and is more prominent in the longer hair cells at the apex of the cochlea and in the third row (Thorne *et al.*, 1987). Several of our recent experiments have demonstrated that the presence of the infracuticular network is not necessary for shortening to occur.

In the guinea pig the presence of the infracuticular network is not always correlated with outer hair cell shortening. In isolated guinea pig outer hair cells which have been fixed, permeabilized and stained with phalloidin, a central core of actin is present in some normal cells as well as in some cells that have been induced to shorten by the application of potassium. However, it is not present in some guinea pig hair cells where potassium-induced shortening has been documented, and it has been observed in guinea pig hair cells which did not respond. Moreover, an infracuticular network has not been observed in chinchilla outer hair cells or in gerbil outer hair cells. In isolated chinchilla outer hair cells an infracuticular network has never been observed in fixed, permeabilized normal cells or potassium-shortened cells.

Further evidence that the cuticular plate and infracuticular network does not play a role in shortening comes from guinea pig outer hair cells, where mechanical damage has been induced during dissociation to rip the cuticular plate and infracuticular network off from outer hair cells. Although, the apical region of these cells now shows no labeling with fluorescent phalloidin (which stains actin filaments), these cells still shorten.

Evidence exists that some component of the cytoplasm is necessary for shortening, and ultrastructural analysis of potassium shortened cells suggests an association of the contractile apparatus with the lateral wall (Ulfendahl and Slepecky, 1988).

Calcium involvement

Calcium activation of motility is a common property of muscle and non-muscle cells although the source of calcium differs. Skeletal muscle depends primarily on calcium liberated from sarcoplasmic reticulum, whereas smooth muscle and non-muscle cells may require calcium influx, depending on the amount of calcium sequestering membrane systems present in the cell. Using permeabilized cells, calcium has been implicated in the shortening response of outer hair cells (Flock *et al.*, 1986; Zenner, 1986).

Our recent results with intact cells suggest that the source for calcium activation of outer hair cell shortening is internal. The role of calcium was probed with pharmacological agents which are known to affect contraction in muscle. Caffeine is a substance which activates contraction in muscle cells by releasing calcium from intracellular storage sites. In non-muscle cells caffeine releases calcium from endoplasmic reticulum. Caffeine applied to intact isolated outer hair cells causes these cells to shorten. The caffeine effect does not result from an influx of calcium, since the caffeine-induced shortening occurs even when extracellular calcium has been lowered. In muscle and non-muscle cells local anesthetics such as tetracaine antagonize caffeine- and potassium- induced responses. In hair cells, the caffeine-induced shortening and the potassium-induced shortening can be blocked by pretreating outer hair cells with tetracaine.

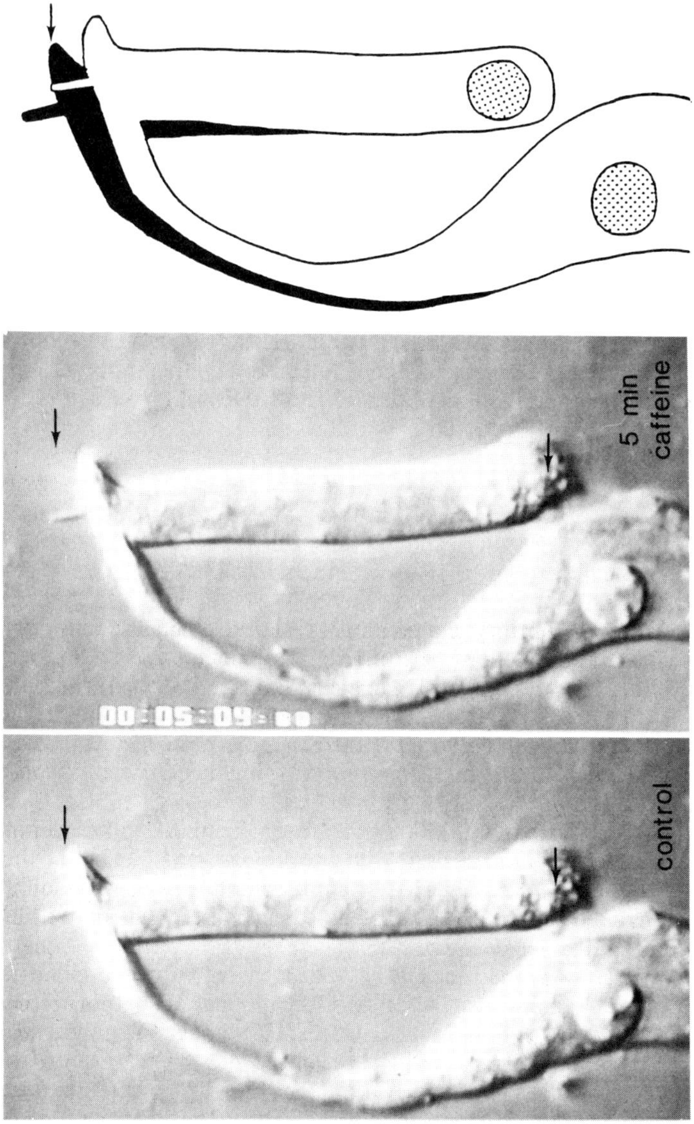

Figure 1. A normal outer hair cell (control) shortens after exposure to 5 mM caffeine. When the image of the shortened cell is superimposed over the image of the control cell, the amount of shortening and the effect of the supporting cell can be observed.

Summary

The mechanism causing the slow sustained shortening of outer hair cells in response to potassium depolarization, activation of voltage sensitive channels, and neurotransmitter substances has yet to be determined. However evidence is accumulating to suggest that hair cell shape changes are similar to other forms of cell motility occuring in muscle and non-muscle cells. Calcium-binding regulatory proteins are present in hair cells and co-localize with actin. Pharmacological agents which affect calcium activation of muscle contraction induce and inhibit outer hair cell shortening. Morphological and ultrastructural analysis of normal and shortened hair cells suggest similarities with other forms of muscle and non-muscle cell motility. Muscle-like cytoskeletal, contractile and regulatory proteins are present in outer hair cells. Cytoplasmic components are necessary for shortening and the contractile apparatus is associated with the lateral wall cell membrane. Shortening is not correlated with the presence of a visible infracuticular network of actin filaments extending as a central core into the cytoplasm. Calcium is involved in the activation of shortening.

These results suggest that in hair cells, contractile and regulatory proteins may interact in a calcium-dependent manner to cause stimulus induced hair cell shape changes which might alter the sensitivity of the auditory system.

References

Brownell, W.E., Bader, C.R., Bertrand, D. and deRibaupierre, Y. (**1985**). "Evoked mechanical responses of isolated cochlear outer hair cells," Science **227**, 194-196.

Drenckhahn, D., Kellner, J., Mannherz, H.G., Gröschel-Stewart, U., Kendrick-Jones, J. and Scholey, J. (**1982**). "Absence of myosin-like immunoreactivity in stereocilia of cochlear hair cells," Nature **300**, 531-532.

Flock, Å., Bretscher, A. and Weber, K. (**1982**). "Immuno-histochemical localization of several cytoskeletal proteins in inner ear sensory and supporting cells," Hearing Res. **6**, 75-89.

Flock, Å., Flock, B. and Ulfendahl, M. (**1986**). "Mechanisms of movement in OHCs and a possible structural basis," Arch.Otorhinolaryngol. **243**, 82-90.

Schacht, J. and Zenner, H.P. (**1986**). "The phosphoinositide cascade in isolated outer hair cells: Possible role as a second messenger for motile responses," Hearing Res. **22**, 94.

Slepecky, N., Ulfendahl, M. and Flock, Å. (**1988a**). "Shortening and elongation of isolated outer hair cells in response to application of potassium gluconate, acetylcholine and cationized ferritin," Manuscript submitted for publication.

Slepecky, N., Ulfendahl, M. and Flock, Å. (**1988b**). "Effects of caffeine and tetracaine on outer hair cell shortening suggest intracellular calcium

involvement," Hearing Res. In press.
Thorne, P.R., Carlisle, L., Zajic, G., Schacht, J. and Altschuler, R.A. (**1987**). "Differences in the distribution of F-actin in outer hair cells along the organ of Corti," Hearing Res. **30**, 253-266.
Ulfendahl, M. and Slepecky, N. (**1988**). "Ultrastructural correlates of inner ear sensory cell shortening," J. Submicroscopic Cytology. In press.
Zenner, H.P. (**1986**). "Motile responses in outer hair cells," Hearing Res. **22**, 83-90.

The fine structure and organization of tip links on hair cell stereovilli

J.O. Pickles, J. Brix*, O. Gleich*, C. Köppl*, G.A. Manley*, M.P. Osborne and S.D. Comis

Department of Physiology, University of Birmingham, Birmingham, B15 2TJ, UK, and
**Institut für Zoologie, Technische Universität München, D-8046 Garching, FRG.*

Introduction

We have recently described a set of links between the stereovilli of hair cells in the mammalian cochlea. The links emerge from the tips of the shorter stereovilli in the bundle, and extend upwards to join the side-wall of the adjacent taller stereovillus (e.g. Pickles *et al.*, 1984; Comis *et al.*, 1985). The tip links may be particularly interesting, because the evidence suggests that they are likely to be involved in sensory transduction, coupling the stimulus-induced movement to the transducer channels, perhaps situated at one or both of their points of insertion into the stereovilli (e.g. Hudspeth 1985; Pickles, 1985). In the present experiments, we have further investigated the fine structure of the tip links, in order to see how the structure might be related to a possible role in transduction. We have also investigated the organization of the links in stereovilli from a variety of species, since if they are involved in transduction, we might expect them to be universally present on mechanoreceptor hair cells of acousticolateral origin and to be oriented parallel to the excitatory-inhibitory axis of the cell.

Methods

For transmission electron microscopy, guinea pigs were anaesthetised, the bullae extracted, and perfused with 2.5% glutaraldehyde and 2% tannic acid in 0.05 M BES buffer, adjusted to pH 7.4 with NaOH (method modified from Little and Neugebauer, 1985). After extraction of the modioli, the specimens were fixed for 0.5 h in the same buffer but including in addition 2% tannic acid, followed by postfixation in 1% OsO_4 in the same buffer for 5 min, and soaking in 2% tannic acid in distilled H_2O, at pH 7.0. Dehydration was accomplished with ethanol and the material stained *en bloc* with uranyl acetate and phosphotungstic acid, before embedding in an Epon Araldite epoxy resin mixture. Sections were stained in methanolic uranyl acetate and lead citrate before examination.

For scanning electron microscopy in lizards, pigeons and starlings, the subjects were anaesthetised and were perfused either intravenously or directly through the oval or round windows with fixative (pigeon: 2.5% glutaraldehyde in 0.1 M phosphate buffer; starling and lizard: 1% glutaraldehyde and 15% saturated picric acid in 0.1 M phosphate buffer). Specimens were stored in 2% glutaraldehyde in 0.05 M or 0.1 M phosphate buffer until further treatment. They were then dehydrated in acetone, dried by the critical point technique with liquid CO_2, and sputter-coated with platinum to a nominal depth of 25 nm. Specimens were examined in a JEOL 120 CXII microscope with a scanning attachment, and images were observed by a secondary electron detector.

In order to measure the electrophysiological responses of the chick basilar papillae, chicks (1 - 14 days old) were anaesthetised, and the basilar papillae removed via an intracranial approach. The papillae were mounted in bird ringer or buffered saline (pH 7.4, 285 mOsm) in a recording chamber, with electrodes on either side of the sensory epithelium. The tectorial membrane was moved directly by means of a piezoelectric pusher (Burleigh), usually at 200 Hz and a peak to peak amplitude of 70 nm, the microphonic being detected with the help of a spectrum analyzer (Hewlett-Packard 3580A). Responses were tested every 5 min; after responses had been shown to be stable for 20 min, enzyme solution was introduced into the chamber, and responses were monitored at 10 min intervals for a further 40 - 60 min. The papillae were then fixed in 2.5% glutaraldehyde and processed for scanning electron microscopy as above.

For enzyme experiments in the guinea pig, temporal bones were extracted as above, the cochleae perfused with 2.5 % glutaraldehyde, and the cochleae opened under fixative, giving a total time in fixative of 5 min. The opened modioli were immersed in enzyme solution at 4°C for 10 or 20 min, and then processed for scanning electron microscopy as above.

Results

The fine structure of tip links

In sections stained with uranyl acetate and lead citrate, a fine relatively straight filament was visible in the centre of the tip link (Fig. 1). The central filament was surrounded by darkly-staining material with a variable appearance. In some sections, the central filament appeared to be negatively stained. The central filament, including the heavily darkly-staining material immediately surrounding it, was measured as having a diameter of 5.5 nm ± 0.4 nm (sem, n = 16).

At its upper end, the central filament ran to the centre of a density on the sidewall of the taller stereovillus, the density forming a bridge between the external membrane of the stereovillus and the internal actin paracrystal. At its lower end, the filament ended on what usually appeared as a conical extension of the membrane of the stereovillus (Fig. 2). Below this, there was a clear area, and below that, there was a dense cap over the ends of the filaments of the actin paracrystal (Fig. 2). In some cases it was just possible to see filaments

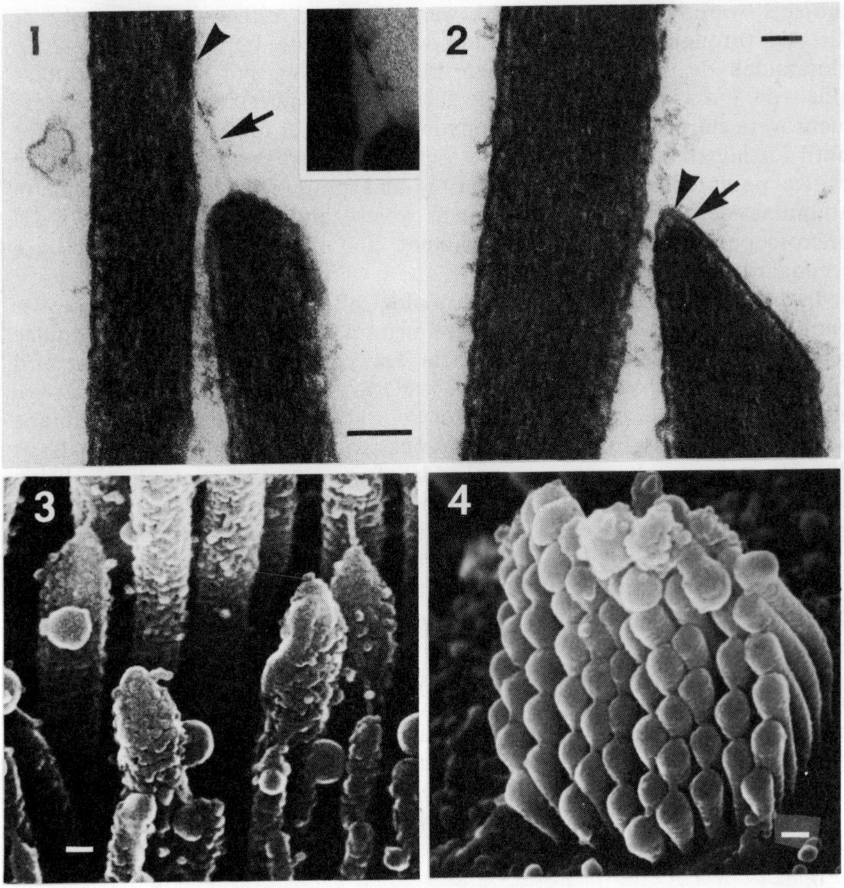

Figure 1. Tip link with central filament (arrow), and upper dense point of attachment (arrowhead). Insert: same, more densely printed. Guinea pig outer hair cell. Scale bar: 100 nm.
Figure 2. Dense cap (arrow) over actin filaments just under tip link. Filaments (arrowhead) are just visible, connecting density to surface membrane just under tip link. Guinea pig inner hair cell. Scale bar: 100 nm.
Figure 3. Chondroitinase-digested inner hair cell, showing some tip links remaining, but thinner than in control cochleae. Insert: detail. Guinea pig. Scale bars: 200 nm and 50 nm.
Figure 4. Hair bundle from the lizard Podarcis sicula, showing columns of stereocilia joined by tip links (arrows). Scale bar: 500 nm.

running between the dense cap and the overlying membrane near the point of insertion of the central filament of the tip link.

The material of variable appearance surrounding the central filament of

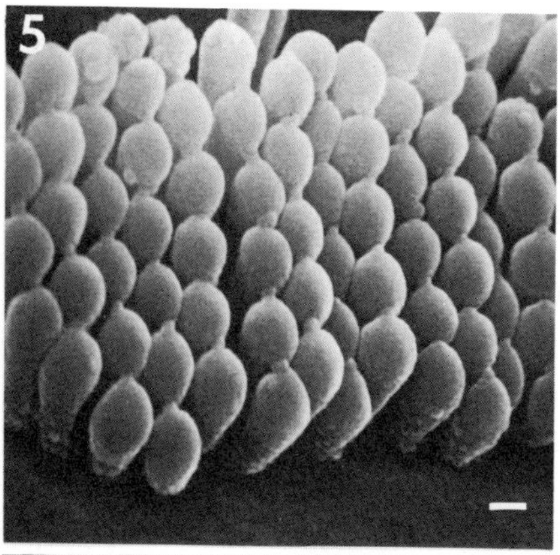

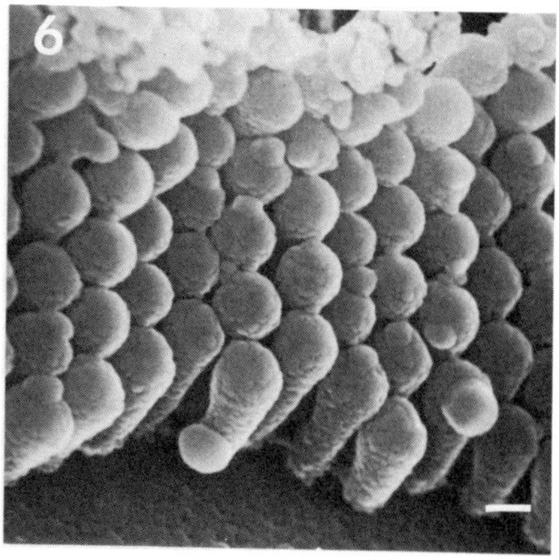

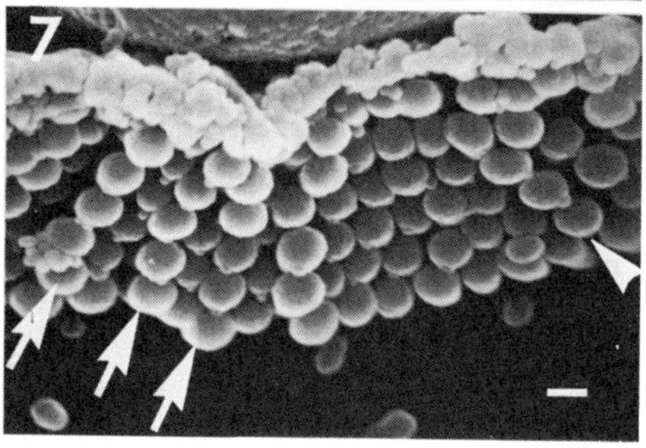

Figure 5. Hair bundle in starling, showing tip links, with stereocilia organized into columns running at right angles to the rows (i.e. along the axis of bilateral symmetry). Basal end of papilla, near abneural edge. Scale bar: 500 nm.
Figure 6. Tip link organization in pigeon. Abneural edge, middle of papilla. Scale bar: 500 nm.
Figure 7. Anomalous bundle in pigeon, with tip links over left and some of right of bundle oriented towards the right (arrows), and with those on the extreme right running towards the left (double-headed arrows). This hair cell was oriented 30 degrees differently from its neighbours. The latter were oriented such that their rows of stereovilli ran at right angles to the arrows on the left of the figure, with their tip links running parallel to the arrows. The large structure at the top is a bleb, probably associated with the hole in the cuticular plate. Middle of papilla, neural edge. Scale bar: 200 nm.

the tip link appeared to be continuous with the variable material surrounding the external membranes of the stereovillus. It may therefore consist of glycocongugates. This hypothesis was tested by enzyme digestion in the guinea pig. Opened cochleae were incubated in chondroitinase (Sigma C-3509, 1 unit/ml) for 10 min at 4°C. While some of the tip links were missing, those that did survive were usually finer than in control cochleae (Fig. 3), suggesting that a surrounding coat had been removed, and that it was susceptible to chondroitinase. On the other hand, incubation in crude protease (Sigma Type I P-4630, 200 μg/ml for 10 min) or trypsin (Sigma Type III-S, T-2395, 1000 72 μg/ml for 20 min) removed the links as soon as it produced other observable changes on the surface of the stereovilli. The links therefore may well contain a protein component, perhaps in the central filament, although we have no further information on the composition of the filament.

A common procedure for the isolation of viable hair cells from the mammalian cochlea involves incubation in collagenase (e.g. Zajic and Schacht, 1987). Digestion of the isolated chick basilar papilla in collagenase (Sigma type IV C-5138, 1 mg/ml) for up to 1 hr at 20°C had little effect on the evoked microphonic current, and was associated with survival of the tip links, although changes in the membrane texture sometimes made them difficult to see. This suggests that the links may not be composed of collagen.

The spatial organization of tip links

We have previously reported that in the guinea pig, tip links have a horizontal component in their orientation which is parallel to the axis of bilateral symmetry of the hair cell, or in other words parallel to the excitatory-inhibitory axis (Pickles *et al.*, 1984; Comis *et al.*, 1985). This was true in both inner and outer hair cells, i.e. in bundles of very different conformation. The presence and spatial organization of tip links was further investigated in hair cells of the bird and lizard basilar papillae, which have conformations quite different from that of the mammalian cochlea.

In the lizards *Podarcis sicula* and *Podarcis muralis* the tip links ran parallel to the axis of bilateral symmetry, i.e. in the direction from the shortest stereovilli to the tallest (Fig. 4). The stereovilli and their associated tip links in fact formed columns, running parallel to the axis of symmetry, sometimes clearly separating out into groups (Fig. 4). The same columnar organization was found in the starling (Fig. 5), pigeon (Fig. 6) and chick basilar papillae.

Where anomalous tip link orientations were found, they were generally associated with the following: (i) the stereovilli had been obviously disorganized in preparation, so that the links had been distorted, and (ii) there were other abnormalities in the bundle. In some cases moreover extraneous material lay over the surface of the bundle, making it difficult to identify the tip links. In only a few hair cells (an average well under 1%) was it possible to find anomalously-oriented tip links in an otherwise normal bundle. Mostly there were other abnormalities as well. In the case illustrated in Fig. 7, the tip links on the whole of the left half and on part of the right half ran towards the right; those on the extreme right of the bundle ran towards the left. This bundle was also anomalous in that the bundle as a whole was tilted with respect to its neighbours, with the orientation of the rows as a whole being some 30° different from those on either side. The orientation was such that the tip links over most of the bundle (i.e. over the left half and most of the right half) ran in a direction nearly parallel to the tip links on the adjacent hair cells.

Discussion

The results show that tip links have two components, namely a fine central filament, and a variable surrounding coat. We do not have information on the nature of the filament, although it is presumably protein. It has the same diameter as actin filaments within the paracrystal of the stereovilli in our material. Like actin, the filament is negatively-staining, and is susceptible to osmium tetroxide (Comis *et al.*, 1985). A fine filament would be ideal for concentrating the stimulus-induced movements onto a small area of membrane, suitable for opening the 1 - 4 transducer channels associated with each stereovillus (Russell, 1983; Holton and Hudspeth, 1986).

We do not know at which end of the link the transducer channels might be situated. The density at the upper point of attachment, or the conical extension of the stereovillar membrane at the lower point of attachment, are both possible sites, under the hypothesis that the tip links are involved in transduction (Pickles *et al.*, 1984). We note that the membrane around the lower point of insertion, at the tip of the shorter stereovillus, is anchored by filaments onto the dense cap on the underlying actin paracrystal, so that stimulus-induced shear can be concentrated on the membrane at that point.

The finding that tip links are present in a wide range of species supports the notion that they have an important functional role. They have so far been reported for the mammalian cochlea and vestibular system, including the guinea pig, rat and man (Pickles *et al.*, 1984; Rhys-Evans *et al.*, 1985) and the fish vestibular system (Little and Neugebauer, 1985). Here, the observations have been extended to include birds (chick, starling and pigeon) and reptiles (lizards). Investigation of these species had advantages, in that the hair bundles have a compact form, with the stereovilli being tightly packed into a hexagonal array. In such bundles, the orientation of the tip links parallel to the hair cell axis of symmetry is particularly obvious. The fact that the stereovilli tend to split into columns which run parallel to the axis of bilateral symmetry (i.e. along the excitatory-inhibitory axis) suggests that the mechanical connections along this axis are stronger than those in the other directions. This again emphasises the possible importance of the axis in hair cell function.

The laying down of the axis of the hair cell during ontogeny, and the development of the tip links and their organization (Neugebauer, 1986), are particularly interesting issues. Anomalously-oriented tip links may give suggestive evidence here. We have as yet only preliminary evidence on this point. We have previously reported in a group of guinea pigs where hair cells were found with anomalous axes, that tip links nevertheless tended to run at right angles to the long axis of the individual rows of stereovilli (Pickles *et al.*, 1986). This suggests that tip link organization is more closely related to the hair cell itself rather than to its surroundings. Here, however, we report a case where anomalous organization of the tip links was associated with an anomalous orientation of the bundle as a whole. This suggests that the orientation of the tip links can be affected by the surroundings of the cell, as well as by factors internal to the cell.

Summary

Tip links on hair cells of the guinea pig cochlea have a fine (6-nm) central core, surrounded by a variable outer coat. The fine central filament is related to densities at its points of attachment on the stereovilli (stereocilia). We report here tip links for a wider range of systems, including birds (starling, pigeon and chick) and lizards. With very few exceptions, the tip links run parallel to the axis of bilateral symmetry of the hair cell, and the stereovilli are organized into columns parallel to this axis. When the organization of the tip links does not fit into this scheme, there are generally other anomalies in the hair bundle.

Acknowledgements

The work reported here was supported by the Medical Research Council (UK), and the Deutsche Forschungsgemeinschaft within the programme of the SFB 204 "Gehör". The expert technical assistance of L.M. Tompkins and T.L. Hayward is gratefully acknowledged.

References

Comis, S.D., Pickles, J.O. and Osborne, M.P. (**1985**). "Osmium tetroxide postfixation in relation to the crosslinkage and spatial organization of stereocilia in the guinea pig cochlea," J.Neurocytol. **14**, 113-130.

Holton, T. and Hudspeth, A.J. (**1986**). "The transduction channel of hair cells from the bull-frog characterized by noise analysis," J.Physiol. **375**, 195-227.

Hudspeth, A.J. (**1985**). "The cellular basis of hearing: the biophysics of hair cells," Science **230**, 745-752.

Little, K.F. and Neugebauer, D.Ch. (**1985**). "Interconnections between the stereovilli of the fish inner ear II," Cell Tissue Res. **242**, 427-432.

Neugebauer, D.Ch. (**1986**). "Interconnections between the stereovilli of the fish inner ear. III," Cell Tissue Res. **246**, 447-453.

Pickles, J.O. (**1985**). "Recent advances in cochlear physiology," Prog. Neurobiol. **24**, 1-42.

Pickles, J.O., Comis, S.D. and Osborne, M.P. (**1984**). "Cross-links between stereocilia in the guinea pig organ of Corti, and their possible relation to sensory transduction," Hearing Res. **15**, 103-112.

Pickles, J.O., Comis, S.D., Osborne, M.P. and Pepper, C. (**1986**). "Guinea pigs with backwards outer hair cells," Abstracts, 23rd Meeting Inner Ear Biology, p. 13, Berlin, DDR.

Rhys-Evans, P.H., Comis, S.D., Osborne, M.P., Pickles, J.O. and Jeffries, D.J.R. (**1985**). "Cross-links between stereocilia in the human organ of Corti," J.Laryngol.Otol. **99**, 11-19.

Russell, I.J. (**1983**). "Origin of the receptor potential in inner hair cells of the

mammalian cochlea: evidence for Davis' theory," Nature **301**, 334-336.
Zajic, G. and Schacht, J. (**1987**). "Comparison of isolated outer hair cells from five mammalian species," Hearing Res. **26**, 249-256.

Comments

Slepecky:

In your diagram you show the tip links parallel to the direction of bilateral symmetry, which is also parallel to the direction of hair cell excitation in the radial direction. This arrangement of stereocilia may be true for the basal region of the cochlea, but at the apical region the axes of bilateral symmetry of the stereocilia bundle is not exactly radial, and the fibers of the tectorial membrane curve. Does the orientation of the tip links vary with the shape of the stereocilia bundle, along the length of the cochlea?

Reply by Pickles:

There is almost certainly a longitudinal component to the travelling wave in the cochlear duct, so it should not be surpising that the axis of bilateral symmetry of the hair cells does not always run in a direction which is radial across the duct.

There are problems in analyzing the three-dimensional organization of stereovillar bundles in the apex of the mammalian cochlea, since the stereovilli are rather long and are easily disturbed during the preparation. However, it should be noted that in species such as birds, the angle of the hair cell axis changes in a regular and systematic manner across the width of the papilla, undergoing a change in orientation of up to 90°. In these cases, the columns formed by the tip links, and the tip links themselves, nevertheless continue to run parallel to the axis of bilateral symmetry of the bundle, in spite of the change in orientation.

Functional parallels between hair-cell populations of birds and mammals

Geoffrey Manley, Otto Gleich, Jutta Brix and Alexander Kaiser

Institut für Zoologie der Technischen Universität München, Lichtenbergstr. 4, 8046 Garching, FRG

Introduction

The evolution of land vertebrates has produced an extremely interesting variety of structure and function of the hearing organ. We find not only large differences in the overall dimensions of the basilar papilla, but also in the structure, arrangement and innervation of the hair cells. Large, specialized hearing organs developed during the mesozoic adaptive radiation of the reptiles within two evolutionary lines: the mammals and the archosaurs (crocodilians and birds). Since a number of reptilian groups which also originated during the same adaptive radiation still show simple, hearing organs, it is reasonable to assume from the paleontological evidence that the common, early mesozoic, ancestor of these groups had a rather simple, unspecialized hearing organ. The complexities we see today in the inner ears of mammals and crocodilians are thus independent developments from a common stock. The similarities we discuss below are the result of parallel evolution and show convergence in some important features. In this report, we discuss two points. Firstly, we summarize the evidence concerning both the structural differences but also the similarities between the hearing organs of birds and mammals. Secondly, we point out that our recent physiological studies provide the first evidence for the supposition that functional parallels exist between the hearing organs of birds and mammals.

Structural differences between the anatomy of the avian and of the mammalian hearing organ

The structure of the bird basilar papilla (see below, Fig. 1) is different to that of mammals (Organ of Corti). Although the total number of hair cells can be similar, the sensory epithelium is not so stretched out and coiled. Rather, although also showing the familiar base-to-apex width gradient, it is generally shorter than 5 mm (some owls being a remarkable exception) and, at the most, somewhat bent and twisted along its length (Schwarzkopff and Winter, 1960). The hair cells of the avian papilla are not so clearly divided into two populations as in the mammalian hearing organ, where there is one single row of inner hair cells (IHC) and mostly three rows of outer hair cells (OHC). Avian papillae do show structural variety of the hair cells, the tall hair cells (THC) looking very different to the short hair cells (SHC). However, the extremes grade into one another, so that a strict division of hair cells into different types should perhaps be regarded as merely convenient for descriptive purposes.

The combination of a relatively large number of hair cells and a short papilla lead to the fact that in a transverse section of the avian papilla at the apical end, there can be up to about 50 hair cells; at the basal end there are about 10 hair cells. The cells on the neural side are columnar in shape (Tall hair cells, THC), those on the abneural edge are bowl-shaped (short hair cells, SHC; Takasaka and Smith, 1971). Unlike in the crocodilians, however, these cell types in birds are not clearly-definable separate classes, but form a morphological continuum. Hair cells with intermediate shape have been termed intermediate hair cells. In some papillae, a fourth type similar to SHC has been recognized (lenticular hair cells; Smith, 1985). Unlike in the mammalian hearing organ, not all hair-cell types are necessarily found throughout the avian papilla. In addition, unlike in mammals, all avian hair cells are firmly connected to the tectorial membrane.

A further difference, which has only come to light through recent investigations, concerns the hair-cell orientation. In mammals, both IHC and OHC have their axis of stimulation (perpendicular to the stereovillar bundle) oriented at or close to a right angle to the edge of Corti's organ. Although early reports suggested that the situation in birds is the same (e.g. Takasaka and Smith, 1971), this was an error. In the chick (Tilney *et al.*, 1987), pigeon and starling (Gleich and Manley, 1988) and the barn owl (Fischer *et al.*, 1988) papillae, hair-cell orientation in the center of the apical part is rotated up to 90° towards the apex. The hair cell orientation changes back to 0° (i.e., abneural) towards both edges of the papilla.

Structural similarities between the two types of papillae

In spite of these considerable differences in morphology, there are striking parallels, both in the arrangement and structure of hair cells and in the patterns of afferent and efferent innervation. These convergences suggest that the phylogenetic development and organization of avian and mammalian hearing organs were strongly influenced by certain common features. We suggest that these features are some of the fundamental mechanisms of stimulus processing in vertebrate hair cells and in hair-cell mosaics.

The structural similarities between IHC and OHC on the one hand and THC and SHC on the other can be summarized as follows:

1) The relative placement of the different cell types in the respective papillae is almost the same. Both IHC and, in general, THC are not found over the free basilar membrane. Except for apical THC, they are situated within the neural side of the papilla, which overlies the superior cartilaginous plate in birds and

the spiral lamina in mammals (Smith, 1985).
2) The hair cells lying on the neural side of the papilla are regarded as being the less specialized in both vertebrate classes (Chandler, 1984, Takasaka and Smith, 1971).
3) Like IHC, THC are usually exclusively innervated, that is, their afferents synapse only with one single hair cell (Liberman, 1982; also see data below). Although Whitehead and Morest (1985) found many afferents which penetrated between two THC and innervated both, this pattern is very seldom in our data. In addition, both IHC and THC are innervated by the bulk of the afferent fibers. In contrast, SHC, like OHC, are innervated non-exclusively by a relatively small percentage of the afferent fibers (mammal 5 to 10%, starling 14%), which have small synaptic endings (von Düring *et al.*, 1985; Spoendlin, 1979).
4) The efferent innervation of both OHC and SHC is markedly stronger than that to THC or that to the afferent fibers of IHC, and the synaptic endings are much larger (Firbas and Müller, 1983; Hirokawa, 1978; Spoendlin, 1979; Takasaka and Smith, 1971). Also, in both cases, the innervation density of efferents is higher in the basal than in the apical half of the papilla.
5) The ontogenetic development of the afferent and efferent innervation follows very similar patterns in birds and mammals (Whitehead and Morest, 1985; Pujol *et al.*, 1978).
6) With regard to their sensitivity to noise damage, both SHC and OHC tend to be the first to show morphological changes (Cotanche *et al.*, 1987; Liberman and Kiang, 1978; Robertson, 1982).

A functional parallel in the two types of cochleae

The morphological parallels outlined above have, to date, not been matched by equivalent findings of similarities in the physiological responses of, for example, primary nerve fibers. Although the response activity of bird primary afferents certainly does resemble that of mammalian afferents in many respects, these similarities are, in general, features of all vertebrate auditory organs (tonotopicity, frequency selectivity, etc.). There are both quantitative and qualitative differences in the activity patterns of primary auditory neurons of birds and mammals (Manley *et al.*, 1985; Schermuly *et al.*, 1983; Schermuly and Klinke, 1985). Even though otoacoustic emissions with features similar to those of mammals have been reported from a bird species (Manley *et al.*, 1987b) and the related Caiman (Klinke and Smolders, 1984), they have also been found in a frog (Palmer and Wilson, 1981). Thus, such phenomena should perhaps be attributed more to general properties of hair cells than to unique properties of hearing organs with specialized hair-cell populations. We report here an investigation of the innervation patterns of active afferent fibers in two avian species, where the results indicate an unexpected and remarkable parallel to the situation in mammals.

We have recently mapped the tonotopic arrangement of the basilar papilla of two bird species, using HRP in the chicken (Manley *et al.*, 1987a) and the

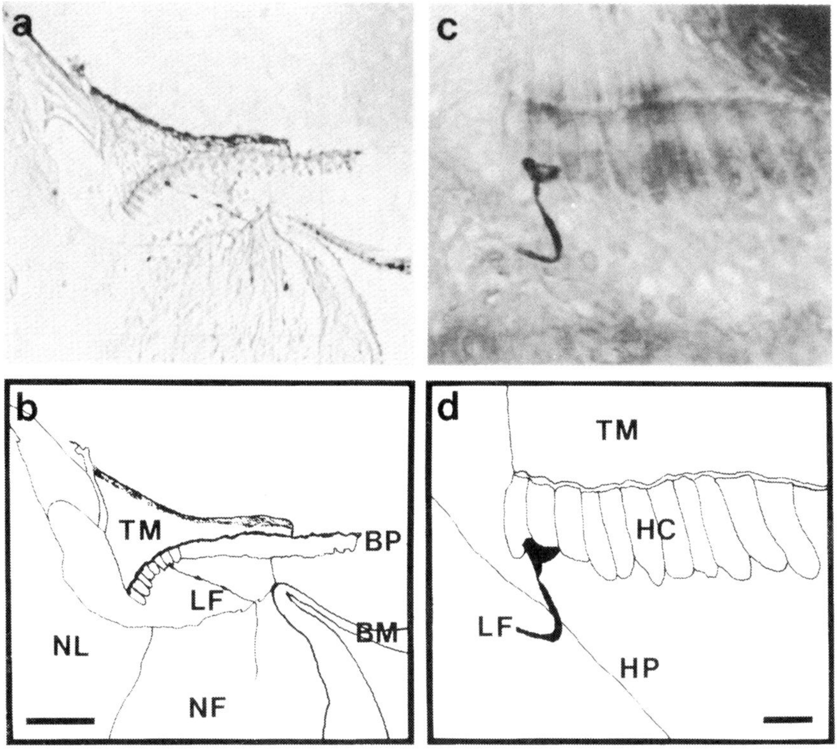

Figure 1 **a**,**b**: *Light micrograph (***a***) and corresponding schematic drawing (***b***) of a 15 μm transverse section through the starling basilar papilla (bar=50 μm). A single, cobalt-stained afferent auditory nerve fiber (CF=0.4 kHz: threshold=45 dB SPL) runs to the seventh THC from the neural edge (left). The fiber can be followed from the synapse through the habenula perforata and a short distance towards the cochlear ganglion. The receptor epithelium ruptured from the basilar membrane during the histological procedure. For the same reason, the abneural part of the basilar papilla is missing.*
c,**d**: *Higher-magnification micrograph (***c***) and schematic drawing (***d***) of a HRP-stained afferent auditory fiber in the same frequency range from a chick's basilar papilla synapsing with the second THC (bar=10 μm).*
Abbreviations: BM basilar membrane, BP basilar papilla, HP habenula perforata, HC hair cells, LF labeled fiber, NF nerve fibers, NL neural limbus, TM tectorial membrane.

cobalt technique in the starling (Gleich, in preparation; Köppl and Gleich, 1988). In each case, we stained single auditory-nerve cells or fibers in the cochlear ganglion. Following the investigation of the frequency response characteristics of individual fibers, either HRP or cobalt hexamminechloride

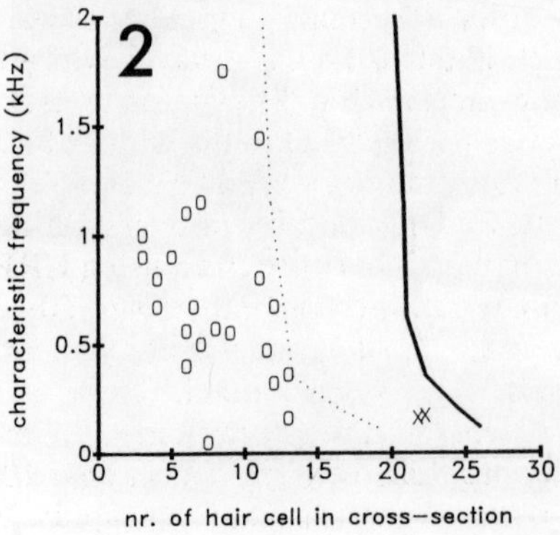

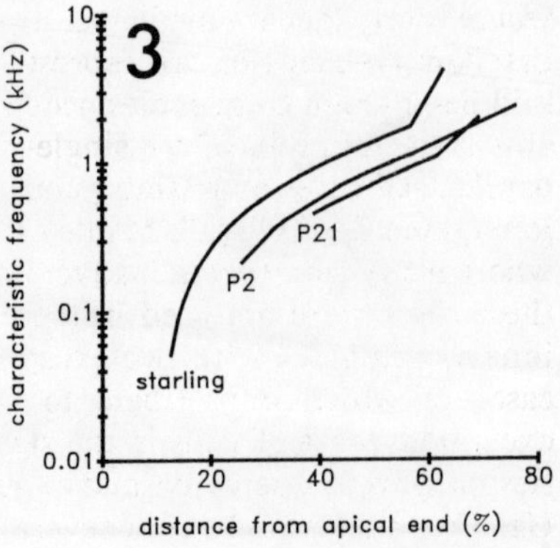

Figure 2. Distribution of labeled and physiologically-characterized fibers in the basilar papilla of the starling with respect to their relative distance from the neural edge of the papilla. The CF is plotted against the location of the innervated hair cell as counted from neural to abneural in a transverse section. The solid line indicates the abneural border of the sensory epithelium; the dotted line shows the location of hair cells with a 1:1 ratio of length to width. It is evident that, with two exceptions, all labeled fibers terminate on THC (O). The two apical cells in the abneural region (×) innervated one and six hair cells, respectively (see text).

Figure 3. Second-order polynomial regressions of the distribution of CF of labeled auditory nerve fibers in the basilar papillae of the starling and in chicks of two different age groups (2nd postnatal day P2 and 21st day P21). Starling: n=34; r^2=0.79; chick, P2: n=13; r^2=0.98; P21: n=8; r^2=0.93.

was injected iontophoretically through the electrode. After a survival time of at least two hours, the animals were perfused through the heart and the cochlear ducts processed to develop the stain. The cochleae were embedded in Spurr, examined and measured both as whole-mount preparations and as serial sections. The position of the fibre terminations were measured from the apical end, as the strong twisting of the basal end makes an accurate correction for the curvature more difficult. As different cochleae differ in length (partly as a result of different ages in the chicks), the locations of the stained terminals (Fig. 1) are given in the figure as a percentage of the distance from the apical end. Further details on techniques are given in the papers cited.

The tonotopic arrangement in both the starling and the chick is unremarkable; the frequency distribution in the starling can be represented as 0.33 mm/oct, in the chicken as about 0.6 mm/oct. Both of these values are obtained from linear regressions over the available range of data. As we have noted elsewhere, however, the distribution of octaves is not uniform in vertebrate hearing organs (Manley *et al.*, 1988). In both the chick and the starling, less space is devoted to the lowest-frequency octaves. In the starling, where more data are available, a second-order polynomial regression reveals that low frequencies are represented with about 0.1 mm/ octave, whereas middle-to-high frequencies occupy 0.5 mm/octave (Fig. 2). What is remarkable is the locations of the single-fibre stains with respect to the width of the papilla. All cases of unambiguous single fibre staining were of fibers which innervated THC (Fig. 3; Manley *et al.*, 1987a). Only in cases of overstaining, where many fibers were inadvertently stained (this only occurred using HRP, these cases were not used in the above analysis), did we find stained fibers innervating SHC. With two exceptions (of a total of 54), we did not find any cases in which only fibers to short hair cells were stained. These two exceptions were of cells in the starling, which had unusual response properties; they were insensitive and extremely poorly tuned to frequencies near 100 Hz. They innervated one or several cells on the abneural side of the papilla. In our material it was not possible to classify the innervated hair cells as intermediate or short according to the criteria of Takasaka and Smith (1971). However, they were certainly not tall hair cells. Afferent fibres with similar response properties and innervation patterns have been reported in the pigeon, where they appear to belong to a population specialized for the reception of infrasound (Klinke and Schermuly, 1986).

We thus conclude that, in both species, all the neural recordings were from single afferent fibers which innervate single THC. This is an unexpected parallel to the situation in mammals, where single-fibre stains of primary afferents in the cat and guinea pig were exclusively of fibers innervating IHC (Liberman and Oliver, 1984; Robertson, 1984). The only documented cases of recordings from afferent fibers to OHC indicated that, under experimental conditions at least, these fibers do not respond to sound (Robertson, 1984). Taken together, the anatomical and physiological data indicate that it is reasonable to expect that some of the mechanisms underlying the function of the hair-cell mosaics of birds and mammals will be very similar, if not identical. This expectation increases the usefulness of investigations in avian species with respect to the understanding of the function of complex hearing organs and, more specifically, to the elucidation of function in the mammalian cochlea.

References

Chandler, J.P. (**1984**). "Light and electron microscopic studies of the basilar papilla in the duck, Anas platyrhynchos: I. The hatchling." J.Comp.Neurol. **222**, 506-522.

Cotanche, D.A., Saunders, J.C., and Tilney, L.G. (**1987**). "Hair cell damage produced by acoustic trauma in the chick cochlea." Hearing Res. **25**, 267-286.

Düring, M. von, Andres, K.H., and Simon, K. (**1985**). "The comparative anatomy of the basilar papillae in birds." Fortschritte der Zoologie **30**, 681-684.

Fischer, F.P., Köppl, C., and Manley, G. (**1987**). "The basilar papilla of the barn owl: *Tito alba*: A quantitative morphological SEM analysis," Hearing Res. (in press)

Gleich, O., and Manley, G.A. (**1987**). "Quantitative morphological analysis of the sensory epithelium of the starling and pigeon basilar papilla." Hearing Res. (in press)

Hirokawa, N., (**1978**). "The ultrastructure of the basilar papilla of the chick," J.Comp.Neurol. **181**, 361-374.

Klinke, R., and Schermuly, L. (**1986**). "Inner ear mechanics of the crocodilian and avian basilar papillae in comparison to neuronal data." Hearing Res. **22**, 183-184.

Klinke, R., and Smolders, J. (**1984**). "Hearing mechanisms in caiman and pigeon." in *Comparative physiology of sensory systems*, edited by L. Bolis, R.D. Keynes and S.H.P. Maddrell (Cambridge Univ. Press, Cambridge) pp. 195-211.

Köppl, C., and Gleich, O. (**1987**). "Cobalt labelling of single primary auditory neurons - an alternative to HRP." Hearing Res. **32**, 111-116.

Liberman, M.C. (**1982**). "Single-neuron labeling in the cat auditory nerve." Science **216**, 1239-1241.

Liberman, M.C., and Kiang, N.Y.S. (**1978**). "Acoustic trauma in cats." Acta Otolaryngol., Suppl. **358**, 1-63.

Liberman, M.C., and Oliver, M.E. (**1984**). "Morphometry of intracellularly labeled neurons of the auditory nerve: correlations with functional properties." J.Comp.Neurol. **223**, 163-176.

Manley, G.A., Brix. J., and Kaiser. A. (**1987a**). "Developmental stability of the tonotopic organization of the chick's basilar papilla." Science **237**, 655-656.

Manley, G.A., Schulze, M., and Oeckinghaus, H. (**1987b**). "Otoacoustic emissions in a song bird." Hearing Res. **26**, 257-266.

Manley, G.A., Gleich, O., Leppelsack, H.-J., and Oeckinghaus, H. (**1985**). "Activity patterns of cochlear ganglion neurones in the starling." J.Comp. Physiol. **157**, 161-181.

Manley, G.A., Brix, J., Gleich, O., Kaiser, A., Köppl, C., and Yates, G. (**1988**). "New aspects of comparative peripheral auditory physiology." in *Auditory System - Structure and Function*, edited by J. Syka (Plenum Publ. Corp., N.Y.) in press.

Palmer, A.R., and Wilson, J.P. (**1981**). "Spontaneous and evoked acoustic emissions in the frog Rana esculenta." J.Physiol. **324**, 66P.

Pujol, R., Carlier, E., and Devigne, C. (**1978**). "Different patterns of cochlear innervation during the development of the kitten." J.Comp.Neurol. **177**, 529-536.

Robertson, D. (**1982**). "Effects of acoustic trauma on stereovillar structure and spiral ganglion cell tuning properties in the guinea pig cochlea." Hearing Res. **7**, 55-74.

Robertson, D. (**1984**). "Horseradish peroxidase injection of physiologically characterized afferent and efferent neurones in the guinea pig spiral ganglion." Hearing Res. **15**, 113-121.

Schermuly, L., and Klinke, R. (**1985**). "Change of characteristic frequency of pigeon auditory afferents with temperature." J.Comp.Physiol. **156**, 209-211.

Schermuly, L., Göttl, K-H., and Klinke, R. (**1983**). "Little ototoxic effect of Furosemide on the pigeon inner ear." Hearing Res. **10**, 279-282.

Schwarzkopff, J.J., and Winter, P. (**1960**). "Zur Anatomie der Vogel-Cochlea unter natürlichen Bedingungen." Biol.Zentralblatt **79**, 607-625.

Spoendlin, H. (**1979**). "Neural connections of the outer hair cell system." Acta Otolaryngol. **87**, 381-387.

Takasaka, T., and Smith, C.A. (**1971**). "The structure and innervation of the pigeon's basilar papilla." J.Ultrastruct.Res. **35**, 0-65.

Tilney, M.S., Tilney, L.G., and DeRosier, D.J. (**1987**). "The distribution of hair cell bundle lengths and orientations suggests an unexpected pattern of hair cell stimulation in the chick cochlea." Hearing Res. **25**, 141-151.

Whitehead, M.C., and Morest, D.K. (**1985**). "The development of innervation patterns in the avian cochlea." Neuroscience **14**, 255-276.

Comments

Evans:

How far can you push this intriguing analogy between mammalian and bird cochleas? Fuchs has recently shown electrical tuning of tall hair cells in the avian cochlea. Does this mean we should expect to find, eventually, electrical tuning in mammalian inner hair cells (for which at present there is contrary evidence) or are there real differences between mammalian and avian mechanisms of frequency selectivity?

Fuchs, P.A., & Mann, A.C. (1986). "Voltage oscillations and ionic currents in hair cells isolated from the apex of the chick's cochlea." J. Physiol. 371, 31P.

Reply by Manley et al.:

Our paper describes data which do not directly address the question of the mechanisms of frequency selectivity in birds and mammals, unless we imagine that the outer hair cells in mammals and the short hair cells in birds are necessary for creating appropriate mechanical conditions for the tuning of inner and tall hair cells, respectively. At present, we know too little to seriously discuss this possibility. We (Manley *et al.*, 1985) emphasized that, although many characteristics of the activity of primary auditory nerve fibres of birds strongly resemble equivalent measures in mammals, there are also consistent differences in both the tuning-curve symmetry and the presence of preferred intervals in spontaneous activity. In the red-eared turtle, such preferred intervals are correlated with membrane-potential oscillations in the hair cells and can be regarded as a neural indicator of the presence of electrical tuning in the hair cell. In the starling, such preferred intervals are characteristic of low-frequency (< 1,5 kHz) fibres. Preferred intervals have also been reported in some reptile preparations at low frequencies. Although there are few data on low-CF fibres in mammals in the literature, Geisler (pers. comm.) carefully investigated many low-CF fibres of a mammal and found no evidence for preferred intervals in the spontaneous activity. On the other hand, our data from reptiles suggests that the presence of preferred intervals is correlated with fibres only innervating one single hair cell. The avian tall-hair-cell fibres only innervate one hair cell. In mammals, there is evidence (Pujol, pers. comm.) that the innervation pattern of the middle- and basal- turn hair-cell regions is not necessarily continued in the low-frequency apical -turn regions. If apical-turn radial fibres in mammals do not simply innervate one hair cell, then the absence of preferred intervals in primary fibres does not necessarily mean that the hair cells are not electrically tuned. Thus, while we should not necessarily **expect** to find electrical tuning in mammalian hair cells, the present data do not completely rule it out. Nevertheless, there are common patterns across many groups of terrestrial vertebrates, which would suggest that certain fundamental features of frequency selectivity remained unchanged in the evolution along the various lines. One such common pattern is the consistent tendency for the amount of space in the hearing organ devoted to low-frequency octaves to be substantially less than the space devoted to high-frequency octaves (see Manley *et al.*, 1988). In lizards, the low-CF area (below approx. 0.8 to 1.0 kHz) is anatomically separated from the one or two high-CF areas. In at least some of these cases, the presence or absence of strong anatomical gradients suggest a micromechanically-based frequency analysis only in the high-CF area.

Wilson:

Do you think that the graded sensitivity of hair cells across the basilar papilla could be due to differing mechanical input levels to the stereocilia?

Reply by Manley:

The graded sensitivity may well be due to a change in the mechanical input to the hair cells, although this is somewhat counter-intuitive. Almost all of the tall hair cells are not found on the free basilar membrane, so that one might expect their mechanical input to be *reduced* compared to the short hair cells. However, our recent anatomical data indicate strong changes in orientation of hair cells across the apical half of the papilla of the starling (Gleich and Manley, in press). Clearly, we simply know too little about hair-cell stimulation at present.

Section 3

Analyzing and modeling the periphery

Experimental results and theoretical interpretations are presented in eleven papers on cochlear (non)linearity, otoacoustic emissions (active behavior), interaural interaction, and, again, spectral channel vs temporal neural information. The papers and discussions show that as yet no communis opinio has been reached on the question of to what extent each of these complicated effects play a role in, e.g., auditory frequency selectivity.

Micromechanics remove the need for active processes in cochlear tuning

Paul J. Kolston

Department of Electrical and Electronic Engineering, University of Canterbury, Christchurch, New Zealand.
&
Faculty of Mathematics and Informatics, University of Technology, Delft, The Netherlands.

Introduction

Recent measurements of basilar membrane (BM) motion in the guinea pig have shown that the radial position of the Mossbauer source greatly influences the measured response (Sellick *et al.*, 1983a). This is not surprising, considering that the structure of the cochlear partition is quite different in the arcuate and pectinate zones of the BM. It seems reasonable, therefore, to assume that an accurate cochlear model must allow for a radial variation in response.

This paper describes a cochlear model whose partition is divided into two zones, with the inclusion of the outer hair cells (OHCs) greatly modifying the mechanics of the arcuate zone. The model exhibits a large response peak in the arcuate zone without requiring negative damping in the cochlear partition. The model is called the OHCAP model, to emphasise the importance of the OHCs and the Arcuate and Pectinate zones of the BM.

The OHCAP model

The usual macromechanical assumptions are made in the formulation of the OHCAP model (see Viergever (1986) for a review). The fluid flow within the scalae is assumed to be one-dimensional, meaning that all pertinent dependent variables depend on only one independent variable, the longitudinal coordinate. A schematic of one section of the cochlear partition appears in Fig. 1, which shows the two zones of the BM and the organ of Corti. Shear

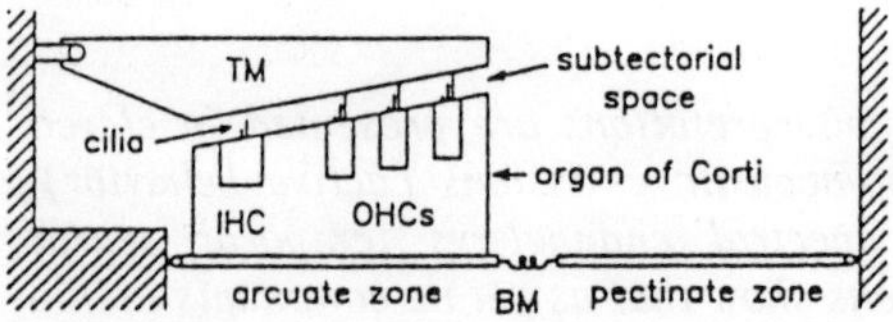

Figure 1: Cross section schematic of the cochlear partition. The basilar membrane is divided into its two zones. The OHC stereocilia alter the impedance of the arcuate zone.

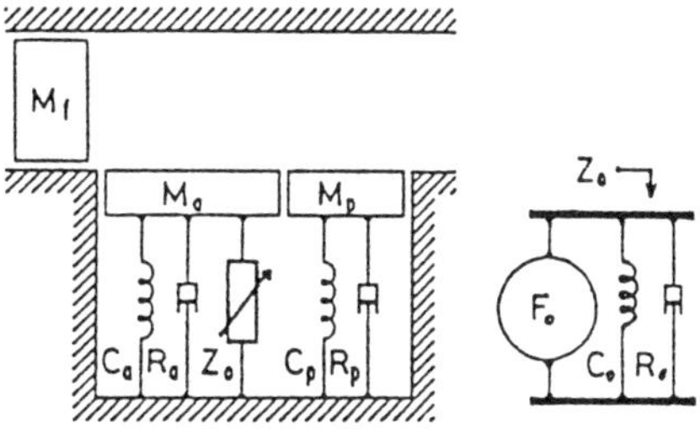

Figure 2. Simplified partition schematic, with lumped elements representing the arcuate and pectinate zones (subscript a and p respectively). The OHC stereocilia impedance is represented by Z_0 consisting of a force generator (F_0), compliance (C_0) and resistance (R_0) in series.

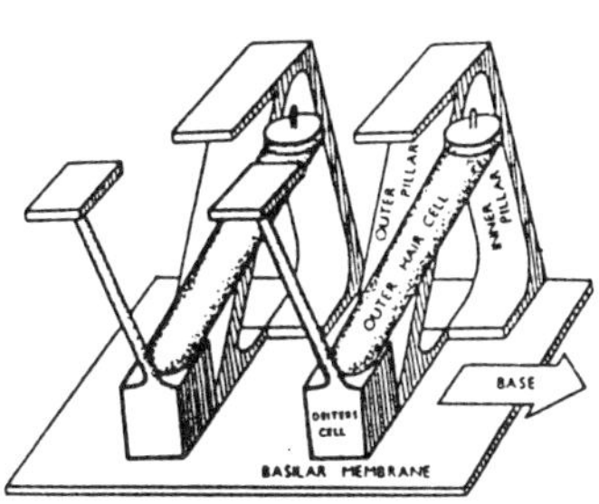

Figure 3. Drawing of the geometric arrangement of the supporting cells and the outer hair cells (OHCs) in the organ of Corti (modified from Voldrich, 1983). Each OHC is assumed to receive stimulus from adjacent sections of the pectinate zone and use this to control its stereocilia bending impedance.

motion in the subtectorial space occurs when there is vertical motion of the arcuate zone. Therefore the OHC stereocilia alter the impedance in the arcuate zone, since they present an impedance to subtectorial shear motion.

Figure 1 can be redrawn in simplified form as in Fig. 2. The complete OHCAP model is formed by cascading a number of these (Fig. 2) sections. The fluid mass between the sections is represented by M_f. The mass, compliance and resistance of the arcuate zone ot the BM are represented by the components M_a, C_a and R_a, and similar in the pectinate zone by M_p, C_p and R_p. The OHC model consists of the force generator F_0 in series with the compliance C_0 and the resistance R_0. The effective impedance (in the arcuate zone) of this series network is designated Z_0. For stimuli frequencies much less than the characteristic frequency (CF) Z_0 is considerably smaller than the impedance of the BM fibres, and so the response in the arcuate zone is mainly determined by C_a. For stimuli frequencies less than half an octave below the CF the arcuate response in the real cochlea rapidly increases, resulting in a large peak at the CF (Sellick *et al.*, 1983a). This peak is produced in the OHCAP model by the functional form of Z_0: small for low frequencies but increasing (rapidly) for frequencies near the CF. Z_0 is (approximately) imaginary and positive, and so its increase cancels the BM stiffness, resulting in an increase in arcuate motion. The frequency dependence of Z_0 is controlled by the corresponding OHC. Each OHC extracts a controlling signal with the required frequency dependence from the velocity of two adjacent sections of the pectinate zone.

Figure 3 shows a schematic of the geometric arrangement of the OHCs, the Deiters' cells and their phalangeal processes (Voldrich, 1983). The base of each OHC is supported by the top of a Deiters' cell, while the top of each OHC is in close proximity to a phalangeal process from an adjacent Deiters' cell. Each Deiters' cell base lies on the edge of the pectinate zone. It is postulated that the top of the OHC senses the velocity of the adjacent (basal) Deiters' cell (V_b), while the bottom of the OHC senses the velocity of its supporting Deiters' cell (V_a). The OHC filters the signal V_a to obtain a signal $V_{a'} = V_a \cdot K_z\,(i\omega M_z + R_z)$; where K_z is a real constant, and M_z and R_z are the parameters of the OHC filter.

For stimulus frequencies much less than the CF $V_{a'}$ and V_b have very similar magnitude and phase. When the stimulus frequency is less than half an octave below the CF of both $V_{a'}$ and V_b, the phase of $V_{a'}$ deviates from that of V_b. The OHC subtracts V_b from $V_{a'}$ and uses the result (V_d) to control F_0. By making F_0 directly proportional to V_d the correct functional form for Z_0 is obtained.

Response of the OHCAP model

The OHCAP model used 50 sections (Fig. 2) per cm, and was numerically analysed in the frequency domain. The parameter values are listed below (all dimensions are in cgs units. Δ = distance from stapes):

scala width = 0.16, scala height = 0.08, fluid density = 1.0
$M_z = 1.35 \times 10^{-4}$, $R_z = 4.0 \times 10^{-1}$, $K_z = 0.80 \times 10^{-4}$, $M_{a,p} = 1.0 \times 10^{-2}$,
$C_{0,p} = 3.3 \times 10^{-9}\, e^{4.4\Delta}$, $R_{a,p} = 4.0 \times 10^{0}\,(1 + 40\, e^{-3.6\Delta})$,
$C_a = 1.1 \times 10^{-9}\, e^{4.4\Delta}$, $R_0 = 2.0 \times 10^{2}\,(1 + 40\, e^{-3.6\Delta})$.

The input to the OHCAP model is a constant eardrum velocity, and the response is the BM velocity (plotted relative to an arbitrary reference). A second-order differentiator is used to model the middle ear. No attempt is

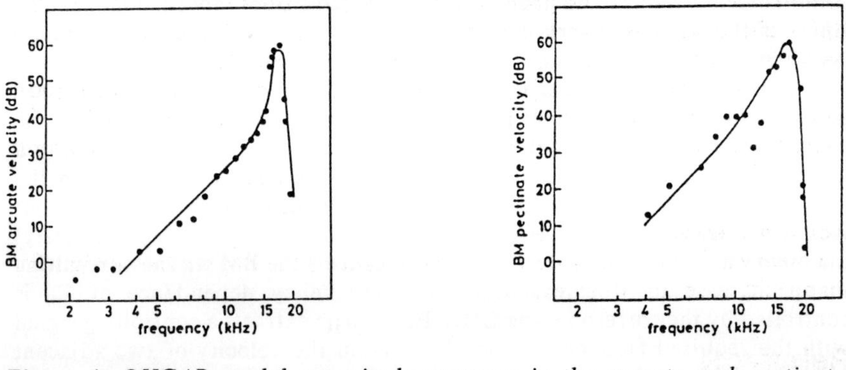

Figure 4: OHCAP model magnitude response in the arcuate and pectinate zones, for a point 2 mm from stapes. Dots show the responses measured by Sellick et al. (1983a).

made to justify this model physiologically - it was chosen so that the OHCAP model low frequency magnitude response slope corresponds to that measured experimentally by Sellick *et al.* (1983a).

The solid lines in Fig. 4 show the model magnitude response in the arcuate and pectinate zones, for a point 2 mm from the stapes (note that the phase response is very similar to that exhibited by an earlier version of the OHCAP model (Kolston, 1988). Sellick *et al.* (1983a) measured BM isovelocity magnitude curves in 11 different guinea pigs, taking care to note the radial position of the Mossbauer source on the BM (the corresponding phase curves were not reported). Typical measured response curves for sources in the arcuate and pectinate zones are shown by the dots in Fig. 4 (animals 116 and 90 respectively). The measured pectinate response exhibits a large notch at 12kHz, which is most probably an artifact of the experimental procedure (Sellick *et al.*, 1983b).

Discussion

It is probably true that cochlear models which assume only one mode of vibration for the cochlear partition cannot exhibit the correct selectivity without the inclusion of energy-producing active processes (Viergever and Diependaal, 1986). In the OHCAP model the real part of the OHC stereocilia bending impedance is always positive, and so the OHCs only apply positive damping to the BM. This shows that, by allowing a radial variation in BM motion, a cochlear model can exhibit a large and broad response peak (in the arcuate zone) without the use of negative damping.

Evans and Wilson (1975) made concurrent BM and nerve fibre measurements. They found that the neural response had a large peak, implying a cochlea with minimal trauma. However the BM response, measured using a capacitive probe, had little or no peak. These observations are consistent with the OHCAP model, since for any capacitance measurement - where the probe diameter is comparable to the width of the BM - the capacitance variation (and hence "response") will be due to the pectinate zone, as the motion there is much greater (Fig. 4).

It is postulated that the OHC force generation is physiological vulnerable, so that simulation of cochlear trauma is achieved by a reduction in F_0. This reduces the sensitivity at the CF, which is consistent with trauma changes observed in the real cochlea.

Acknowledgement

I wish to thank Egbert de Boer, Max Viergever and Rob Diependaal for many stimulating discussions.

References

Evans, E.F. and Wilson, J.P. (**1975**). "Cochlear tuning properties: concurrent basilar membrane and nerve fibre measurements". Science, **190**,

1218-1221.
Kolston, P.J. (**1988**). "Sharp mechanical tuning in a cochlear model without negative damping," J.Acoust.Soc.Am. (accepted for publication).
Sellick, P.M., Patuzzi, R. and Johnstone, B.M. (**1983a**). "Comparison between the tuning properties of inner ear cells and basilar membrane motion," Hearing Res. **10**, 93-100.
Sellick, P.M., Yates, G.K. and Patuzzi, R. (**1983b**). "The influence of Mössbauer source size and position on phase and amplitude measurements of the guinea pig basilar membrane," Hearing Res. **10**, 101-108.
Viergever, M.A. (**1986**). "Cochlear macromechanics - a review," in *Peripheral Auditory Mechanisms*, edited by J.B. Allen, J.L. Hall, A. Hubbard, S.T. Neely and A. Tubis. (Springer, Munich) pp 63-72.
Viergever, M.A. and Diependaal, R.J. (**1986**). "Quantitative validation of cochlear models using the Liouville-Green approximation," Hearing Res. **21**, 1-15.
Voldrich, L. (**1983**). "Experimental and topographic morphology in cochlear mechanics," in *Mechanics of Hearing*, edited by E. de Boer and M.A. Viergever. (Delft University Press) pp 163-168.

Comments

Kim:

Your modeling approach of separately treating the arcuate and pectinate zones of the basilar membrane is very interesting.

A distinct feature of cochlear biomechanics is that the frequency selectivity and the sensitivity at the characteristic frequency (CF) co-vary such that, when the physiological condition of the cochlea is disrupted, the sharply-tuned tip of a tuning curve is lost and the sensitivity at the CF is reduced by about 40 dB. In the views of some investigators (e.g. Kim *et al.*, 1980; Davis, 1983; Neely and Kim, 1983), this is interpreted that the amplitude of cochlear-partition motion is amplified one hundred fold relative to the motion in a severely disrupted cochlea, this interpretation is based on results from active cochlear models where the 100-fold amplification is achieved by the help of an active (i.e., energy-adding) process in the cochlear partition. I would like to ask you the following:

1. What are the pieces of evidence that favor a passive cochlear model over an active cochlear model?

2. How can a passive cochlear model account for: a) an absolute sensitivity of basilar-membrane displacement on the order of 10 Ångstrom at 20 dB SPL (Sellick *et al.*, 1982); and b) 40 dB change in sensitivity between a healthy and a disrupted condition?

Reply by Kolston:

I agree that the sensitivity at the OHCAP model, with the given set at parameters is tens at decibels less than that measured exerimentally. A higher sensitivity can be achieved by appropriate alteration to the parameters, and so I believe that the model should not be disregarded, on the basis at sensitivity, until accurate measurements at basilar membrane mass, stiffness and resistance are known (in its 2 zones).

The paper does show that realistic selectivity, and change at sensitivity and selectivity with trauma, can be exhibited by a passive cochlear model. The OHCs enhance the response by reducing the reactive component as is the case in active models. An enhancement of over 50 dB is possible (Kolston and Viergever, 1988, Mechanics of Hearing Conference, Keele), and so the magnitude of the sensitivity change with trauma is in accordance with experimental data.

I think that I have to debate the active vs passive question somewhat philosophically. I look at the very different radial structure of the cochlear partition and think to myself, why? Nature has decided that this anatomical feature is necessary and so I intuitively like a cochlear model which provides a reason for it. In order to achieve (simultaneously) a realistic magnitude and phase response in a passive model, the basilar membrane must be divided into its 2 zones, and the organ of Corti must influence the mechanics of the arcuate zone only. These assumptions are *not* necessary in active cochlear models, and so such models do not conform with cochlear partition anatomy. Furthermore, active models possess inherent stability (i.e. parameter sensitivity) problems. These can be removed by introducing strong non-linearities (see Neely's paper), but the presence at such non-linearities near threshold is uncertain.

Wilson:

The ingenious model of Kolston appaears to reproduce the shape of the tuning characteristic of the basilar membrane satisfactorily, but it does this by reducing the response at low frequencies whilst leaving the amplitude of the peak approximately unchanged. This is contrary to all available basilar membrane data in which the peak is greatly increased in amplitude (as well as in sharpness of tuning) in modern measurements whilst the low frequency response is unchanged. On this and other evidence an active process still appears to be necessary.

Reply by Kolston:

The OHCAP model reproduces the tuning characteristic by enhancing the response near the peak, and not by reducing the response at low frequencies.

Level dependence of frequency tuning in human ears

J.P. Wilson, R.J. Baker, M.L. Whitehead

Department of Communication and Neuroscience, University of Keele, Staffs ST5 5BG, UK

Introduction

One of the striking features of otoacoustic emissions (OAEs) is their nonlinear behaviour. This is manifest in their compressively nonlinear growth with stimulus level; in the generation of intermodulation distortion products, particularly the cubic difference tone, $2f_1$-f_2; and in their ability to be suppressed by a neighbouring tone, from which a suppression tuning curve can be derived. These non-linear effects can all be demonstrated down to levels near subjective threshold. Another less well investigated type of non-linear behaviour is an apparent change of latency of the click- or tone burst-evoked OAE with level (Kemp & Chum, 1980; Wilson, 1980; Grandori, 1985). As click intensity is increased the latency to the envelope maximum decreases, as might be expected for a filter whose bandwidth was becoming greater. More surprisingly, however, the latency to a particular identifiable feature in the waveform increases. One interpretation of this phenomenon is that the tuning frequency of auditory filters is slightly level-dependent, decreasing with increasing intensity. There may be some evidence for this in the slight dependence of the pitch of a pure tone upon sound level. The present paper attempts to quantify these changes in OAEs by two different methods and to relate them to published pitch changes.

Experiment I: Latency changes of click-evoked OAEs

Rectangular clicks of 0.1 ms duration and a pulse rate of 20 per second were fed via an attenuator and amplifier to a B & K 4134 microphone used as a generator, without d.c. bias, at a maximum level of 300 V peak. Zero bias was used to reduce the effects of amplifier noise and necessitated halving the required attenuator settings to allow for the square-law characteristics. The sound was coupled to the ear by a damped Y-tube with a sensitive microphone connected to the other arm (System 1/2" SM, filter C, of Wilson, 1980). The output was fed to a Tektronix 5113 storage 'scope triggered from the pulse generator and the responses filtered by the internal 1 kHz low-pass and

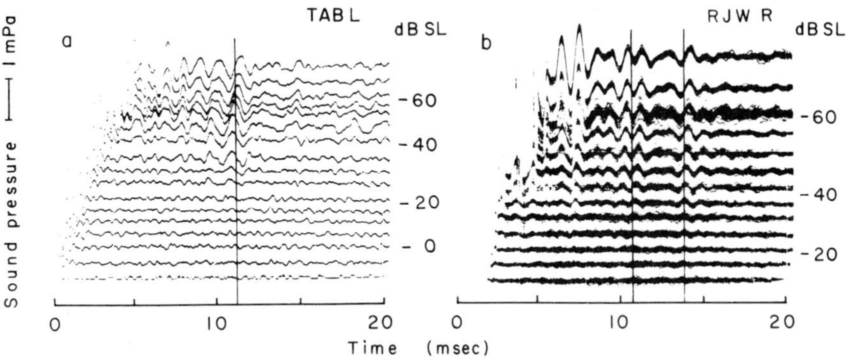

Figure 1. Click-evoked OAEs showing ear canal sound pressure as a function of time after the click offset. The click sound level has been incremented in steps of 5 dB from below threshold (see right hand scales) to a maximum set by the voltage limit of the microphone (300 V peak), duration 0.1 msec. (a) Individual responses are slightly contaminated by an SOAE at 1.6 kHz. (b) Superimposed traces from a different subject. Note how repeatable features in the waveform become more delayed with respect to the vertical lines as level is increased.

high-pass filters to reduce noise, and displayed at 5 dB increments of level up to the 300 V maximum. Measurements were made at 45 trace positions from 32 ears of 18 subjects. Fig. 1(a) shows individual responses from one subject contaminated slightly by a spontaneous emission at 1.6 kHz. In order to reduce the influence of this and other noises, multiple traces were superimposed (shown for a different subject in Fig. 1(b)). The most distinctive peak or dip detectable at the lowest level was chosen for study and its latency measured at each sound level. In some cases two or more suitable features were measured on the same trace. In each case the period of the wave in the neighbourhood of the peak or dip was also measured so that a frequency could be assigned to it. Although it was apparent that this period also changed in a similar way with level, it was a much less precise measurement than the latency. Frequency changes were therefore estimated from latency changes assuming a constant starting phase at the end of the stimulus. In order to minimise the effects of any linear after-ringing of the stimulus in the ear canal, features with latencies less than 8 ms were not used. For this reason and because of the filtering used, this experiment is limited to the lower frequencies. The results of all these measurements are plotted in Fig. 2 as a function of level, where 70 dB represents 300 V peak. As all the subjects used in this analysis had subjective thresholds for the pulse train lying between 65 and 75 dB below this level, it is reasonably accurate to label this point 70 dB SL. It should not, however, be assumed to relate in a simple way to the sensation level at the frequencies concerned. In all cases it is apparent that frequency appears to decrease systematically with level. Some data were also

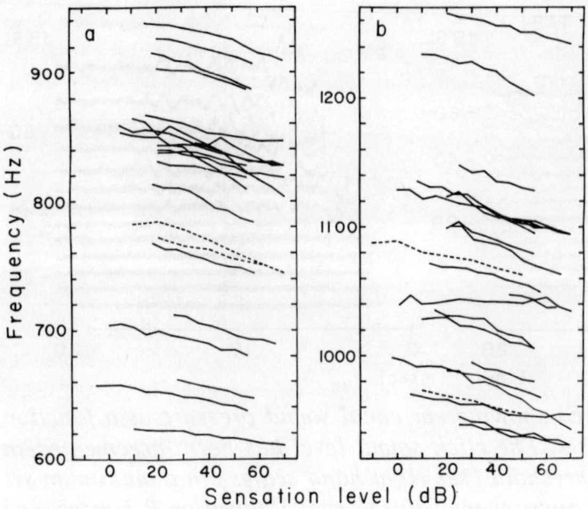

Figure 2. Frequency-level relations for 45 features from the responses of 32 ears of 18 subjects. Frequency regions have been obtained from the period of the wave around the peak or dip whose delay has been measured to obtain the frequency change. The dashed curves have been measured using tone burst stimulation (see text). In all cases except one there is a high negative correlation between frequency and level.

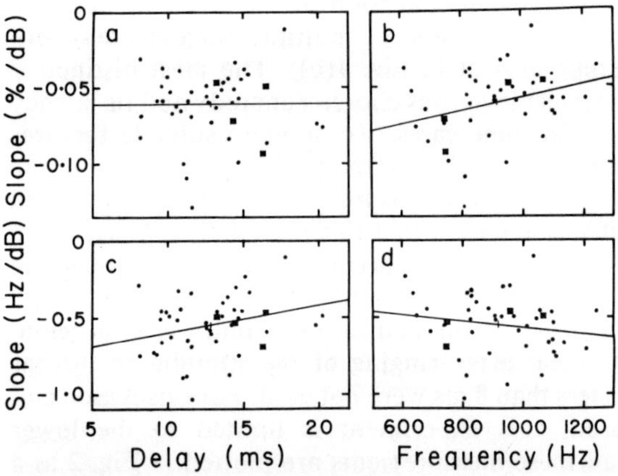

Figure 3. The slopes of the regressions calculated from Fig. 2 plotted as a function of delay (a,c) and frequency (b,d) and expressed as percent per decibel (a,b) and Hertz per decibel (c,d). The mean values -0.061 %/dB, -0.55 Hz/dB give the level dependence. Only (b) is significantly different from a zero slope (p < 0.05).

available using tone-burst stimulation where the stimulation frequency was set to a frequency of strong emission in the subject. These included 4 cycles at 710 and 752 Hz and 8 cycles at 750 and 1100 Hz, starting and finishing on a zero crossing. When these were plotted using the termination of the tone burst as time-zero they showed similar delay/level behaviour to the click-evoked responses. They have therefore been included in the analysis and are identified by dashed lines in Fig. 2 and by squares in Fig. 3. As the conditions of stimulation were different, including using d.c. bias on the driver microphone, the absolute levels are not directly comparable.

In order to test for possible dependencies upon frequency or upon latency, regressions were calculated for each curve and the slopes plotted in Fig. 3(c and d) as a function of latency and frequency respectively. The average correlation between frequency and level was 0.96. In addition the percentage changes in frequency (i.e. negative changes in latency) are plotted in Fig. 3(a and b). The negligible slope of the regression in Fig. 3(a) confirms the impression that on average the whole time scale of the response is expanded uniformly even though individual subjects show some idiosyncratic behaviour. Since it has been noted earlier (Wilson, 1980) that high frequency evoked emissions appear to have shorter delays than low frequency ones, a regression of estimated frequency upon delay was also calculated ($r = -0.46$, $N = 45$) and found to be significant at $p < 0.01$. The only regression of slope versus level found to be significant at $p < 0.05$, however, was (b) the percentage change per dB as a function of frequency. Extrapolating this regression would give a slope of zero %/dB at 2,380 Hz. In view of the limited range of frequencies tested it is reasonable to summarise the results as mean slopes of -0.55 ± 0.19 Hz/dB and -0.061 ± 0.022 %/dB.

In order to check some of the assumptions inherent in the above analysis and to provide further evidence of level dependence of OAE frequency a second experiment was undertaken using continuous tonal stimulation.

Experiment II. Changes of frequency of interference minima between the stimulus and a continuously stimulated OAE

The same stimulating and recording microphone assembly was used as in Experiment I. Now, however, continuous tonal stimulation was applied from a low-distortion voltage-controlled oscillator (Brookdeal 9471) together with 200 V d.c. bias and using only high-pass filtering (3 pole, -3 dB at 1 kHz) on the output. Calibration of the recording microphone in a closed coupler allowed the stimulus and response to be expressed in dB SPL. The response was analysed with a quadrature pair of Brookdeal 401 lock-in amplifiers and displayed as a Nyquist plot on the storage 'scope and a pen recorder (Fig. 4). Frequency of the stimulus tone was adjusted with a multiturn pot to obtain the exact minima, which were measured on a digital frequency meter. The points of minimum represent the frequencies at which the OAE is in opposite phase to the stimulus in the ear canal, and are therefore maximally cancelling it. These points were chosen because they can be measured much more pre-

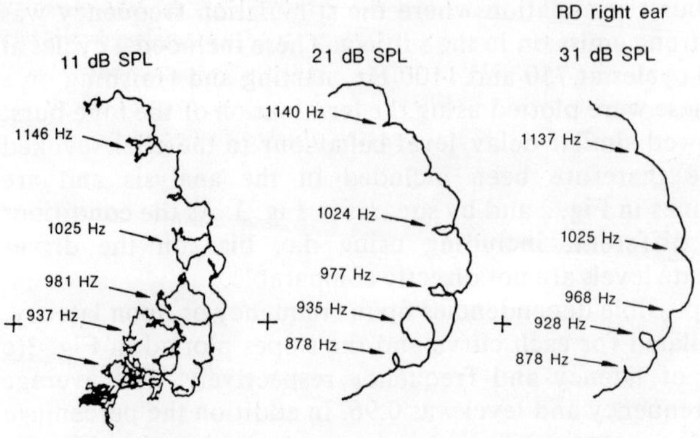

Figure 4. Nyquist plots of ear canal sound pressure for a range of frequencies of continuous tone stimulation at three different sound levels in one subject. The distance from the origin (+) represents the vector sum of the sound stimulus and the continuously re-emitted OAE. Note how the loops or cusps become smaller with level due to compressive nonlinearity of the OAE, and the marked frequencies become lower with level.

cisely than any other frequency. The assumption in this experiment is that any change in the frequency of a minimum might represent a change in tuning frequency of the underlying auditory filter.

The above measurements were repeated at 2, 3 or 5 dB intervals over the range limited at low levels by the intrusion of noise and at high levels by the compressive non-linearity of the OAE, which became relatively too small to produce a measurable minimum. Measurements were made on 78 minima from 14 normal-hearing ears of 11 subjects (different from those of experiment I). In several cases SOAEs were present in the region of measurement and became locked to the stimulus. Sample responses are illustrated in Fig. 4 for one subject. The frequencies of minimum are plotted as a function of SPL (*re* 20 μPa) in Fig. 5 for the same subject. In each case the frequency of minimum decreases systematically with sound level.

Regressions of frequency upon level were calculated for each minimum in each subject and generally gave high correlations but, unlike the click data, 8 % of these were positive, 24 % had no significant slope, and 68 % were negative. The slopes of the regressions are plotted in Fig. 6(a) as a function of frequency. In Fig. 6(b) the slopes have been expressed as percentage frequency change per decibel, also as a function of frequency. Compared to the first experiment (Fig. 3(d and b) the trends are similar although the mean values of the slopes are less. The slopes of the regressions, however, are not significantly different from zero. It is also clear that the wide spread of values above 3 kHz considerably influences the result. Both the very low values come from the same subject in the region of a strong bistable SOAE. Overall the mean values of slope are -0.38 ± 0.09 Hz/dB and -0.028 ± 0.004 %/dB. If the

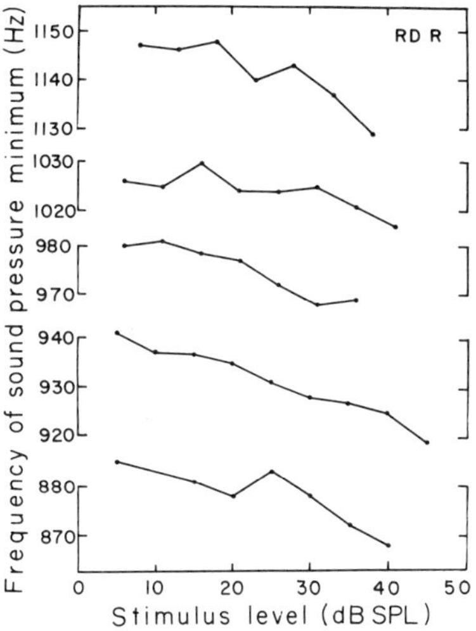

Figure 5. Frequencies of five minima for the same subject as Fig. 4 plotted as a function of stimulus level. Slopes of the regressions of these curves are plotted in Fig. 6.

analysis is restricted to 1.25 kHz in order to make a more direct comparison with the first experiment the slopes become -0.32 ± 0.34 Hz/dB and -0.031 ± 0.034 %/dB respectively.

Discussion

In qualitative terms the two experiments are in agreement and do not provide any evidence that the underlying assumption (that the auditory filters are decreasing in their frequency of tuning with increasing sound level) is incorrect. A similar trend is observed in the data of Rutten & Buisman (1982). The effect does not appear to be strongly frequency dependent within the range tested, although the results are equivocal at high frequencies. On

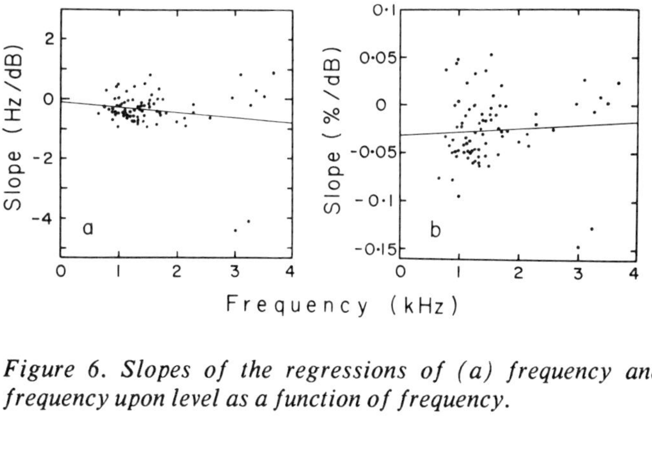

Figure 6. Slopes of the regressions of (a) frequency and (b) percentage frequency upon level as a function of frequency.

general grounds one would expect any system to approach linearity at the lowest levels and there does on average appear to be less downward slope at the lowest levels in Figs. 2 and 5.

There would appear to be three types of experiment with which these results can be compared and contrasted: (1) the psychophysical pitch shift with level, (2) the influence of signal level on single auditory nerve fibre tuning and (3) the frequency shift of spontaneous OAEs (SOAEs) under conditions of suppression.

(1) The psychophysical pitch shift has been the topic of considerable controversy probably partly due to large individual differences. The widely quoted Stevens' rule that with increasing intensity pitch shifts downwards below 1 kHz and upwards above, appears to be derived chiefly from data gathered at higher sound levels. For levels as low as those used in the present study, however, many of the individual curves for low frequencies actually start out with a slight positive slope until about 60 dB SPL where the direction reverses (Morgan et al. 1951, Ward 1970, Terhardt 1974, Verschuure and van Meeteren 1975, Jesteadt and Neff 1982). This is less apparent in the data of Burns (1982). The most comprehensive study on a single subject (van den Brink, 1979) consistently shows a positive slope of pitch versus intensity over the range of frequencies used in the present study and between 10 and 60 dB SPL. Over octave intervals from 500 Hz to 4 kHz these values average 0.036, 0.046, 0.078 %/dB. Similar values of 0.03, 0.07, 0.05, 0.04 %/dB can be calculated from Verschuure and van Meeteren (1975) at 300, 500, 1 k and 2 kHz respectively, for low sound levels. For a simple place model a decrease in frequency of tuning of the underlying auditory filters implies an increase in pitch, so that these values correspond well with the present findings. We would like, therefore, to suggest a new (WBW) pitch-intensity rule that "Pitch usually increases with sound level up to about 60 dB SPL". Above 60 dB SPL the Stevens' rule appears to apply with pitch decreasing for low frequencies and increasing for high frequencies. With these relationships in mind much of the previous psychoacoustical data appears less idiosyncratic.

(2) Physiological recordings of iso-response contours to pure tones have not been determined with sufficient precision to be compared with the present data. Reverse correlation techniques using noise stimulation in cats (Evans, 1977), however, do show shifts of CF at high levels consistent with Stevens' rule.

(3) The shift downwards in frequency of an SOAE induced by a higher frequency suppressor tone (Wilson and Sutton, 1981, Fig. 2a,c) may be a related phenomenon where in the present case the stimulus is also acting as "suppressor". Intriguingly, the slope of frequency shift at 3 kHz is comparable to the present data (-0.66 Hz/dB, -0.022 %/dB) and appears to flatten-out above 60 dB SPL.

References

Brink, G. van den (**1979**). "Intensity and pitch," Acustica **41**, 271-273.

Burns, E.M. (**1982**). "Pure-tone pitch anomalies. I.Pitch-intensity effects and diplacusis in normal ears," J.Acoust.Soc.Am. **72**, 1394-1402.

Evans, E.F. (**1977**). "Frequency selectivity at high signal levels of single units in cochlear nerve and cochlear nucleus." In: *Psychophysics and Physiology of Hearing*, edited by. E.F.Evans and J.P.Wilson, (Academic, London) pp. 185-192.

Grandori, F. (**1985**). "Nonlinear phenomena in click- and tone-burst-evoked otoacoustic emissions from human ears," Audiol. **24**, 71-80.

Jesteadt, W. and Neff, D.L. (**1982**). "A signal detection theory measure of pitch shifts in sinusoids as a function of intensity," J.Acoust.Soc.Am. **72**, 1812-1820.

Kemp, D.T. and Chum, R. (**1980**). "Properties of the generator of stimulated acoustic emissions," Hearing Res. **2**, 213-232.

Morgan, C.T., Garner, W.R., and Galambos, R. (**1951**). "Pitch and intensity," J.Acoust.Soc.Am. **23**, 658-663.

Rutten, W.L.C., and Buisman, H.P. (**1983**). "Critical behaviour of auditory oscillators near feedback phase transitions." In: *Mechanics of Hearing*, edited by E.de Boer and M.A.Viergever (Nijhoff, Delft) pp.91-99.

Terhardt, E. (**1974**). "Pitch of pure tones: its relation to intensity." In: *Facts and Models in Hearing*, edited by E.Zwicker and E.Terhardt (Springer, Berlin) pp.353-360.

Verschuure, J., and van Meeteren, A.A. (**1975**). "The effect of intensity on pitch," Acustica **32**, 33-43.

Ward, W.D. (**1970**). "Musical perception." In: *Foundations of Modern Auditory Theory*, edited by J.Tobias (Academic, New York) pp.407-447.

Wilson, J.P. (**1980**). "Evidence for a cochlear origin for acoustic re-emissions, threshold fine-structure and tonal tinnitus." Hearing Res. **2**, 233-252.

Wilson, J.P., and Sutton, G.J. (**1981**). "Acoustic correlates of tonal tinnitus." In: *Tinnitus*, edited by D.Evered and G.Lawrenson (Pitman Medical, London) pp.82-107.

Changes in spontaneous otoacoustic emissions produced by acoustic stimulation

Susan J. Norton[1], John B. Mott[2] and Stephen T. Neely[2]

[1]*University of Kansas Medical Center, Kansas City, Kansas, U.S.A*
[2]*Boys Town National Institute, Omaha, Nebraska, U.S.A.*

Introduction

Spontaneous otoacoustic emissions (SOAEs) are low-level narrowband signals measured in the ear canal in the absence of external stimulation. Although their exact origin is unknown, SOAEs appear to be closely linked to active biomechanical elements which improve the sensitivity of the cochlea to low-level sounds. Investigating the effects of external stimuli on SOAEs, measured in human ears, offers a potent yet non-invasive tool for studying cochlear mechanics. Previously we reported experiments in which SOAEs were measured in the presence of ipsilateral (Norton, Champlin and Mott, 1987) and contralateral (Mott, Norton, Neely and Warr, 1987) tones. In this paper, we present new data on the effects of binaural stimulation.

Effects of Monaural Acoustic Stimulation

The standard ipsilateral exposure was a 30 s, 105 dB SPL tone. Following stimulation, the SOAE was absent for up to four minutes. When the SOAE became measurable, it was reduced in frequency and amplitude. The effect was tuned with stimuli 1/8 to 5/8 oct below the SOAE producing the largest shifts. As exposure level and duration decreased, the magnitude and duration of the post-exposure reductions decreased; however the tuning did not change.

The standard contralateral stimulus was a 40 s, 80 dB SPL tone. During stimulation, SOAE frequency increased and SOAE amplitude decreased, increased or remained unchanged. The contralateral effect was also frequency selective, and tuned much like the ipsilateral effect. SOAE shifts began within 150 ms of stimulus onset; and the SOAE recovered to baseline values within 150 ms of stimulus offset.

Methods

Subjects were two normal-hearing adults with one or more stable SOAEs which varied by less than 1 Hz and 1 dB within a single day, and by less than 5

Table 1.

Subject	Freq (Hz)	Amp (dB SPL)	Amp re Noise Floor (dB)
S1	2026	11.7	23.34
S2	3998	3.0	21.17

Hz and 5 dB over a period of days. The characteristics of these SOAEs are summarized in Table 1.

Emissions were measured using the Etymotic Research ER-10 insert microphone and sinusoidal stimuli were delivered using the Etymotic Research ER-2 insert earphones. The preamplified microphone output was fed to a H-P 3561A signal analyzer. The SOAE was sampled over successive 2-s time windows. A 1024-point FFT was computed for each sample with the center frequency equal to the SOAE frequency, an analysis span of 200 Hz, and a .25-Hz resolution. Stimulus level, duration and presentation were under computer control, as was the operation of the signal analyzer.

For each SOAE the frequencies of the ipsilateral (30 s, 105 dB SPL) and contralateral (30 s, 80 dB SPL) tones producing the greatest changes were determined. These stimuli were then presented binaurally.

Results

The data, given in terms of frequency and amplitude shift from baseline as a function of post-exposure time, are shown in Figs. 1 through 3. In the figures, the light solid line shows baseline data, the fluctuation of the SOAE in the absence of any stimulation. The heavy solid line shows the effect of

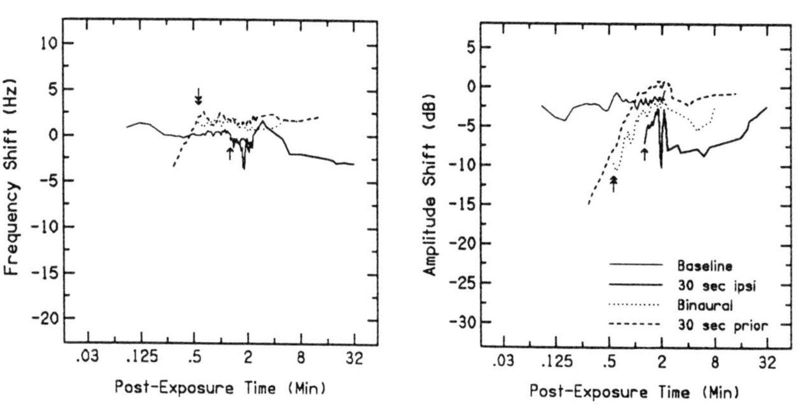

Figure 1. Effects of concurrent and prior binaural stimulation on post-exposure SOAE recovery for S1.

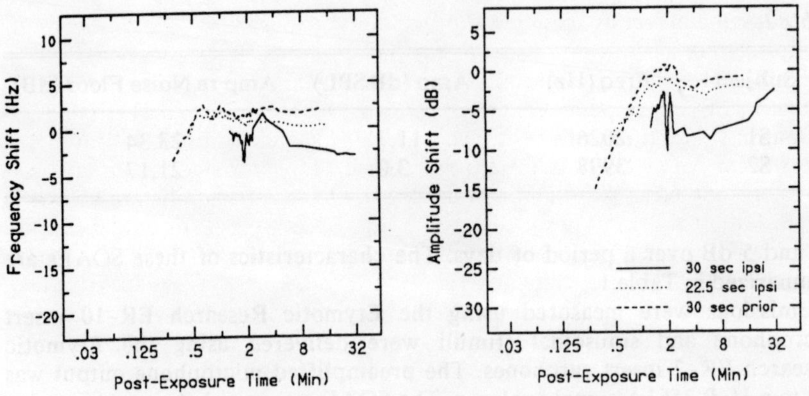

Figure 2. SOAE recovery as a function of exposure duration compared to binaural stimulation for S1.

ipsilateral exposure alone. The remaining dashed and dotted lines show the effects of various manipulations.

For S1, the optimal ipsilateral and contralateral stimuli were both 5/8 oct below the SOAE. For this subject the timing of the stimuli was varied; the contralateral stimulus was presented either concurrent with, or 30 s prior to and during, the exposure. Fig. 1 shows that following the ipsilateral exposure the SOAE was absent for almost two minutes. It reappeared (arrow) at its pre-exposure frequency reduced in amplitude. With concurrent binaural stimulation, shown by the dotted line, recovery began about 1.5 min earlier (double arrow). With prior contralateral stimulation, shown by the dashed line, recovery began 1.75 min earlier. In addition to earlier recovery, there was less amplitude reduction with binaural stimulation. Binaural stimulation

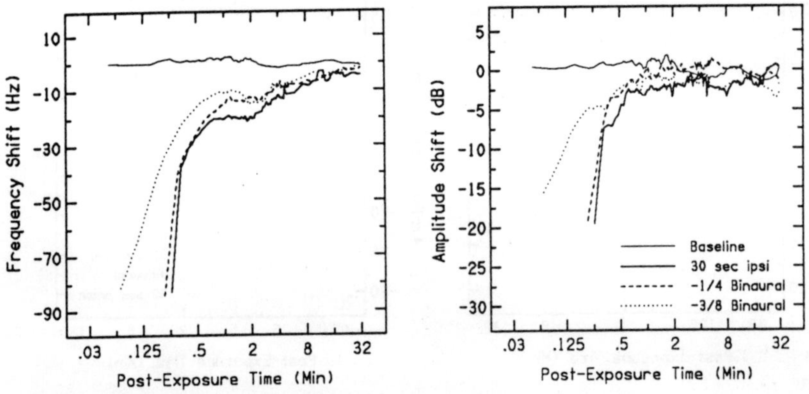

Figure 3. Effects of contralateral stimulation at and below the exposure frequency on SOAE recovery for S2.

had the same effect as reducing the ipsilateral exposure to 22.5 s, shown by the dotted line in Fig. 2.

For S2, the optimal ipsilateral and contralateral stimuli were 1/4 and 3/8 oct below the SOAE, respectively. Therefore, the effects of binaural stimulation with an ipsilateral tone 1/4 oct below the SOAE and contralateral tones 1/4 and 3/8 oct below the SOAE were measured. The contralateral stimulus was always presented prior to and during the exposure. The results are shown in Fig. 3. Following the exposure alone the SOAE was absent for only 0.25 min, and reappeared reduced in frequency and amplitude. Binaural stimulation with the ipsilateral and contralateral stimuli at the same frequency (dashed line) produced only a small improvement in recovery. However, when the contralateral stimulus was at 3/8 oct below the SOAE frequency (dotted line), the SOAE showed less initial frequency shift and recovery began earlier.

Discussion

Contralateral stimuli at or below the frequency of an ipsilateral exposure were found to mitigate the effects of the exposure such that the frequency and amplitude reductions were smaller and recovery began earlier. These effects mimic those obtained by decreasing the duration of the exposure.

These results are consistent with the reductions in guinea pig N1 threshold shifts (Cody and Johnstone, 1982; Rajan and Johnstone, 1983) and human behavioral TTS (Hirsh, 1958; Ward, 1965) observed using similar paradigms.

Like Johnstone, we attribute our results to activation of efferent fibers arising in the medial region of the superior olivary complex. We propose that efferent activity causes local changes in tuning, possibly by modification of cochlear partition stiffness or outer hair cell (OHC) membrane properties, rendering the exposure less effective. Because these fibers terminate almost exclusively on OHCs, these data support cochlear models presuming that the OHC subsystem is involved in emission generation (Kim, 1986). These data also argue that TTS is due to changes in cochlear micromechanics, particularly to the OHC subsystem.

Acknowledgments

This work was supported by NINCDS grants R15NS23202 and K08NS01036 [SJN], and F32NS07811 [JBM].

References

Cody, A.R. and Johnstone, B.M. (**1982**). "Temporary threshold shift modified by binaural acoustic stimulation", Hearing Res. **6**, 199-205.

Hirsh, I.J. (**1958**). "Monaural temporary threshold shift following monaural and binaural exposures", J.Acoust.Soc.Am. **30**, 912-914.

Kim, D.O. (**1986**). "Active and nonlinear cochlear biomechanics and the role of the outer-hair-cell subsystem in the mammalian auditory system", Hearing Res. **22**, 105-114.

Mott, J.B., Norton, S.J., Neely, S.T. and Warr, W.B. (1987). "Changes in spontaneous otoacoustic emissions produced by acoustic stimulation of the contralateral ear", Abst.Assoc.Res.Otolaryngol. **10**, 21.

Norton, S.J., Champlin, C.A. and Mott, J.B. (1987). "The behavior of spontaneous otoacoustic emissions from human ears following exposure to intense pure-tone stimuli", Abst.Assoc.Res.Otolaryngol. **10**, 21.

Rajan, R. and Johnstone, B.M. (1983). "Crossed cochlear influences on monaural temporary threshold shifts", Hearing Res. **9**, 279-294.

Ward, W.D. (1965). "Temporary threshold shifts following monaural and binaural exposure", J.Acoust.Soc.Am. **38**, 121-125.

Modification of the external-tone synchronization and statistical properties of spontaneous otoacoustic emissions by aspirin consumption

Glenis R. Long, Arnold Tubis, Kenneth L. Jones and Savithri Sivaramakrishnan

Purdue University, West Lafayette, Indiana, 47907, U.S.A.

Introduction

Studies of the statistical properties of spontaneous otoacoustic emissions (Bialek and Wit, 1984; Wit, 1986) indicate that some spontaneous emissions are manifestations of noisy self-sustained or limit-cycle oscillations of a nonlinear-active cochlea, not the selective amplification of narrow bands of noise. Additional evidence in support of this conclusion may be obtained from data on the interaction of spontaneous emissions with external tones. As the swept frequency of a low level external tone approaches that of an emission, a type of beating between the tone and the emission is detected, which disappears when the external tone is sufficiently close to the emission

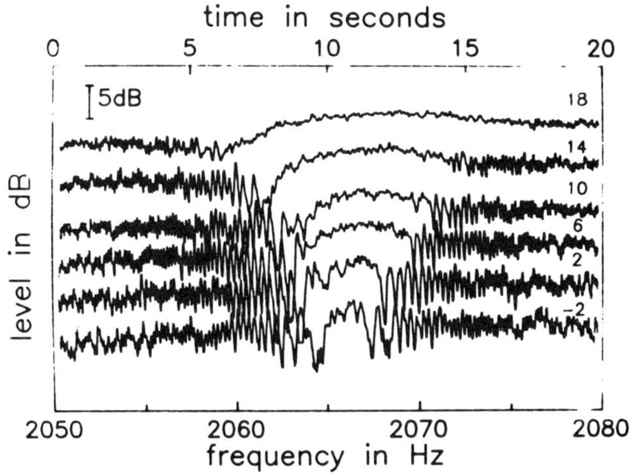

Figure 1. RMS level of the filtered (31.6 Hz bandwidth) ear-canal signal in the right ear of CH when tones (levels in dB SPL indicated above the traces) were swept from 2050 Hz to 2080 Hz past a 2067 Hz, 8 dB SPL emission. Traces shifted vertically to avoid overlap.

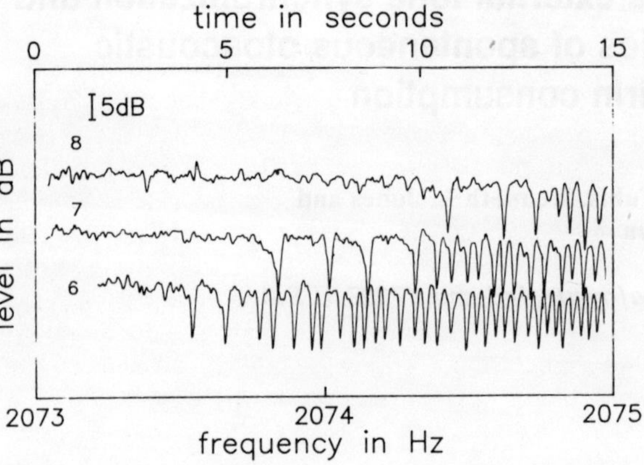

Figure 2. RMS level of the filtered (10 Hz bandwidth) ear-canal signal in the right ear of CH when tones (levels indicated above the trace) were swept from 2073-2075 Hz in 15 sec. The emission was near 2072 Hz at 7 dB SPL.

so as to entrain (frequency-lock) it (Kemp, 1979; Wilson and Sutton, 1981; Zwicker and Schloth, 1984; Long, Tubis and Jones, 1986a). Kemp (1979) had his subjects report "synchronization" thresholds (the levels at which the probes stopped sounding rough or beating and became tone-like) in addition to the "detection" thresholds for tonal probes. The two thresholds were similar near the threshold minima but very different at threshold maxima. An objective correlate of synchronization thresholds was found by Zwicker and Schloth (1984) when they filtered ear-canal pressure recordings to detect both the external tone and the spontaneous otoacoustic emission. They determined the frequencies at which beating between the external tone and the emission ended for a range of stimulus levels and thus obtained synchronization tuning curves for the entrainment of a spontaneous otoacoustic emission by an external tone. Close examination of ear-canal measures of the interactions between swept low level external tones and spontaneous otoacoustic emissions (Long, Tubis and Jones, 1986a), reveal that one can detect transitions from normal beating to both periodic and aperiodic asymmetric beating on either side of the region of entrainment Figures 1 and 2). Otoacoustic synchronization tuning curves and psychoacoustic measures of "roughness" or "tone-like" thresholds from the same observers (Long, Tubis and Jones, 1986a) indicate that the subjects are indeed detecting the transitions from entrainment to beating.

A similar pattern of entrainment is a general feature of externally-driven limit-cycle oscillators (e.g. Stratonovich, 1963; Machlup and Sluckin, 1980: Hanggi and Riseborough, 1983). The output of a computer simulation of the response of a Van der Pol oscillator to a frequency-swept external sinusoidal driving stimuli at different levels are illustrated in Figure 3. The oscillator is assumed to satisfy the equation,

$$d^2x/dt^2 + \omega_0^2 x - (a - bx^2) dx/dt = F \sin\omega(t)t, \qquad (1)$$

where a and b are positive, ω_0 is the limit-cycle angular frequency, $\omega(t)$ is the external driving angular frequency, and $x_0^2 = 4(a/b)$ is the square of limit-cycle displacement amplitude in the absence of external driving. The results in the figure were obtained using the first approximation averaging method of Krylov and Bogoliubov (cf., Hanggi and Riseborough, 1983). Similar results have been obtained for ear-canal pressure in a model of the full auditory periphery with a linear cochlea except that one site on the cochlear partition has nonlinear active damping of the parabolic type in equation (1) so as to simulate a spontaneous emission. This model was not used for Figure 3 because the time needed to calculate such long frequency sweeps in the complete model is excessive on the present version of the model which is implemented on a personal computer. These models reveal three characteristic interaction patterns depending on the relative frequencies and levels of the limit-cycle oscillation and the external driving force. When the external driving frequency is very different from the frequency of the limit cycle the result is a simple beating. As the driving frequency approaches that of the limit cycle this changes to "asymmetrical beating" or "partial synchronization" in which the emission is very nearly entrained over many cycles but periodically has rapid phase changes of about a whole period. Further approach of the driving frequency to the natural limit-cycle frequency leads to synchronization (i.e., frequency locking or entrainment) of the oscillator by the external tone. The associated frequency ranges of these three interaction regimes are level dependent, with the frequency-level relationship at the border of the entrainment region constituting a simple tuning curve.

In related studies of the entrainment of spontaneous otoacoustic emissions by cubic difference tones generated in the cochlea by two external tones, van Dijk and Wit (1987) showed that for some levels of the cubic difference tone, the period of the filtered ear canal signal fluctuated between those of the natural emission and the combination tone. The statistical distribution of the period was found to be in qualitative agreement with the response of a single Van der Pol oscillator in the presence of noise to a sinusoidal driving force

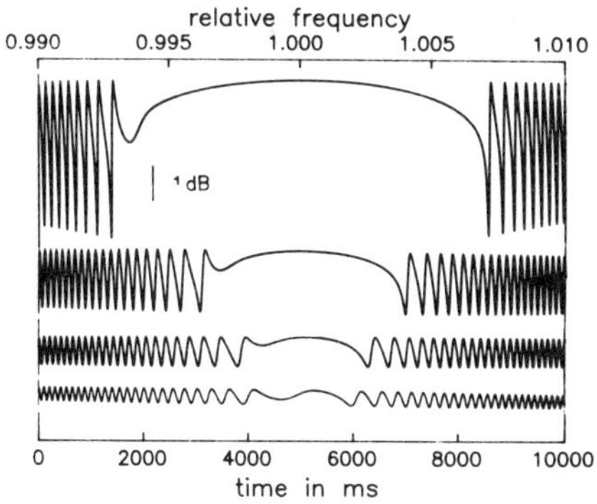

Figure 3. Computer simulation of the response of Van der Pol oscillator to driving forces of amplitudes 1.0, 0.5, 0.25 and 0.125 swept from 0.99 to 1.01 of the limit-cycle frequency ($x_0 = 0.2$).

(Stratonovich, 1963; Hanggi and Riseborough, 1983). The pattern of shifts in period seen by van Dijk and Wit (1987) is very similar to aperiodic asymmetric beating seen in our measures of the filtered ear canal stimulus (Figure 2).

Our understanding of the mechanisms leading to the production of spontaneous otoacoustic emissions will be enhanced if we can explore how the characteristics of individual emissions such as their interactions with external tones and their statistical properties, change as their characteristics (such as frequency and level) are modified over time. Wit (1986) reported that the statistical properties of the filtered ear-canal signal centered at the frequency of an emission when monitored during partial suppression of the emission by an external tone, changed from that expected of a noisy self-sustained oscillation to that of noise (Wit, 1986). We wish to determine if this effect is specific to suppression of the stimulus by an ipsilateral tone. Consumption of aspirin provides one mechanism for modifying the level of (normally very stable) spontaneous otoacoustic emissions over time in a relatively predictable manner (McFadden and Plattsmier, 1984; Long, Tubis and Jones, 1986b). In this paper we explore the modification of the statistical properties and synchronization of spontaneous emissions by external tones during aspirin consumption.

Methods

The ear-canal pressure was measured using an Etymotic ER-10 low noise microphone. Stimuli were applied to the ear using an Etymotic ER-2 tube phone which attaches to the ER-10 assembly. FFT analysis of the spontaneous emissions was performed by a Wavetek 5820A spectrum analyzer with spectrum averaging (typically an average of 32 samples) for improved signal-to-noise ratio. Analysis of the RMS level of the sound pressure in the ear canal when an external tone was added, was provided by a Bruel and Kjaer 2010 hetrodyne analyzer which outputs a DC voltage proportional to the RMS level within a filter (typically 31.6 Hz) centered around the frequency of the stimulus. This DC voltage was stored on a Tektronix 2230 digital storage oscilloscope and transferred to a Nova 4 computer for further analysis. Most measures were made by sweeping a constant level tone over 30 Hz (centered on an emission) in 20 s at stimulus levels from 30 to -4 dB SPL. At times the sweep was reduced to 10 or 20 Hz to provide better resolution of the bandwith of entrainment. The stimulus was calibrated in the subjects' ear canal prior to the start of each experiment. Spontaneous emissions were monitored before, during and after measurement of the interaction of the external tone and the emission.

The statistical distribution of the ear-canal signal in a 10 Hz band centered either around the frequency of the spontaneous emission or an adjacent region with no measurable emissions, were analyzed by a Zenith 158 computer and a Modular Instruments Incorporated M202 A/D converter (50kHz sampling rate). The signal was filtered and amplified by a Wavetek/Rockland 743A

Brickwall filter (200Hz bandwith) before further filtering by a Bruel and Kjaer 2020 heterodyne filter (10 Hz bandwith). A histogram was built up of amplitudes sampled for 135 seconds. This was later reanalyzed by binning 8 adjacent amplitude samples.

Each of the subjects (two female graduate students) were seated in a soundproof room and took no active part in the collection of data reported in this paper. Measurements were obtained from the right ear of each subject (near 2070 for CH and 1630 for JN) before, during and after consumption of three 325 mg tablets every 6 hours for 18 hours.

Results

The general pattern of the results of sweeping a tone past an emission can be seen in Figure 1. The pattern of simple beating, changing to asymmetrical beating, entrainment, asymmetrical beating, and simple beating depends on the level of the stimulus such that the bandwidth of entrainment depends on the stimulus level. Slower sweeps at the edge of entrainment displayed in Figure 2 show aperiodic asymmetric beating moving to asymmetric periodic beating and finally to simple beating. The time/frequency at which the transition from beating to entrainment and vice versa, can be estimated from plots like those in Figure 1 and synchronization tuning curves obtained. The amplitude of the beating is maximal when the ear-canal stimulus level is similar to that of the emission. This factor, combined with the signal to noise ratio, determines the range of levels for which the transition from beating can be accurately measured. Small changes in emission frequency are often associated with changes in level (cf., McFadden and Plattsmier, 1984; Long, Tubis and Jones, 1986). This complicates comparison of the synchronization

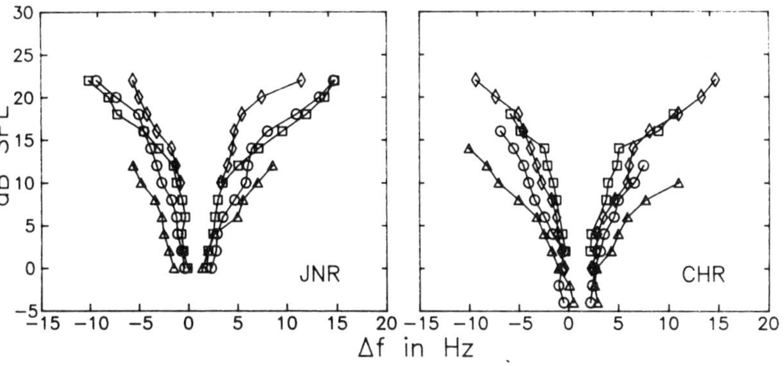

Figure 4. Transition from beating to entrainment as a function of the level of the stimulus and level of one emission from each of two subjects. The emission for JN was near 1630 Hz at levels of 12 dB (○), 9 dB (□), 5 dB (△) and 13 dB (◇). CH's emission was near 2070 Hz at levels of 7 dB (□), 5 dB (○), 3 dB (△), and 8 dB (◇).

of tuning for different emission levels. Consequently, the synchronization tuning curves presented in Figure 4 are normalized with respect to the frequency of the spontaneous emission determined closest in time to the measurement of the synchronization tuning curve (a smaller drift in frequency is often seen during the data collection session). As the level of the emission is reduced the frequency region over which it can be entrained at a given level of the external tone increases. The synchronization tuning curve returns to its pre-aspirin shape upon recovery of the emission.

Measurements of the statistical properties of the ear-canal signal in the frequency region centered on the emission and in adjacent regions without emissions, prior to aspirin consumption, give results comparable to those of Bialek and Wit (1984) and Wit (1986): Gaussian distributions for the regions without emissions and double peaked distributions for the regions containing an emission (Figure 5). Reduction of the levels of the emissions reduces the size of the dip in the double peaked pattern but does not convert the pattern to the Gaussian pattern.

Discussion

These results imply that aspirin consumption, at the levels used in this study, weakens the active cochlear response, but does not change the essential characteristics of spontaneous otoacoustic emissions. The decrease in the amplitude of a spontaneous emission is correlated with: 1) a decrease in the peak-to-valley ratio of the double-peaked statistical distribution of ear-canal pressure in a frequency band centered at the emission frequency; and 2) a broadening of the external-tone frequency locking tuning curve for the emission. It can be shown that this pattern of results follows theoretically for the Van der Pol oscillator of Equation (1) (e.g., if the parameter a is reduced as a simulation of the effect of aspirin consumption).

The effects of aspirin consumption on spontaneous emissions are in apparent contrast to the effects of ipsilateral-tone suppression found by Wit (1986) described in the introduction. Because of the partial entrainment of the emission by the ipsilateral tone (van Dijk and Wit, 1987), and the filtering of the ear canal signal to exclude the frequency of the external tone, the proportion of time that the emission was present in the filtered signal would have been reduced as the level of the entraining stimulus increased (i.e., as "suppression" increased). The remaining noise component of the filtered signal could have lead to the Gaussian-like statistical distribution (van Dijk, private communication).

The results of this paper, along with the work of Bialek and Wit (1984), Wit (1986), and van Dijk and Wit (1987), give confirmation that a non-linear active cochlear response underlies spontaneous otoacoustic emission and that the essential features of this response can be qualitatively modeled using a Van der Pol oscillator.

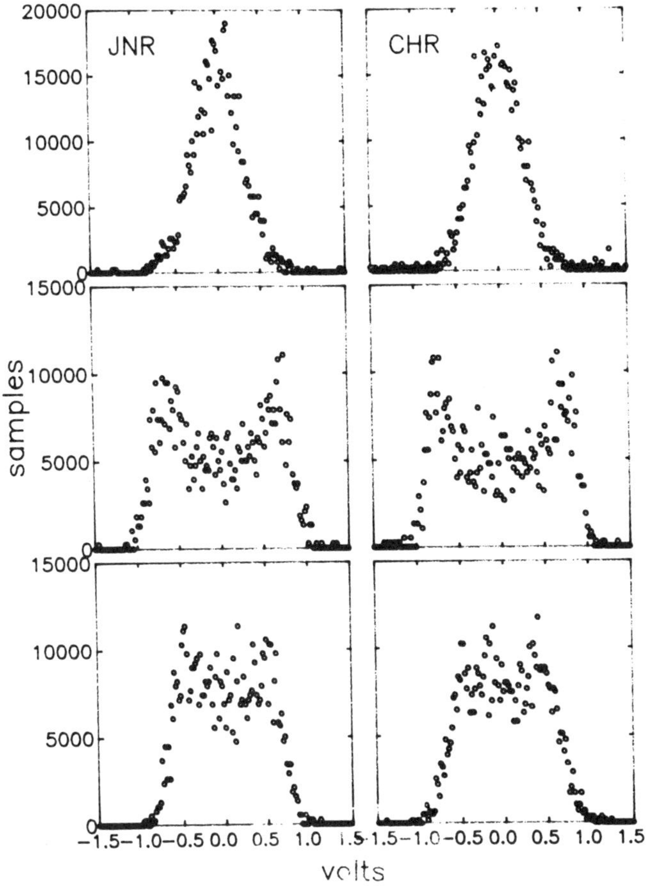

Figure 5. Statistical properties of the filtered ear canal signal centered at a frequency with no spontaneous emission (top). At the frequency of a spontaneous emission, before (center), and during aspirin consumption (bottom). The signals were amplified before sampling to cover a similar range of voltages. JN's emission was 13 dB SPL without aspirin and 3 dB SPL during aspirin consumption. CH's emission was 7 dB SPL without aspirin and -2 dB SPL during aspirin consumption.

Acknowledgements

This work was supported by NINCDS Grant NS 22095 and Purdue University. The authors with to thank Elizabeth Marrs, Lidia Lee and William J. Murphy for help analyzing the data and making the figures.

References

Bialek, W.S., and Wit, H.P. (**1984**). "Quantum limits to oscillator stability: Theory and experiments on acoustic emissions from the human ear," Phys. Lett. **104A**, 1973-1978.

Hanggi, P., and Riseborough, P. (**1983**). "Dynamics of nonlinear dissipative oscillators," Am.J.Physics **51**, 347-351.

Kemp, D.T. (**1979**). "Evidence for a new element in cochlear mechanics," Scand.Audiol.Suppl. **9**, 35-47.

Long, G.R., Tubis, A., and Jones, K. (**1986a**). "Synchronization of spontaneous oto-acoustic emissions and driven limit cycle oscillators," J.Acoust. Soc.Am. **79**, S5.

Long, G.R., Tubis, A., and Jones, K. (**1986b**). "Changes in spontaneous and evoked otoacoustic emissions and the corresponding psychoacoustic threshold microstructure induced by aspirin consumption," in : *Peripheral Auditory Mechanisms*, edited by J.B. Allen, J.L. Hall, A.E.Hubbard, S.T. Neely and A. Tubis (Springer Verlag, Berlin), pp.213-218.

Machlup, S., and Sluckin, T. J. (**1980**). "Driven oscillations of a limit cycle oscillator," J.Theor.Biol. **84**, 119-134.

McFadden, D., and Plattsmier, H.S. (**1984**). "Aspirin abolishes spontaneous oto-acoustic emissions," J.Acoust.Soc.Am. **76**, 443-448.

Stratonovich, R.L. (**1963**). *Topics in the Theory of Random Noise*, Volume II (Gordon and Breach, New York), pp. 222-276.

van Dijk, P., and Wit, H.P. (**1988**). "Phase-lock of spontaneous oto-acoustic emissions to a cubic difference tone," This volume, pp xx-xx.

Wilson, J.P., and Sutton, G.J. (**1981**). "Acoustic correlates of tonal tinnitus," in *Tinnitus*, edited by D. Evered and G. Lawrensen (Pitman, London), pp. 82-107.

Wit, H.P. (**1986**). "Statistical properties of a strong spontaneous otoacoustic emission," in *Peripheral Auditory Mechanics*, edited by J.B. Allen, J.L. Hall, A.E.Hubbard, S.T.Neely, and A.Tubis (Springer,Berlin) pp. 221-228.

Zwicker, E. and Schloth, E. (**1984**). "Interrelation of different oto-acoustic emissions," J.Acoust.Soc.Am. **75**, 1148-1154.

Comments

Lewis:

Interaction between a pair of oscillators can lead to at least two interesting phenomena in addition to entrainment (or stable phase locking). The simplest of these is a stable limit-cycle behavior, in which the phase relationship repeatedly passes through a fixed sequence. The other phenomenon is chaotic behavior, in which the phase relationship progresses deterministically through a sequence in which no value (relative phase) is ever repeated. In fact chaotic behavior is difficult to distinguish from noise. It would be interesting to look for these phenomena in your data and your models.

Phase-lock of spontaneous oto-acoustic emissions to a cubic difference tone

P. van Dijk and H.P. Wit

Institute of Audiology, P.O.Box 30.001, 9700 RB Groningen, The Netherlands

Introduction

When two oscillators with slightly different frequencies are coupled, they tend to synchronize. This phase-lock phenomenon has probably first been described by Christiaan Huygens (1893). In a letter to his father, dated 16 februari 1665, he reports that two pendulum clocks, slightly "out of step", tend to synchronize each other when attached to the same wall. Phase-lock is a property typical for selfsustaining oscillators. By studying it, parameters describing the behaviour of an oscillator can be determined.

Spontaneous oto-acoustic emissions (SOAE) can be phase-locked by presenting an external tone to the earcanal with a frequency equal to that of the emission (Bialek and Wit 1984, Long 1986). A disadvantage of this method is the presence of the synchronizing sine wave in the recorded microphone signal. Therefore, we investigated phase-lock of SAOE's to the $2f_1$-f_2 cubic difference tone (CDT) generated in the ear by two tones of frequencies f_1 and f_2. Interaction between SOAE's and a CDT was reported before by Wit *et al.* (1981), Rabinowitz and Widin (1984) and Pasanan *et al.* (1987). In this paper we show that the mechanism of this interaction is phase-lock (in the presence of noise) of a selfsustaining oscillator to a sinusoidal driving force.

Methods

Two earphones were used to present the tones of frequencies f_1 and f_2 and intensities L_1 and L_2 to the ear canal. The ear canal signal was measured with a sensitive microphone (Wit *et al.* 1981) and recorded on one channel of a Sony PCM-F1 recorder for various values of f_1 and f_2 and various levels L_1 and L_2 of these primaries. Simultaneously, a reference tone of frequency $2f_1$-f_2 was recorded on the other channel of the recorder. This reference was generated externally, using the primaries.

Off line, power spectra of recorded microphone signals were determined, using a Unigon 4512 real-time FFT analyser.

For further analysis, recorder signals were bandpass filtered by a B&K

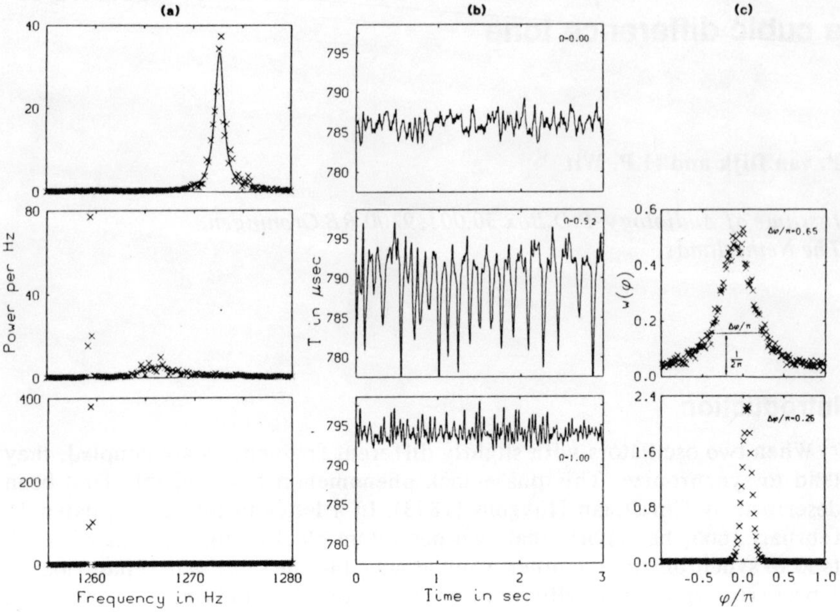

Fig.1. Frequency spectra (a), instantaneous period (b) and phase distributions (c) for subject RL(R). Top to bottom: no stimulus, L_1=L_2=6dB HL, L_1=L_2=16dB HL.

2020 heterodyne filter with a bandwidth of 31.6 Hz. The center frequency was chosen in such a way that both the SOAE-frequency f_0 and the synchronizing frequency $f_s=2f_1-f_2$ fell within the passband.

For the filtered signals the time T between successive positive zero-crossings was measured with a HP5326A timer. After DA-conversion, T was recorded as a function of time. The same instrument was used to determine a long-term average value <f> for the frequency of the emission. Note that $\langle f\rangle=\langle 1/T\rangle$.

Secondly, the phase distribution for the filtered microphone signal with respect to the $2f_1-f_2$ reference sine wave was determined. For this purpose $2f_1-f_2$ triggered an EG&G 4203 signal analyser and a histogram was obtained for the times Δt between the zero-crossings of the reference and the filtered emission signal. These histograms were normalized by computer to give a distribution $w(\phi)$, where $\int_{-\pi}^{\pi} w(\phi)d\phi=1$ and ϕ is defined by $\phi=2\pi f_s\Delta t$.

Results

As an example figure 1 shows results for subject RL. The left column shows spectra for three different levels of the CDT. In the absence of stimuli

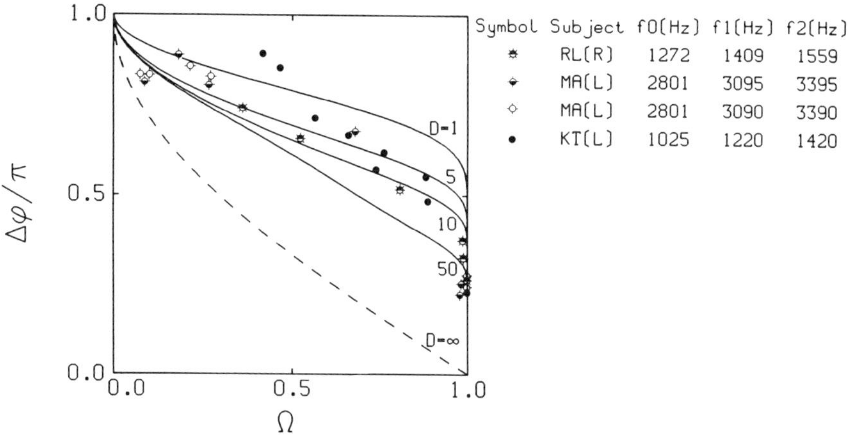

Fig.2 $\Delta\phi$ as function of Ω for 3 subjects. Dotted and solid lines represent calculated curves for the Van der Pol oscillator.

(upper panel) only a Lorentzian peak produced by the emission can be seen. If the CDT is sufficiently loud, only a very narrow peak is present at frequency $f_s=2f_1-f_2$, because the emission is constantly phase-locked to the CDT tone generated inside the ear. At intermediate levels both peaks are present in the spectrum. The emission is not constantly locked at f_s but occasionally jumps to f_0.

This is illustrated in the middle column of fig. 1, where the instantaneous period T is given as a function of time. In the upper panel of this column, T fluctuates around $T_0=1/f_0$ and in the lower panel around $T_s=1/f_s$. In the middle panel the zerocrossing time jumps between T_0 and T_s; this results in an average frequency $\langle f \rangle$ between f_0 and f_s. If we define $\Omega=(\langle f \rangle-f_0)/(f_s-f_0)$, then Ω increases from 0 to 1, with increasing level of the CDT.

The filtered microphone signal can be approximated by $y=A_0\cos(\omega_s t+\phi(t))$. For a sufficiently strong CDT, ϕ fluctuates around a constant value. For weaker CDT, ϕ occasionally "drifts off", resulting in an $\langle f \rangle \neq f_s$. And without the CDT, ϕ continuously drifts off with such a "velocity" that $\langle f \rangle = f_0$.

The normalized phase distributions in the rigth column of fig 1 can be interpreted as probability distributions $w(\phi)$ for ϕ. The witdhs $\Delta\phi$ of these distributions at $w(\phi)=1/2\pi$ are given as numbers in the graphs. With increasing level of the $2f_1-f_2$ CDT, $\Delta\phi$ decreases, and at the same time Ω grows from 0 to 1. By eliminating the (not exactly known) level of the CDT, $\Delta\phi$ can be given as a function of Ω. Fig 2 gives results obtained in this way for various subjects, stimulus levels and frequencies.

The behaviour as described above is characteristic for a selfsustaining oscillator in the presence of noise, driven by an external tone.

Theory

From a mathematical point of view, the simplest selfsustaining oscillator is the Van der Pol oscillator. In the presence of noise and driven by an external tone, the equation describing its behaviour is (Stratonovich, 1963):

$$\ddot{x} - \epsilon\omega_s \dot{x}\left[1 - \frac{4}{3A_0^2}\left(\frac{\dot{x}}{\omega_s}\right)^2\right] + \omega_0^2 x = -\omega_s^2\,\eta(t) - \omega_s^2 E \sin\omega_s t \qquad (1)$$

The term between the brackets contains the parabolic resistance term, typical for the Van der Pol equation. The right-hand side is made up of a noisy function $\eta(t)$ and an external tone of frequency ω_s. We define $\kappa_\eta(\omega)$ as the power spectral density for $\eta(t)$ and introduce $K=\omega_s^2 \cdot \kappa_\eta(\omega_s)$. For $K \ll \epsilon\omega_s A_0^2$ and $E/A_0 \ll \epsilon$ the above equation can be solved by $x=A_0\sin(\omega_s t + \phi(t))$, where $\phi(t)$ turns out to behave identically to the phase of the emission signal as described above. As for experiments, we can define Ω and $\Delta\phi$. The theoretical curves in Figure 2 have been calculated for various $D=(2A_0^2/K)\cdot(\omega_0-\omega_s)$. For subject RL, $\Delta\phi$ increases faster with decreasing Ω than theory predicts. For the other subjects good resemblance between experiment and theory can be observed. Typically $D\approx5$, for $f_s-f_0\approx10$ Hz. This corresponds to a spectral density of the noise equal to $\kappa_\eta(\omega_s)/A_0^2 = 4\cdot10^{-7}$ Hz^{-1}.

All displayed results represent experiments with $\omega_s<\omega_0$. For $\omega_s>\omega_0$ similar results have been obtained, but description of the emission generator with a simple Van der Pol equation does not seem to completely account for the data. More research is needed to clarify this asymmetry.

References

Bialek, W., and Wit, H.P. (**1984**). "Quantum Limits to Oscillator Stability: Theory and Experiments on Acoustic Emissions from the Human Ear," Physics Lett. **104A**. 173-178.

Huygens, C. (**1893**). Letter to his father, februari 26, 1665. In *Oeuvres Completes de Christiaan Huygens*, Volume 5, edited by the Société Hollandaise des Sciences (Martinus Nijhoff, The Hague), p. 243.

Long, G. (**1986**). " Synchronization of Spontaneous Otoacoustic Emissions and Driven Limit-Cycle oscillators," J.Acoust.Soc.Am. **81**, Suppl. 1, S8.

Pasanen, E.G., Wier, C.C., and McFadden, D. (**1987**). "Reciprocal Relation between the Growth of an Emitted Cubic Distortion Product and the Suppression of a Spontaneous Otoacoustic Emission," J.Acoust.Soc.Am. **81**, Suppl. 1, S8.

Rabinowitz, W.M., and Widin, G.P. (**1984**). "Interaction of Spontaneous Otoacoustic Emissions and External sounds," J.Acoust.Soc.Am. **76**, 1713-1720.

Stratonovich, R.L. (**1963**). *Topics in the Theory of Random Noise, Volume II* (Gordon and Breach, New York), Chap. 9.

Wit, H.P., Langevoort, J.C., and Ritsma, R.J. (**1981**). "Frequency Spectra of Cochlear Acoustic Emissions ("Kemp-echoes")," J.Acoust.Soc.Am. **70**, 437-445.

Transient responses in an active, nonlinear model of cochlear mechanics

S. T. Neely

Boys Town National Institute
Omaha, Nebraska, USA

Introduction

The latency of transient evoked auditory brainstem responses (ABRs) is known to be both frequency and intensity dependent (Eggermont and Don, 1980). The latency of the ABR decreases as either the level or the frequency of the evoking stimulus increases. This same trend of decreasing latency with increasing level or frequency has also been observed (although less clearly established) in transient evoked otoacoustic emissions (OAEs) (Norton and Neely, 1987). The purpose of this paper is to investigate how nonlinearities in cochlear mechanics can cause both ABR and OAE latencies to be level dependent. Our method is to look at results from an active, nonlinear model of cochlear mechanics.

Models provide us with a way of testing our understanding of the peripheral auditory system. In this paper, the term model refers to a set of mathematical equations, based on physical principles, which describe (at some level of abstraction) the dynamics of a physical system. Nonlinear models have been useful in understanding the generation and propagation of distortion products such as combination tones (Kim *et al.*, 1973). Active models have been useful in suggesting how the ear can achieve its sharp tuning and high sensitivity (Neely and Kim, 1986). The term active refers to the inclusion of elements within the model which are local sources of mechanical energy. Although it is generally accepted that both active and nonlinear elements have significant roles in cochlear mechanics, it has been difficult to implement a model which contains both elements (Diependaal and Viergever, 1983; Duifhuis *et al.*, 1986; Zwicker and Lumer, 1986).

Model

One-dimensional fluid equations are used to model cochlear macro-mechanics. The micromechanics are modeled with basilar membrane (BM) and tectorial membrane (TM) having no longitudinal coupling (Allen, 1980). The model contains active elements in the form of pressure sources (repre-

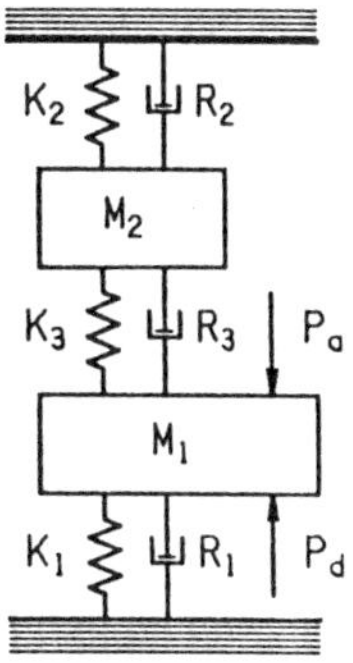

Figure 1. Lumped component model of cochlear micromechanics. The mass M_1 represents a cross-section of the organ of Corti which is attached to rigid bone by stiffness and damping components K_1 and R_1. The BM is "driven" by fluid pressure difference P_d and active pressure source P_a. The mass M_2 represents a cross-section of the tectorial membrane (TM) which is attached to rigid bone by K_2 and R_2. The two masses are coupled by K_3 and R_3. The relative motion between BM and TM represents displacement d_c.

senting outer hair cells) which are controlled by relative displacement between the BM and the TM. These active elements provide the cochlear model with sharp tuning (comparable to neural tuning) and high sensitivity (comparable to the direct measurements of Sellick, *et al.*). Except for the nonlinearity and a change of notation, the form of the equations and their physical interpretation are the same as Neely and Kim (1986).

A time-domain implementation gives us the flexibility of including nonlinear elements in the model. The model is made nonlinear by restricting the feedback force (due to the active elements) to stay within a limited range.

Equations of motion

Let a_b, v_b, and d_b represent the BM acceleration, velocity, and displacement perpendicular to its resting plane and let a_t, v_t, and d_t represent the acceleration, velocity, and displacement of the TM. For convenience, we will use v_c, d_c to describe the relative motion between the two membranes, which represents the displacement and velocity of the hair bundles of the outer hair cells.

$$v_c = v_b - v_t \quad \text{and} \quad d_c = d_b - d_t$$

Let P_d represent the fluid pressure difference across the basilar membrane, and let P_a represent an additional (active) pressure component due to forces within the outer hair cells. Then the first two equations of motion take the general form of two coupled, second-order systems with external forces applied only to the first system:

$$P_d - P_a = M_1 a_b + R_1 v_b + K_1 d_b + R_3 v_c + K_3 d_c$$

$$0 = M_2 a_t + R_2 v_t + K_2 d_t - R_3 v_c - K_3 d_c$$

The correspondence of the parameters in these equations with physical components is illustrated in Fig. 1.

The active pressure P_a is controlled by d_c, but was limited to small values in the following way:

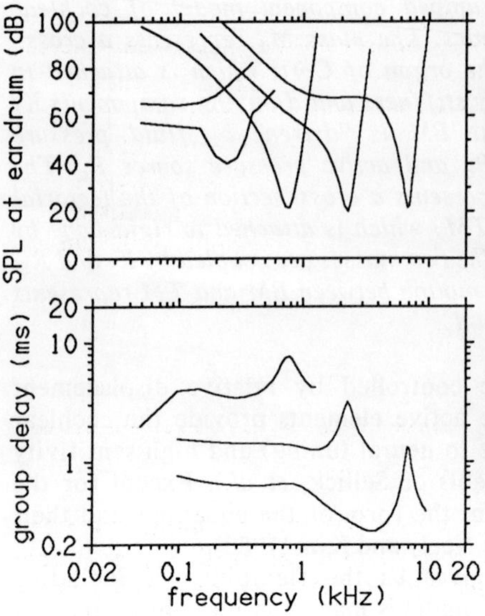

Figure 2. Iso-velocity tuning curves and group delay based on relative velocity between BM and TM. These curves are computed by taking a Fourier transform of the model response to a wideband click stimulus using a linearized version of the model. The iso-velocity curves indicate the sound pressure level at the eardrum needed to obtain a velocity of 4 μm/s at 5 places: 0, 20, 40, 60, 80, and 90% of the length L of the cochlear partition. Group delay is computed (for the first three places) as minus the slope of the phase with respect to frequency.

$$P_a = -K_4\, d_c\,, \text{ for } -d_m < d_c < d_m\,,$$

where d_m is a small, fixed displacement value. When d_c exceeded this range, the value of P_a was not allowed to become less than $-K_4\, d_m$ nor greater than $K_4\, d_m$.

Parameter selection

The parameter values were selected to obtain neural-like tuning and a frequency-to-place map similar to a typical human cochlea. The iso-velocity tuning curves shown in Fig. 2 are for a linearized version of the model. The curves in Fig. 2 are similar in shape to typical neural threshold tuning curves for the cat. The frequency-to-place map of the model is compared with one for human cochleae (Wright, 1984) in Fig. 3. Parameter values for the model are listed in Table I.

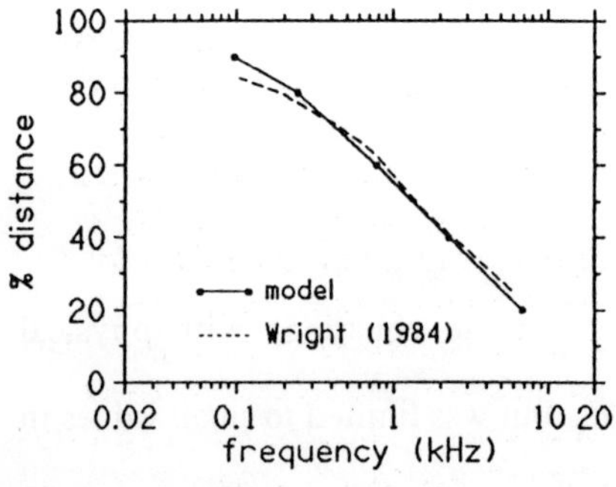

Figure 3. Cochlear frequency-place map. The dashed line is a fit to data of Wright (1984) for a human cochlea. The symbols show the frequency of maximum velocity v_c at the 5 places along the cochlear partition shown in Fig. 2.

Table I: Model parameter values (cgs units)

name	value	name	value
$K_1(x)$	$4{\cdot}10^8\ e^{-3x}$ dyn·cm^{-3}	L	3.5 cm
$R_1(x)$	$960\ e^{-1.4x}$ dyn·s·cm^{-3}	H	0.1 cm
$M_1(x)$	0.004 gm·cm^{-2}	W	0.1 cm
$K_2(x)$	$2{\cdot}10^8\ e^{-3.2x}$ dyn·cm^{-3}	d_m	10^{-7} cm
$R_2(x)$	$2000\ e^{-1.4x}$ dyn·s·cm^{-3}		
$M_2(x)$	0.037 gm·cm^{-2}		
$K_3(x)$	$2.25{\cdot}10^8\ e^{-3.2x}$ dyn·cm^{-3}		
$R_3(x)$	0		
$K_4(x)$	$4.5{\cdot}10^8\ e^{-3.1x}$ dyn·cm^{-3}		

Whole nerve response

In order to compare the model results with ABR data from human subjects, a representation of whole nerve response (WNR) was required. Assuming that the relative velocity v_c between BM and TM provides the input signal to the inner hair cells, we took a half-wave rectified version of v_c, smoothed by an RC low-pass filter with a time constant of 0.5 ms, and combined (with equal weighting) all places along the cochlear partition to obtain the model's estimate of WNR.

Results

The time course of eardrum pressure and our simplified WNR was observed in response to tone-burst stimuli at different levels and frequencies. The stimuli were Blackman-windowed tone-bursts with frequencies of 0.5, 1, 2, and 4 kHz. Burst durations were 4, 2.8, 2, and 1.4 ms, respectively. The stimulus, WNR, and OAE are shown in Fig. 4 for a 1 kHz tone-burst at 40 dB SPL.

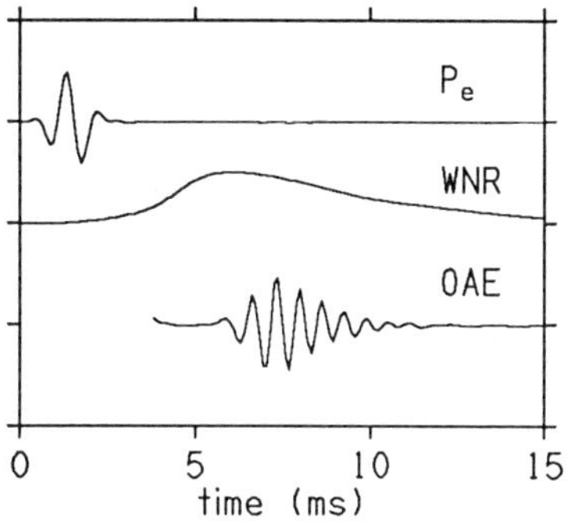

Figure 4. Response of the model to a 1 kHz tone burst. The first trace shows the pressure waveform at the eardrum. The second trace shows an indication of whole nerve activity computed by passing a half-wave rectified version of the velocity v_c through an RC low-pass filter and summing the result over the entire length of the cochlear partition. The third trace also shows pressure at eardrum, but this time magnified to show an otoacoustic emission.

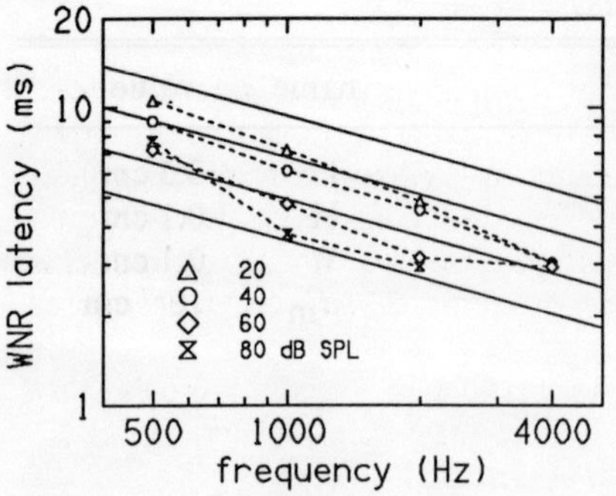

Figure 5. Latency of the whole nerve response (WNR) as a function of tone-burst frequency. The symbols show results of the model at 4 frequencies and 4 levels using the whole nerve measure shown in Fig. 4. Latency is measured from onset of the stimulus to the peak of the WNR. The solid lines represent a fit to ABR wave V at the same stimulus levels, in a group of human subjects minus 5 ms.

The model showed a clear, burst-like OAE in the eardrum pressure waveform (as in Fig. 4) at all four frequencies, but for only one level at each frequency. At the 3 lower frequencies the OAE was only clearly present at 40 dB SPL. At 4 kHz the OAE was only clearly present at 60 dB SPL. The peak of the WNR was well defined for all stimulus frequencies and levels except for 4 kHz at 80 dB SPL.

The latency of the WNR is shown in Fig. 5 at 20, 40, 60, and 80 dB SPL. The model results are compared in Fig. 5 with latency estimates based on human ABR latencies (Gorga *et al.*, 1988). The solid lines in Fig. 5 provide good fits to wave V latency of tone-burst evoked ABRs minus 5 ms (Neely *et al.*, 1988). The 5 ms correction compensates for the additional neural synaptic (1 ms) and propagation (4 ms) delays in the ABR.

The latency of the WNR in the model decreases with increasing level in the same manner as the human ABR data, but the effect is smaller in the model. The ABR data shows a consistent decrease in latency at all frequencies of about 28% for a 20 dB increase in stimulus level. The model results show about 19% decrease in latency per 20 dB increase in level at 1 kHz, and less for other frequencies. The decrease in the WNR latency to the 1 kHz tone-burst as the level increased from 20 to 80 dB SPL is about 6.4 ms, which is more than twice the total duration of the stimulus (2.8 ms).

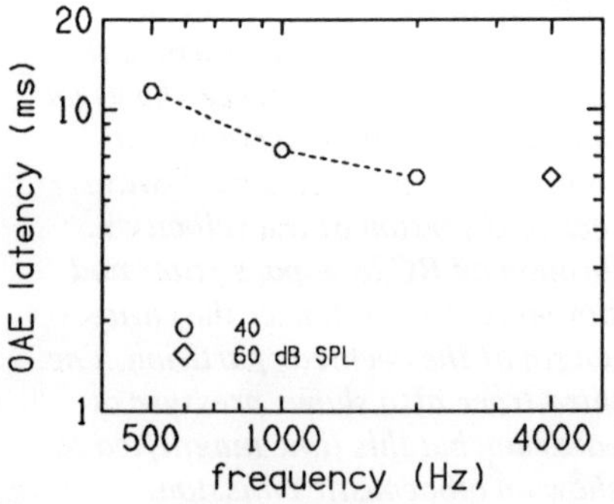

Figure 6. Latency of the otoacoustic emission as a function of tone-burst frequency. The latency is measured from the onset of the stimulus to the peak of the OAE burst in the eardrum pressure waveform.

Discussion

The model is essentially a nonlinear, time-domain version of one presented previously (Neely and Kim, 1986). The active elements in the model provide a feedback force to the basilar membrane which is controlled by displacement of the hair bundle of the outer hair cells. The model is made nonlinear by limiting the feedback force in a peak clipping fashion. Although the model is both active and nonlinear it is still stable in the sense that transient responses decay with time.

The numerical method used for temporal integration was the same used by Allen and Sondhi (1979). Diependaal *et al.* (1987) have shown that a fourth-order Runge-Kutta method would be more efficient.

Iso-velocity curves were used to simulate neural tuning in Fig. 2 instead of iso-displacement curves because this made it easier to achieve higher sensitivity at high frequencies. The choice of iso-displacement or iso-velocity affects the choice of model parameters, but does not greatly influence the results.

The speed at which transient responses travel in the cochlea is mainly determined by the stiffness of the cochlear partition. The model has been set up in such a way that the active elements create a feedback force which decreases the stiffness of the cochlear partition, thereby decreasing the speed of propagation. As stimulus level increases, the relative contribution of this feedback force is smaller and the effective stiffness of the cochlear partition is greater. Thus the latency of the WNR varies in the model primarily because the effective stiffness of the cochlear partition increases as the level of the stimulus increases.

The presence of the nonlinearity in the model increases the amplitude of the OAE significantly for certain stimulus levels. Even though the non-linearity decreases the energy contribution of the active elements at high stimulus levels, it increases the amount of energy which is reflected back out through the middle ear. The model results support the view that nonlinearities in the cochlea are essential to the generation of OAEs (Kemp, 1979).

The latency of the OAE in the model varies with frequency in the same manner as the WNR. The change in OAE latency with level could not be determined by the model results since the OAE was only clearly present at one level for each frequency. Interestingly, the latency of the model OAE latency was not twice the latency of the WNR as expected from comparison of OAE and ABR latencies in human subjects.

The model WNR includes the effect of two nonlinearities. The first nonlinearity is at the outer hair cell and controls the amount of feedback force. The other nonlinearity is at the inner hair cell as a means of deriving a measure of excitation of the afferent nerve fibers. The deviation of the model results from measurements OAE and ABR in human subjects indicates a need to modify one or both of these nonlinearities.

Summary

A cochlear model with active elements representing a feedback force generated by outer hair cells is made nonlinear by limiting the amplitude of this force. One effect of this nonlinearity is that the effective stiffness of the cochlear partition is greater at high levels thereby decreasing the latency of transient responses with increasing level. This effect is clearly seen in a whole nerve response derived from the model. This type of nonlinearity also greatly increases the amplitude of the otoacoustic emission as compared to a linear model.

Acknowledgments

This research was supported by a grant from the National Institutes of Health NS20652. Peter Bodmer provided assistance with computer programming and preparation of the figures.

References

Allen, J. B. (**1980**). "Cochlear micromechanics - A physical model of transduction," J.Acoust.Soc.Am. **68**, 1660-1679.

Allen, J. B. and Sondhi, M. M. (**1979**). "A cochlear micromechanical model of transduction," in *Psychophysical, Psychological, and Behavioural Studies in Hearing*, edited by G. van den Brink and F. A. Bilsen (Delft Univ. Press, Delft, The Netherlands), pp 85-95.

Diependaal, R. J., and Viergever, M. A. (**1983**). "Nonlinear and active modeling of cochlear mechanics: A precarious affair," in *Mechanics of Hearing*, edited by E. de Boer and M. A. Viergever, (Delft Univ. Press, Delft, The Netherlands), pp 153-160.

Diependaal, R. J., Duifhuis, H., Hoogstraten, H. W., and Viergever, M. A. (**1987**). "Numerical methods for the solving one-dimensional cochlear models in the time domain," J.Acoust.Soc.Am. **82**, 1655-1666.

Duifhuis, H., Hoogstraten, S. M., van Netten, S. M., Diependaal, R. J., and Bialek, W. (**1986**). "Modelling the cochlear partition with coupled Van der Pol oscillators," in *Peripheral Auditory Mechanisms*, edited by J. B. Allen, J. L. Hall, A. Hubbard, S. T. Neely, and A. Tubis, (Springer-Verlag, Munich), pp 290-297.

Eggermont, J. and Don, M. (**1980**). "Analysis of click-evoked brainstem potentials in humans using high-pass noise masking. II. Effect of click intensity," J.Acoust.Soc.Am. **68**, 1671-1675.

Gorga, M. P., Reiland, J. K., Beauchaine, K. A., and Jesteadt, W. (**1988**). "Auditory brainstem responses to tone bursts in normal hearing subjects," J. Speech Hear. Res. (in press).

Kemp, D. T. (**1979**). "Evidence for mechanical nonlinearity and frequency selective wave amplification in the cochlea," Arch. Otorhinol. **244**, 37-45.

Kim, D. O., Molnar, C. E., and Pfeiffer, R. R. (**1973**). "A system of nonlinear differential equations modeling basilar-membrane motion," J.Acoust.Soc.

Am. **54**, 1516-1529.

Matthews, J. W. (**1980**). *Mechanical modeling of nonlinear phenomena observed in the peripheral auditory system.* Doctoral thesis, Washington University, St. Louis.

Neely, S. T. and Kim, D. O. (**1983**). "An active cochlear model showing sharp tuning and high sensitivity," Hearing Res. **9**, 123-130.

Neely, S. T. and Kim, D. O. (**1986**). "A model for active elements in cochlear biomechanics," J.Acoust.Soc.Am. **79**, 1472-1480.

Neely, S. T., Norton, S. J., Gorga, M. P. and Jesteadt, W. (**1988**). "Latency of auditory brainstem responses and otoacoustic emissions using tone-burst stimuli," J. Acoust. Soc. Am (in press).

Norton, S. J. and Neely, S. T. (**1987**). "Tone-burst evoked otoacoustic emissions in normal hearing subjects," J.Acoust.Soc.Am. **81**, 1860-1872.

Sellick, P. M., Patuzzi, R., and Johnstone, B. M. (**1982**). "Measurement of basilar membrane motion in the guinea pig using the Mössbauer technique," J.Acoust.Soc.Am. **72**, 131-141.

Wright, A. A. (**1984**). "Dimensions of the cochlear stereocilia in man and in guinea pig," Hearing Res. **13**, 89-98.

Zwicker, E. and Lumer, G. (**1986**). "Evaluating traveling-wave characteristics in man by an active nonlinear cochlea preprocessing model," in *Peripheral Auditory Mechanisms*, edited by J. B. Allen, J. L. Hall, A. Hubbard, S. T. Neely, and A. Tubis, (Springer-Verlag, Munich), 250-257.

Comments

Evans:

I am also puzzled how your model, depending upon a saturating nonlinearity, can account for the level dependency of the single fibre/gross evoked potential onset latency seen over its very wide dynamic range (60 dB+) as in your Fig. 5.

Reply by Neely:

The saturating nonlinearity included in the model does not completely limit the dynamic range of operation of the active elements. As level is increased beyond the saturation level of the transducer, the amount of energy fed into the system by the active elements no longer increases, but remains constant at higher levels.

Zwicker:

There seems to be a basic difference between human responses and results of your model. In human, the evoked otoacoustic emissions remain constant with decreasing evoked level towards and below threshold when expressed in values relative to the amplitude of the evoker. Why does your model show otoacoustic emissions only at a small level range of the evoker?

Reply by Neely:

I agree with you that the model should generate OAE's over a wider range of intensities. Further refinement of the model is required to improve its representation of OAE's.

Wilson:

In your model you explain the latency of the OAE as being twice the basilar membrane travel time due to the addition of reverse traveltime. There does not yet appear to be any convincing evidence that a reverse travelling wave can occur. Support for it appears to arise out of a confusion between a travelling wave and a wave travelling through a medium for a transmission line where energy is passed on from one point to the next and can be stopped and reflected by a short- or open-circuited transmission line. In the basilar membrane, however, the driving force is provided by the pressure difference between scala vestibuli and scala tympani and the motion depends on local mass & stiffness and on coupling to neighbouring segments. The apparent direction of motion is expressed by the relative phases of neighbouring sections which invariably show greater lag towards the low frequency end. Furthermore if the basilar membrane were rigidly fixed (short-circuited) or cut across (open-circuited) there would be little change to the travelling wave pattern on either side with a modified response only in the region of the discontinuity.

An alternative type of model was proposed by Wilson (1980a), an electrical version (Wilson, 1980b) and a computer version (Sutton and Wilson, 1893) both demonstrating a qualitatively & quantitatively correct simulation of OAE generation using realistic model parameters. Although this originally suggested volume changes of OHCs as the source of OAEs, the model would apply equally well to BM position changes induced by cell length changes or stereociliary motion. The net volume displacement of the BM at any instant moved with incompressible fluid, be equal to the instantaneous volume displacement of the stapes. Thus the response arises from all sections of the BM involved in the travelling wave. For a regularly mapped cochlea a large degree of phase cancellation would occur. The basis of the model is that some regions may have slight deviations in the frequency/phase map which would cancel much less effectively leading to a large contribution from this region. The cancellation process leads to a sharpened filter characteristic which therefore has greater delay.

Sutton, G.J. and Wilson, J.P. (1983). "Modelling cochlear echoes: the influence of irregularities in frequency mapping on summed cochlear activity." In: Mechanics of Hearing, eds. E. de Boer and M.A. Viergever. (Delft University Press) pp. 83-90.

Wilson, J.P. (1980a). "Model for cochlear echoes and tinnitus based on an observed electrical correlate." Hearing Res. 2, 527-532.

Wilson, J.P. (1980b). "Model of cochlear function and acoustic re-emission." In: Psychophysical, Physiological and Behavioural Studies in Hearing, G. van den Brink and F.A. Bilsen eds. (Delft University Press) pp. 72-73.

Reply by Neely:

I disagree with your statement that BM position changes will lead to "instantaneous volume displacement of the stapes". Basilar membrane disturbances are propagated with finite velocity due to BM compliance.

I agree that there is some confusion about the notion of a travelling wave. This term is most often used to describe the *steady-state response* of the BM to sinusoidal stimulation. In this paper, the model results are for *transient responses* of the cochlea. The response of the BM is a transient also appears to be a packet of waves, but the envelope of this wave packet also travels. The transient wave packet can be split and partially reflected by discontinuities in BM compliance. The reverse propagation proceeds with the same (place dependent) velocity as the forward propagation.

The dynamics of cochlear perturbations following brief acoustic and efferent stimulation -otoacoustic and CM data

D.T.Kemp and M. Souter

Institute of Laryngology and Otology, Functional Analysis Section, Department of Audiology, Gray's Inn Road, London WC1X 8EE

Introduction

Evidence for some central control of cochlear mechanics via the efferent system has been with us for some time (Guinan, 1987). This and the critical importance of cochlear mechanics for hearing leads to the suspicion that any aspect of the cochlea's receptor function could be under the influence of a complex control system. There is a need to establish under what stimulus parameters and particularly over what time scales cochlear responses are other than locally determined.

One very important dynamic feature of cochlear function is its ability to produce a full response to a weak acoustic stimulus following a more intense sound of similar frequency. This requires (amongst other things) that basilar membrane motion quickly reverts to its low-level/high-Q behaviour, from its more damped mode of vibration during the intense sound (Johnstone *et al.*, 1986). If after a loud sound re-establishment of the normal low-level vibration pattern took some time then the cochlear mechanical contribution to forward masking would extend beyond the physical filter ringing time. One aspect of efferent control of over the cochlea could relate to the management of active mechanical processes in rapidly changing acoustic stimulation situations, perhaps helping optimise sensitivity and dynamic range (Bonfils and Puel, 1987). In that case one would expect the dynamics of post stimulus suppression, and of efferent induced cochlear disturbances to have some common features.

What is the best way to observe the auditory control system in action? Overstimulation can easily reveal fatigue recovery processes, but only at the cost of disabling the normal functional control mechanism. To gain an insight into the functional dynamics of the cochlea's regulatory mechanism, the system must be stressed but within normal stimulus limits and by the smallest amount compatible with the need to detect some perturbation of the system. The induced fluctuations in the cochlea's response to a probe tone will then reveal most faithfully the dynamics of the underlying control mechanism.

In this paper we present a preliminary investigation of the characteristics and time course of changes in otoacoustic and round window CM responses to a continuous probe tone caused by short suppressor tone bursts between 60 and 95 dB SPL. We compare these to the changes induced by electrical excitation of the efferent system. Acoustically induced perturbations were extensively studied in the otoacoustic response from a human ear, and in 3 sedated guinea pig ears using a 2 stimulator, 1 microphone otoacoustic probe.

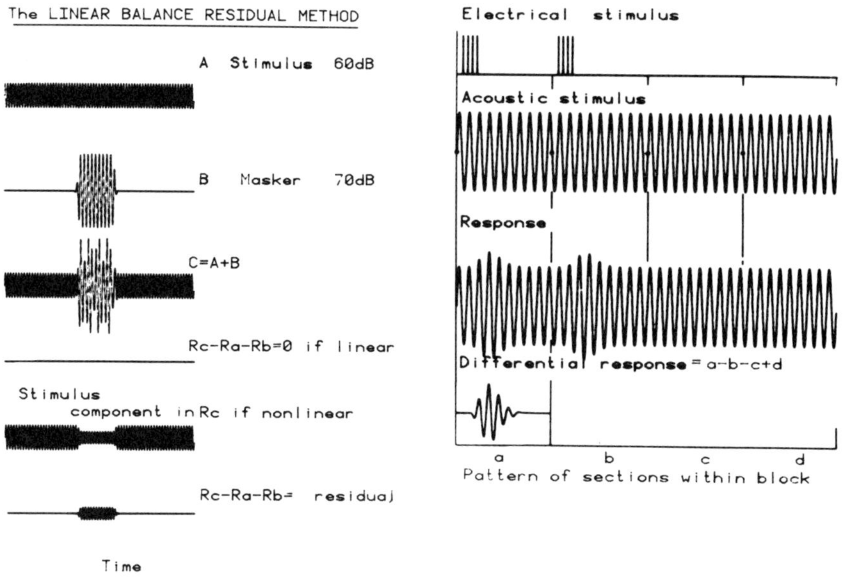

Figure 1. The method used to study cochlear pertubation dynamics, both acoustic and efferent induced. Left: the basic principle. Continuous acoustic tone stimulus A, masker B and combination stimulus C = A + B result in responses Ra, Rb, and Rc respectively. With no direct nonlinear interactions and no system pertubation, Rc - Ra - Rb = 0, i.e. there is complete cancellation with this formula applied to the data. If Ra is directly suppressed (or enhanced) during B, or if the system's response to A is otherwise changed by B, then there will remain a residual signal (bottom) representing this and its after effect. Right: the practical method achieved by computer stimulus synthesis and synchronised digital recording. A four section stimulus block (a,b,c,d) was presented cyclically, and all response waveform sections summed into memory according to (a - v - c + d). The regular stimulus response (and the stimulus itself in the acoustic mode) cancels due to half integral stimulus waves/section relationship. Artifacts and responses associated with the two perturbing stimuli in sections a and b only (here electric COCB pulses in a and b) are eliminated by subtraction. This leaves only a waveform representing the perturbation in the response to A caused by B.

Both acoustic and efferent induced perturbations were observed in the CM and OAE responses in one guinea pig maintained under neurolept anaesthesia and immobilised with Flaxodil. The efferent induced perturbation data has been confirmed in a further 10 guinea pigs (Kemp and Souter, 1988).

Observations of cochlear perturbation dynamics

A null or differential signal recovery approach is highly desirable when searching for the very small perturbations which are nonetheless significant in an efficient, operational closed loop system. The method used (illustrated in Figure 1) was designed to only register CHANGES in the response to the stimulus tone response linked to the stressing agent. It achieves good signal to noise ratio without narrow band filtering, thus preserving temporal resolution. Components of perturbations lasting longer than the stimulus section duration (usually 100 ms) and other slow adaptations are not registered by this method.

With this detection system an imbalance or residual signal can arise from two causes, a) direct interference by the disturbing agent with the stimulus response production, which can only occur whilst the interfering agent persists at the stimulus reponse site, ie simple nonlinear suppression, and b) indirect interference, which requires that the interfering agent temporally changes the primary response mechanism's characteristics in some way.

Acoustically induced perturbations- otoacoustic data

Figure 2 gives experimental examples of otoacoustically traced, acoustically induced, cochlear perturbations in a human and a guinea pig ear. The 50 (25) ms duration masker directly suppresses cochlear mechanical activity leading to a reduction in the OAE sound field in the ear canal. This reduction causes a residual in the balanced summation at the stimulus frequency.

In agreement with known OAE latencies, the external manifestation of the direct suppression OAE residual is delayed with respect to the masker envelope by some 1.5-2 ms for guinea pig and 5-8 ms for human ears, at the frequencies used here. For the higher suppressor levels, in both human and guinea pig ears the residual extends for 20-30 ms beyond the main body, producing a "suppression tail". Spectral analysis of the tail shows it to be comprised of just the stimulus frequency, indicating that the suppression continued well beyond the masker, even after allowing for the known OAE latency.

The residual is not strictly a response but the inverse; the "missing" or suppressed part of the OAE response during the suppressor. For less than 100% suppression, intermodulation products are also produced. Those distortion products depending on odd powers of Fs accummulate in the summation. These beat with the stimulus frequency OAE residual causing envelope modulations at twice the difference frequency to be seen in Fig. 2.

By changing the summation logic and stimulus sequence the whole OAE

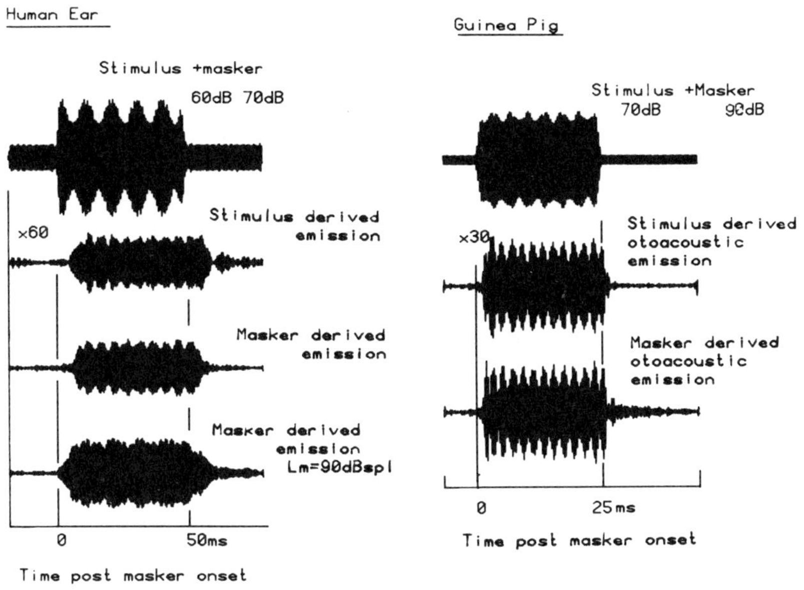

Figure 2. Otoacoustic observation of acoustically induced cochlear pertubations in a human and guinea pig ear. Top: shows for time reference purposes the waveform envelope of the continuous probe stimulus (left: 1600 Hz at 60 dB human data; right: 4000 Hz guinea pig data added to the suppressor/-masker burst (1500 Hz at 70 dB SPL Human; 3700 Hz at 90 dB SPL GP). The frequency difference results in envelope beats. The cosine rise and fall time of the suppressor was 0.8 ms. Bottom shows the perturbation residual (see Fig. 1) due to a suppressor burst of 90 dB SPL. Note the latency with reference to the suppressor and also the slowly fading termination of the residual. Above this trace (human data only), a weaker suppressor (70 dB) results in a smaller post masker residual tail. Second down on both sides, as a control, the otoacoustic emission to a 60 dB stimulus-only burst of the same duration and timing as the suppressor above. Latency is as for masker derived perturbations. There is a slowly decaying tail in this response, but this is due to the recruitment of spontaneous emissions.

(not the residual) can be derived for a short burst of stimulus tone as seen in Figure 2. This is a useful control. A tail is sometimes seen after this OAE in the human ear but it is caused by the spontaneous emissions synchronously reestablishing themselves in the quiet which now follows the stimulus. Spectral analysis typically shows several frequencies to be present. In the perturbation detection method used throughout this study the stimulus is continuous and it continuously suppresses/entrains all close spontaneous activity. Guinea pigs, which tend not to have spontaneous acoustic activity, show the suppressor derived perturbation tail, but not the stimulus derived spontaneous activity tail. We are sure that the phenomenon disussed below is a genuine stimulus response suppression and not a desynchronisation/-resynchronisation phenomenon.

The true extended suppression effect increased rapidly in magnitude and duration with suppressor level above a "threshold" of about 70 dB SPL. In contrast the direct interaction OAE component progressively saturated, with increasing suppressor level to become equal to the total OAE reponse of 26 dB SPL. Figure 3 (left) shows for a human ear that negligible extended suppression occurred with a 45 dB SPL 1600 Hz stimulus and 60 dB suppressor, a stronger direct effect was caused by a 70 dB suppressor with little extended effects, but with greatly extended effects for 80 dB suppressor.

The time constant of post suppressor suppression decay was obtained from a linear fit to the log slope of the tail envelope. These results are summarised in Figure 3(right). For a given stimulus, the time constant increases with increasing masker intensity. Increasing stimulus level caused a proportionately greater DECREASE in time constant.

Efferent induced perturbations- otoacoustic and CM data

The second part of this study involved the observation of efferent induced perturbations of the cochlear response to a single continous stimulus tone. These measurements were conducted on a fully aneasthetised guinea pig using differential signal processing on both the ear canal and round window CM signals simultaneously.

The existence of the acoustically induced otoacoustic suppression tail effect was confirmed. A higher acoustic level and a lower frequency was also introduced into this experiment to correspond to conditions independantly selected for obsererving efferent evoked effects. With a 94 dB, 12.5 ms, 2.2 kHz suppressor and 2 kHz at 80 dB stimulus a direct suppression and an extended suppression tail residual was seen in both otoacoustic and CM responses. The time constant was 10 ms in both cases. The initial tail size in this case was 1/6th of the directly suppressed primary OAE, equal to 50 dB SPL. It was also a similar proportion of the directly suppressed CM which in turn amounted to 1/3 of the total stimulus frequency CM. The phase of the CM residual was consistent with suppression and not enhancement.

For the efferent induced perturbation experiments, the masking burst series of observations was replaced by a series of four 10 V, 0.2 μs electric shocks, each separated by 2.5 ms, corresponding to the 400/second rate commonly used in efferent stimulation experiments. This excitation was applied to the COCB via a bipolar electrode run along the floor of the 4th ventrical. The acoustic stimulus tone was unchanged.

Efferent induced perturbations were observed in both the otoacoustic and CM responses to the stimulus tone, (see Figure 4). In both the perturbation extended beyond the duration of the electrical excitation but then decayed with a time constant of order 25-30 ms. In the acoustic data, where the response was not contaminated with an electrical artifact, it was possible to

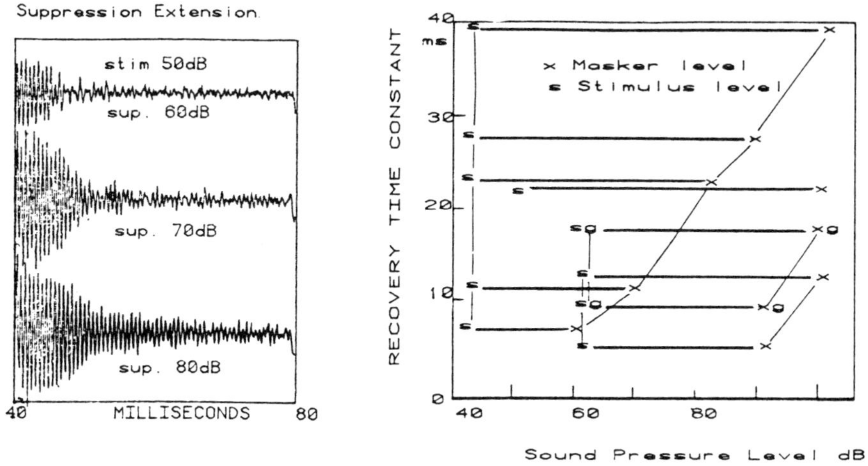

Figure 3. Left: A more detailed view of the post suppressor residual decay in a human ear. Data commences at suppressor termination. The initial bulge is the end of the latent direct suppression component. Right: A summary of oto-acoustic post masker residual decay time constants in a human and a guinea pig ear. Each horizontal line represents an average time constant measurement. It joins points marking the stimulus level (s) and the masker level (x). Points marked (g) denote guinea pig data. Note time constant increases with masker level (s fixed) and decreases with increasing stimulus level (x fixed).

determine the onset latency as about 10 ms. In both CM and acousic data, the rise continued for about 10 ms after the electrical excitation (4b,c,d)

The magnitude of the otoacoustic perturbation was 6 times smaller than the direct suppression residual caused by the 95 dB acoustic masker burst, but was of the **same** order of size as the post acoustic suppression tail effect. The decay time constant was of the order of 30 ms, somewhat longer than seen in the acoustically evoked perturbation.

A similar residual envelope was seen in the round window CM response (see Figure 4c). This was only 1.5 times smaller than the acoustically evokable direct CM suppression, and some 3 times larger than the post acoustic suppression tail. The CM was thus more strongly effected after the efferent stimulation than after the acoustic burst, whereas otoacoustic activity was similarly affected by both agents. The direct acoustic suppression residual was just 25% of the total CM.

Phase through the residual duration showed a steady change of about 20 degrees in the CM and OAE. The analysis also showed that the CM perturbation residual was an ENHANCEMENT, as already known from previous work. The acoustic perturbation was primarily due to a phase

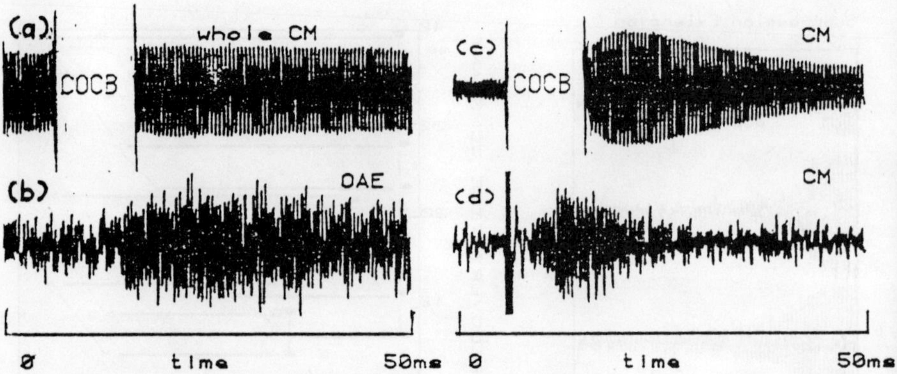

Figure 4. Efferent evoked perturbations. a) for reference is the raw CM signal. The duration of 4 shock COCB stimulation is marked. b) the otoacoustic perturbation caused (average of 512 sections) and c) the corresponding CM perturbation (average over 128, gain 8×a). Finally (d) shows the CM perturbation from one 5 V 0.1 ms shock/section, average of 128, gain 128×c). Data was high pass filtered at 600 Hz, 12 dB/oct.

change, not a suppression as in the acoustically induced effect. Thus despite similarities the efferent evoked perturbation was in a different sense to the acoustically evoked changes.

Since the intensity of the electrical excitation had initially been arbitarily set and as the longer time constants found were previously associated with with stronger disturbances we explored the effects of lower shock voltages and fewer shock impulses. With single shocks the efferent induced perturbation was reduced by a factor of 8. With reduced shock intensity the perturbation effect shortened as the decay time constant decreased (Fig. 4d). It was possible by selecting the degree of efferent stimulation to match several aspects of the acoustic and efferent induced perturbations but not all simultaneously.

Conclusions

Brief, moderate suppressor tone bursts lasting only tens of milliseconds can perturb cochlear mechanics for 20 and more milliseconds after their termination. We have demonstrated this in otoacoustic emissions suppression after effects which have an expontial decay with a time constant between 5 and 40 ms (20 ms GP). We have also shown that when brief electrical stimulation is applied to the efferent system at the COCB, a similar scale of effect can be produced.

The reduced mechanical response to sound following acoustic suppressor bursts points to a mechanical contribution to the forward masking phenomenon extending beyond cochlear filter ringing. Circumstantial evidence that efferent activity could be involved in otoacoustic forward suppression phenonmena is increased by this study because we have shown that the latency, time scale and decay contants of efferent evoked otoacoustic perturbations are generally compatable with such an involvement. The common time scale of the two different perturbation mechanisms examined here may relate to a basic property of outer hair cells.

Acknowledgements

This research was supported by the Hearing and Speech Trust. We also thank Prof Ian Russell for his help with the efferent stimulation technique.

References

Bonfils P, and Puel, J.L (**1987**). "Functional Properties of the crossed part of the medial olivo-cochlear bundle," Hearing Res. **28**, 125-130.

Guinan, J.J. (**1987**). "Effects of efferent neural activity on cochlear mechanics, " Scand.Audiol. Suppl. **25**, 53-61.

Johnstone, B.M., Patuzzi, R. and Yates, G.K. (**1986**). "Basilar membrane measurements and the travelling wave," Hearing Res. **22**, 147-154.

Kemp, D.T. and Souter, M. (**1988**). "A new rapid component in the cochlear response to brief electrical efferent stimulation." Hearing Res. (in press).

Comments

Wilson:

As you mention, the residual response can be due to true suppression or to a change of phase. If it is the latter, this could in turn be due to a change of tuning frequency as we describe in our own paper at this meeting.

Reply by Kemp:

With suppression in the same ear the residual appears to be mostly due to a reduction of amplitude whereas with COCB stimulation it appears to be mostly a phase change.

Power law features of acoustic distortion product emissions

P.F. Fahey[1] and J.B. Allen[2]

[1]*University of Scranton*
Scranton, PA 18510
[2]*AT&T Bell Laboratories*
Murray Hill, NJ 07974

Introduction

Acoustic intermodulation distortion products (DP's) that have their sources in the cochlea can be detected psychophysically; at the auditory nerve; and in the external auditory meatus. Wherever the distortion products are measured they have many distinctive features in common; so, it is assumed that the source of the psycophysically detected DP is the same as the source of the DP's that are physically detected at the auditory nerve and in the external auditory meatus. By impairing the function of the cochlea with drugs or anoxia, it can be shown that the source of the DP's is the nonlinear mechanical response of the cochlea (e.g., Kim, 1980 and Fahey and Allen, 1986). Indeed, a healthy cochlea has an intrinsically nonlinear component in its mechanical response.

Since some intermodulation DP's have frequencies below the input frequencies of the primary tones and some have frequencies above the input frequencies, DP's are a very useful tool in studying the nonlinear cochlear response. The most extensively studied DP has been the one at frequency, $f_D = 2f_1-f_2$. This DP is the most substantial DP and its dependence upon level has been the best characterized. Unfortunately, it has been mostly studied over a range of levels where it is near saturation. In this region the level dependence appears to be linear rather than cubic. That is, the behavior of this DP as a function of level does not seem to correlate with the first term that would produce it in the power series expansion of the nonlinearity. This has led to the notion that the cochlear mechanical nonlinearity is "essential" (Goldstein, 1967), i.e., not expandable in a power series (at least at certain levels.).

The data that we will present here will show that the nonlinearity that is the source of the DP's detected in the external auditory meatus is indeed describable by power law scaling over much of the region of level and frequency space where the DP's are generated. Hence, the nonlinearity of the cochlea should be an analytic function with a Taylor's series expansion in level.

Results

The data presented here is representative of the DP's detected in the external auditory meatus of about 20 adult cats. The animal preparation and the experimental setup have been described elsewhere (Fahey and Allen, 1986 and Allen, 1983). The DP's are generated in the cochlea, so it is useful to consider the cochlea as a Thevenin equivalent pressure source (with its associated Thevenin equivalent impedance) that drives a load impedance (namely the sound source impedance.). The results in this paper are presented as Thevenin equivalent source pressures rather than as raw ear canal pressures. The Thevenin equivalent source pressure can be thought of as a property of the cochlea (because the raw ear canal pressures have been normalized for the properties of the sound delivery system and the input impedance of the animal preparation.) In our particular experimental setup the specific acoustic impedance of the sound delivery system and the input impedance of the animal preparation are both approximatedly equal to the specific acoustic impedance of air over much of the frequency range; hence, the Thevenin equivalent source pressure is approximately equal to twice the ear canal pressure at the distortion product frequency.

All of the data presented here will be organized in the same way. So, after one understands the data and implications of the first figure; the data and the implications of the succeeding figures will be obvious. It has already been shown that level dependence of DP's measured when the frequencies of the primary tone inputs, f_1 and f_2, are held constant are very difficult to interpret because of nonmonotonic level dependence (due to interference effects, Zwicker, 1983). Therefore, to get truer feeling for the level dependence of DP's it is necessary to look at families of DP curves measured at different input levels (Fahey and Allen, 1986). The data here will consist of families of DP curves measured as f_1 is allowed to vary (consequently varying f_D) while holding f_2 constant. Each succeeding curve will be measured at a different level of input amplitude. In each figure either a_1, the amplitude of the tone at frequency f_1, or a_2, the amplitude of the tone at frequency f_2 will be the parameter that varies between adjacent curves. Also in each figure the level that is varying (either a_1 or a_2) will be decreasing in steps of 3 dB between adjacent curves. In each figure the starting levels of a_1 and a_2 will be at approximately 94 dB SPL (re 20 microPascal).

Each figure will consist of (a) the measured Thevenin equivalent pressure of the distortion product and (b) the Thevenin equivalent pressure normalized by either a_1 or a_2 raised to an appropriate power. The power to which either a_1 or a_2 is raised will be the power that a_1 or a_2 would have in a series expansion of the nonlinearity. This will mean that if the DP is describable with a power series expansion the curves that are distinct in part (a) of the figure will then overplot in part (b) of the figure.

The DP's that are presented here are at: $f_D=2f_1-f_2$, the amplitude of this DP should vary (at the lowest levels) as $a_1^2a_2$; $f_D=2f_2-f_1$, the amplitude of this DP should vary as $a_2^2a_1$; $f_D=3f_1-2f_2$, whose amplitude should vary as

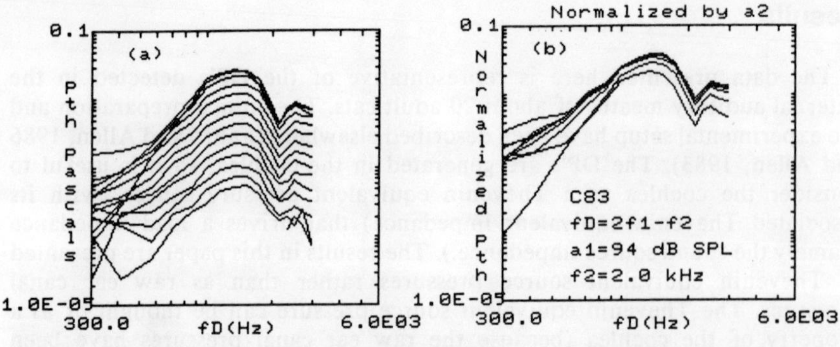

*Figure 1. (**a**) The DP at $f_D=2f_1-f_2$ is shown as a function of f_D. a_1 is held constant at 94 dB SPL and each successive curve is measured at a value of a_2 that is 3 dB lower than the previous curve. The beginning value of a_2 was 94 dB SPL. In panel (**b**) the data normalized by a_2 is plotted and it is obvious that the scaling is linear in a_2.*

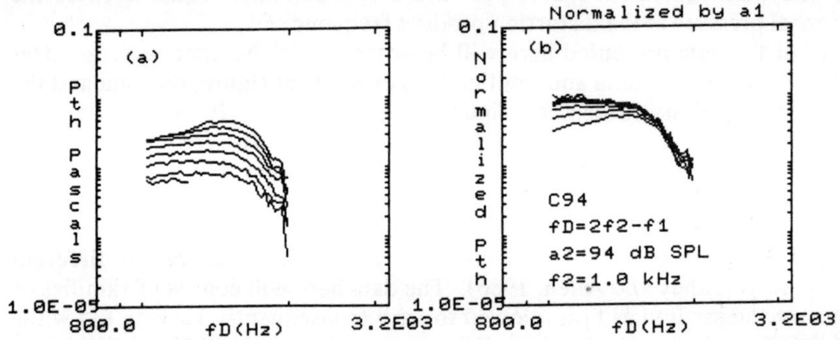

*Figure 2. (**a**) The DP at $f_D=2f_2-f_1$ is shown as a function of f_D. a_2 is constant and is at 94 dB SPL (re 20 microPascal). Each successive curve is at a 3 dB lower level of a_1. The five lowest curves in (**a**) are spaced at roughly 3 dB intervals in level. Hence, when the left panel curves are normalized by a_1 and replotted in (**b**) the right panel, the curves that were spaced 3 dB apart now plot on top of one another.*

$a_1^3a_2^2$; and $f_D=3f_2-2f_1$, whose amplitude should vary as $a_2^3a_1^2$. These scaling rules would be expected to hold best at low levels of the distortion product because as level increases more terms in the power series expansion become important and then the scaling no longer follows just the lead term. In fact, in every figure it is obvious that the scaling holds at just the lowest levels and at the higher levels the DP's begin to saturate.

In Fig. 1 (a) the level of the "lower cubic distortion product" whose frequency, f_D, is at $2f_1-f_2$ is plotted as a function of f_D. f_2 is held constant at 3-kHz and a_1 is constant at 94 dB SPL. In each succeeding curve a_2 is

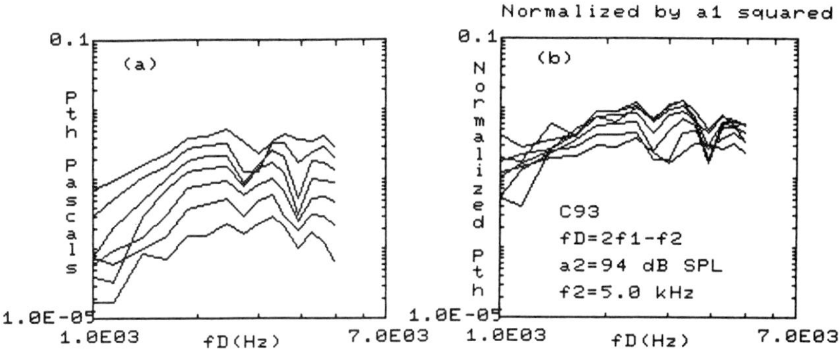

*Figure 3. (**a**) The DP at $f_D=2f_1-f_2$ is shown as a function of f_D. a_2 is held constant at 94 dB SPL while a_1 is varied in 3 dB steps. The data in (**a**) is rescaled by a_1^2 and replotted in (**b**). It is evident that the rescaling is effective for the lower four curves in (**a**).*

decreased by 3 dB from the preceding curve. It is apparent that the curves at lower level appear to be 3 dB apart and at the higher levels there seems to be a saturation in the level. If the curves in Fig. 1 (a) are normalized by a_2 (raised to the first power) and plotted in Fig. 1 (b) the curves in (a) that were 3 dB apart now plot on top of one another. This shows that the scaling followed a_2, as expected. The curves that were in the saturation region in Fig. 1 (a) obviously plot in (b) below the curves that scaled with a_2.

In Fig. 2 (a) the level of the "upper cubic distortion product", $f_D=2f_2-f_1$, is plotted as a function of f_D. f_2 is constant at 1 kHz. For this distortion product the frequency, f_D, is higher than both of the input pure tone frequencies. In Fig. 2 a_2 is held constant at 94 dB SPL and a_1 is decreased in 3 dB steps from one curve to the next. Note that lower curves in (a) are approximately 3 dB apart as would be expected from a power law nonlinearity. In (b) the curves in (a) are normalized by a_1 (raised to the first power.) Now the curves that in (a) were 3 dB apart in (b) overplot. The bottom 3 curves in (b) that do not overplot the others were in the region of saturation in (a).

In Fig. 3 (a) the DP at $f_D=2f_1-f_2$ is plotted as a function f_D with a_2 held constant at 94 dB and a_1 decreased in 3 dB steps. The data in (a) normalized by a_1^2 is replotted in (b). Here the scaling is good but certainly not as exact as in the first two figures. As the level in (a) becomes low the scaling becomes better.

In Fig. 4 (a) the DP at $f_D=2f_2-f_1$ is plotted as a function of f_D with f_2 held constant at 1 kHz and a_1 constant at 94 dB SPL. The data in (a) is normalized by a_2^2 and replotted in (b). Here the bottom four curves in (a) essentially overplot (the last curve in (a) was left out of (b) because its noisiness somewhat obscured the overplotted curves.) The scaling of the DP is as expected of a cubic term in the nonlinearity.

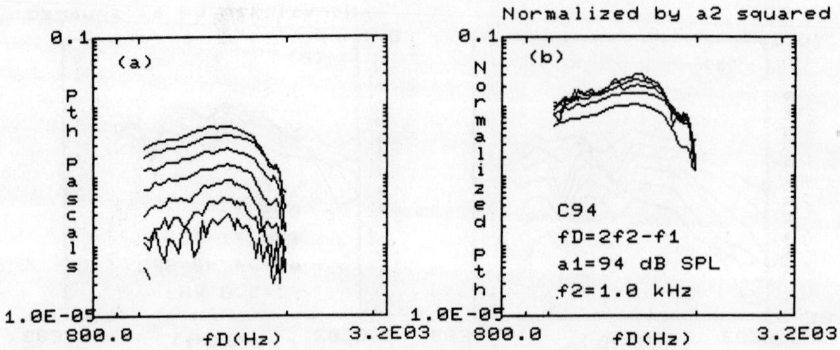

*Figure 4. (**a**) The DP at f_D=$2f_2$-f_1 is shown as a function of f_D. Now a_1 is constant at 94 dB SPL. In (**a**) the top curve is at a_2=94 dB SPL and each successive curve is at a value of a_2 that is 3 dB lower. The data in (**a**) is replotted in (**b**) after normalizing by a_2^2 (the lowest curves in (**a**) were not replotted to minimize the clutter).*

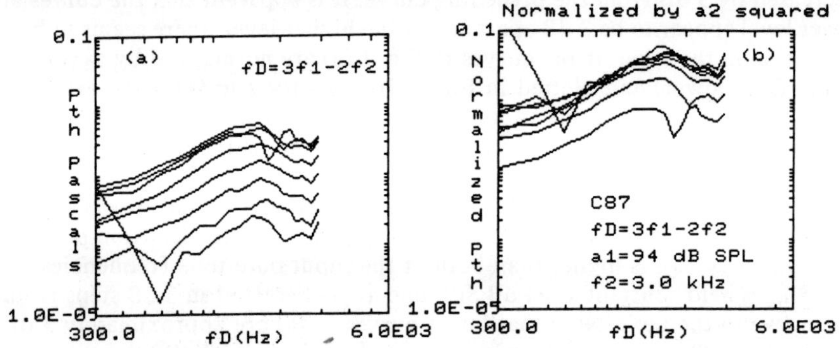

*Figure 5. (**a**) The DP at f_D=$3f_1$-$2f_2$ is plotted as a function of f_D. a_1 is constant at 94 dB SPL and a_2 is varied in 3 dB steps, starting at a_2=94 dB SPL. In (**b**) the data from (**a**) is replotted after normalizing by a_2^2 It is evident that the bottom four curves in (**a**) are overplotted in (**b**). Hence, when a_2 only is varied this distortion product (at low levels) scales as a_2^2.*

In the next four figures the distortion product is of fifth order rather than of third order as in the first four figures. In Fig. 5 f_D=$3f_1$-$2f_2$ and a_1 is held constant at 94 dB SPL and f_2 is constant at 2 kHz. The data in (a) is replotted in (b) after normalization by a_2^2. The lower curves in (a) overplot one another in (b), showing the expected power law scaling.

In Fig. 6 the DP at f_D=$3f_2$-$2f_1$ is plotted with a_2 held constant at 94 dB SPL and f_2 constant at 1 kHz. a_1 is decremented in 3 dB steps between adjacent curves. In (b) the data in (a) is replotted after normalization by a_1^2. The lower curves in (a) are approximately 6 dB apart so that in (b) these curves overplot.

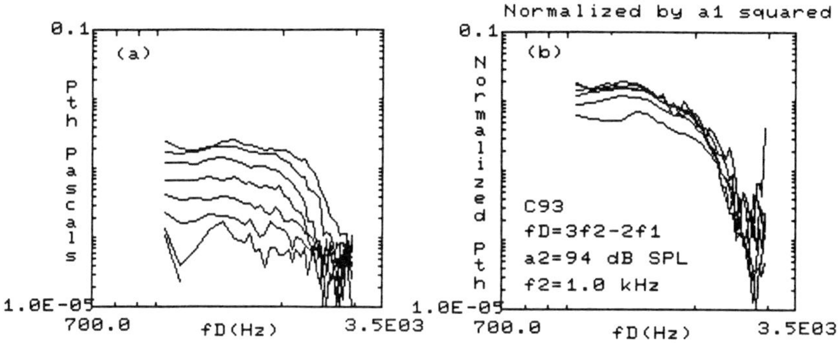

*Figure 6. (**a**) The DP at $f_D=3f_2-2f_1$ is shown as a function of f_D. Here a_2 is constant at 94 dB SPL. In (**a**) the top curve is at $a_1=94$ dB SPL and each successive curve is at a value of a_1 that is 3 dB lower than the previous curve. The data in (**a**) is replotted in (**b**) after normalizing by a_1^2. While the data above $f_D=2.5$ kHz is too noisy to be revealing, the data below $f_D=2.5$ kHz generally scales as a_1^2 except for the top two curves in (**a**) that are in the saturation.*

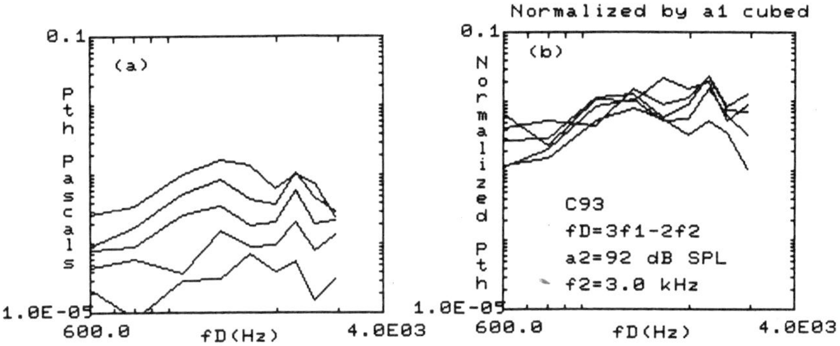

*Figure 7. (**a**) the DP at $f_D=3f_1-2f_2$ where a_1 is decreased in 3 dB steps is shown. The data in (**a**) is normalized by a_1^3 and replotted in (**b**). While the scaling is far from exact due to the bumpiness of the data, the normalization by a_1^3 is the best normalization available.*

The scaling is as expected from a fifth order nonlinearity.

In Fig. 7 the DP at $f_D=3f_1-2f_2$ is plotted with a_2 and f_2 held constant and a_1 varied in 3 dB steps. The data in (a) is normalized by a_1^3 and replotted in (b). The scaling of the distortion product as a_1^3 is good although not exact.

Finally in Fig. 8 this set of data is completed with a_2 varied in 3 dB steps as a_1 and f_2 are held constant and the DP at $f_D=3f_2-2f_1$ is plotted versus f_D. The data in (a) is normalized by a_2^3 and replotted in (b). The expected power law scaling does seem to hold for the last two curves.

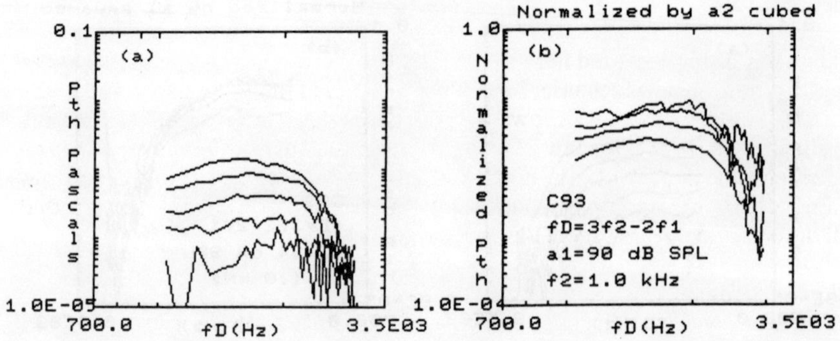

*Figure 8. (**a**) The DP at $f_D=3f_2-2f_1$ is plotted as a function of f_D. a_1 is constant at 90 dB SPL and a_2 is varied in 3 dB steps. The data of (**a**) is normalized by a_2^3 and replotted in (**b**). At the lowest levels of the distortion product it scales as a_2^3. Unfortunately, there is not enough data to show this scaling unambiguously.*

Discussion

The data presented here show that over certain ranges of level and frequency DP's show the level dependence that would be expected from a power law nonlinearity. Since the distortion products also show saturation as level increases, it is obvious that a series expansion of the nonlinearity would have to contain terms of several orders and that the higher order terms would cancel the lower order in the saturation region. Indeed higher order terms imply higher order intermodulation distortion products and these have been observed by us and by others.

The answer to the question of why did the early observations of the "lower cubic distortion product" ($f_D=2f_1-f_2$) show such unusual and distinctly "noncubic" level dependence is now apparent. The higher order terms in the nonlinearity, such as the fifth and the seventh, etc., also generate "cubic" distortion products and these DP's mix with the DP's from the cubic term. The higher the level of the input the more the higher order terms mix to determine the level of an individual DP. It is obvious from data presented here that the fifth order DP's are substantial and at high levels are certain to obscure the "cubic" behavior in the "cubic" distortion products. Missing from the data presented here are DP's measured where a_1 (=a) and a_2 (=a) are varied together and the data then normalized by a^3 for "cubic" DP's or a^5 for "quintic" DP's. Generally we have found that when both tones are decremented in 3 dB steps we very quickly runs out of dynamic range and consequently we will be doing these measurements with smaller (about 1 dB) level decrements in order to test the scaling under these conditions.

Conclusion

Data has been presented here to show that it is reasonable to assume that the cochlear nonlinear mechanical response (detected noninvasively from the external auditory meatus) shows a level dependence that suggests that the nonlinearity has a power law (Taylor's series) expansion. The determination of the nonlinear part of the input-output function of the cochlea will put strong constraints upon the structure of the partial differential equation that will describe cochlear response to mechanical input.

Acknowledgement

This work was partially supported by an NIH AREA research grant to PFF.

References

Allen, J.B. (**1983**). "Magnitude and Phase Frequency Response to Single Tones in the Auditory Nerve," J.Acoust.Soc.Am. **73**, 2071-2092.

Fahey, P.F. and Allen, J.B. (**1986**). "Characterization of Cubic Intermodulation Distortion Products in the Cat External Auditory Meatus," In *Peripheral Auditory Mechanisms*, eds. J.B. Allen, J.L. Hall, A. Hubbard, S.T. Neely, and A. Tubis (Springer-Verlag, Berlin).

Goldstein, J.L. (**1967**). "Auditory Nonlinearity," J.Acoust.Soc.Am. **41**, 676-689.

Kim, D.O. (**1980**). "Cochlear Mechanics: Implications of Electrophysiological and Acoustical Observations," Hearing Res. **2**, 297-317.

Zwicker, E. (**1983**). "Level and phase of the ($2f_1$-f_2)-cancellation tone expressed in vector diagrams," J.Acoust.Soc.Am. **74**, 63-66.

Comments

Duifhuis:

Since the auditory nonlinearity is of the compressive type, the Taylor series expansion provides an inefficient approximation. All its nonlinear terms are expansive, and behave in several aspects quite differently from compressive terms. The historical terms "cubic" and "quintic" DP are misleading.

I maintain that a single compressive power-law nonlinearity provides a biophysically more realistic approximation. Note that an 'exact' fit of any function over a finite range is possible by the sequence $\Sigma a_i x^{\nu_i}$, where $0 < \nu_1 < \nu_2 < ... < K$, with K any positive number (this goes back to Bernstein, 1922). Taylor's expansion is the special case with ν being integers and K approaching infinity. Setting K to 1 shows that an approximation with compressive terms is mathematically equally appropriate. Interestingly, the prediction for the amplitude behavior of low-order distortion products turns out to be completely independent of the power of the nonlinearity for the amplitude ranges covered above. However, for the non-tested complementary ranges the predictions are clearly different, as indicated in Table C1. Thus, I disagree with the first sentence of your conclusion.

Table C1. Predictions of amplitudes of the lowest odd-order combination tones in the Taylor expansion and in a one term Bernstein approximation.

	$a_1 < a_2$			$a_1 > a_2$		
component	Taylor	Bernstein	test	Taylor	Bernstein	test
$2f_1-f_2$	$a_1^2a_2$	$a_1^2a_2^{\nu-2}$	a_1^2 Fig.3	$a_1^2a_2$	$a_1^{\nu-1}a_2$	a_2 Fig.1
$2f_2-f_1$	$a_1a_2^2$	$a_1a_2^{\nu-1}$	a_1 Fig.2	$a_1a_2^2$	$a_1^{\nu-2}a_2^2$	a_2^2 Fig.4
$3f_1-2f_2$	$a_1^3a_2^2$	$a_1^3a_2^{\nu-3}$		$a_1^3a_2^2$	$a_1^{\nu-2}a_2^2$	a_2^2 Fig.5
$3f_2-2f_1$	$a_1^2a_2^3$	$a_1^2a_2^{\nu-2}$	a_1^2 Fig.6	$a_1^2a_2^3$	$a_1^{\nu-3}a_2^3$	

Bernstein, S.N. (1922). "Sur l'ordre de la meilleure approximation des fonctions continues par des polynomes," Académie Royale de Belgique, Classe des Sciences, Mémoires, Deuxième Série, Tome IV, 1-103.

Reply by Fahey:

We feel that your point is well taken that not all expansions of a function are equally efficient approximations. At higher levels for a saturating nonlinearity the Taylor series requires many terms to match the data and it is difficult to calculate. Your suggestion that the Bernstein expansion is more efficient is probably true at higher levels, although several terms are required to match the data. At lower levels the Bernstein expansion has a very steeply rising slope that becomes infinite at zero input. It is at low levels the Taylor series expansion about zero requires the fewest terms and is the superior expansion (unless the nonlinearity really does have infinite slope at zero).

A major advantage that a Taylor series has over any other power series is that its output is more intuitive when the inputs are sinusoidal. Most of us know that, using trigonometric identities, a term like (sin $y)^N$ produces an N-th harmonic, the (N-2)-th harmonic, etc., and that the relative levels of these

harmonics are given by the amplitudes of the Taylor series. To calculate the relative levels of the harmonics output from the Bernstein series is a very involved calculation as you have already shown.

Now referring to the table in your comment, it is obvious that the one term Taylor series and the one term Bernstein make the same prediction to the data in the paper. Hence the data presented in our paper do not give us a basis for distinguishing the two. But cat ear canal data taken under the conditions where a1>a2 and also a2>a1 but where both a1 and a2 are varied together show that the one term Bernstein approximation (that the DP varies as a^ν, where $\nu<1$) is completely inadequate. The one term Taylors series is also inadequate over much of the data range but it does work at the very lowest levels (Weiderhold *et al.*, 1986). It should be noted that both the two term and the three term Taylor series are consistent with the table C1 in the comment as long the one primary level is much greater than the other.

Zwicker:

There has been agreement so far that the nonlinearity in $(2f_1-2f_2)$-difference tones can *not* be described by a regular simple power law. Goldstein's (1967) and Helle's (1969) data have shown this effect as clearly as my own data (Zwicker, 1955). Most convincing to me is still the content of Fig. 11 of the last mentioned paper which is reproduced here together with data created 19 years later (Zwicker and Fastl, 1973) and data produced 10 years later as well as 10 days ago. Corresponding to a regular cubic power law, the data should follow the dashed lines. This may be the case only for very low levels, while the slope of the data points and the slope of the dashed lines diverge as much as a factor 10. Although the absolute values of the cancellation level may diminish with age, the slope as a function of primary levels remains the same.

"The answer to the question of why did the early observation of the lower cubic distortion product ($f_D = 2f_1-f_2$) show such unusual and distinctly noncubic level dependence is" that the earlier researchers measured in a larger level range than Fahey and Allen. Any irregular nonlinearity like a symmetrical dislocation of a straight line around the origin produces $(2f_1-f_2)$-distortion products which follow a regular cubic power law as long as only one of the primaries is changed in level regions smaller than the level of the other primary. Nonlinear input-output functions which are irregular around the origin are linearized by large inputs of one primary. Most of the data discussed by Fahey and Allen belong to such conditions. The other data are ignored. Therefore, the conclusion "that the nonlinearity has a power law (Taylor's series) expansion" can not be accepted until data with levels L_1 = const and L_1 - 20 dB $\leq L_2 \leq L_1$ + 20 dB and vice versa are available. The data given so far indicate the contrary.

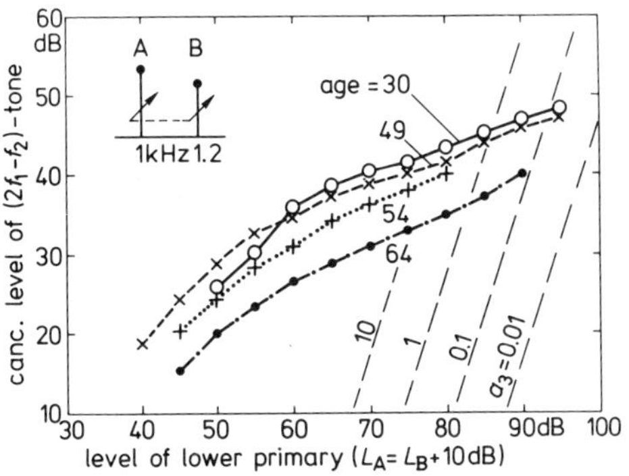

Figure C1. Level of the $(2f_1-f_2)$-difference tone, needed to cancel the audible difference tone, as a function of the level of the lower primary which is 10-dB larger than the upper primary. Four sets of data for different age of the subject (the author) are given. The dashed lines indicate the dependencies assuming a cubic power law.

Helle, R. (1969). "Amplitude and Phase des in Gehör gebildeten Differentztones dritter Ordnung", Acustica 22, 74-87.

Zwicker, E. (1955). "Der ungewöhnliche Amplitudengang der nichtlinearen Verzerrungen des Ohres", Acustica 5, 67-74.

Zwicker, E. and Fastl, H. (1973). "Cubic difference sounds measured by threshold- and compensation-method", Acustica 29, 336-343.

Reply by Fahey:

The data in our paper make it obvious that we certainly do not believe that the $2f_1$-f_2 DP is explainable by only a cubic term of a power series, nor do we make such a claim. Indeed, half of the data presented is of a fifth order intermodulation DP. A point that we should have emphasized is that the $2f_1$-f_2 DP and the $2f_2$-f_1 DP (both called cubic DP's) are produced by all of the odd order terms (above the linear term) in a Taylor series expansion of the nonlinearity. For a saturating nonlinearity the DP's from these terms have phases that produce cancellations. To explain the data in the figure in Zwicker's comment (and also the cat ear canal data acquired by ourselves and others (see references in the paper) one must sum many terms in a Taylor's expansion. This is not an easy task, but a scheme to organize the sumation is detailed in Weiner and Spina (1980).

Let us also clear up a common misunderstanding. Nonlinear input-output functions which are irregular, are not linearized by large input from one primary. Indeed, Figs. 3 through 8 show very marked nonlinear behavior even though one of the primaries is larger than the other over much of the range of the primary that is changing.

We think that it is important to note that the following equivalent of a power law expansion of a nonlinear input-output function is a very common laboratory procedure. Drive the nonlinearity with a pure sine wave. Now express the output in a Fourier series. You have just done the equivalent of a power series expansion of the input-output function if you rewrite the harmonics in the output spectrum in terms of powers of the fundamental and collect the coefficients multiplying the same power.

Finally, we wish to make this very important point. We know of no data on distortion products (either animal or psycophysical) that requires the invocation of an essential nonlinearity into the cochlear response.

Weiderhold, M.L., Mahoney, J.W., and Kellogg, D.L. (1986). "Acoustic Overstimulation Reduces $2f_1$-f_2 Cochlear Emissions at All Levels in Cat," In: Peripheral Auditory Mechanisms, eds. J.B. Allen, J.L. Hall, A. Hubbard, S.T. Neely, and A. Tubis (Springer-Verlag, Berlin).

Weiner, D.D., and Spina, J.F. (1980). Sinusoidal Analysis and Modeling of Weakly Nonlinear Circuits. (Van Nostrand Reinhold Company, New York).

Schroeder:

The conclusion in this paper, as I (and others) read it, is - to put it bluntly - wrong. Even nonanalytic functions, such as infinite clippers exhibit the observed amplitude dependence, as I have shown in an earlier paper (Schroeder, 1975). In fact, the shoe is on the other foot: namely to find mathematical functions that do *not* have the observed amplitude dependence - there may not be any, in which case the authors' conclusion is void of content.

Schroeder, M.R. (1975). "Amplitude behavior of the cubic difference tone". J. Acoust. Soc. Am. 58, 728-732.

Reply by Fahey (shortened by editor):

It should be recognized that some of the discussion is moot for we all agree that the nonlinearity in question is instantaneous, monotonic, saturating and has no infinities and discontinuities.

Binaural processing without neural delays

Shihab Shamma, Naiming Shen[a], and Preetham Gopalaswamy[a]

Electrical Engineering Department[a], Systems Research Center, & the University of Maryland Institute for Advanced Computer Studies, University of Maryland College Park, MD 20742
Mathematical Research Branch, National Institute of Diabetes Digestive and Kidney Diseases, National Institutes of Health Bethesda, MD 20982

Introduction

In binaural sound processing, the central auditory system compares the signals impinging on the two ears, detecting and utilizing various imbalances (e.g. sound level, time of arrival, and phase) to perform such perceptual tasks as sound localization in space and signal-to-noise enhancement. In this sense, binaural hearing is analogous to binocular vision in endowing perception with an extra spatial dimension based primarily on disparity measures in the stimulus projection upon the sensory organs. Numerous computational and phenomenological models have been proposed to account for and elucidate the available experimental psychoacoustical and neurophysiological data (see Blauert, 1983; Colburn and Durlach, 1978).

Correlation-based models have been successful in accounting for the widest range of binaural phenomena, and in providing a theoretical framework for investigating the physiological bases and neural networks that can perform these functions. The primary computational structure in all these models is the array of coincidence detectors which effectively compute a running cross-correlation measure of the cochlear outputs from corresponding or *equal* characteristic frequency (CF) locations on the two ears. Combining such functions from all output pairs at other CFs, a two-dimensional cross-correlation image results in which one axis represents the CFs of the cochlear outputs, and the other represents different lags or delays. Details of these output patterns would then reflect the sound spectral and lateralization information along its two axes (Colburn and Durlach, 1978).

In searching for the neural substrate of the correlation algorithms, the most common assumption has been to associate the various lags required in the above computations with *neural* delays (Jeffress, 1948), e.g. neuronal pathways of differing lengths or latency effects. Fig.1a illustrates a typical network based on these principles.

The success of such correlation-based models in accounting for many experimental findings, and the convenience of their mathematical formulations, have indirectly lent support to, and acceptance of the notion of

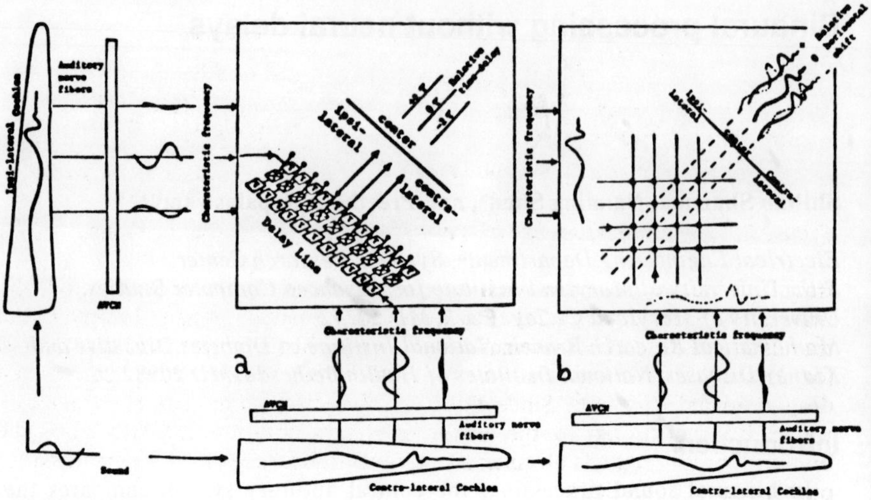

Figure 1. Schematics of the (a) Jeffress model and (b) the stereausis network.

organized neural delay lines despite the lack of firm physiological evidence of their existence.

The stereausis network

There is at present little evidence in support of any particular neural network to implement the correlation models. Thus, in advocating a specific network, one may at best show that the relevant physiological, anatomical, and physiological data are consistent with various aspects of the model, and that the fundamental organizational principles of the auditory system are observed. These include the tonotopic order of the auditory pathways, and the utilization of the fine temporal structure of the auditory-nerve responses, which is preserved by the *Bushy cells* of the AVCN, by the cells of the NTB, and by the inputs of the SOC nuclei.

The *stereausis* network[1] proposed here (Fig.1b) satisfies the above criterea, and takes a fundamentally different approach to the computation of inter-aural-time-differences. Instead of comparing the cochlear outputs of one ear with the *delayed* versions from the other ear (e.g. the Jeffress model, Fig.1a), the network here detects and encodes the *spatial* disparities between the *simultaneous* travelling waves at the two ears (Figs.2). For example, a low frequency tone produces in each cochlea a spatially distributed travelling wave which is projected relatively intact onto the responses of the spatially ordered array of auditory-nerve-fibers. At any instant in time, the central binaural processor receives two spatial *images* (or snap-shots) of the

1. Because of the fundamental similarity that emerges between the binaural network proposed here and the type of computations used for stere-op-sis in vision, we shall refer to it as the stere-au-sis network.

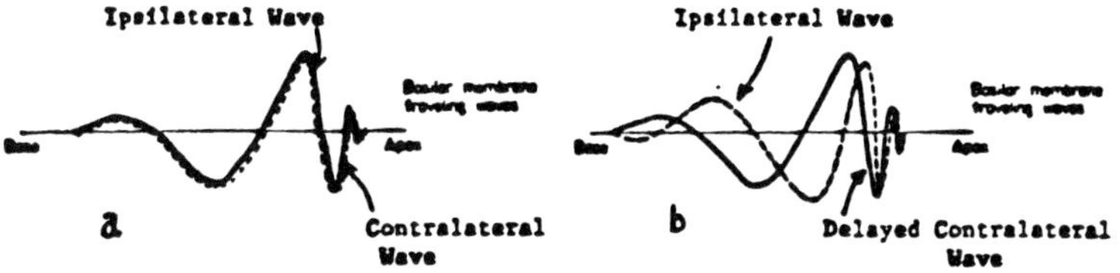

Figure 2. Travelling waves of (a) a centered and (b) a lateralized tone.

travelling waves, one from each ear (Figs.2). When the tone is centered, the images are identical (Fig.2a); For binaurally unequal signals, however, the travelling waves differ systematically. Thus, when the tone is phase-shifted (or delayed) in one ear relative to the other, the images appear correspondingly shifted (Fig.2b)[2]. Since this *spatial* disparity between the travelling waves is proportional to the *temporal* delays between the two ears, the binaural processing of all interaural-time-differences can be reduced to purely spatial operations.

Therefore, to measure the horizontal disparity between the simultaneous binaural patterns of Figs.2, the network of "coincidence" detectors in Fig.1b would compare, at various relative horizontal shifts, the instantaneous images from the two ears. Along the center diagonal of the network, the images are registered (i.e. the inputs are of equal CFs). Along the other diagonals, the images are compared at progressively larger relative horizontal shifts. Consequently, for a centered tone (Fig.2a), the location of the best match occurs along the center diagonal; for a lateralized tone (Fig.2b) the match is maximal off the diagonal.

A different, but entirely equivalent view of the network operation emerges if we observe that the "coincidence" detectors off the major diagonal systematically correlate the responses from fibers of *unequal* CFs. The significance of this arrangement for the cross-correlation computations is that, because of the finite velocity of the travelling waves, delayed versions of the responses at a given CF can be obtained from off-CF fibers in the local neighborhood of the CF, and not necessarily through further neuronal delays (Pfeifer and Kim, 1975; Shamma, 1985b). In essence, the basilar membrane acts as the needed delay line. This possibility seems to have been first proposed by (Schroeder, 1977).

The network of Fig.1b was simulated using a two-dimensional array of operators, each generating a measure of comparison ($c_{ij} = C(x_i,y_j)$) between its inputs. Equivalent results are obtained for $c_{ij} = x_i + y_j$, $c_{ij} = x_i y_j$, or $c_{ij} = g(x_i - y_j)$ where $g(x) = max(x,0)$. The inputs to the binaural network are the spatiotemporal response patterns of the auditory-nerve (Shamma, 1985b), computed using a detailed biophysical model of the basilar membrane and of hair cell function (Shamma *et al.*, 1986). The output patterns of the network

2. Note that the relative shifts are in the fine structure of the travelling waves, and not in the envelopes which remain stationary since their horizontal displacement depends only on the frequency of the tone.

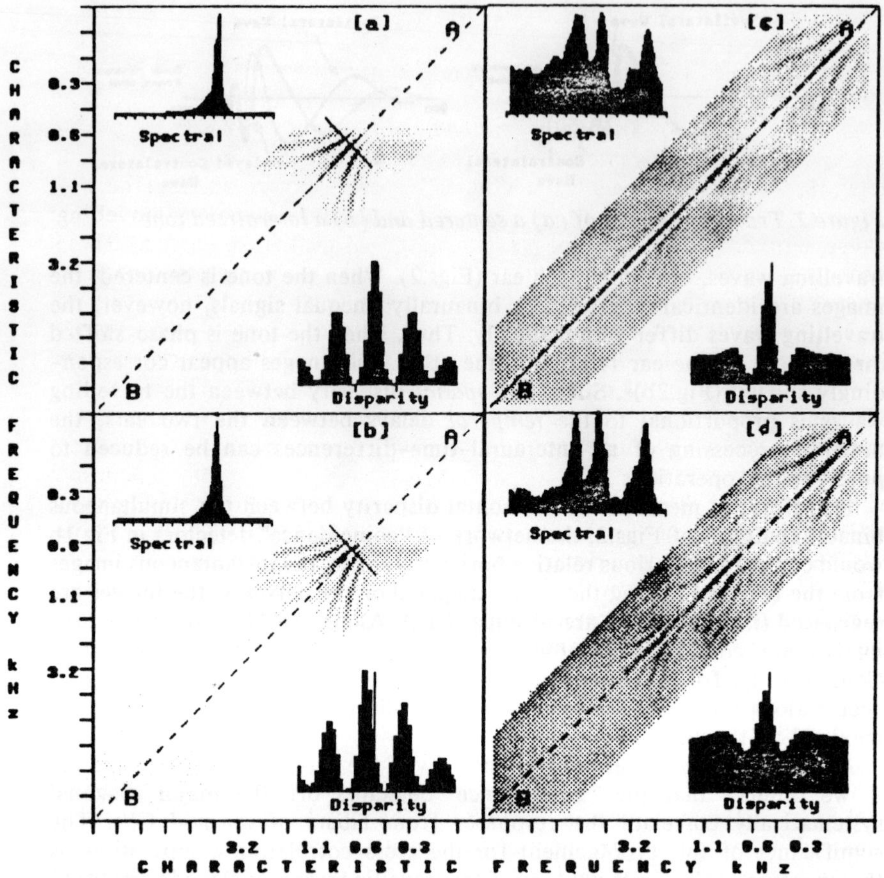

Figure 3. Outputs of the stereausis network for (a,b) a single tone and (c,d) noisy speech vowel [a]. The spectral plot is activity along the major diagonal of the network. The disparity plot is the activity of the network along the orthogonal axis to AB.

are further processed by a 2-dimensional lateral inhibitory network (Shamma, Shen and Gapalaswamy, 1987) in order to sharpen the peaks and edges of the response. The output is then integrated over a short time interval (e.g. 5 ms) so as to enhance further the final displays. As we shall illustrate below, the location of the pattern peaks in the plane of the network, and the sharpness of its profiles, can be directly related to such psychophysical attributes as the lateralization of the sound source, its frequency, and the degree of its compactness in space.

Examples of the network operation

Two examples of the network operation are discussed here: The lateralization of a low frequency tone, and the enhancement of speech signals in noise background. For a spatially centered low frequency tone, the travelling waves are maximally matched along the major diagonal of the binaural network, where consequently a dominant peak in the response occurs. However, because of the multiple peaks within the envelope of the travelling waves, secondary correlation peaks also appear off the major diagonal. These responses exhibit two features related to the amplitude and phase characteristics of the cochlear filters: (1) The output activity is concentrated around the CF location specific to the tone (CF = 600 Hz in this case). Varying the frequency of the tone would cause the output to move along the *spectral axis* of the network, i.e. along or parallel to the center diagonal. (2) The secondary maxima of the network outputs appear to converge towards the primary maximum. This is due to the rapidly increasing slope of the phase function of the travelling wave, and the accompanying decrease of the spatial separation of its peaks, near the point of resonance. When the tone is binaurally delayed ($\pi/3$ interaural-phase-shift), the response pattern shifts accordingly, and the relative height of the primary to secondary peaks decreases gradually (Figs.3b). At π shift, the two peaks are equal and on either side of the midline. With further shifts, the previously secondary image moves further towards the center, becoming the dominant peak. The periodic behavior of these patterns and the appearance of multiple confusing images at π phase-shifts correspond closely to the lateralization of continuous low frequency tones performed by human and animal subjects (Durlach and Colburn, 1978; Sayers, 1964).

The outputs due to a noisy speech stimulus (vowel [a] in 0.1-10 kHz noise; S/N $\approx$ -6 dB) are shown in Figs.3c-d. When both signal and noise are centered, all responses are maximally correlated along the diagonal, and hence the speech spectrum is contaminated (Fig.3c). When the noise is interaurally delayed or reversed, its maximal correlation peaks move off the diagonal leaving behind the peaks due to the speech signal alone (Fig.3d).

The stereausis network can account for a variety of other stimulus conditions and percepts, e.g. detection of interaural-level-differences, time-level trading, and lateralization utilizing onset cues and envelope modulations of high frequency sounds (Shamma, Shen and Gapalaswamy, 1987).

Physiological considerations

The *stereausis* network is essentially a correlation-based model, and hence much of the neurophysiological evidence available in support of such central mechanisms is consistent with its operation (Sullivan and Konishi, 1986; Yin and Kuwada, 1984). However, unlike the strict alignment of the inputs' CF in the Jeffress model, the stereausis network exhibits a certain amount of CF-overlap reflecting the balance between basilar membrane originated delays, and the inevitable delays, imbalances, and inaccuracies that are inherent in real neuronal transmission. Experience during development would presumably achieve the fine tuning of the final map.

The *stereausis* network is closely related to the computational algorithms proposed to account for stereopsis in vision, e.g. (Marr and Poggio, 1979). Together with the Lateral Inhibitory Network (LIN) proposed earlier for monaural spectral estimation (Shamma, 1985a), these results point to the essential similarity between early vision and auditory processing, and to the role of the cochlea in transforming the uni-dimensional sound signal into the spatial response features that the CNS can realistically detect and process.

Acknowledgments:
This work is partially supported by an NSF initiation award.

References

Blauert, J. (**1983**). *Spatial Hearing* (MIT Press, Cambridge, MA).

Colburn, S. and Durlach, N.I. (**1978**). "Models of binaural interactions," in: *Handbook of Perception, IV*, edited by E.C.Carterette and M.P.Friedman (x,y), pp. z-z.

Durlach, N.I. and Colburn, S. (**1978**). "Binaural phenomena," in: *Handbook of Perception, IV*, edited by E.C.Carterette and M.P.Friedman (x,y), pp. 365-466.

Jeffress, L. (**1948**). "A place theory of sound localization," J.Comp.Physiol. Psych. **61**, 468-486.

Marr, D. and Poggio, T. (**1979**). "A computational theory of human stereo vision," Proc.R.Soc.Lond. **204**, 301-328.

Pfeifer, R.R. and Kim, D.O. (**1975**). "Cochlear nerve fiber responses: Distribution along the cochlear partition," J.Acoust.Soc.Am. **58**, 867-869.

Sayers, B. (**1964**). "Acoustic-image lateralization judgement with binaural tones," J.Acoust.Soc.Am. **36**, 923-926.

Schroeder, M.R. (**1977**). "New Viewpoints in binaural interactions," in: *Psychophysics and Physiology of Hearing*, edited by E.F.Evans and J.P. Wilson (Acadamic Press), pp. 455-467.

Shamma, S., Shen, N. and Gapalaswamy, P. (**1987**). *Stereausis: Binaural processing without neural delays.* Systems Research Center Tech.Rep.(SRC TR 87-165), University of Maryland, College Park.

Shamma, S.A. (**1985**). "Speech processing in the auditory system.II: Lateral inhibition and the processing of speech evoked activity in the auditory-nerve," J.Acoust.Soc.Am. **78**, 1622-1632.

Shamma, S.A. (**1985**). "Speech processing in the auditory system.I: Representation of speech sounds in the responses of the auditory-nerve," J.Acoust.Soc.Am. **78**, 1612-1621.

Shamma, S.A., Chadwick, R., Wilbur, J., Rinzel, J.and Moorish, K. (**1986**). "A biophysical model of cochlear processing: intensity dependence of pure tone responses," J.Acoust.Soc.Am. **80**, 133-145.

Sullivan, W. and Konishi, M. (**1986**). "Neural map of interaural phase difference in the owl's brainstem," Proc Nat.Acad.Sci. **83**, 8400-8404.
Yin, T. and Kuwada, S. (**1984**). "Neuronal mechanisms of binaural interactions," in: *Dynamic aspects of neocortical function*, edited by G.Edelman, W.Gall and W.Cowan (A Neurosciences Institute Publication; Wiley, New York), pp. 263-314.

Comments

Henning:

Models for localisation based on interaural correlation of signals at the ears have certain difficulties whatever the mechanism by which the cross-correlation is carried out. For example the figure below shows two sets of stimuli for the left and right ears that have identical cross-correlations but which lead to very different lateralisation performance as Gaskell (1983) has pointed out.

The stimuli consist of pairs of clicks; in the top row there is an interauaral delay, Δt, in the first arriving pair and a simultaneous pair arrive after a larger delay, D. For a sufficiently large Δt, the stimulus is heard as coming from the left. The resulting cross-correlation, r(τ) is shown on the second row.

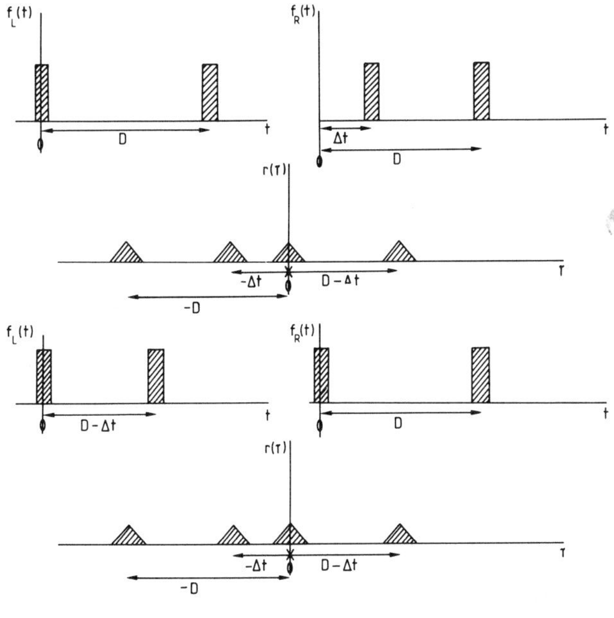

Figure C1.

However, a stimulus with the same cross-correlation (3rd row) is heard in the centre of the head.

These psychophysical observations can be made with durations, D, ranging from 1 to 2 ms down to 100 μs or so. Since they would give rise to identical output from the (presumably relatively peripheral) device you propose, it seems unlikely that processing subsequent to your device could recover the difference observers clearly hear.

Gaskell, H. (1983) "The precedence effect," Hearing Res. 13, 277-303.

Schroeder:

I am delighted to see my old ideas (Schroeder, 1977) resurrected by the present authors. At the Keele symposium I was rash enough to suggest that the basilair membrane, very naturally, furnishes some of the differential delay necessary in binaural processing. Now is an excellent time to reexamine this proposal in view of our refined understanding of basilar membrane mechanics, including particularly, active processes.

Hafter:

In your talk you said that one advantage of your model is that it does not require a neural delay line with micro-second accuracy in its transmission characteristics. I don't see how placement of the delay line in the travelling wave reduces the demands for such accuracy in the paths from cochlea to binaural comparison.

One aspect of your model that I find especially appealing is that it suggests a direct test. For cells sensitive to large interaural differences of time, there must be a correlated and measurable difference between the characteristic frequencies of the inputs from the two ears.

Rate coding predictions for frequency and amplitude JND's of simple tones in the presence of noise

Adoram Erell

Department of Electronic Systems, Faculty of Engineering
Tel Aviv University, Ramat Aviv 69978, Israel.

Introduction

Detection and discrimination of simple tones in the presence of noise present a challenge to the rate (or place) theory. Recent physiological studies indicate that rate suppression and the distribution of thresholds within the fiber population allow the rate model to account for psychophysical critical ratios (Young and Barta, 1986) and intensity JND of broad band noise (Delgutte, 1986). The present study was undertaken to examine the ability of the rate theory to account for frequency discrimination in noise. The rate coding predictions are derived using a neural-counting detection model, incorporating the distribution of fiber thresholds and rate suppression. The effect of signal variability, which has been assumed in previous studies to be negligible (Siebert, 1968, Miller *et al.*, 1987), is also evaluated. The model predictions are then compared to published psychophysical data.

Model

The model for the neural rate response is outlined in Fig.1. The cochlear filters are linear and follow the standard triangular frequency response on a log-log scale (Siebert, 1968; Srulovicz and Goldstein, 1983). The filter slopes were determined from data on cats obtained by Goldstein *et al.* (1971).The cochlear to neural transduction is modelled by a memoryless nonlinearity. Following Delgutte (1986), the fiber population is assumed to be divided into four uniform groups, differing by their thresholds, spontaneous rates and

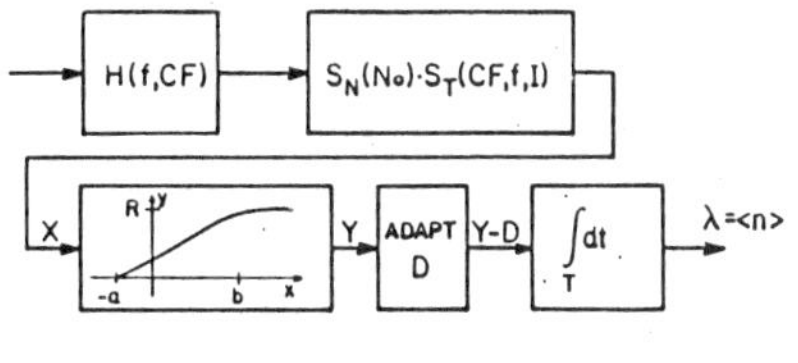

Figure 1. A single fiber model, composed of a linear filter, attenuation due to suppression, memoryless non-linearity, rate decrement due to adaptation and time integration. λ represents the average spike count in the interval T.

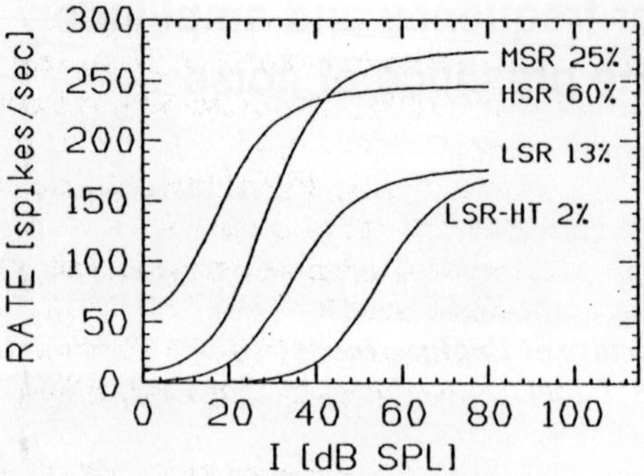

Figure 2. Simulated tone-evoked rate intensity functions for the four fiber types: high, medium and low spontaneous rate fibers, and a low spontaneous rate, high threshold fiber. Their assumed percentages in the population are also denoted.

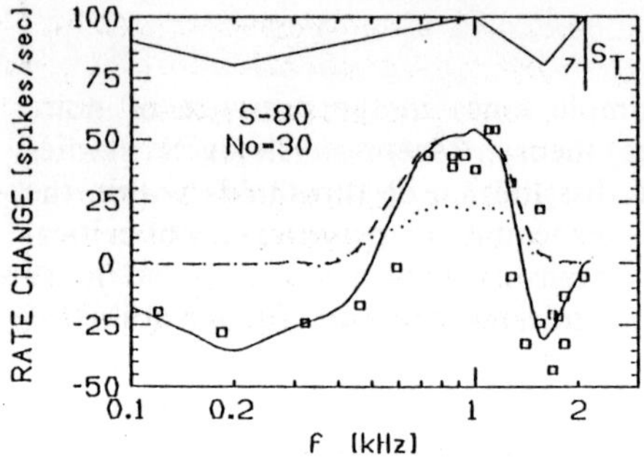

Figure 3. The response of a 1 kHz, LSR fiber as a function of tone frequency. The dotted line is the response in the absence of suppression. The dashed line is with S_N=10 dB. The open squares represent transformed (from 2.9 kHz to 1 kHz) data from Rhode et al. (1978). The solid line was obtained by adjusting the ad hoc attenuation function, S_T (shown at the top), to fit the data.

saturation properties. These characteristics are determined by the transduction function, which was chosen so that the simulated rate-intensity functions, shown in Fig.2, would fit the corresponding data from Delgutte (1986). Noise rate suppression is introduced by two independent factors. S_N is a CF independent attenuation which represents a suppression due to the noise frequency components lying within the suppression areas. It was determined by fitting data from Costalupes *et al.* (1984) on the ratio of maximum tone-evoked rate-increments in the presence of noise to their values in quiet. A second attenuation factor, S_T, represents suppression of noise due to a tone within the suppression area, and was determined by fitting relevant data from Rhode *et al.* (1978), as shown in Fig.3. Long term adaptation due to the continuous background noise is represented by a constant decrement D, also determined from the data of Costalupes *et al.* (1984). The resulting model rate profiles fit data from Costalupes (1985) on tone-evoked rate increments in the presence of noise.

Neural noise and signal variability are introduced as follows. With respect to the stochastic nature of the neural response it is assumed here that the spike counts are independent Gaussian random variables whose variance follows a phenomenological function, adopted from Delgutte (1986). Signal variability was evaluated using simulation. The model output for a given signal is a sequence of λ_i as a function of CF_i, where λ_i represents the average spike count in the i-th fiber. In the presence of noise, different noise samples produce somewhat different rate profiles. The variance of a given fiber response, λ_i, about the mean (where the average is over many, statistically independent, noise samples) may be defined as the contribution of the signal variability to the overall statistical fluctuations of the fiber response. This part of the variability is correlated between fibers, as long as their respective frequency responses are overlapping. The standard deviation of a single fiber response due to the signal variability was evaluated for a 100 ms signal, and the resulting value was about an order of magnitude smaller than the standard deviation due to the neural noise.

A hypothetical central processor estimates the tone frequency (or amplitude) from the noisy rate profiles. It is assumed that the processor performs via template matching, where the template follows the mean tone-evoked rate increment profile and the matching is achieved by minimizing a χ^2 function. The reasoning behind this assumption is that, in the absence of signal variability, this processor is almost equivalent to a maximum likelihood estimator. The effect of the neural noise on the performance was thus evaluated using a Cramer-Rao' limit, similar to Siebert's (1968) method. The effect of signal variability on the performance was estimated by actual template matchings to a number of simulated rate profiles, each one corresponding to a different, statistically independent, noisy signal. The central processor was assumed to combine the estimates from the four fiber groups using a rule which is optimal with respect to the neural noise. Following Siebert (1968), the overall standard deviation, σ_f (or σ_A), is directly compared to the JND in a 2I2AFC experiment.

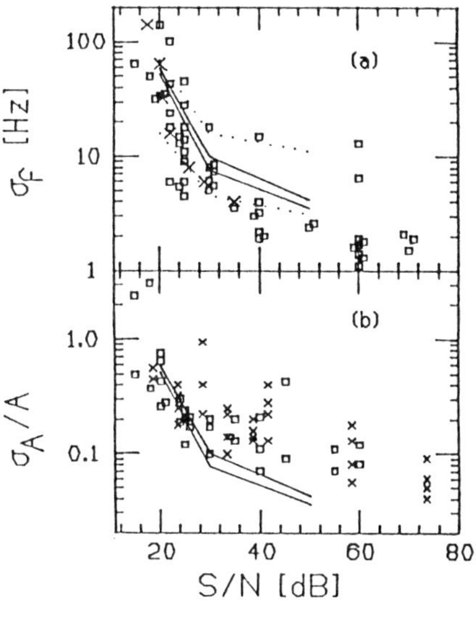

Figure 4a: Frequency JND for a 1 kHz, 100 ms tone in the presence of 10 dB SPL/Hz (lower solid curve) and 30 dB (upper solid curves) noise. The upper dotted curve is for 30 dB noise, without suppression, and the lower dotted curve is for 10 dB noise, without signal variability. The data are adopted from Henning (1967a) (□) for 32 dB noise, and from Cardozo (1974) (×) for 10 dB noise. S/N is defined here as the ratio in dB between the signal intensity (in SPL) and the noise spectral power density. 4b: Amplitude Weber fractions under similar conditions. The data are from Hanna et al. (1986) (×) and from Henning (1967b) (□).

Results and conclusions

The predictions for σ_f (or JND) in the presence of noise are presented in Fig.4a. The combined effects of threshold distribution, rate suppression, and signal variability make the discrimination level almost invariant with noise level. The suppression is most significant at high noise, high S/N values, whereas the signal variability affects mostly the low noise, low S/N values. In any case, the signal variability has a significant effect, which is somewhat surprising in view of the fact that for a single fiber response it is considerably smaller than the neural variance. This result is a direct consequence of the fact that the fibers' responses are correlated with respect to the signal noise, whereas they are uncorrelated with respect to the neural noise; thus, the processing of a large number of fibers within a critical band effectively reduces the latter, but not the former.

Comparing the model with psychophysical JND, it may be concluded that the model successfully predicts the invariance of the data with noise level, but it is borderline in accounting for the absolute level of discrimination at high S/N ratios. I feel that it is impossible to reach a negative conclusion with regard to the adequacy of the rate model based on such a borderline result. However, it is interesting to note that, repeating the analysis for amplitude JND, the resulting predictions are below, rather than above, the data (Fig.4b). In fact, there is a discrepancy of a factor of five between the model and the data with respect to the ratio of frequency to amplitude Weber fractions. This ratio can be traced in the model to the *filters'* slopes, suggesting that they should be steeper by a factor of five. This result may indicate either sharper cochlear filters in man relative to cat, or the existence of an additional high resolution filtering process beyond the cochlear level.

References

Cardozo, B.L. (**1974**). "Some notes on frequency discrimination and masking". Acustica **31**, 330-336.

Costalupes, J.A., Young, E.D. and Gibson, D.J. (**1984**). "Effects of continuous background noise on rate response of auditory nerve fibers in cat". J. Neurophysiol. **6**, 1326-1344.

Costalupes J.A., (**1985**). "Representation of tones in noise in the responses of auditory nerve fibers in cats". J.Neuroscience, **5**, 3261-3269.

Delgutte, B. (**1986**). "Peripheral auditory processing of speech information: implications from a physiological study of intensity discrimination" in the Proceedings of the NATO Advanced Research Workshop on "The Psychophysics of Speech Perception", Utrecht, June 30-July 4, **1986**.

Goldstein, J.L., Baer, T. and Kiang, N.Y.S. (**1971**). "A theoretical treatment of latency, group delay and tuning characteristics for auditory-nerve responses to clicks and tones" in *Physiology of the Auditory System*, edited by M.B. Sachs (National Educational Consultants, Baltimore), pp 133-141.

Hanna, T.E., Von Gierke, S.M. and Green, D.M. (**1986**). " Detection and

intensity discrimination of a sinusoid," J.Acoust.Soc.Am. **80**, 1335-1363.
Henning, G.B. (**1967a**). "Frequency discrimination in noise". J.Acoust.Soc. Am. **41**, 774-777.
Henning, G.B. (**1967b**). "Amplitude discrimination in noise". J.Acoust.Soc. Am. **41**, 1365-1366.
Miller, M.I., Barta, P.E. and Sachs, M.B. (**1987**). "Strategies for the representations of a tone in background noise in the temporal aspects of the discharge patterns of auditory nerve fibers". J.Acoust.Soc.Am. **81**, 665-679.
Rhode, W.S., Geisler, C.D. and Kennedy, D.T. (**1978**). "Auditory nerve fiber responses to wide band noise and tone combinations," J. Neurophysiol. **41**, 692-704.
Siebert, W.M. (**1968**). "Stimulus transformations in the peripheral auditory system". in *Recognizing Patterns*, edited by P.A. Kohlers and M. Eden (M.I.T., Cambridge, MA), pp 104-133.
Srulovicz, P. and Goldstein, J.L. (**1983**). "A central spectrum model: a synthesis of auditory nerve timing and place cues in monaural communication of frequency spectrum," J.Acoust.Soc.Am. **73**, 1266-1276.
Young, E.D. and Barta, P.E. (**1986**). "Rate responses of auditory nerves to tones in noise near masked threshold". J.Acoust.Soc.Am. **79**, 426-442.

Comments

Duifhuis:

How do you interpret the dramatic increase of $\Delta f/f$ for pure tones exceeding a few kHz (Henning, 1966; Moore, 1973)? In this frequency range, the steepness of the tuning curve slopes, if anything, still increases with increasing CF. Several theoreticians, including myself, have seen this as an important point favouring the time coding, which rolls off in this frequency range.

Henning, G.B. (1966). "Frequency discrimination of random-amplitude tones", J. Acoust. Soc. Am. 39, 336-339.
Moore, B.C.J. (1973). "Frequency differece limens for short duration tones", J. Acoust. Soc. Am. 54, 610-619.

Reply by Erell:

I agree that the frequency dependence of the frequency JND is so far the best evidence in favour of the temporal *versus* the place model. In my study I tried to test wether the rate-place scheme would fail also to account for the absolute value of the JND in noise. Although I found that it did not, I by no means consider my results as supportive of the rate theory.

A computional model of low pitch judgement

Ray Meddis and Michael Hewitt

Department of Human Sciences
University of Technology, Loughborough, UK

Introduction

Licklider's (1959) theory of pitch perception was presented long before we had the computational means to evaluate it thoroughly. Recently, a number of new theories have been proposed (Moore, 1982; Van Noorden, 1982) which seek to explain similar phenomena. These theories share the property of using time intervals among auditory nerve spikes for the purpose of specifying perceived pitch. As such they are 'timing' theories which are to be contrasted with 'place theories'. Timing theories owe their existence to pitch phenomena which are less easily explained by place theories. Accordingly, a minimum requirement of timing theories is that they should give a good detailed explanation of existing data on pitch perception.

Below, we present a computational realisation of the salient aspects of Licklider's hypothesis composed of a simple peripheral auditory model (middle ear transmission, mechanical filtering, and spike generation using a hair cell model) which feeds into a module which detects and aggregates time intervals among the spikes. The model has been exposed to a variety of stimuli chosen to simulate classical investigations of pitch phenomena involving responses to harmonic and inharmonic tone complexes. In most situations the model appears to behave as intended but some discrepancies indicate that additional principles may be needed.

The model

The version of the model to be described deals only with steady state tone complexes whose component frequencies and amplitudes are specified. The model is composed of a number of cascaded modules:

1. Middle ear transmission. All frequencies below 1 kHz are attenuated. The reduction is a linear function of frequency with 0 dB at 1 kHz and -25 dB at 100 Hz.

2. 63 bandpass filters with centre frequencies equally spaced along a Bark scale between 0.25 and 16 Bark are used to create 63 separate channels of

filtered input. The attenuation for each frequency component is computed from expressions given by Moore and Glasberg (1983).

3. The output from each filter is fed into a hair cell model (Meddis, 1986) which generates a fluctuating probability of spike occurrence.

4. These probabilities are used to generate a probability density distribution of interspike time intervals within each channel. The computations assume that each channel has, in fact, a large population of hair cells generating identical probabilities and that all time intervals are counted - not just between successive spikes - including time intervals between spikes in different fibres from the same channel.

5. The distributions from the individual channel periodogram are summed to produce a summary distribution or 'compound periodogram'. This is the distribution used for predicting pitch judgements. For the purpose of this study, we have assumed that pitches heard correspond to peaks in the distribution within the 'pitch region'.

The implementation described does not incorporate nonlinear mechanical effects. Interspike refractory effects have little influence on the model performance for steady state stimuli and they have also been omitted.

Simulations

Figure 1 shows the response of the model to an harmonic three tone complex (4th 5th and 6th harmonics of a 200 Hz fundamental). The periodograms for the individual channels show a clear separation in the response to the tone components. Note that the periodograms look very similar to the filtered inputs but that this is only the case for steady state sinusoids. The compound periodogram at the top of the figure is the rescaled sum of all of the periodograms shown. It clearly posesses a peak in the region of 5.0 msec corresponding to the period of the fundamental (200 Hz). It is the location of this peak which is used to specify the frequency of the pitch percept as perceived by the model.

Pitch ambiguity.

The major peak in Fig. 1 also has two lower peaks at either side which we assume are normally ignored when pitch matching. However, some studies have specifically explored these alternative responses. Schouten *et al.* (1962) used the 9th, 10th and 11th harmonics of a 199 Hz fundamental and obtained reports of alternative pitches at 220, 178, 160 and 154 Hz. When the model is exposed to the stimulus, peaks are found at 222, 180, 165 and 154 Hz. We assume that the discrepancies can be explained by the absence of nonlinear mechanical effects in the model.

De Boer (1956) obtained pitch matches to inharmonic stimuli generated by adding a fixed frequency increment (dF) to each component ((n-1).g, n.g, (n+1).g) of a harmonic complex (fundamental frequency, g). He found that the pitch matches could be predicted by the function (n.g+dF)/n with sudden discontinuities when the centre frequency passed half way between the nth

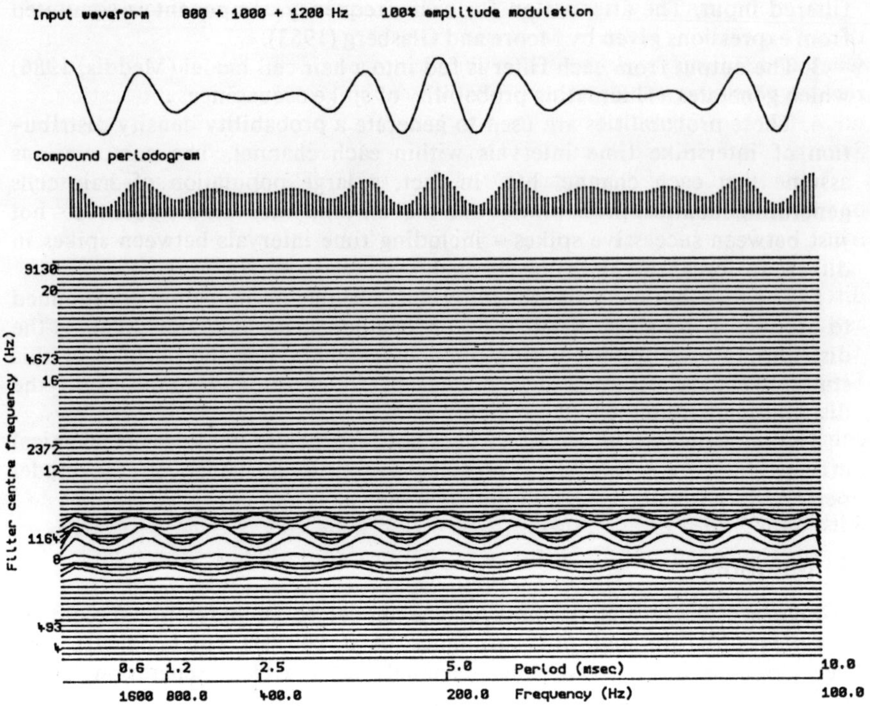

Figure 1. Output of the model in response to a three harmonic tone complex. The lower half of the figure shows the individual periodograms for each channel (see text).

and the (n+1)th harmonic. At this point the matched frequency fell to ((n-1).g+dF)/(n-1) before continuing to rise with further increases in dF.

The model performed exactly as expected on this test. As dF increased, the largest peak in the periodogram shifted slowly upwards in frequency. However, it became smaller in height as it did so. The alternative pitch peak at a longer period (lower pitch) also shifted upwards but grew in size. When the centre frequency of the complex was midway between the two harmonic starting values, the two pitch peaks were equally high and equidistant from the fundamental period.

Dominance.

Plomp (1967) investigated the relative dominance of individual harmonics in 12 tone complexes by shifting a lower set of harmonics 10% down while shifting the remaining (higher) harmonics 10% upwards in frequency. He asked subjects to say whether the resulting stimulus had a higher or a lower pitch than the original harmonic complex.

The same stimuli were presented to the model and the relative heights of the two peaks on either side of the fundamental were used to adjudicate whether subjects would hear a higher or lower pitch. The model produced results which matched Plomp's data reasonably well but it is interesting to note that the degree of middle ear loss applied is crucial to a good fit. Switching off the middle ear loss function produced a very poor fit.

Another study of dominance by Moore *et al.* (1985) involved shifting only one harmonic in a 12 tone complex and noting the pitch shift. This experiment was replicated using the model. For a 400 Hz fundamental, the results were very similar to those obtained by Moore *et al.* but at 200 Hz and 100 Hz discrepancies occurred. At 100 Hz the observed pitch shift was less than half as great as Moore *et al.*'s results. The reason for this is still unclear to us.

Existence region.

A systematic study of 'pitch salience' was made using 3 harmonic tone complexes. Salience was measured in terms of the ratio of the height of the major summary periodogram pitch peak to the height of the neighbouring trough. Above 100 Hz, it was possible to fit equal salience contours to Ritsma's (1962) existence region. Below this frequency, pitch salience failed to decrease as Ritsma indicates that it should do. Indeed, it continued to increase as the stimulus CF decreased.

Ritsma used continuous stimuli and at low frequencies these are often heard analytically rather than as having a single low pitch. The model described above has no mechanism for 'hearing out' stimulus components. We are currently adding mechanisms which will vary the weights assigned to individual channels when generating the compound periodogram. The purpose of this amendments is to permit the simulation of certain selective attention phenomena but we anticipate that this will weaken the low pitch percept for low frequency stimuli. We expect that this will be the case for continuous stimuli but not gated or pulsed stimuli when the shortness of the stimulus will prevent analytical listening from taking place.

References

De Boer, (**1956**). *On the 'residue' in hearing*, Ph.D. thesis, University of Amsterdam.

Licklider, J.C.R. (**1959**). "Three auditory theories," in *Psychology: a study of a science*, vol 1, edited by S.Koch (Mcgraw Hill).

Meddis, R. (**1986**), "Simulation of mechanical to neural transduction in the auditory receptor," J.Acoust.Soc.Am. **79**, 702-711.

Moore, B.C.J. (**1982**). *An introduction to the psychology of hearing*, (Academic, London).

Moore, B.C.J., Glasberg, B.R. (**1983**). "Suggested formulae for calculating auditory filter bandwidths and excitation patterns," J.Acoust.Soc.Am. **74**, 750-753.

Moore, B.C.J., Glasberg, B.R., and Peters, R.W. (**1985**). "Relative dominance

of individual partials in determining the pitch of complex tones," J.Acoust. Soc.Am. 77, 1853-1860.
Noorden, L. van (**1982**). "Two channel pitch perception," in *Music, Mind and Brain*, edited by M.Clynes (Plenum).
Plomp, R. (**1967**). "Pitch of complex tones," J.Acoust.Soc.Am. 38, 548-560.
Ritsma, R.J. (**1962**). "Existence region of the tonal residue. I," J.Acoust.Soc. Am. **34**, 1224-1229.
Schouten, J.F., Ritsma, R.J. and Cardozo, B.L. (**1962**). "Pitch of the residue," J.Acoust.Soc.Am. **34**, 1418-1425.

Comments

Horst:

The capability of single nerve fibers to encode the fundamental period of complex stimuli in the inter-spike intervals has been studied by Horst et al. (1986). Their data show that this capability rather increases than decreases for increasing harmonic number. This indicates that the pitch extraction mechanism is selective in using temporal information. Do you have suggestions how to implement this?

Horst, J.W., Javel, E. and Farley, G.R. (1986). "Coding of spectral fine structure in the auditory nerve. I. Fourier analysis of period and interspike interval histograms." J. Acoust. Soc. Am. 79, 398-416.

Reply by Meddis:

In our model, each harmonic complex, generates a number of peaks in the periodogram which are candidates for pitch matches. For low harmonic numbers, these peaks are few and well separated. For high harmonic numbers, there is a proliferation of candidate peaks which are closely packed and difficult to separate. The peak trough ratio declines as a consequence and the 'salience', as measured by the model, is reduced. While it is true that individual fibres carry more information about the fundamental frequency for high harmonic numbers, this benefit is outweighed by the above effect.

Patterson:

There is a striking similarity between your compound periodogram and Wightman's (1973) smeared autocorrelation. This is not suprising as both models are developments of Licklider's (1951) pitch theory. But it does suggest that the authors should compare their timing model with Wightman's spectral model in terms of predictive accurarcy and computational efficiency.

The revised version of Wightman's model (Patterson and Wightman, 1976) provides excellent fits to the residue pitch data cited by Meddis and Hewitt in support of their timing model. Indeed, given Patterson's (1973) demonstration of the residue's lack of phase sensitivity, and the phase insensitivity of the individual autocorrelations in Meddis and Hewitt, it seems unlikely that these two place and timing models will make may different predictions, if any. Wightman's model would also be by far the more efficient computationally.

Perhaps the authors should turn their attention to timbre perception which is far more phase sensitive than pitch perception (Patterson, this volume), and which would probably enable them to demonstrate a predictive advantage over Wightman's model.

Reply by Meddis:

The superficial similarity between Wightman's model and our own is misleading. Where the individual components of a harmonic complex are not all resolved, our model is sensitive to phase changes among the components. This sensitivity is shown by changes in the pattern of peaks in the periodogram. The dominant (pitch) peak remains unaffected by phase changes but the subsidiary peaks do change. We interpret this phase sensitivity to reflect timbre perception although we have not yet studied this effect systematically.

Section 4
Neurophysiology and neural information

The section starts with three experimental papers on hearing and related systems in lower vertebrates. The next three are concerned with coding properties in primary auditory nerve fibers in mammals that respond to simple, tonal stimuli. Then four papers consider responses to signals with complex signals. These are followed by two that examine responses to speech stimuli. Two studies focus on more central responses, viz. an experimental paper (inferior colliculus) and a theoretical which addresses neural interaction. The last two papers in this section study more central responses, now again in lower vertebrates.

Effects of noise on temporal coding in the frog

P.M. Narins and I. Wagner

Department of Biology
University of California Los Angeles
Los Angeles, CA 90024, USA

Introduction

Anurans (frogs and toads) produce a small repertoire of sterotyped sounds which are used for species and perhaps individual identification. Moreover, they rely on acoustic communication in surprisingly high levels of broadband, ambient noise to perform many of their life functions, namely mate attraction, territorial defense, feeding, etc. It is of interest therefore, to characterize the response of the amphibian auditory periphery to tone-in-noise combinations.

The effect of adding wideband noise on the responses of amphibian auditory nerve fibers to pure tones at the fiber's characteristic frequency (CF) has been investigated (Narins, 1987). Under conditions of continuous background noise the saturation discharge rate of the fiber progressively decreases as the level of noise is raised. In addition, background noise apparently causes the rate-level functions for low-threshold amphibian auditory nerve fibers to undergo a horizontal shift to higher intensities. This phenomenon has also been reported for mammalian eighth nerve fibers (Young *et al.*, 1983; Costalupes *et al.*, 1984). Furthermore, in frogs, the amount of shift appears to be inversely proportional to the best threshold of the fiber, so that the net effect is a shift in the operating point of the fiber in the presence of background noise. The adaptive advantage of this finding for frogs living in high-level ambient noise is obvious; under such conditions the dynamic range of the most sensitive fibers is shifted to higher intensities so that intensity coding by discharge rate is not sacrificed (Narins, 1987; Narins and Zelick, 1988).

In the frog inner ear, the low-frequency, suppressible fibers and the mid-frequency, non-suppressible fibers from the amphibian papilla (a.p.) and the high frequency, non-suppressible fibers from the basilar papilla (b.p.) all exhibit phase-locked responses to pure tones (Narins and Hillery, 1983; Hillery and Narins, 1987). The purpose of the present investigation is to further quantify the "existence region" of phase- locking for both a.p. and b.p. fibers and to examine the ability of single eighth nerve fibers to phase-lock to sinusoidal stimuli in the presence of wideband masking noise. Studies in other vertebrates have examined the effects of background noise on the phase-locking ability of auditory nerve fibers to pure tones (squirrel monkey: Rhode *et al.*, 1978; cat: Sachs *et al.*, 1983; goldfish: Fay and Coombs, 1983). We now extend the previous work to include amphibians, and provide a quantitative description of the effects of noise on vector strength (VS) as determined from period histograms (Goldberg and Brown, 1969) obtained in response to test frequencies (TFs) below, at, and above a fiber's CF.

Methods

Adult male treefrogs (*Eleutherodactylus coqui*) were collected from their natural habitat in the Caribbean National Forest in eastern Puerto Rico. The animals were anesthetized with an intramuscular injection of pentabarbitol sodium (Abbott, 50 mg/ml; 0.1 mg/g body weight) prior to surgery. The eighth nerve and its point of entry into the dorsal medulla were then exposed, and single units were isolated for study. Each animal was used for two recording sessions, one for each ear, and allowed to fully recover between and after the experiments. The animals' post- operative condition was typically so robust that they could be routinely returned to the original collecting site during the next field season.

Stimuli were presented using a closed sound system which was equalized (Biamp EQ270A) before each experiment, resulting in a consistently flat frequency response (± 2 dB, 0.05-6.40 kHz). Continuous broadband noise was produced by low-pass filtering the output of a digital, recirculating, 32-bit shift register, clocked at 1 MHz (Narins *et al.*, 1979). The noise level was controlled manually; its RMS level at 0 dB attenuation (maximum system output) was 84 dB SPL (bandwidth: 100 Hz), corresponding to 64 dB/Hz spectrum level over the system bandwidth . For convenience, total noise levels are expressed in attenuation values in dB relative to the maximum system output.

Typically, FTCs were obtained with a frequency resolution of 40 points/octave, and 1 dB intensity resolution. Next, phase-locking of the fiber was quantified in response to two stimuli: (a) a continuous tone initially presented at 110 dB SPL for a duration sufficient to evoke a preset number of spikes (mimimum: 200; usually > 500). Before each subsequent tone presentation, its intensity was reduced in 10 dB steps, until the fiber showed no evoked response to the tone, and (b) a continuous tone presented at 10 dB above TF-threshold, embedded in continuous broadband noise at an initial level of 40 dB attenuation, and increasing in 5 dB increments with each subsequent presentation until reaching the maximum system output level, namely 0 dB attenuation. For both stimuli, the tone frequency was first adjusted to the unit's CF. The entire range of stimulus intensities described above was tested, before the frequency of the stimulus tone was incremented or decremented in octave or 1/2 octave steps around the CF, attempting to cover as much of the phase-locking "existence region" as possible during the time the fiber could

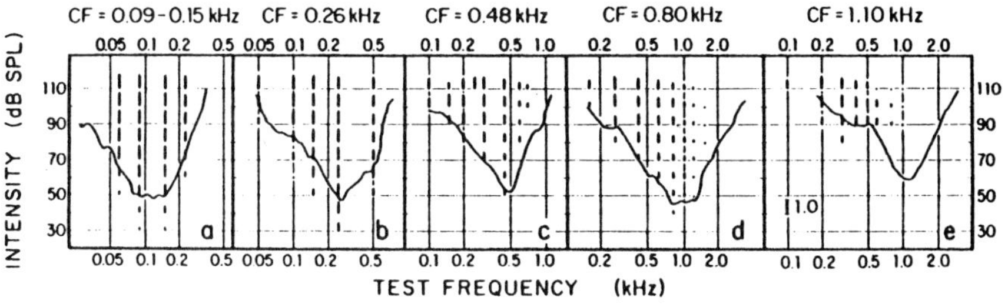

Figure 1. Pure tone responses of five representative amphibian papillar fibers, arranged by increasing CF. Vertical bars superimposed on the FTCs represent vector strength determined at the frequency and intensity corresponding to the base of each bar. Calibration scale shown in (e) obtains for all fibers: VS=1.0.

be "held".

Results and discussion

Figure 1 shows a set of responses to tones for five a.p. fibers, arranged by CF. Superimposed upon each fiber's FTC is an array of vertical bars representing the VS magnitudes obtained in response to a discrete set of continuous tones presented at distinct frequencies and intensities. The area covered by these vertical bars is known as the "phase-locking existence region" (PLER). Several observations can be made regarding these data: (1) all a.p. fibers tested (N=45) exhibited a well-defined PLER over at least part of their response area, as defined by their FTC; (2) the region of strongest phase-locking (highest VS) was consistently below 0.5 kHz, independent of the fiber's CF.

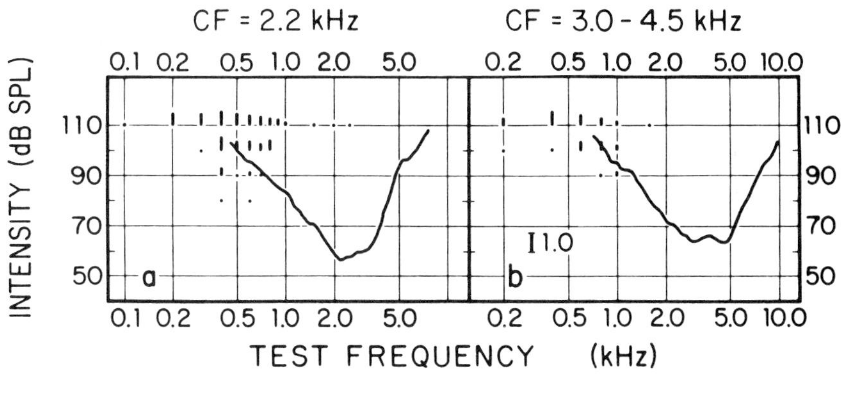

Figure 2. Same as Fig.1 for two representative basilar papillar (b.p.) fibers from E. coqui. Note the highly compressed dynamic range of the phase-locked responses. Format, notation, calibration and scale bars: same as Fig. 1.

Noise effects on temporal coding

The pure tone responses from two representative b.p. fibers from E. coqui are illustrated in figure 2. No b.p. fiber tested (N=24) exhibited phase-locked firing to a stimulus tone at its CF. However, all b.p. fibers with FTCs encompassing frequencies below 1.0 kHz showed some degree of phase-locked responses to low TFs, albeit with a highly compressed dynamic range.

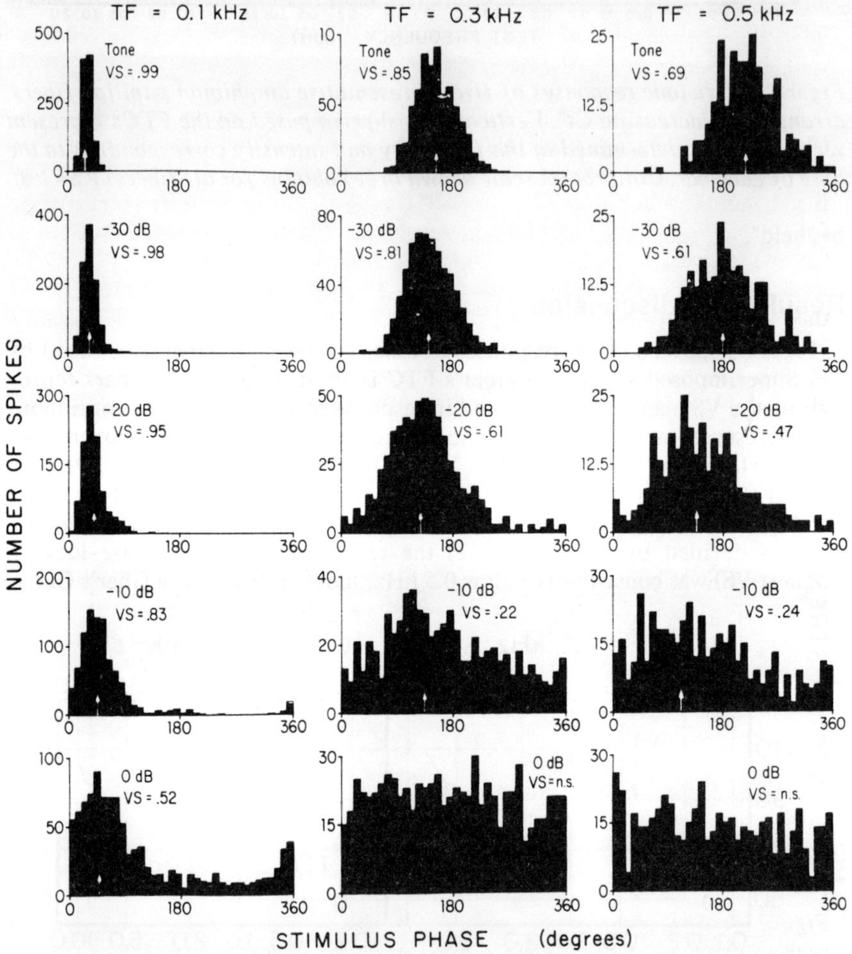

Figure 3. Period histograms for a single auditory fiber (CF = 0.3 kHz, CF-threshold = 53 dB SPL) to TFs below, equal to and above CF, presented 10 dB > TF-threshold (top row). The response to the tone as broadband noise is added at progressively higher levels (from top to bottom) is also shown. Arrows indicate the preferred phase of firing. n.s.= not significant.

To examine the effects of simultaneous broadband noise on the ability of a fiber to phase-lock to a pure tone, a fiber's response to tone-plus- noise combinations was quantified. The continuous tone was always delivered 10 dB above TF-threshold, whereas the noise level was increased in 10 dB steps from below a level evoking a response (usually 30-40 dB attenuation) to maximum system output (0 dB attenuation). Figure 3 illustrates the response of an a.p. fiber to tone-plus-noise combinations, for TFs less than, equal to and greater than CF. Vector strength clearly deteriorates with increasing masking noise level, but in this case, TFs<CF appear to be less susceptible (lower rate of VS fall-off with increasing noise) to the effects of masking noise than are TFs>CF.

Figure 4 shows the quantitative relationship between VS and masking noise level for a series of TFs for two representative a.p. fibers. In Fig. 4a, the rate of VS fall-off with increasing levels of masking noise at or near CF (0.2 kHz) is greater than at other TFs. In fact, the VS vs. masking noise level function for the CF-tone *crossed* the corresponding functions for TFs > CF. The following criterion to identify "crossing" functions was adopted: if the VS vs. masking noise function determined at a TF 1 octave greater than CF crossed the function derived at a TF 1 octave less than CF, this was considered a valid "cross". Forty-three percent of the a.p. fibers tested satisfied this criterion. Fig. 4b illustrates the response of another a.p. fiber with a CF = 0.3 kHz which also exhibited "overlapping" functions, but in this case, VS fall-off initiated at higher absolute masking noise levels due to the fiber's elevated

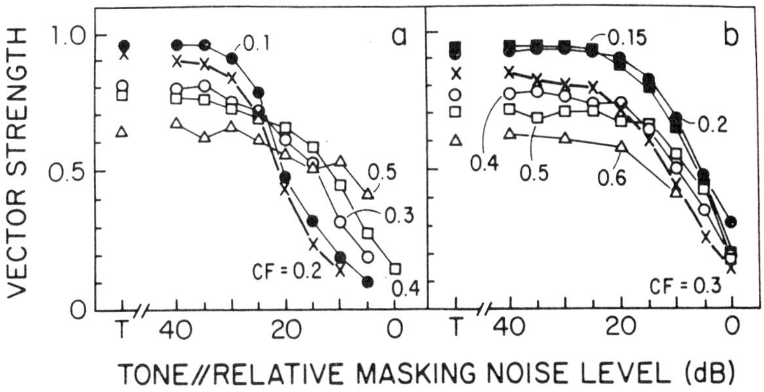

Figure 4. Vector strength dependence on masking noise level for two representative low-frequency a.p. fibers, for a variety of TFs. (a) The functions for this fiber (CF-threshold = 49 dB SPL) exhibit a rate of VS fall-off which is greater for the CF+noise combination (crosses) than for all TFs > CF (open symbols). (b) An example of a less-sensitive a.p. fiber (CF-threshold = 62 dB SPL) also illustrating "overlapping" functions, albeit for higher absolute noise levels.

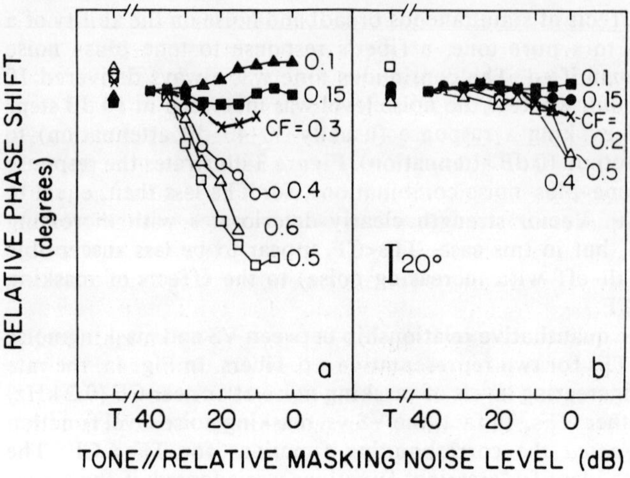

Figure 5. The effect of masking noise on the preferred phase of firing for two a.p. fibers. (a) CF-threshold=53 dB SPL, and (b) CF-threshold = 78 dB SPL. The response to the tone alone is indicated above "T". The parameter is the TF (kHz) presented in each case at 10 dB > TF-threshold. The curves indicate the shift of the preferred phase (re that measured in response to the TF+broadband noise at 40 dB attenuation) produced by the tone in increasing levels of broadband noise. Filled symbols, crosses, and open symbols represent the phase shift functions <, = and > the fiber's CF, respectively. Calibration bar in (b) applies to both fibers.

CF-threshold. Less-sensitive fibers (i.e., those with CF-thresholds ≥ 70 dB SPL) rarely exhibited "crossing" behavior.

Figure 5 illustrates the shifts in the preferred firing phase induced by masking noise for a representative pair of a.p. fibers. A consistent finding in this study is that for low-frequency, low-threshold fibers (e.g., Fig. 5a) the preferred firing phase for TFs < CF was largely noise-level-independent. This is in marked contrast to the preferred firing phase for TFs > CF, which always exhibited a pronounced phase lead with increasing levels of wideband masking noise. The same result obtains for relatively insensitive fibers (e.g., Fig. 5b), although the effects of the masker are not seen until higher absolute noise levels.

In summary, our findings suggest that: (a) there is a threshold below which masking noise has little or no effect on VS; then with increasing masking noise level, VS appears to decrease monotonically for all TFs; (b) there exist subpopulations of auditory nerve fibers in the frog for which the deterioration of phase-locking to tones in wideband noise depends critically on the relationship of the test frequency to the fiber's CF. Specifically, in one subpopulation (43% of the fibers studied), the rate of VS decrease with increasing levels of masking noise is greater for CF-tones than it is for TFs > CF. The net result is a "crossing" of the VS versus masking noise functions (e.g., Fig. 4); (c) there exists a small subpopulation of a.p. fibers for which the rate of VS decrease with increasing levels of masking noise is less for TFs < CF than it is for CF-tones (e.g., Fig. 3); (d) there is a pronounced noise-induced phase lead for TFs>CF, whereas for stimulus tones at or below CF, the preferred firing phase is nearly noise-level independent; (e) the remainder of the sample consists of fibers in which the VS-falloff rates appear to be test-frequency-independent. Finally, we find that i) addition of wideband masking noise to a CF-tone or ii) increasing the CF-tone level in the absence of noise produced (qualitatively) similar effects on the preferred firing phase of auditory nerve fibers (Fig. 5). Thus, at first appearances, amphibian a.p. fibers appear to be energy detectors, i.e., exhibit phase shifts corresponding to total energy within the filter passband defined by the tuning curve. The dependence of the magnitude of the phase shift on the TF is still under investigation.

Acknowledgments

We thank M. Kowalczyk for help with the preparation of the figures. This work was supported by the National Institutes of Health/NINCDS Grant No. NS19725 to PMN.

References

Costalupes, J.A., Young, E.D., and Gibson, D.J. (**1984**)."Effects of continuous noise backgrounds on rate response of auditory nerve fibers in the cat", J. Neurophysiol. 51, 1326-1344.

Fay, R.R., and Coombs, S. (**1983**). "Neural mechanisms in sound detection and temporal summation," Hearing Res. **10**, 69-92.

Goldberg, J.M., and Brown, P.B. (**1969**). "Response of binaural neurons of dog superior olivary complex to dichotic tonal stimuli: some physiological mechanisms of sound localization," J.Neurophysiol. **32**, 613-636.

Hillery, C.M., and Narins, P.M. (**1987**). "Frequency- and time-domain comparison of low-frequency auditory fiber responses in two anuran amphibians," Hearing Res. **25**, 233-248.

Narins, P.M. (**1987**). "Coding of signals in noise by amphibian auditory nerve fibers," Hearing Res. **26**, 145-154.

Narins, P.M., and Hillery, C.M. (**1983**). "Frequency coding in the inner ear of anuran amphibians," in *Hearing-Physiological Bases and Psychophysics*, edited by R. Klinke and R. Hartmann (Springer-Verlag, Berlin), pp. 70-76.

Narins, P.M., Evans, E.F., Pick, G.F., and Wilson, J.P. (**1979**). "A comb-filtered noise generator for use in auditory neurophysiological and psychophysical experiments," IEEE Trans.Biomed.Eng. BME-**26**, 43-47.

Narins, P.M., and Zelick, R. (**1988**). "The effects of noise on auditory processing and behavior in amphibians," in *The Evolution of the*

Amphibian Auditory System, edited by B.Fritzsch, M.Ryan, W.Wilczynski, T.Hetherington and W.Walkowiak (John Wiley and Sons, New York), pp. 511-536.

Rhode, W.S., Geisler, C.D., and Kennedy, D.T. (**1978**). "Auditory nerve fiber responses to wide-band noise and tone combinations," J. Neurophysiol. **41**, 692-704.

Sachs, M.B., Voigt, H.F., and Young, E.D. (**1983**). "Auditory nerve representation of vowels in background noise," J.Neurophysiol. **50**, 27-45.

Young, E.D., Costalupes, J.A., and Gibson, D.J. (**1983**). "Representation of acoustic stimuli in the presence of background sounds: Adaptation in the auditory nerve and cochlear nucleus", in *Hearing-Physiological Bases and Psychophysics*, edited by R. Klinke and R. Hartmann (Springer-Verlag, Berlin), pp. 119-124.

Comments

van Stokkum:

Is it possible to interpret your results in terms of time lock instead of phase lock? Redrawing your Fig. 3 with time instead of phase along the abscissa shows a resemblance between the period histograms. The standard deviation of the latency (as a measure of the timelock) is almost independent of the test frequency for the pure tone and the lowest noise levels.

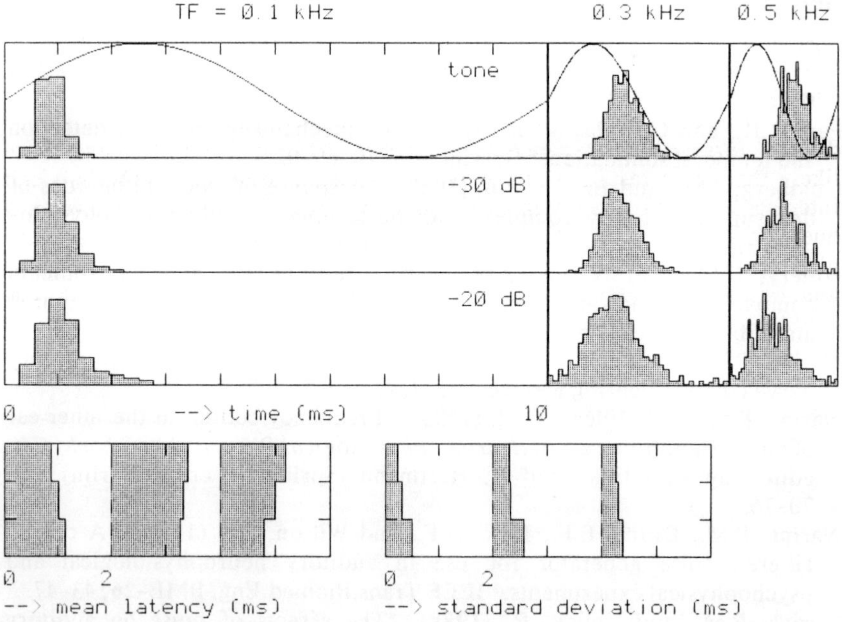

Figure C1.

In your Fig.1 there appear to be different cut-off frequencies for phase locking. How does time lock vary across the units? Is there a relation with the adaptation pattern?

Megela and Capranica (1981) suggested that the temporal characteristics may be related to some anatomical property, e.g. the innervation of hair cells (Lewis *et al.*, 1982, in particular their Fig.5). What mechanism or what structural basis can be responsible for your findings?

Did you find any correlation between phase lock and temperature (cf. the remark by Eggermont in Narins & Hillery, 1983, p.75)?

Lewis, E.R., Leverenz, E.L. and Koyama, H. (1982): "The tonotopic organization of the bullfrog amphibian papilla, an auditory organ lacking a basilar membrane. J. Comp. Physiol. 145, 437-445.

Megela, A.L. and Capricana, R.R. (1981): "Response patterns to tone bursts in peripheral auditory system of anurans. J. Neurophysiol. 46, 465-478.

Reply by Narins:

Replotting our phase data (Fig.3) in terms of time, as you correctly point out, reveals that the standard deviation of the latency distribution is nearly frequency-independent for the pure tone and the lowest masking noise levels. However, the mean latency and the preferred firing phase still show a similar dependence on masking noise level. Thus, irregardless of the uncertainty in the measurement (standard deviation) being relatively constant, the measurement itself (mean latency) still covaries with noise level.

We have not yet plotted our data in terms of "time-locking". Since the intensity effects we have seen in the frog are highly frequency dependent, it is unlikely that rapid adaptation can account for these effects since the rapid adaptation time constant is carrier frequency-independent (Gummer and Johnstone, 1984).

It is difficult to see how hair cell innervation patterns could account for our data on intensity-dependence of preferred phase of firing. It seems more likely that these results would depend on the tectorial membrane-hair cell interface. Current experiments in our laboratory are designed to answer this question as well as to determine the relationship between temperature and phase-locking.

Gummer, A.W. and Johnstone, B.M. (1984). "Group delay measurement from spiral ganglion cells in the basal term of the guinea pig cochlea." J.Acoust.Soc.Am. 76, 1388-1400.

Frequency response of single unit afferents innervating the lateral line system of Acerina cernua

R.J. Wubbels

Laboratory for General Physics, Biophysics Department, Rijksuniversiteit Groningen, Westersingel 34, 9718 CM Groningen The Netherlands

Introduction

The lateral line system enables fishes and amphibians to detect water-movements in their direct vicinity. In fish an important part of the organs of the lateral line system is found in canals under the skin. So is the neuromast in this study. The hairbundles of a neuromast are covered by a cupula. The mechanical tuning properties of the cupula determine the frequency dependence of the microphonic response (van Netten, 1987). This same conclusion may lead us to expect a similar tuning curve for the afferents innervating these haircells. Support for this assumption comes from the fact that different afferent fibres from the same lateral line neuromast show identical frequency responses (Kroese *et al.*, 1978; Münz, 1985).

In this study the frequency response of afferent neurons was measured for the same neuromast for which the mechanical and microphonic tuning properties are known (van Netten, 1987). Experiments were done in vivo. Because the neurons were penetrated from the bottom of the canal (through the eye socket) the entire canal could be left undisturbed. Results presented here are in the range where the response shows linear behaviour.

Methods

Experiments were performed on ruff (Acerina Cernua). The fish was anaesthetized by an intraperitoneal injection (24 mg/kg bodyweight) of Saffan (Glaxovet) and tightly fixed. Artificial respiration was provided by a tap water flow of 0.25 l/min. The right eye was taken out and a small opening made in the bone which separates the eye socket and the canal. In order to keep the water out a dyke was build of silicon impression material (Sta Seal) and glued (histacryl) around the eye socket. A glass sphere (r=1.2 mm) at a distance of about 1 cm of the neuromast supplied the stimuli. This sphere was mounted on a piëzo electrically driven element. Single unit recordings were made with glass micro electrodes (100 - 250 MΩ) and stored on tape to be analysed afterwards.

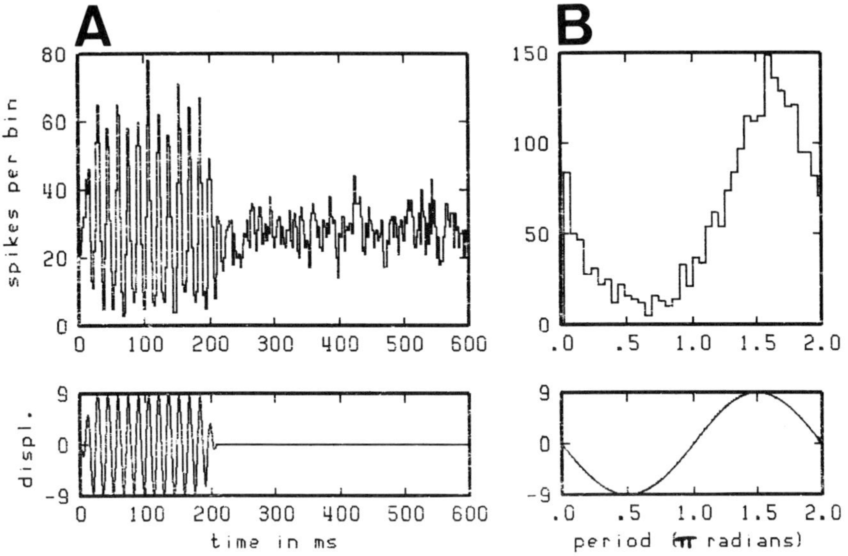

Figure 1. **A** *PST histogram of the response to 183 tone bursts. In each bin (binwidth 2 ms) the total number of spikes is shown for the corresponding part of the stimulus. Stimulating frequency 64 Hz. In the lower figure the stimulus is indicated increasing linearly in the first 20 ms to a maximum amplitude of 9 a.u. After 12 completed cycles the amplitude is decreased within 20 ms. Tone bursts are 656 ms apart (corresponding to 42 cycles at this frequency). Last 56 ms are not shown.* **B** *Period histogram derived from PSTH in A for which cycle 3 to 12 are added (binwidth 0.4 ms). Response is 98 %Mod.*

Stimuli were applied for different amplitudes and frequencies. Each frequency was applied as a tone burst gated with rise and fall times with the amplitude reaching the intended value within two cycles. This amplitude was maintained until the twelfth cycle was completed. A decrease within two cycles completed a tone burst and after a pause of 30 cycles a new tone burst started. The response was recorded for about two minutes.

For each recording a period histogram was made by averaging for the ten periods within each tone burst during which the stimulus amplitude was constant (Fig. 1). The harmonic contents of a period histogram and the phase were determined by means of Fourier analysis. Response amplitude is expressed as 'percent modulation' (%Mod) by dividing 100 times the first harmonic component by the mean activity. Stimulus amplitude is indicated by arbitrary units (a.u.) with 1 a.u. corresponding to 0.25 μm sphere displacement. Gain (dB) is calculated as 20log(%Mod/a.u.).

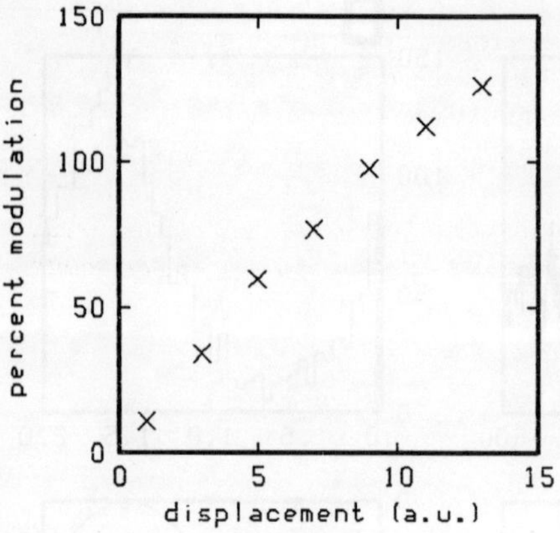

Figure 2. Percent modulation as a function of stimulus amplitude.

Results and discussion

While recording from the same neuron for which Fig. 1 was computed the stimulus amplitude was changed. Modulation was calculated and the results are shown in Fig. 2. The response expressed as %Mod appears to be linear up to 100 % and therefore the gain remains constant. Also the phase does not change in this range. The spike rate during stimulus time is independent of the amplitude and is equal to the spontaneous rate: 87 s^{-1}. However other experiments show that when %Mod is increased further the spikerate is raised as well. Similar data are available for auditory nerve of mammals (Rose *et al.*, 1967) amphibia (Lewis, 1986) and for the (superficial) lateral line of amphibia (Kroese *et al.*, 1978).

In Fig. 3 the frequency response is shown. Data of three different fishes are shown. Comparison with mechanical and microphonic data (van Netten, 1987) leads to the following conclusions. Maximum sensitivity is found at lower frequencies which might be in accordance with predictions of van Netten's model because slightly larger fish were used in this study. Lower frequency values for the gain indicate a slope between 32 and 47 dB/decade and the phase reaches a value between 90 and 180 degrees suggesting an acceleration detector. This conclusion is supported by the shape of PSTH's of responses where on- and offset effects were less attenuated (data not shown here).

Two obvious differences with data of van Netten are worth mentioning. First the phase changes rapidly. Propagation times of underwater waves and of action potentials along the neural membrane are negligible. Synaptic delay is at least in part responsible for this rapid change in phase especially in the high frequency range. Second the high frequency slope for the gain is steeper than the slope found by van Netten. According to his model this slope should become steeper with larger fish nevertheless this cannot be the entire explanation. Another cause may be that for van Netten's experiments part of

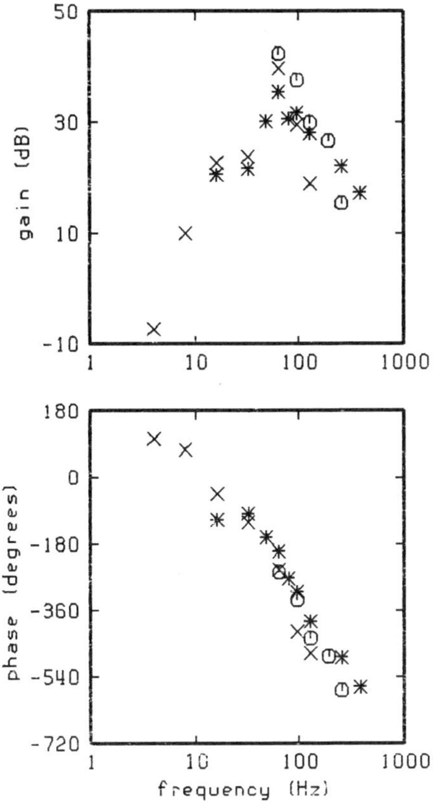

*Figure 3. Frequency response of neurons innervating supra orbital canal neuromast. Data of 3 experiments are indicated by different symbols. Values for the gain shown as * were shifted 15 dB upwards. Positive phase is a phase lead. Apparently in all three experiments fibres innervating the same population of haircells were found.*

the canal had to be opened whereas in these experiments the canal was left entirely intact.

References

Kroese, A.B.A., Zalm, J.M. van der, and Bercken, J. van den (**1978**). "Frequency response of the lateral-line organ of Xenopus Laevis," Pflügers Arch. **375**, 167-175.

Lewis, E.R. (**1986**). "Adaptation, suppression and tuning in amphibian acoustical fibers," in *Auditory Frequency Selectivity*, edited by B.C.J.Moore and R.D.Patterson (Plenum, New York), pp 129-136.

Münz, H. (**1985**). "Single unit activity in the peripheral lateral line system of the cichlid fish Sarotherodon Niloticus L.," J. Comp. Physiol. A **157**, 555-568.

Netten, S.M. van (**1987**). "Laser interferometric study of the mechanosensitivity of the fish lateral line," Ph.D. thesis, Groningen University, Groningen, Netherlands.

Lateral line: neural frequency response

Rose, J.E., Brugge, J.F., Anderson, D.J., and Hind, J.E. (1967). "Phase-locked response to low-frequency tones in single auditory nerve fibers of the squirrel monkey," J. Neurophysiol. **30**, 769-793.

Psychophysics and neurophysiology of frequency selectivity and masking in the goldfish

Richard R. Fay and Sheryl L. Coombs

Parmly Hearing Institute, Loyola University of Chicago
6525 N. Sheridan Rd., Chicago, IL 60626

Introduction

The goldfish is a useful model system for studying the relations between psychophysical performance and coding in auditory nerve fibers (e.g. Fay, 1985). A question of interest concerns the consequences for hearing of the tuning observed in auditory (saccular) nerve fibers.

Tuning curves for saccular fibers in the goldfish are grouped into three "best frequency" clusters at about 200, 500, and 1 kHz (Fay and Ream, 1986). Within the group tuned at 200 Hz, fibers differ in the shapes or profiles of peri-stimulus-time histograms (PSTH) (Fig. 1). Both show a decreasing responsiveness during the 200 ms stimulus that grows with frequency (sometimes termed "adaptation"). For fiber 51, however, the fiber's response declines below ongoing activity for high frequency stimulation. We have termed this effect "suppression" (Fay, 1986), although it may not be the same as "two-tone-rate-suppression" observed in some other vertebrates. One consequence of this frequency-dependent PSTH profile is that the shapes of the excitatory tuning curves for these fibers evolve with time (in 10 to 100 ms) during a stimulus (Fig. 2).

In Fig. 2, thresholds were defined in terms of an increment in spike rate during the first and second 25 ms epoch of a 50 ms tone burst (10 ms rise/fall times). The lower curve in each case shows the tuning of the fiber for the first 25 ms epoch, and the higher curve shows the tuning for the second 25 ms epoch. The shaded areas indicate the difference in sensitivity obtained. By

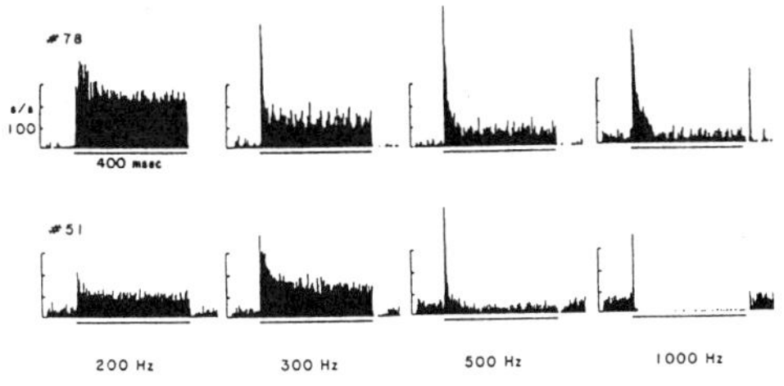

Figure 1. PSTHs for two saccular fibers to tone bursts at 10 to 15 dB above threshold. Both show adaptation; #51 shows strong suppression.

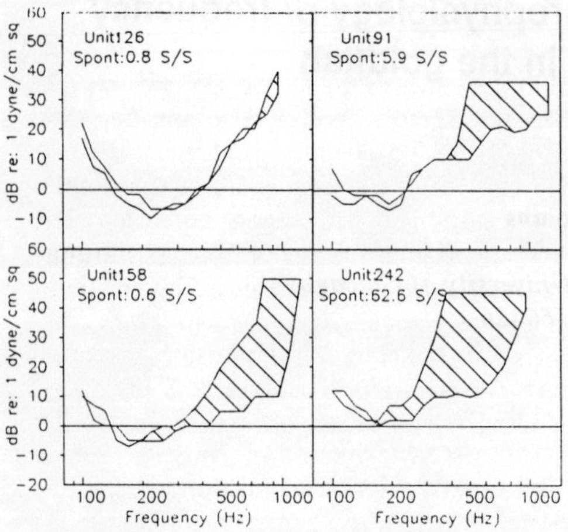

Fig. 2. Tuning curves for fibers showing different degrees of narrowing during the 1st and 2nd halves of a 50 ms tone (see text).

this definition, frequency selectivity narrows over a 20 to 50 ms period. The degree of narrowing and its frequency range vary among fibers.

These experiments investigate possible consequences for hearing of this temporal evolution of frequency selectivity in auditory nerve fibers. Psychophysical experiments measured the detection of a 250 Hz tone burst as a function of the temporal position of the signal within a 200 ms masker. If the peripheral channels responsible for signal detection narrow their tuning curves during the masker, this should result in reduced effectiveness for high frequency maskers. Thus, high frequency "legs" of psychophysical tuning curves (PTC) should be steeper for signals beginning well after masker onset compared with simultaneous masker and signal onsets. Complementary neurophysiological studies repeated these stimulus conditions to provide a look at the neural events corresponding to behavioral thresholds for masked tones.

Psychophysical experiments

Behavioral detection thresholds were measured in four *Carassius auratus* using classical delay conditioning of respiration, as described previously (e.g. Fay, 1985). Animals were restrained in a small tank with an underwater loudspeaker at the bottom. A brief shock causes an unconditioned transient suppression of respiration. A signal preceding the shock by seven sec evokes respiratory suppression after pairings with shock. A tracking procedure with a 5 dB step size was used. Thresholds were based on 17 to 20 tracks.

Stimuli were 200 ms maskers and 20 ms signals with 10 ms rise/fall times. All signals were 250 Hz tone bursts presented 10 dB above detection threshold in quiet. The 200 ms masker was repeated continuously once per sec. The conditioned stimulus was a brief signal during the masker for seven masker bursts. At each masker frequency, thresholds were measured at five masker-signal delay times. When both masker and signal were 250 Hz, the signal was added in-phase.

Psychophysical results

Figure 3A shows that with signal and masker both at 250 Hz, the masker effectiveness was independent of delay, with a mean signal-to-masker ratio of -5.4 dB (giving an increment threshold of 3.7 dB).

Higher thresholds using the 500 Hz and 1 kHz maskers indicate that neural channels tuned in the 250 Hz region are responsible for signal detection. The 500 Hz masker is most effective when signal and masker onsets are simultaneous, and is less so as the signal occurs later during the masker. The slope of this function is about -52 dB per sec. The 1 kHz masker shows a greater effect of signal delay, reaching a maximum when the signal is temporally centered in the masker. Here, the masker is 18 dB less effective than at 0 ms delay. These data are qualitatively like those from human observers in similar experiments (Bacon and Viemeister, 1985).

Figure 3B plots the "upper legs" of the PTC derived from the data of Fig. 3A for the 0 ms and 90 ms signal delays. Also plotted are thresholds from an earlier PTC study (200 Hz signal frequency, continuous masker) by Fay, Ahroon, and Orawski (1978). The PTCs indicate a wider auditory filter when the signal and masker onsets are simultaneous compared with the other masker conditions. The slope of the PTC at 0 ms delay is about 10 dB per octave compared with about 20 dB per octave for the other masker conditions.

These results are consistent with the notion that the auditory filter narrows with time during a stimulus, and are qualitatively parallel with the physiological excitatory tuning curves (Fig. 2) which also show narrowing following stimulus onset.

That masking functions of signal delay have the same qualitative shape as the PSTHs from saccular fibers might suggest that the decline in spike rate

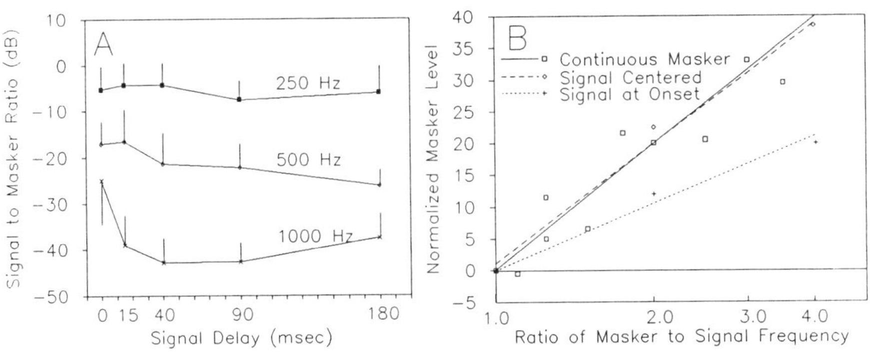

Figure 3. **A** *Psychophysical thresholds for the 250 Hz signal at 10 dB above quiet threshold as a function of signal delay (see text).* **B** *Tuning curves derived from A at 0 and 90 ms signal delays compared with thresholds using a continuous 200 Hz masker from Fay, Ahroon, and Orawski (1978). Vertical bars indicate one standard deviation.*

that evolves during a 200 ms masker renders the masker less effective. The following physiological experiments looked at the conditions under which a masker looses its effectiveness over time.

Neurophysiological experiments

Fibers of the saccular nerve were recorded as described in Fay and Ream (1986). Stimuli and acoustic conditions were the same as in the psychophysical experiments.

A 250 Hz signal was set a few dB above excitatory threshold, and a masker added to cause a robust response of its own, or reduce the response to the signal by 50 percent. PSTHs were obtained with the signal occurring at various times relative to masker onset. In some cells, PSTHs were obtained as a function of masker level to define physiological masked thresholds for the signal.

Neurophysiological results with discussion

Figure 4 shows PSTHs for masked signals at different delay times in two fibers. For the 250 Hz masker, the signal to masker ratio was -5 dB (at behavioral threshold) for fiber 16, and 0 dB (5 dB above behavioral threshold) for fiber 9. Figure 5 shows the effect of signal delay on the spike rates due to the signal (the response to masker and signal presented together minus the response to masker alone). For both fibers, the trend is for the signal effect to be smallest at masker onset, and then to grow as signal delay increases up to 40 to 100 ms. Note that for fiber 16 (Fig. 4), the response to the signal in the presence of the 250 Hz masker is significantly greater than for the signal alone. These two fibers are typical of 28 fibers studied.

In general, these response patterns do not provide ready explanations for the psychophysical results in Fig. 3. For example, the 250 Hz masker is more effective at shorter delays, while behavioral signal detection with a 250 Hz masker is independent of signal delay. However, fiber 9 behaves more consistently with the psychophysical masking data than fiber 16 (note the sharp loss of effectiveness of the 1 kHz masker for signal delays greater than 0 ms). Figure 4 indicates that fiber 16 exhibits strong suppression for 1 kHz stimulation while fiber 9 does not. We have not been able to find a saccular nerve fiber whose response to a signal in the presence of a masker "explains" the psychophysical masking in a simple way. However, we have concluded that at least one class of fibers - those showing strong suppression - are <u>not</u> the neural channels underlying the psychophysical masking effects of Fig. 3. The following data illustrate the effects of suppression on a fiber's frequency selectivity and masking patterns.

Figure 6 shows masking functions of signal delay and the tuning curves that can be derived from them for a strongly suppressing fiber (see also Fig. 7). From functions relating the signal-evoked spike rate to masker intensity, the masker levels resulting in a 50 spikes per second rate to the signal were plotted for different masker frequencies and signal delays in Fig. 6A. As is the case for most all fibers studied in this way, the 250 and 500 Hz masker curves show a drop in masker effectiveness as signal delays grow to 40 ms. The 1 kHz masker curve is typical of all fibers showing suppression, and is qualitatively unlike the behavioral function (Fig. 3) in showing a large <u>growth</u> in masker effectiveness as the signal delay lengthens.

These data give rise to the tuning curves of Fig. 6B. The dashed lines are tuning curves based on spike rate increments to the masker alone; either at masker onset (lower curve), or at "steady state," 100 ms after masker onset (upper curve). When the masker effect is used to define the fiber's frequency response (solid lines), the curves are similar to the excitatory tuning curves at 250 and 500 Hz, but deviate sharply at 1 kHz. For this fiber, a 1 kHz tone is more effective as a masker than it is in evoking spikes "of its own".

This suppression is again illustrated in Figs. 7 and 8. Fiber #19 shows little or no suppression, and #17 is the same suppressing cell as in Fig. 6. For #17, the masker suppresses the response to the signal at masker levels well below

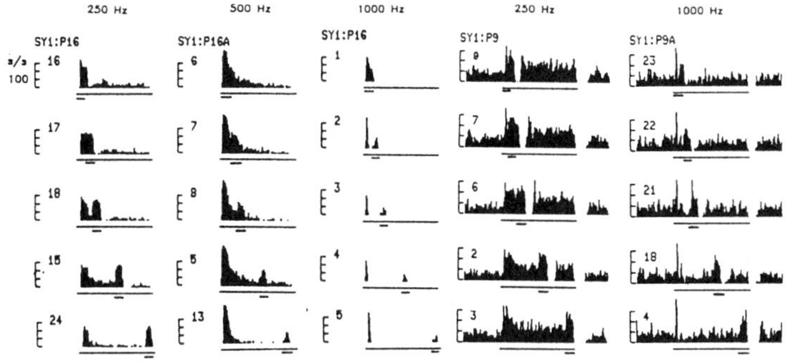

Figure 4. The effects of masker frequency and signal delay on the response to a 20 ms, 250 Hz signal in two fibers (see text).

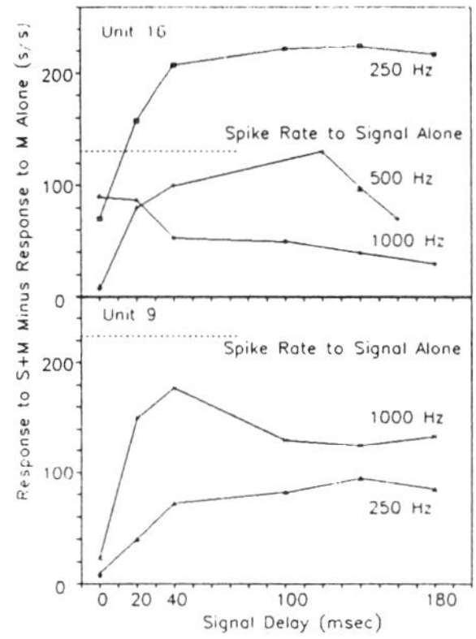

Figure 5. Spike rates due to the signal as a function of signal delay in the presence of maskers of different frequencies (derived from Fig. 4).

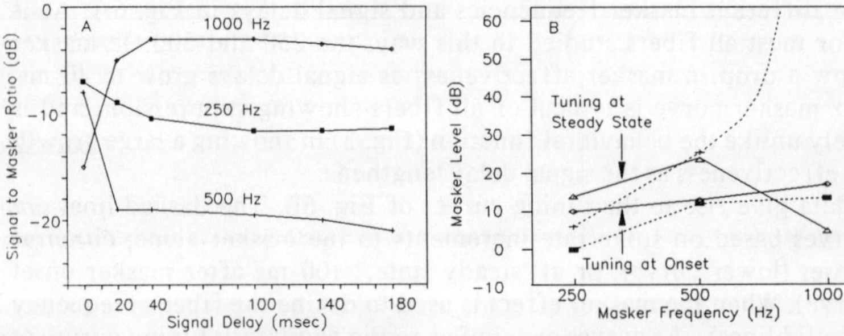

Figure 6. **A** *Masker levels required to reduce the response to the signal to 50 s/s (fiber 17).* **B** *Solid lines are tuning curves defined by the masking effects shown in* **A**. *Dashed lines are tuning curves derived from the rate-intensity functions for the masker alone (level required for an excitatory response of 50 s/s). Solid squares based on the spike rates within 10 ms of masker onset, and "+" based on spike rates at 100 ms following masker onset ("steady state").*

those resulting in masker-evoked spikes. In #19, on the other hand, even masker levels that produce a large number of spikes are poor maskers.

Concluding discussion

Figure 7 suggests our present view of the masking effect of suppression (see also Lewis, 1986). Fiber 19 responds to the 1 kHz masker with a net excitation that grows with masker level. Signal excitation simply adds to this masker excitation, producing additional excitation, at least at low and moderate masker levels. This summation of masker and signal excitation occurs whenever there is a net excitatory masker effect, and give rise to nonmonotonic functions relating masked signal response to masker level (as observed in many fibers studied, including #19 in Fig. 8). Cells like #17 respond to the masker with a net suppression that grows with masker level. In these cases, the masker's suppression subtracts from the excitatory effect of the signal, and the signal is completely masked when the masker's suppression exceeds the signal's excitation level. Suppression (as in #17) produces masking without generating spikes (except at masker onset). The tuning curve as defined by masking is quite broad, and is wider than the tuning curve defined by the cell's excitatory response to masker onset. Thus, cells showing strong suppression cannot account for the finding that PTCs are more sharply tuned 40 to 100 ms following masker onset than at masker onset.

We therefore assume that cells showing little or no suppression (e.g. #19 in Fig. 7 and #78 in Fig. 1) underlie the psychophysical tuning curves of Fig. 3. But we are still left with the question of the physiological basis for the narrowing of the psychophysical auditory filter for signal delays in the 40 to 100 ms range. The answer may lie in considering the processing strategies that could be used in discriminating the envelope of excitation (the shape of

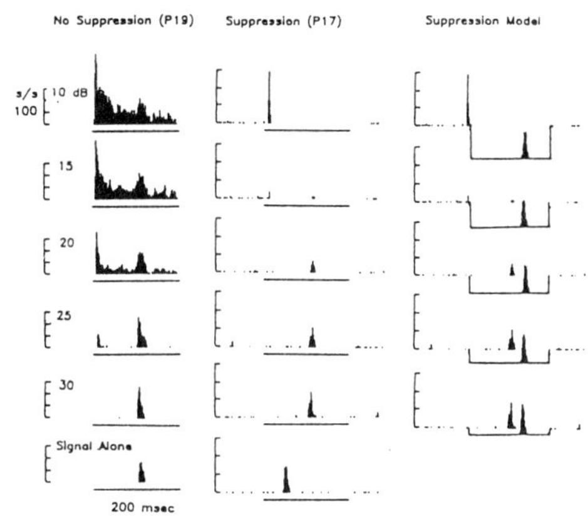

Figure 7. The effect of 1 kHz masker level on response to a signal at 100 ms in two fibers; #19 showing adaptation but little suppression, and #17 showing strong suppression. The right column illustrates how suppression magnitude is measured. The signal excitation alone is added to a baseline adjusted so that the peak of the excitatory response to signal alone matches the peak due to the masked signal.
Note added in proof: The masker levels labeling each PSTH row are incorrect. From the top, the levels should read 30, 25, 20, and 10 dB.

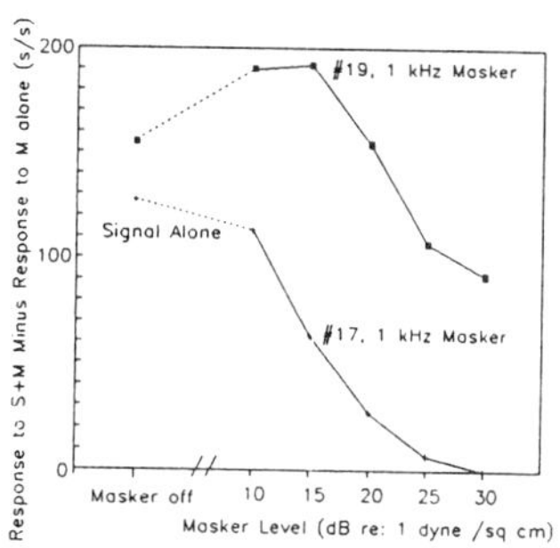

Figure 8. Spike rate to signal as a function of masker level for the fibers of Fig. 7.

the PSTH) caused by masker alone from the masker plus signal envelope. As signal onset is progressively delayed relative to masker onset, the PSTH envelope changes qualitatively from one with one peak (at masker onset) to one with two or more peaks. The signal could possibly be detected as a sort of "roughness" on the PSTH envelope. The difference in roughness between the PSTHs for masker alone and masker plus signal is minimal at 0 ms signal delay. Assuming a limited temporal resolution of envelope features, it seems plausible that the roughness cue would grow larger as the masker onset and signal onset peaks in the PSTH separate in time, and thus that signal detectability would be more efficient at longer signal delays. As is illustrated for the 500 Hz masker in Fig. 4, the "modulation depth" of PSTH envelope features caused by the signal grows larger as spike rate declines throughout the masker presentation. The greater loss of psychophysical masker effectiveness that occurs at higher masker frequencies (Fig. 3; thresholds for the temporally centered signal) could possibly result from the greater adaptation generally observed at higher frequencies.

Acknowledgement

Research supported by a grant from the NINCDS.

References

Bacon, S., and Viemeister, N. (**1985**). "The temporal course of simultaneous tone-on-tone masking," J.Acoust.Soc.Amer. **78**, 1231-235.

Fay, R. (**1985**). "Sound intensity processing by the goldfish," J.Acoust.Soc. Amer. **78**, 1296-1309.

Fay, R., Ahroon, W., and Orawski, A. (**1978**). "Auditory masking patterns in the goldfish (Carassius auratus): Psychophysical tuning curves," J.Exp. Biol. 74, 83-100.

Fay, R. and Ream, T. (**1986**). "Acoustic response and tuning in saccular nerve fibers of the goldfish," J.Acoust.Soc.Amer. **79**, 1883-1895.

Lewis, E. (**1986**). "Adaptation, suppression, and tuning in amphibian acoustical fibers." In *Auditory Frequency Selectivity*, edited by B.C.J. Moore and R. Patterson. (Plenum, New York) pp. 129-136.

Comments

Lewis:

As you know, we found (in the American bullfrog amphibian papilla) phenomena similar to what you show in the center column of Fig. 7. Our data implied a stimulus-dependent DC shift of the generator potential. For single tones at frequencies close to CF that shift was monotonic with stimulus intensity and positive in some axons, nonmonotonic (positive then negative) in others. For higher frequency suppressive tones, the DC shift was monotonic and negative.

Cochlear axon responses to tonal offsets: near-linear effects

E. R. Lewis and K. R. Henry

Electronics Research Laboratory
University of California
Berkeley, California USA 94720

Psychology Department
University of California
Davis, California USA 95616

Introduction

The abilities to localize acoustic sources and to interpret amplitude modulated acoustic signals depend on the ability of the cochlea to encode temporal structure as well as spectral structure. Evidence of temporal-structure encoding is seen in the responses of individual cochlear afferents to complex tones (Javel, 1980; Miller and Sachs, 1983) and to tone bursts (Kiang, 1984, Geisler and Sinex, 1982; Rhode and Smith, 1985). Conspicuous among the latter are onset and offset responses to trapezoid tone bursts. When the amplitudes of such stimuli fall into the normal range of speech (e.g., 50 dB or more above the threshold, at characteristic frequency [CF], of the afferent axon), then individual axons exhibit onset and offset responses to tones far removed from CF. Such responses have been attributed to "splatter" of energy into the tuning band of the axon. Our data suggest that, in some instances, onset and offset responses can be explained in this way.

Theory

The Fourier transform (from which a signal's spectral splatter normally would be determined) is a linear operation that effectively decomposes a signal into its spectral components. That transform is defined by the entire stimulus waveform. Thus, when an onset or offset response occurs before a tone-burst is complete, it is occurring when the spectral splatter is still undefined in terms of the Fourier transform. It can be defined, however, in terms of the Laplace transform and linear decomposition in the time domain rather than the frequency domain. Thus, for example, a trapezoidal tone burst can taken to be the sum of four ramp-modulated sinusoids, each beginning at a different time (Figure 1). At its beginning, or onset corner, each ramp-modulated sinusoid would elicit transient excitation in any spectral filter. Consider an analog spectrum analyzer comprising a large number of parallel narrow-band, linear spectral filter channels, each covering a different part of the spectrum. The onset corner of the ramp-modulated sinusoid would excite a transient response in each channel, and the distribution of responses over the channels would provide a practical measure of the spread (splatter) of energy over the spectrum.

In any linearly operating filter, a ramp-modulated sinusoid will produce two families of response components: (1) for each natural frequency of the filter, a transient excitation equal to that which would have been produced by an impulse occurring precisely at the time of the corner of the stimulus ramp, and (2) at the stimulus frequency, a step-modulated sinusoid and a ramp-modulated sinusoid, each beginning precisely at the time of the corner of the stimulus ramp. The amplitude of the transient excitation of each natural frequency will be directly proportional to the slope of the stimulus ramp and will depend upon the frequency of the stimulus relative to the natural frequency being excited (Lewis and Henry, 1988). For any stable tuning structure, there are two types of natural frequency to consider: (1) those associated with simple exponential decay, and (2) those associated with damped or undamped oscillation. For a type 1 natural frequency (with time constant $1/a_0$), the dependence of the amplitude of transient excitation on stimulus frequency is given by

$2Ma_0\omega_s/[(a_0)^2+(\omega_s)^2]^2$ for sine phase

$M[(a_0)^2-(\omega_s)^2]/[(a_0)^2+(\omega_s)^2]^2$ for cosine phase

and for a type 2 natural frequency (ω_0 rad/sec) with very small damping factor, the dependence is given by

$2M\omega_0\omega_s/[(\omega_0)^2-(\omega_s)^2]^2$ for sine phase

$M[(\omega_0)^2+(\omega_s)^2]/[(\omega_0)^2-(\omega_s)^2]^2$ for cosine phase

where ω_s (rad/s) is the frequency of the ramp-modulated input sinusoid (rad/s), and M is the slope of the ramp. In sine phase, the onset corner of the ramp is coincident with an upward zero-crossing of the modulated sinusoid;

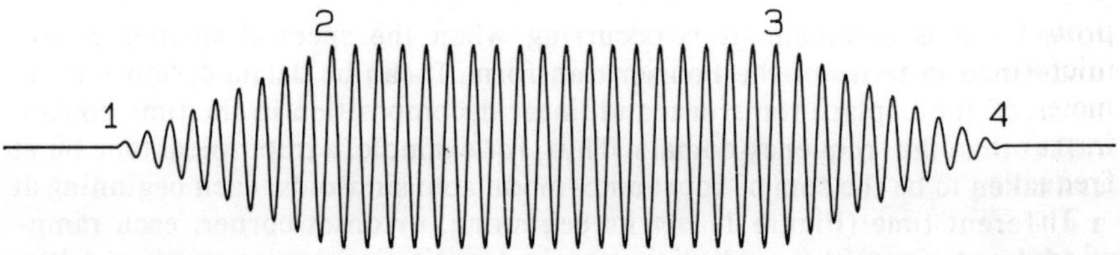

Figure 1. A trapezoid tone burst comprises four ramp-modulated sine waves of equal slopes-- one beginning at each of the four corners (1,2,3 and 4).

in cosine phase it is coincident with the positive peak of the sinusoid.

When the frequency of the stimulus sinusoid is within or close to the pass band of the filter, the transient excitations of the filter's natural frequencies merge with the responses at the stimulus frequencies to produce a "delayed" version of the input waveform (the original ramp-modulated sinusoid). In that case, the transient excitations are manifested merely as the "delay" itself.

If the pass band of the filter is bordered by sustained, steep slopes that are derived from high order dynamics, and the frequency of the stimulus sinusoid is well outside the pass band, then the second family of reponse components may be sufficiently attenuated to allow the transient excitations to stand alone as a discrete marker at the corner of the ramp. Under these circumstances, the trapezoid tone burst will produce four transient excitations, one at each corner. Even though these excitations are time-domain events, they might be considered to be equivalent to acoustic splatter, which is a frequency-domain concept.

Experiment

Spike activity from gerbil cochlear axons responding to trapezoidal tone bursts was recorded. It subsequently was analyzed for the presence of offset responses, and for the dependence of those responses on frequency and offeset ramp slope.

Methods

60 to 200-day old Mongolian gerbils, reared in an acoustically controlled room, were pretranquilized with chlorprothixene and anesthetized with ketamine. The surgical approach was that first published by Chamberlain, 1977. The left pinna and associated muscles were removed, leaving the left ear canal exposed and unimpeded. The left bulla was opened, exposing the round-window antrum; and part of the floor of the antrum was removed to expose the cochlear nerve of the left ear. Single cochlear afferent axons within 0.25 mm of the surface of the nerve were penetrated with glass micropipettes and spike activity was recorded simultaneously with the stimulus and stimulus trigger. The stimulus was a trapezoid tone burst, approximately 20 ms in duration, with the onset corner occuring at random phases of the modulated sine wave. It was monitored with an Etymotic ER7C probe microphone inserted in the ear canal. The output of the probe microphone was analyzed on-line with a Bruel & Kjaer sound pressure level meter and a Hewlett-Packard 3561A Dynamic Signal Analyzer. Both instruments were used to calibrate the stimulus amplitude over the entire frequency range employed in the experiment.

The CF of each unit was determined from on-line auditory presentations of spike responses to 20-ms tone bursts presented at a rate of 5/s. Threshold in each case was taken to be the minimum sound pressure level at CF at which the experimentor could hear clear spike responses to each tone burst. Once CF had been determined, the stimulus amplitude was increased to a level approximately 50 dB above threshold at CF, and the frequency, amplitude and onset and offset slopes were varied in steps.

Results

The offset responses in Figures 2 and 3 conform very nicely to the linear theory (i.e., they seem to be explicable in terms of splatter). This interpretation is based upon the assumption that the responses to corners 3 and 4 are too close in time to be separated, as are those to corners 1 and 2. Because each tone burst was presented at least 50 times, and because the phase of the sinusoid at each corner varied randomly from one presentation to another (over the full range of phases), the data accumulated over the presentations reflect responses to essentially identical sets of stimuli at each corner. Therefore, in Figures 2 and 3, we expect the offset responses to be identical to the onset responses; and they evidently are. Furthermore, as the frequency of the tone burst approaches CF, we expect the offset (and onset) responses to disappear; and they do (see Figures 4 and 5).

However, one of the most intriguing aspects of the results was the apparently idiosyncratic nature of the tone-burst response. In response to tone bursts close to or equal to CF, some axons produced conspicuous offset responses and others produced none at all. Both types of responsiveness were found over the same range of CFs (most axons studied to date had CFs in the range 2 kHz to 6 kHz) and over the same range of thresholds (most axons studied to date had thresholds ranging from less than 10 dB SPL to approximately 25 dB SPL). There was no obvious correlation between offset response at CF and the CF itself, or between the offset response and the threshold at CF.

Thus, for example, among axons penetrated successively with the same electrode, in the same animal, under the same stimulus conditions, some would produce conspicuous offset responses for tone bursts at frequencies in the 2 to 6 kHz range, over wide ranges of amplitudes and ramp slopes. Others would produce no offset responses to stimuli in that frequency range, regardless of ramp slope or amplitude. Offset responses to stimuli at CF imply nonlinearities in the system (see Henry and Lewis, 1988). All axons tested to date showed conspicuous offset responses to tone bursts having frequencies well above CF; some showed conspicuous offset responses to stimuli whose frequencies were below CF (see Figure 6). Notice that in Figure 6, onset and offset responses occurred for approximately 40% of the 50 tone bursts presented; when the stimulus amplitude was raised by 10 dB, the percentage increased to 100% for both onset and offset. This nearly linear relationship between percentage response and stimulus amplitude (for fixed r/d time) was observed commonly and is further evidence in favor of the hypothesis that the responses in question are consequences of splatter.

With some axons, driven at very high stimulus intensities, we were able to obtain offset responses to stimuli with linear rise and decay times long enough to associate the onset and offset responses to specific corners of the trapezoidal envelop. In the case of Figure 7, we see evidence of nonlinearity

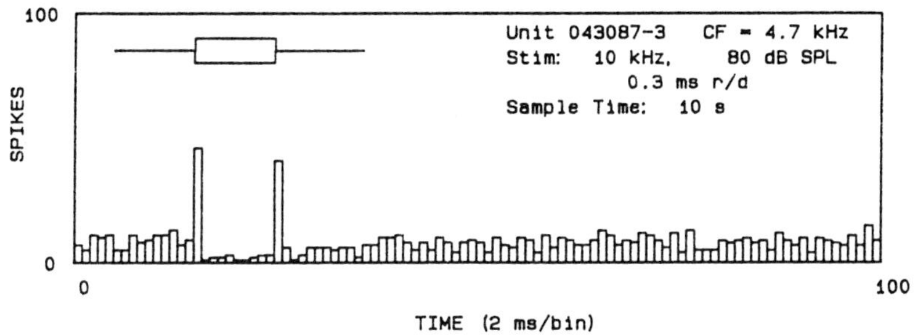

Figure 2. Peristimulus time histogram: spike activity surrounding a trapezoid tone burst. Threshold at CF (4.7 kHz) was approx. 25 dB SPL. Stimulus parameters are given in the upper right (80 dB SPL, 0.3 ms rise and decay times). Timing of the burst is depicted by the figure in the upper left. The entire stimulus period (200 ms) is shown. 10 kHz stimulus.

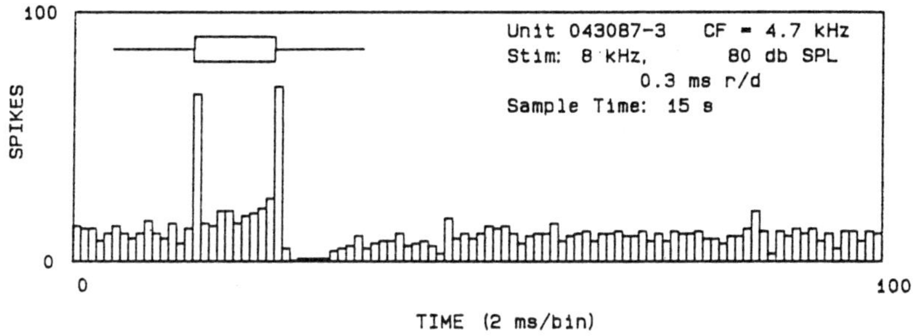

Figure 3. Peristimulus time histogram: same unit as Fig. 2, 8 kHz stimulus.

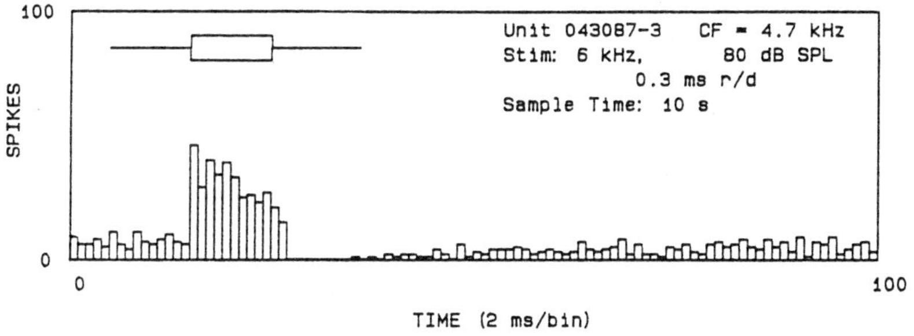

Figure 4. Peristimulus time histogram: same unit as Fig. 2, 6 kHz stimulus.

and something other than splatter at work. Peaks occur in the histogram in response to only two of the four corners; yet the splatter at all four corners should be the same. Furthermore, during much of the tone burst, and for

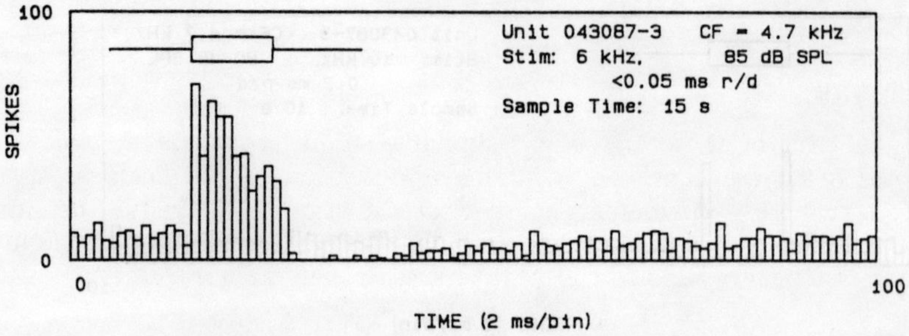

Figure 5. Peristimulus time histogram: same unit as Fig. 2, 6 kHz stimulus, increased amplitude, very short rise and decay times.

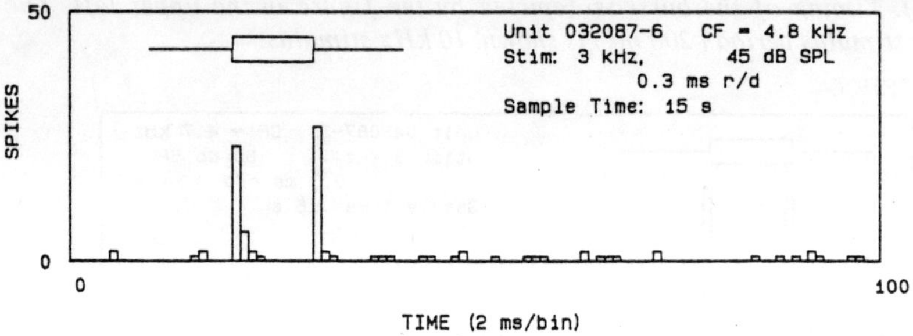

Figure 6. Peristimulus time histogram: onset and offset responses in a unit with low spontaneous activity. Threshold at CF (4.8 kHz) was approx. 25 dB SPL.

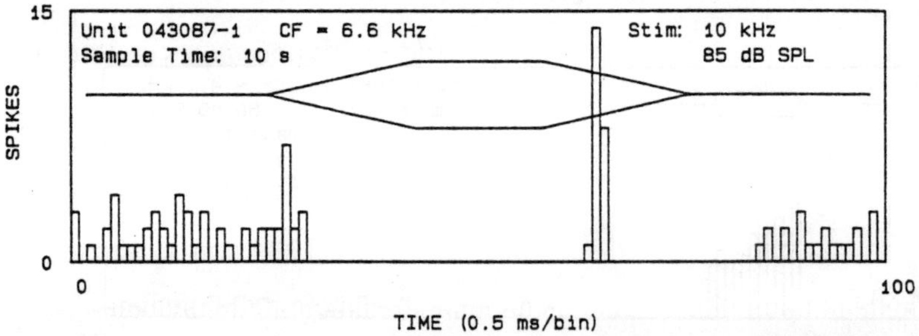

Figure 7. Peristimulus time histogram: Threshold at CF (6.6 kHz) was less than 10 dB SPL. Figure above histogram depicts timing of tone burst. 10 kHz stimulus, with 9 ms rise and decay times. Partial period shown.

several ms afterwards, the firing rate of the axon was reduced well below the spontaneous rate. This is a very common phenomena at high stimulus intensities (Henry and Lewis, 1988).

Conclusion

On the basis of these and other, similar data, we conclude that offset responses often are consistent with linear operation of the cochlea, and therefore can be attributed to spectral "splatter." By virtue of its extraordinarily steep high-frequency rolloff, the cochlea evidently is able to extract splatter energy and convert it to precise time-domain information.

Acknowledgements

We thank Dr. Nigel Woolf for teaching us the gerbil preparation. Research supported by Grant 1 R01 NS 12359 (NINCDS) to ERL and by a Deafness Research Foundation grant to KRH.

References

S.C. Chamberlain (**1977**), "Neuroanatomical aspects of the gerbil inner ear: Light microscope observations," J.Comp.Neurol. **171**, 193-204.

C.D. Geisler and D.G. Sinex (**1982**), "Responses of primary auditory fibers to brief tone bursts," J.Acoust.Soc.Am. **72**, 781-794.

E. Javel (**1980**), "Coding of AM tones in the chinchilla auditory nerve: Implications for the pitch of complex tones," J.Acoust.Soc.Am. **68**, 133-146.

E.R. Lewis and K.R. Henry (**1988**), "Linear transient responses to trapezoidal tone bursts," in preparation.

M.I. Miller and M.B. Sachs (**1983**), "Representation of stop consonants in the discharge patterns of auditory-nerve fibers," J.Acoust.Soc.Am. **74**, 502-517.

W.S. Rhode and P.H. Smith (**1985**), "Characteristics of tone-pip response patterns in relationship to spontaneous rate in cat auditory nerve fibers," Hearing Res. **18**, 159-168.

Comments

De Boer:

In general, I applaud the idea to isolate effects attributable to filtering and to nonlinearity from the responses of auditory-nerve fibres. Such a procedure will allow us to deepen our insight, particularly in the response aspects that are due to physiological events in the cochlea. The use of specialized stimuli for this purpose as advocated by Lewis and Henry would be a useful first step. However, I am much less satisfied by the results reported in the paper and the conclusions drawn. It is certainly not sufficient to describe the responses obtained in terms of a general type of filter. For each nerve fibre measured, the response should be compared to (or interpreted in terms of) the response of a filter that has characteristics appropriate to that fibre - and to that fibre only. Such filters can be obtained from, e.g., a reverse correlation function measured for that fibre, or from a frequency-threshold curve (FTC) in which the response phase is included. Without such a firm basis, the conclusions in the paper cannot be justified.

Reply by Lewis:

De Boer's point is well taken. Although we are able to draw certain robust generalizations about the time-domain responses of linear filters to ramp-modulated sinusoids and other waveforms, the applications of those generalizations are problematic wherever we are uncertain about the actual properties of the filter at hand. For example, we know that if a filter strongly attenuates the tone frequency itself, then the onset corners of the ramp can produce impulse-response-like behavior in the filter. Since this is likely to be true of 8- or 10-kHz tones in a cochlear filter channel with CF at 4.7 kHz, our interpretations of Figs. 2 and 3 probably are strong. On the other hand, shouldn't the same thing be true of a 6-kHz tone? Without the sort of knowledge de Boer describes, our interpretations of Figs 4 and 5 are questionable. The same thing is true of Fig. 6. The conspicuous nonlinearities reflected in Fig.7, however, leave no doubt about the validity of our interpretation there. We can state the following generality that is entirely independent of a filter's properties: if the filter is responding linearly, then its transient response to each of the four corners of the waveform of Fig. 1 must be the same (under conditions of random phase described in the paper).

A new method for estimating stimulus and refractory related functions from auditory-nerve discharges

Neophytos Karamanos and Michael I. Miller

The Institute for Biomedical Computing and
The Department of Electrical Engineering
Washington University School of Medicine
St. Louis, Missouri 63130

Introduction

The responses of single auditory-nerve fibers to acoustic stimuli suffer from refractory effects. That is, the occurrence of a discharge decreases the probability of a succeeding discharge for some short time interval, commonly termed the refractory interval. Auditory-nerve data is commonly used for the generation of post-stimulus time histograms, from which inferences about intracochlear mechanisms are made. Due to the refractory property of the neurons these histograms are distorted, resulting in the fact that inferences concerning intracochlear mechanisms based on them may be erroneous. Consequently, a method for removing refractory-related distortion from auditory-nerve discharge patterns under general stimulus conditions is invaluable.

Towards the goal of resolving this problem, there has been a fair amount done on more general than Poisson models of auditory-nerve discharge from which estimates of the stimulus related function, which are free from refractory distortion, might be generated. Beginning with the work of Siebert and Gray (1963) and Gray (1967), and more recently Gaumond and coworkers, (Gaumond *et al.*, 1982, 1983) there now exists a model of auditory-nerve discharge which allows for the generation of separate estimates of the stimulus function free from refractory effects. The Siebert/Gaumond model describes the intensity of auditory-nerve discharge as the product of two functions, a stimulus related function, denoted as $s(t)$, and a refractory related function, denoted as $r(\tau)$. Using the product model, Gaumond attempted to generate maximum-likelihood estimates of the stimulus and refractory functions. Unfortunately, the maximization of the likelihood function involved a coupled nonlinear pair of equations, which first led Gaumond *et al.* (1983) and then Johnson and Swami (1983) to assume a known *a priori* refractory function, from which the stimulus function could be generated. This method of analysis therefore relies on the basic assumption that there is a single refractory function which is in some sense representative of auditory-neurons, which if separately estimated can be used in removing discharge history effects.

In 1985 (Miller, 1985) we derived the maximum likelihood estimates of both the stimulus and refractory functions under general stimulus conditions. By adopting an iterative algorithm for the generation of the joint maximum-likelihood estimates, we were able to abandon the assumption of a single representative refractory function. Indeed if the refractory function varies across nerve fibers with varying stimulus conditions, then an estimation scheme based on an *a priori* knowledge of $r(\tau)$ from a previous estimation procedure is not acceptable. The iterative solution described by us previously does not, however, take into account the fact that the refractory function $r(\tau)$ is a monotonically increasing function of τ. This paper presents a solution to the same problem with the added monotonicity constraint, and presents experimental results demonstrating the application of these methods to populations of auditory-nerve fibers in response to 1 and 3 kHz tones.

We find that contrary to previous assumptions, auditory-nerve fibers exhibit widely varying refractory functions. We have also found that low spontaneous activity neurons seem to form a separate subgroup in that their refractory functions are markedly less steep than other neurons in the population. In addition, we present evidence that the refractory functions exhibited by nerve fibers vary with average firing rate, with the refractory functions becoming less steep as average firing rate increases.

Parameter estimation via Maximum-Likelihood methods

Markov point process model having a multiplicative intensity:

As discussed earlier, we apply the multiplicative intensity in which auditory-nerve fibers are modeled as a self-exciting point process with intensity given by the product of the stimulus-related function $s(t)$ and refractory-related function $r(\tau)$. We assume that the process is single-memory; that is the refractory function depends only on the time that has elapsed since the occurrence of the most recent spike.

Let [0,T) be the interval over which the process is measured and and define $N_{s,t}$ to be the number of events in an interval $[s,t)$ with $s < t$. Then, the intensity of the process is given by

$$\lambda_t(0;s) = \lim_{\Delta \to 0} \frac{\Pr\{N_{t,t+\Delta} = 1 | N_{0,t} = 0\}}{\Delta} = s(t), \tag{1.a}$$

$$\lambda_t(W;(s,r)) = \lim_{\Delta \to 0} \frac{\Pr\{N_{t,t+\Delta} = 1 | N_{0,t}, W\}}{\Delta} = s(t)r(t - w_{N_{0,t}}), \tag{1.b}$$

where w_i is the ith discharge time, $W = \{w_1, w_2, \ldots, w_{N_{0,t}}\}$ is the complete set of event times over the stimulus [0,T), $w_{N_{0,t}}$ is the time of occurrence of the last event of the process prior to time t, and Pr{ . } denotes probability of the event { . }. From Equation (1.a) we see that prior to the occurrence of the first discharge, the intensity of the process is given simply by the stimulus function $s(t)$. Following a discharge, the intensity becomes a function of the history of the process via the dependence of the refractory function on the previous spike discharge. For this reason, the process is termed self-exciting.

Maximum Likelihood Estimates of s(t) and r(τ)

The maximum likelihood estimates (MLEs) of $s(t)$, $r(\tau)$ are those waveforms which maximize the logarithm of the likelihood function (log-likelihood function). Partitioning the observation interval $[0,T)$ into K equal subintervals $[t_0 = 0, t_1), [t_1, t_2), \ldots, [t_{K-1}, t_K = T)$ with bin widths Δ, with the number of events and stimulus intensity in the kth bin denoted by $x^k, s(k)$ respectively, then the ML estimation problem is to estimate (s,r) by maximizing the log-likelihood with respect to both $s(k)$, $r(\tau)$ subject to the constraints that $0 \leq r(\tau) \leq 1$ and $r(\tau)$ is a monotonically increasing function of τ.

The third constraint that $r(\tau)$ is monotonic expresses the fact that $r(\tau)$ (often called the hazard function for $s(k)$ constant) is in effect a probability distribution representing the probability that a discharge will not be suppressed due to refractory effects. Its monotonic nature is based on the assumption that this probability increases as more time elapses from the occurrence of the previous discharge. As shown previously, (Miller, 1985) the MLE of $s(k)$ is given by

$$\hat{s}_{ML}(k) = \frac{x_k}{\hat{r}_{ML}(k - w_{N_k})\Delta}. \tag{2a}$$

The monotonically constrained MLE of $r(\tau)$ is given by Karamanos (1987):

$$\hat{r}_{ML}(\tau) = \min\left(1, \max_{\{0 \leq j \leq \tau\}} \min_{\{\tau \leq l \leq K-1\}} \frac{\sum_{\tau'=j}^{l} \sum_{k=1}^{K} x_k I_{(k,\tau')}}{\sum_{\tau'=j}^{l} \sum_{k=1}^{K} \hat{s}_{ML}(k) I_{(k,\tau')} \Delta}\right). \tag{2b}$$

The indicator function $I_{(k,\tau)}$ which appears in (2b) is defined as follows:

$$I_{(k,\tau)} = \begin{cases} 1 \text{ if } N_{k-\tau} = 1 \text{ and } N_{(k-\tau+1,k)} = 0, \\ 0 \text{ otherwise.} \end{cases}$$

We note that the two Equations (2a,b) which the ML estimates satisfy are coupled; we have not to date obtained closed form solutions for $\hat{s}_{ML}(k)$, $\hat{r}_{ML}(\tau)$. We therefore introduce an iterative algorithm for solving these equations.

Iterative maximization via the EM algorithm:

The algorithm we utilize for generating the MLE's is known in the literature as the expectation-maximization (EM) algorithm (Dempster, 1977).

Let $(s,r)^i$ be the estimates of $s(k)$, $r(\tau)$ that are obtained during the ith iteration of the algorithm. Then we have proven (Miller, 1985; Karamanos, 1987) that the sequence $\{(s,r)^0, (s,r)^1,....\}$ given as follows converge to the MLE's of $s(k)$, $r(\tau)$:

$$s^i(k) = \frac{1}{P\Delta}[\, x_k + \{1 - r^{i-1}(k-w_{x_k})\}\, s^{i-1}(k)\Delta\,]\,, \tag{3a}$$

$$r^i(\tau) = \max_{\{0\le j\le \tau\}} \min_{\{\tau\le l\le K-1\}} \frac{\sum_{\tau'=j}^{l}\sum_{k=1}^{K} x_k I_{(k,\tau')}}{\sum_{\tau'=j}^{l}\sum_{k=1}^{K}\{x_k + [1-r^{i-1}(\tau')]s^{i-1}(k)\Delta\} I_{(k,\tau')}}\,. \tag{3b}$$

Simulation results

We have statistically evaluated the performance of the ML estimates generated via the EM algorithm by simulating processes with known stimulus and refractory functions, and by generating bias and variance statistics of the estimators. For conducting the simulations we have chosen stimulus parameters, refractory functions and event counts to closely match the experimental data presented in the next section. We used as the stimulus an exponentiated sinusoid with a frequency of 1 kHz. The observation interval was chosen to be 360 ms long, with binwidths of $\Delta = 0.0625$ ms. The periodicity of the stimulus function is incorporated into the estimation problem by generating 8 ms long stimulus estimates folded 45 times in the observation interval, a procedure very similar to the conventional period histogram (see Miller, 1985, for details). For the refractory function we used a monotonically increasing function which was similar in form to many of the refractory functions we and others (Gaumond, 1983) have generated from the experimental data. From these parameters we created Markov point processes with intensity given by Eqns. (1a,b). The algorithm's performance was studied for the case of 1000 events in the data record, with a firing rate of 150 discharges/second. These parameters match well the majority of actual auditory-nerve fibers analyzed in the next section. Shown in Figure 1 are the mean ML estimates of the stimulus functin (left column) and recovery function (right column). The left column of Figure 1 plots the mean ML estimate $\hat{s}(k)$ along with the input $s(k)$ (bold line) and the bias; plotted via the dashed line is the sample mean period histogram. These results illustrate that the MLE $\hat{s}$ of the stimulus function is virtually unbiased. The most striking result is that the period histogram is extremely biased with an average value of one half of the true $s(k)$ function. The other result seen clearly in this simulation is that the MLE of the stimulus function is simply a scaled version of the period histogram, which is consistent with the results we find

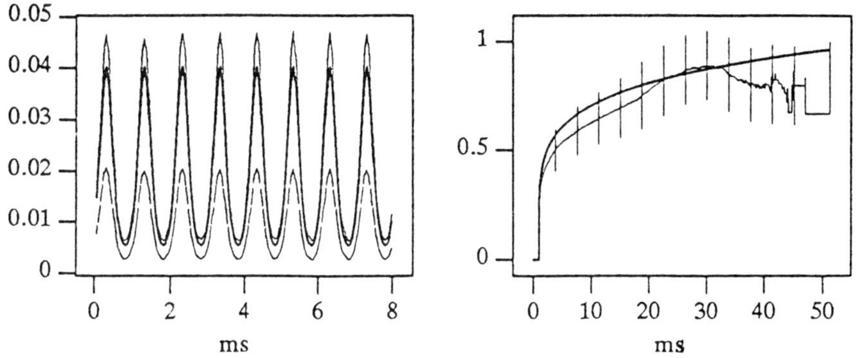

Figure 1. Simulation mean. Plotted in the left column is the mean of the MLE $\hat{s}(k)$ (solid line) superimposed over the true underlying stimulus function $s(k)$ (bold line) and conventional period histogram (dashed line). The right column shows the mean of the MLE $\hat{r}(\tau)$ (solid line) superimposed over the true recovery function $r(\tau)$ (bold line; the solid bars show the standard deviation of the recovery estimators.

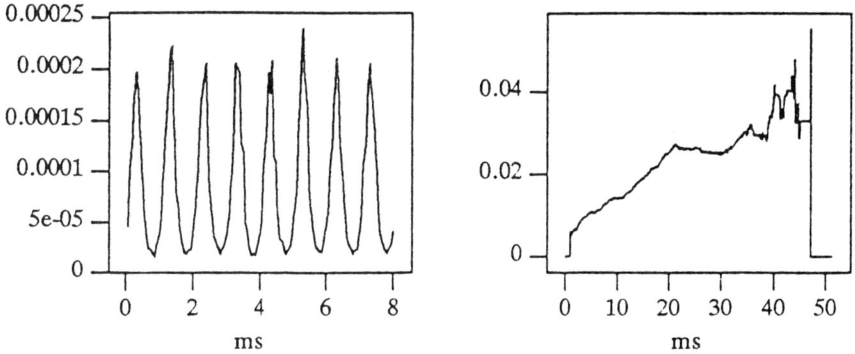

Figure 2. Simulation variance. The left column shows the variance of the MLE $\hat{s}(k)$ of the stimulus; the right column shows the variance of the MLE $\hat{r}(\tau)$ of the recovery.

for the experimental data. The right column of Fig. 1 shows plots of the mean of the MLE $\hat{r}(\tau)$ along with the true $r(\tau)$ (bold line) and its bias. The vertical bars correspond to the sample standard deviation of the refractory function estimator. This result illustrates that the refractory function MLE is also virtually unbiased, with fairly small standard deviation.

Shown in Figure 2 are the variances of the MLE's $\hat{s}(k)$ (left column) and $\hat{r}(\tau)$ (right column). From these and other simulations (Karamanos, 1987) we conclude that the ML estimates are virtually unbiased with fairly low standard-deviations.

Experimental results

In this section we show experimental results demonstrating the application of the ML method to actual auditory-nerve fiber data. The responses of populations of auditory-nerve fibers excited with a 1 and 3 kHz tone have been examined. The tone stimuli were 400 ms in duration and were repeated once per second. Eight *ms* period-histogram representations of the periodic stimulus function $s(k)$ were generated, with the data digitized to 128 bins within the *8 ms* long records.

Figures 3 and 4 shows the MLE's derived from a neuron with characteristic frequency (CF) of 5.91 kHz and a spontaneous activity of 110.70 spikes/sec. Figure 3 shows the conventional period histogram (left column) and the MLE of $s(k)$ (right column). We note that the MLE of $s(k)$ is simply a scaled by a factor of ≈ 2 version of the period histogram. Interestingly, this is a result that we found to be true for the entire population of auditory nerve responses to both the 1 and 3 kHz tone stimuli; MLE's of the stimulus functions are scaled versions of the period histograms of response.

Figure 4 shows the nonmonotonic MLE of $r(\tau)$ (left column generated via algorithm proposed in Miller, 1985); right column shows the monotonic estimator. As seen in Figure 4, the monotonic MLE of $r(\tau)$ is 0 for about 1.5 ms expressing the absolute refractory interval. While the refractory function shown in Figure 4 is similar to that published by other investigators (Gaumond, 1983) as a "typical" function in that it smoothly increases to 1 in ≈ 40 ms, we have found that the refractory function estimates may vary dramatically across the population of neurons. In fact the stimulus parameter corresponding to average firing rate has an important effect on the shape of

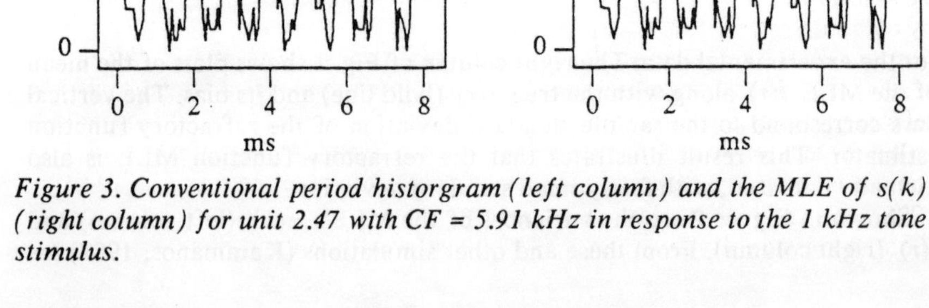

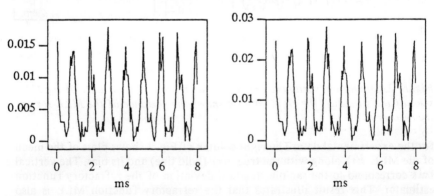

Figure 3. Conventional period historgram (left column) and the MLE of s(k) (right column) for unit 2.47 with CF = 5.91 kHz in response to the 1 kHz tone stimulus.

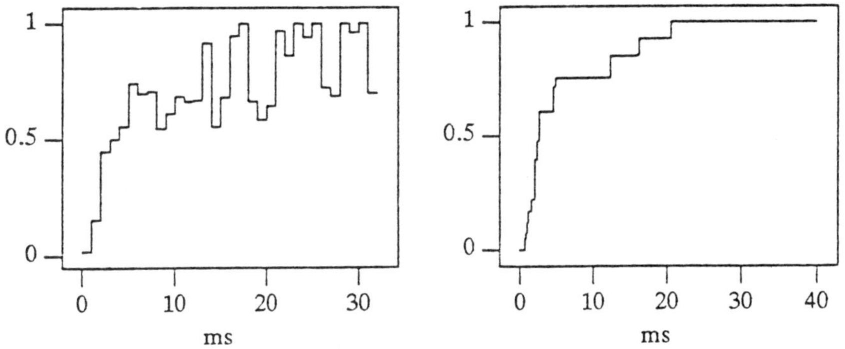

Figure 4. Non-monotonic (left column) and monotonic (right column) MLEs of $r(\tau)$ for unit 2.47 with CF = 5.91 kHz in response to the 1 kHz tone stimulus.

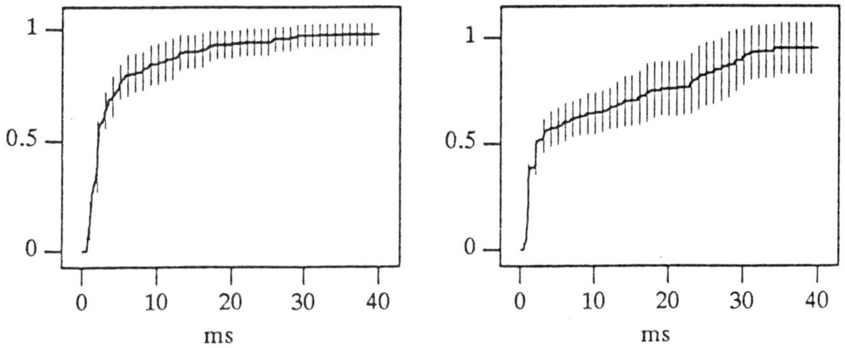

Figure 5. Averages of the recovery functions for firing rates of 15-30 (left column) and 50-60 (right column) spikes/second in response to the 1 kHz tone stimulus. The standard deviations of the sample averages are plotted superimposed via the vertical bars.

the function. To illustrate this, shown in Figure 5 are the sample average refractory functions derived from 16 neurons in response to the 1.0 kHz tone whose firing rates were in the range of 15-30 spikes/second (solid line, left column) and 26 neurons with firing rates in the range of 50-60 spikes/second (solid line, right column). The sample average for each group was generated by computing the MLE of the refractory function for each neuron, and then simply averaging the estimators. In each plot the sample standard deviations of the respective group are superimposed as vertical bars. Notice how the refractory functions are lower for the higher firing rates.

We have also found an extremely strong dependence of the refractory functions on the spontaneous activity classification of the neurons (Liberman, 1978). We define the low spontaneous activity neurons to be those with spontaneous activity less than 1 spike/second. All the data shown thus far are from neurons with medium or high spontaneous activities. Shown in Figure 6 is the MLE of the refractory function generated from a single low spontaneous activity neuron measured in response to a 3 kHz tone. Notice how shallow the refractory function (left column) is in comparison to the high spontaneous activity neurons shown in previous figures. We have replotted the refractory estimates over a longer range of τ, $0 \text{ ms} \leq \tau \leq 100 \text{ ms}$ (right column), so as to illustrate that for low spontaneous activity neurons recoveries may be substantially lower than 1 for $\tau > 50\text{-}100$ ms. Shown in Figure 7 are the refractory MLE's from the 12 low spontaneous activity neurons measured in response to the 1 kHz tone. The solid lines are the sample averages of the 12 refractory function estimates; the bars are the sample standard deviations.

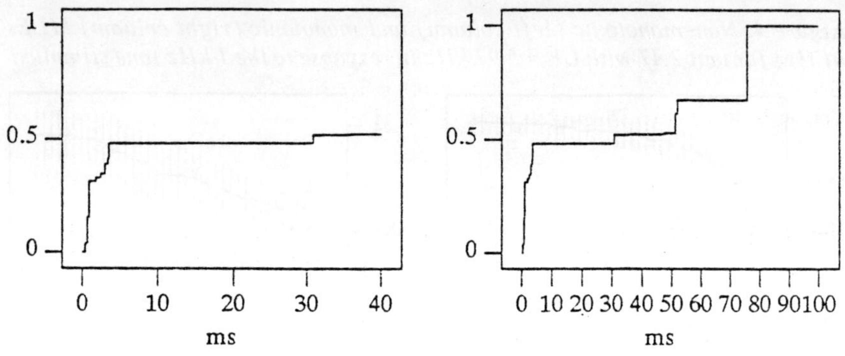

Figure 6. The MLE of the recovery function for the low spontaneous activity nerve fiber in response to a 3 kHz tone stimulus. Shown plotted in the left column is the first 40 ms of the recovery, with the first 100ms shown plotted on the right.

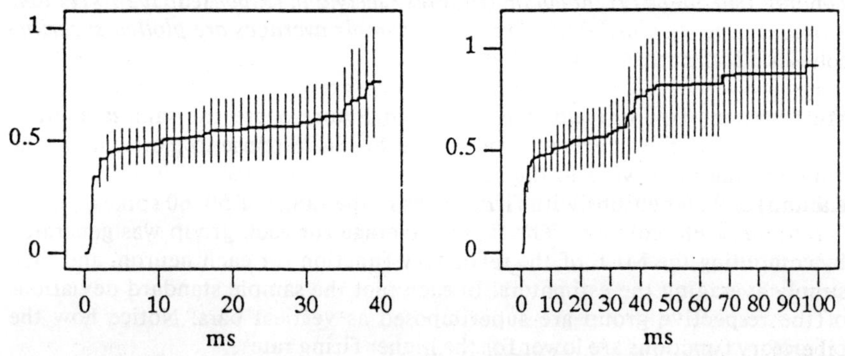

Figure 7. Average of the recovery functions for the population of low spontaneous activity nerve fibers in response to the 1 kHz tone stimulus. Shown plotted in the left column is the first 40 ms of the recovery, with the first 100 ms shown plotted on the right.

Conclusion

We conclude that the refractory functions of auditory neurons show wide variations. There seems to be a systematic decrease in the steepness of the refractory function across neurons in a population as average firing rate increases. Interestingly, low spontaneous activity neurons exhibit refractory functions which are markedly lower than all other neurons in the same population, and may be substantially less than 1 for recovery intervals up to and greater than 50 ms. Perhaps the most important result to come out of this study is the fact that auditory-nerve refractory functions cannot be assumed to be represented by a single common function, but must be jointly estimated along with the stimulus function for each neuron.

Acknowledgement

This work was supported by the National Institutes of Health Research Grant No. RR1380 and by the National Science Foundation via a Presidential Young Investigator Award No. ECE-8552518.

References

Siebert, W.S. and Gray, P.R. (**1963**). "Random process model for the firing pattern of single auditory neurons," in: Res.Lab. of Elect.-M.I.T., Quart. Prog. Rep. **71**, 241-246.

Gray, P.R. (**1967**). "Conditional probability analyses of the spike activity of single neurons,"" Biophys.J. **7**, 759-777.

Gaumond, R.P., Molnar, C.E., and Kim, D.O. (**1982**). "Stimulus and recovery dependence of cat cochlear nerve fiber spike discharge probability," J. Neurophysiology **48**, 856-873.

Gaumond, R.P., Kim, D.O., and Molnar, C.E. (**1983**). "Response of cochlear nerve fibers to brief acoustic stimuli: role of discharge history effects," J. Acoust.Soc.Am. **74**, 1392-1398.

Johnson, D.H. and Swami, A. (**1983**). "The transmission of signals by auditory-nerve fiber discharge patterns," J.Acoust.Soc.Am. **74**, 493-501.

Miller, M.I. (**1985**). "Algorithms for removing recovery related distortion from auditory-nerve discharge patterns," J.Acoust.Soc.Am. **77**, 1452-1464.

Karamanos, N. (**1987**). *A New Method for the Analysis of Auditory-Nerve Discharge Patterns*, Master's Thesis for the Sever Institute of Technology, Washington University at St. Louis, St. Louis, Mo., November 1987.

Dempster, A.D., Laird, N.M., and Rubin, D.B. (**1977**). "Maximum likelihood from incomplete data via the EM algorithm," J.Royal Stat.Soc. **B39**, 1-37.

Liberman, M.C. (**1978**). "Auditory-nerve responses from cats raised in a low-noise chamber," J.Acoust.Soc.Am. **63**, 442-455.

Comments

Evans and Cooper:

1. Your figure 3 is used to demonstrate the approximate proportionality between 'recovered' and 'unrecovered' probabilities of firing through the period of stimulation. It should be noted that this relationship is only to be expected under conditions of stimulation approaching steady-state. In contrast, other workers have shown quite dramatic effects associated with refractoriness in response to more transient stimuli such as clicks (e.g. Gray, 1967; Gaumond et al., 1982, 1983; Johnson and Swami, 1983). Work in our laboratory (unpublished data) has demonstrated that the effects of refractoriness can be varied in the responses of a single cochlear nerve fibre by simply changing the stimulus repetition rate. This in Fig. 1, at a click repetition rate of 100/s (A), the recovered PSTH is proportional to the unrecovered PSTH. However, decreasing the click rate to 10/s (B) allows the effects of refractoriness to be demonstrated clearly.

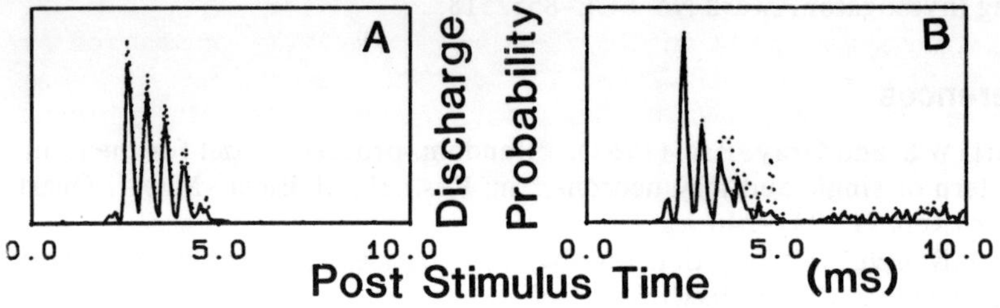

Figure C1. Response of fibre (CF 2.1 kHz) to click train stimulation approx. 20 dB above threshold. (A) click repetition rate 100/s, (B) 10/s. Solid line shows unrecovered PSTH response, dotted line response recovered by a technique similar to Gaumond's (1982).

2. You infer that refractoriness is an increasing function of discharge rate by observation with respect to neural 'place'. Such a suggestion seems to conflict with the results of Gaumond *et al.* (1982, 1983) which show the form of the recovery function in a single fibre to be independent of driven rate. We have direct evidence from continuous white noise stimulation of sibngle fibres in the guinea-pig cochlear nerve which further supports Gaumond's findings.

3. Your finding with respect to low spontaneous rate fibres is very appealing in that it may correlate with Liberman's (1978) report of smaller than average terminal diameters in such fibres. However, one should be cautious about your interpretation. Presumably, in order to achieve sufficiently high discharge rates here the effective stimulus levels had to be quite high. On the basis of your argument (that refractoriness is an increasing function of driven rate - *contra* Gaumond), the effects related to spontaneous rate will be difficult to separate from those due to level of stimulation. In order to clear up the conflict with Gaumond's work, it would be necessary to compare the time-course of recovery in both low and high spoontaneous rate fibres at the same rates of discharge.

Reply by Karamanos and Miller:

1.We agree completely with the fact that only for steady-state stimuli is there a linear scale between the period histogram and stimulus function s(k). In fact, we also find in analyzing non steady-state speech stimuli that this simple scale does not hold; rather there is a significant non-scale like distortion at the onset of response which is consistent with that which you and others show.

2. Our results do not conflict with Gaumond *et al.* in that Gaumond has never estimated the stimulus function and recovery functions simultaneously at frequencies where the neurons are showing phase-locking. As we emphasized in the introduction, measurements of this kind have never been made in that the algorithm for simultaneously estimating these two functions did not exist before 1985 (Miller, 1985), and our recent implementation of the algorithm (Karamanos, 1987).

3. Let me simply point out that the stimulus level was constant for the entire population of neurons. Therefore, there is no confounding effect of an increase in discharge rate of the low spontaneous (low-spac) fibers forcing the recovery measure lower. In fact, the low-spac fibers of Figs. 6,7 would be expected to have lower firing rates, implying that if there were a discharge rate effect (as in Fig. 5) the low-spac neurons would have steepened recovery function estimators. This would imply that low-spac neurons would have even lower recovery function estimators than shown here.

Lewis:

The dynamics of potassium and sodium channel populations suggest the possibility of damped oscillation of spike initiator excitability following a spike. We see suggestions of this in PSTHs from Mongollan Gerbil cochlear axons. It also was reported frequently in the early literature on axon physiology. Did your analysis reveal anaything of this sort before you imposed the monotonicity constraint?

Reply by Karamanos & Miller:

We have found the standard deviations of our non-monotic maximum-likehood $r(\tau)$ estimators generated from our 1000 spike histograms to be quite substantial for long lags τ. This led us to incorporate the monotonicity constraint which reduces the variability considerably, and captures a major systematic trend in the recovery properties of the neurons. In order to see the effect you have mentioned we would have to collect much longer spike trains with substantially larger numbers of data points.

Dynamic tuning properties in the guinea pig

V.F. Prijs

E.N.T. Department, University Hospital,
P.O. Box 9600, 2333 RC Leiden, The Netherlands

Introduction

One of the phenomena in hearing in which non-linearity plays and important role is the frequency selectivity of the cochlear structures. Since the properties of cochlear mechanics change with intensity, a Frequency Threshold Curve (FTC) (which is obtained over a large range of intensities) is different from the filter tuning curve at one stimulus level. Moreover, the FTCs are commonly obtained for a steady state condition, a situation in which the unit responses are adapted. For responses to complex stimuli, as in daily life situations, and for on responses like the Compound Action Potential (CAP), the influence of adaption is much less or zero, and the responses will be described by the dynamic properties of the cochlea. Since in some respect the latter properties differ from the steady state response behaviour (Smith and Brachman, 1980; Horst, Javel, and Farley, 1985; Yates, 1987), a deviation in tuning properties can also be expected. In this paper a series of experiments is described in which dynamic tuning properties are obtained from histograms to short tone bursts, while the consequences for a model for the CAP is discussed.

Methods

For six guinea pigs dynamic and static properties were investigated in 32 fibres. Accidentally three of the animals suffered from high frequency loss which possibly could be induced by noise exposure during transport. Premedication was given by atropine sulphate (25 μg/kg body weight, i.m.), followed by a combination of Thalamonal® and Nembutal (45μg and 16 μg/kg bodyweight, i.m. and i.p. respectively) with a supplement of 100% and 10% respectively each 1.5 or 2 hours.

Registration of the Compound Action Potential (CAP) was achieved with a silver ball electrode on the round window. Single-fibre recording was intracranially performed with 2.7 M KCl filled glass micropipets (40-80MΩ in situ).

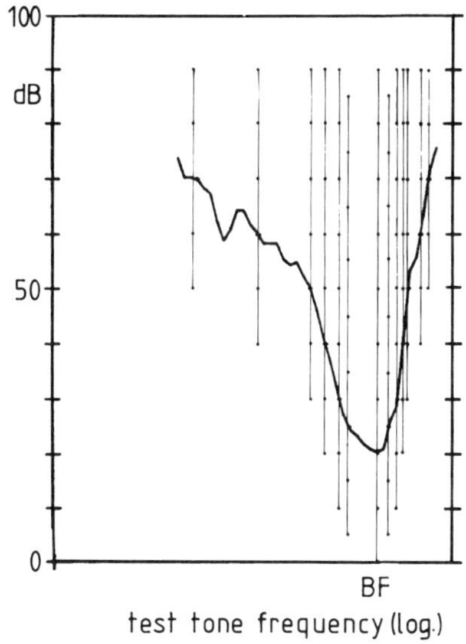

Figure 1. FTC, determined with a tracking algorithm. From the FTC, the test frequencies are computed (vertical lines); having thresholds at 0, 5, 10, 20, 30, 40, 50 dB above tip threshold, test tones are represented by dots.

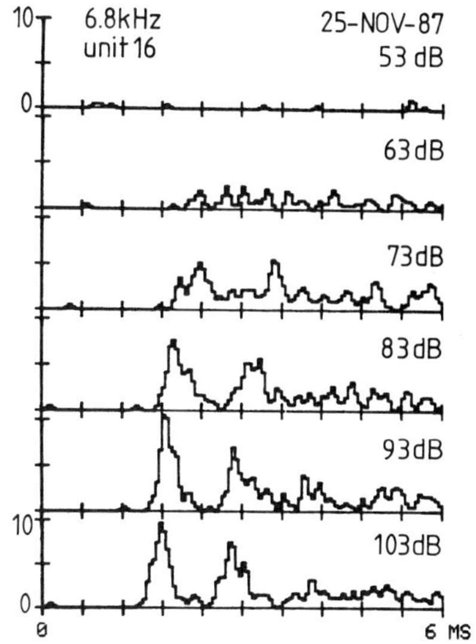

Figure 2. PSTHs (total spikes) to a cycle of test tones at one frequency (at BF) and increasing intensities (10 dB steps). Bin width is here 50 μs, the test tones are presented 64 times. PSTHs are smoothed.

The stimulation and registration equipment used is described in detail in Harrison and Prijs (1984).

When a fibre was encountered, a frequency threshold curve (FTC) was determined with a threshold tracking method, using a rate-increase criterion of 20% from spontaneous activity, with an under limit of 20 spikes/sec (1 in 50ms). Hence from the FTC, test frequencies were computed so that their threshold lay at 0, 5, 10, 20, 30, 40, and 50 dB above tip threshold. (See Fig. 1.) At these frequencies tone bursts with a trapezoidal envelope, 2 cycles rise- and fall time and 4 ms plateau duration were presented in increasing steps of 10 dB. Presentation of probe tones was performed with an inter-stimulus interval of 107 ms so little or no adaptation was effected in the onset responses. Post Stimulus Time Histograms (PSTH) were determined to 64 presentations of the test tones using 50 or 100 μs bins. (See Fig.2.) At each test frequency after the tone-burst cycle of different intensities the (static) rate-intensity function was determined for semicontinuous tone stimulation (window 1000-2000 ms). Test frequency was alternated between below and above best frequency (BF) in order from low to high threshold. From the PSTHs dynamic rate intensity functions were determined with a window of

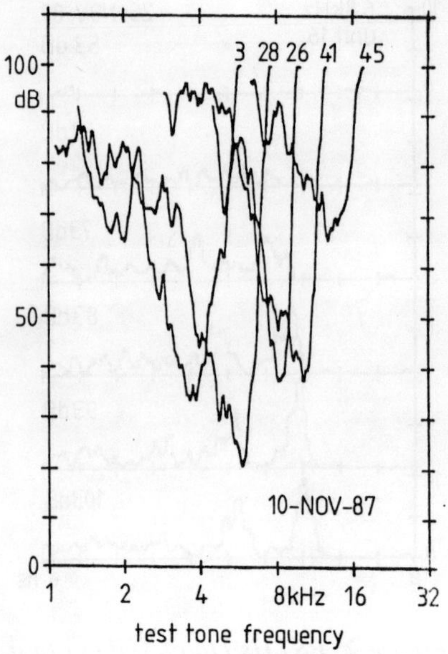

Figure 3. A series of FTCs from five fibres in one animal; the place of the high frequency slopes are evenly spread over the (logarithmic) frequency range.

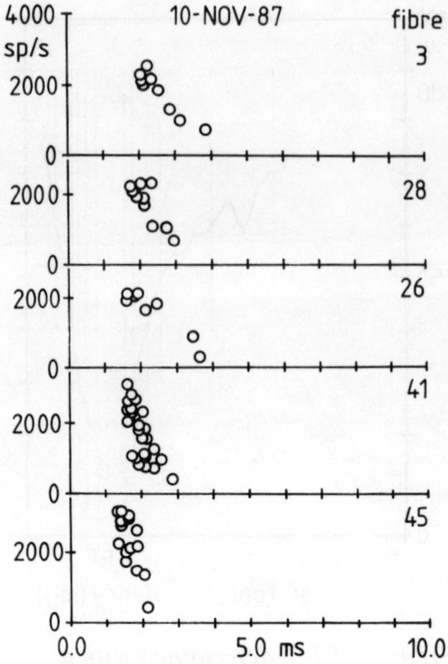

Figure 4. Amplitude-latency relations for the five fibres for which FTCs are shown in Fig.3. Amplitude and latency are determined from PSTHs.

200 μs. The maximum amplitude (in spikes/sec) and corresponding latency were determined. In a small group of fibres (8) the amount of (static and dynamic) rate functions was sufficient to distillate iso-rate curves named static (SFTC) and dynamic (DFTC) frequency threshold curves, respectively.

Results

The FTCs of the normal hearing guinea pigs had normal threshold and Q_{10dB}. The same results were found for the other animals in the frequency region where their thresholds were normal, while the FTCs for BFs at the edge of the loss showed tips shifted to higher intensities, and a decrease of tail threshold, sometimes below tip threshold. In the region of high frequency-loss FTCs without any tip section were encountered. The BFs of the fibres tested ranged from 1.1 - 19 kHz.

The PSTHs showed, especially for high frequencies two peaks (see Fig. 2) for lower frequencies the second peak as was less pronounced. The peaks were narrower for higher frequencies, caused by better synchronization and resulted in higher amplitudes. The amplitude of the first peak and the corresponding latency showed a relation typical for a fibre, i.e., more

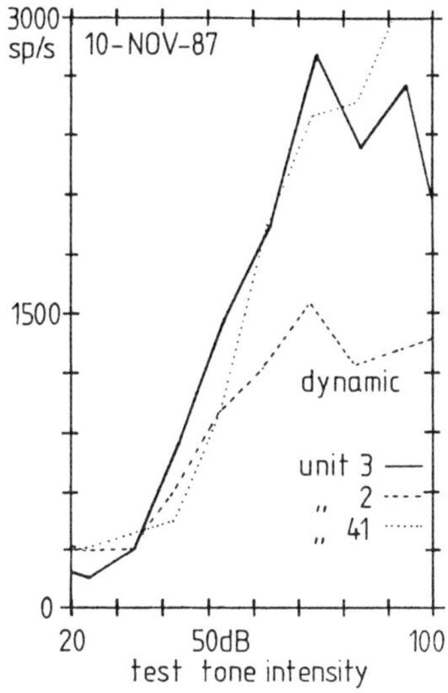

Figure 5A. Rate-Intensity Functions for three fibres with different spontaneous activity. The rates are determined from the PSTHs in response to tone bursts.

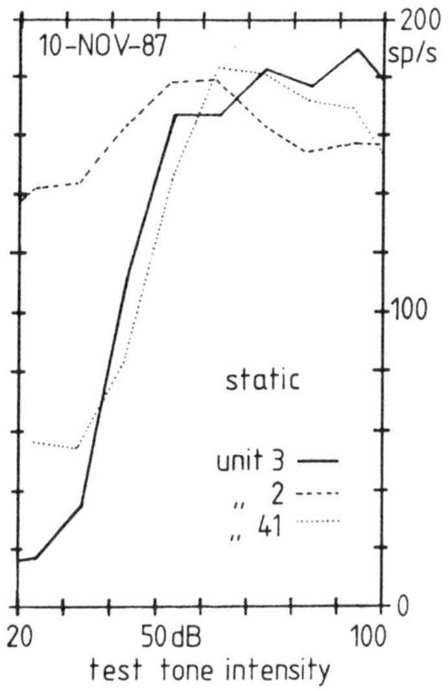

Figure 5B. Rate-Intensity Functions for the same fibres as in 5A (same animal). The rates are determined from semi-continuous (2000 ms) tones (on effect excluded).

determined by tuning properties than stimulus frequencies. Fig.3 shows FTCs for five fibres in a normal hearing animal, and in Fig.4 the amplitude and latencies of the largest peaks in the PSTHs are presented. In Fig.3, as in all figures, the level of the electrical stimulus is given, so no correction is made for the acoustic transducer (Standard Telephones and Cables 4026A; see Harrison and Prijs, 1984) which shows a large reduction for frequencies above 10 kHz. When fibres with bad tuning are stimulated with frequencies in the middle of their responding frequency region, the amplitude-latency relation is most in agreement with those of fibres with the same high frequency slope.

The rate-intensity functions computed from the PSTHs (dynamic R(I)) show on the average a 10 - 15 dB larger dynamic range than the R(I) determined under the quasi-static condition. (See Fig. 5A and 5B.). Where the maximum static rate lies for all fibres around 200 sp/s, the maximum dynamic rate differs for BF and spontaneous activity. (Fibres 3, 2, and 41 have BFs of 3.7, 4.5, and 10.4 kHz, respectively.) In fibres, revealing bad tuning abnormal steep rate-intensity functions (15-20 dB dynamic range) were found in both conditions. When it was possible dynamic and static FTCs were calculated from the rate-intensity functions. Figure 6 shows the FTC determined with a tracking algorithm and via the R(I)s. As in other fibres there are no striking differences between the three FTCs, albeit that for high

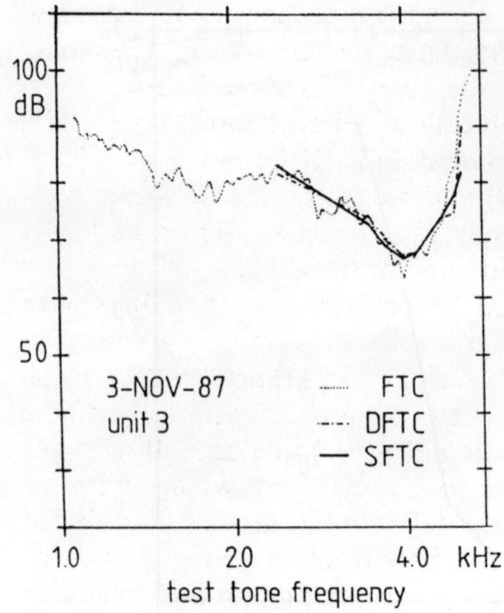

Figure 6. Frequency threshold curves, determined with a tracking algorithm (FTC), via dynamic rate-intensity functions (DFTC) via static rate-density functions (SFTC).

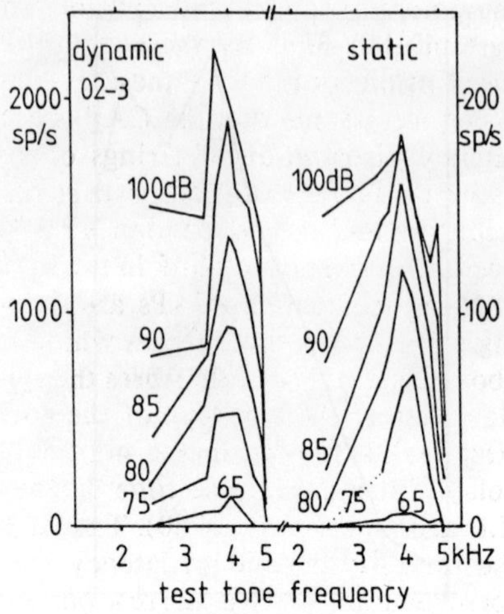

Figure 7. Response areas for the fibre with corresponding FTCs in Fig.6. The dynamic properties show a better preservation of tuning at and higher stimulus levels.

BFs the SFTC turns out to be somewhat narrower than the FTC and DFTC. The response areas show clearly the effect of a larger dynamic range: tuning is better preserved at higher intensities in the dynamic situation.

Discussion

As can be concluded from the experiments described, the Frequency Threshold Curve is not different for static and dynamic stimuli. This result is in agreement with adaptation theories (Smith and Brachman, 1982; Eggermont, 1985) and the experiments of Smith and Brachman (1980) and Yates (1987) where there is no difference in threshold and little difference at levels just above threshold for adapted and onset responses. The differences in FTCs that have been found can be attributed to other aspects inherent to differences in stimulation and FTC determination, e.g., the spread in frequency domain in case of toneburst stimulation and some hysteresis effect in case of the tracking algorithm. Also according to forementioned work it was to be expected that the dynamic aspect of tuning is prominent in the excitation pattern. The non-linearities in frequency selectivity for single tone stimuli express themselves in these patterns: the saturation of the mechanical system, as seen in hair cell responses (Russel and Sellick, 1978; Patuzzi and Sellick, 1983) and the stimulus frequency dependent slopes of the rate intensity functions (not shown here; see Sachs and Abbas, 1974). The maximum dynamical rate is determined by saturation of the hydromechanical system as well as by the synchronization of the responses. So in a model description for the CAP these dynamic tuning properties should be involved. When we assume that the CAP is a convolution of a unit contribution and a latency distribution of firings or a Compound PST (Goldstein and Kiang, 1958; de Boer, 1975; Bappert, *et al.* 1980) and we know that the unit contribution and its independence of BF (Prijs,1986), the description of PSTH becomes an important link in the in the modelling of the CAP.

In most situations CAPs are determined by contributions of fibres with high BF, i.e., of those fibres which less or no phase following (in guinea pigs above 3 kHz). For those fibres the synchronization in PSTH is the result of the steepness of the envelope of the cochlear filter response. The latency of the first peak is the result of a minimal synaptic delay (0.8 ms), travelling wave delay, filter delay, rise time of the tone burst, and refractory mechanisms (Lütkenhöner, *et al.*, 1980). The latter three contributions are responsible for the intensity dependent latency shift of the first peak in PSTH as well as corresponding shift in narrow band latencies (Prijs and Eggermont, 1981). In the pathological cochleas, where we found a high threshold tip and a lower threshold tail, the latency of the first peak still has a value corresponding to tip frequency, while the lowest threshold (in the tail) has a much lower frequency. These findings could explain the extremely short latencies, found for narrow band responses in deteriorated human cochleas (Eggermont, 1980). The second peak in the PSTH is due to repetitive firing (Lütkenhöner, 1980) and gives rise to the N_2 in the CAP. Since this second peak is large enough to account for the N_2 and moreover, the single-unit contribution to the CAP does not show a second negative peak it should be concluded that the N_2 in the guinea pig is the result of second firings and not of a nucleus contribution.

Acknowledgements

This study was supported by the Heinsius Houbolt Fund and by the Netherlands Organization for Scientific Research (NWO).

References

Bappert, E., Hoke, M., and Lütkenhöner, B. (**1980**). "Deconvolution of compound action potentials and non-linear features of the PST histogram." *Proc. Symp. Nonlinear and Active Mechanical Processes in the Cochlea.* Hearing Res. **2**, 573-580.

Boer, de E. (**1975**). "Synthetic whole nerve action potential for the cat." J.Acoust.Soc.Amer. **58**, 1030-1045.

Eggermont, J.J. (**1980**). "Narrow-band AP studies in normal and recruiting human ears." In: *Psychophysical, Physiological and behavioural studies in Hearing*, edited by G. van der Brink and F.A. Bilsen. (Delft University Press, Delft) pp. 166-170.

Eggermont, J.J. (**1985**). "Peripheral auditory adaptation and fatigue: A model oriented view," Hearing Res. **18**, 75-71.

Goldstein, H.M.Jr., and Kiang, N.Y.-S (**1958**). "Synchrony of neural activity in electric responses evoked by transient acoustic stimuli," J.Acoust.Soc. Amer. **30**, 1030-1045.

Harrison, R.V. and Prijs, V.F. (**1984**). "Single cochlear fibre responses in guinea pigs with long-term endolymphatic hydrops," Hearing Res. **14**, 179-184.

Horst, J.W., Javel, E., and Farley, G.R. (**1985**). "Extraction and enhancement of spectral structure by the cochlea," J.Acoust.Soc.Am. **78**, 1898-1901.

Lütkenhöner, B., Hoke, M. and Bappert, E. (**1980**). "Effect of recovery properties on the discharge pattern of auditory nerve fibres." In: *Cochlear and brainstem evoked response audiometry and electrical stimulation of the VIIIth nerve*, edited by M.Hoke, G.Kauffmann, E.Bappert, Scand.Audiol. Suppl. **11**, pp. 25-43.

Patuzzi, R., and Sellick, P.M. (**1983**). "A comparison between basilar membrane and inner cell receptor potential input-output functions in the guinea pig cochlea," J.Acoust.Soc.Am. **74**, 1734-1741.

Prijs, V.F. (**1986**). "Single-unit response at the round window of the guinea pig," Hearing Res. **21**, 127-133.

Russel, I.J., and Sellick, P.M. (**1978**). "Intra cellular studies of hair cells in the mammalian cochlea," J.Physiol. **284**, 261-290.

Sachs, M.B., and Abbas, P.J. (**1974**). " Rate versus level functions for auditory-nerve fibres in cats: Tone-burst stimuli," J.Acoust.Soc.Am. **56**, 1835-1847.

Smith, R.L. and Brachman, M.L. (**1980**). "Response modulation of auditory-nerve fibres by AM stimuli: effects of average intensity," Hearing Res. **2**, 123-133.

Smith, R.L. and Brachman, M.L. (**1982**). "Adaptation in auditory-nerve fibres: a revised model," Biol.Cyber. **44**, 107-120.

Yates, G.K. (**1987**). "Dynamic effects in the input/output relationship of auditory nerve," Hearing Res. **27**, 221-230.

Comments

Evans:

On other grounds, I am happy with your conclusion, but not from your data! Your Fig.6 is clearly obtained from a guinea pig cochlea in poor physiological condition, as judged by the high threshold and broad tuning of the cochlear fibre. Opponents of your conclusion could well argue that because many cochlear non-linearities are eliminated by cochlear pathology, you have not shown appropriate evidence. Do you obtain good correspondence between static and dynamic tuning in cochlear fibres from normal cochleas in good condition?

Reply by Prijs:

I agree with your point of poor physiological condition. I had to emphasize that also in normal cochleas identical results were found. Figure 6 was presented because it was the most complete set of data.

Physiological mechanisms of masking

Bertrand Delgutte

*Research Laboratory of Electronics,
Massachusetts Institute of Technology, Cambridge, Massachusetts,
and Eaton-Peabody Laboratory,
Massachusetts Eye and Ear Infirmary, Boston, Massachusetts.*

Introduction

The idea that psychophysical masking patterns produced by acoustic stimuli are closely related to their patterns of excitation along the cochlea (Wegel and Lane, 1924; Fletcher, 1940; Zwicker, 1970), has been useful in hearing theory. This correspondence is based on the view that masking is due to the spread of the excitation produced by the masker to the place of the tone signal along the cochlea. Studies of two-tone suppression in auditory-nerve fibers (Sachs and Kiang, 1968) challenged this classical view because masking might be due to the suppression of the neural responses to the signal by the masker, even if the masker does not excite neurons tuned to the signal frequency (Javel *et al*., 1983; Pickles, 1984; Sinex and Havey, 1986)[1]. This possibility that suppression contributes to masking when the signal and the masker are simultaneously presented led Houtgast (1974) to propose that nonsimultaneous masking techniques (such as pulsation thresholds) might better reflect the pattern of excitation produced by the masker than simultaneous masking. In this paper, we compare masked thresholds of auditory-nerve fibers obtained by simultaneous and nonsimultaneous techniques in order to separate the contributions of two-tone rate suppression and spread of excitation to tone-on-tone masking. The results show that physiological masking is both excitatory and suppressive, with the relative importance of the two mechanisms being dependent on the masker level and the frequency separation between signal and masker.

Figure 1 illustrates how spread of excitation and suppression might mask the response of an auditory-nerve fiber to a tone signal. Each panel shows discharge rate as a function of signal level both in the presence and in the absence of a fixed masker. In Fig. 1A, the masker is excitatory because it produces an increase in discharge rate over spontaneous. Two-tone rate suppression does not occur because the rate in response to the signal plus the

---

1. Either of two response measures might be suppressed, the average rate of discharge, or the synchrony of discharges to the signal frequency. This paper concerns the role of two-tone RATE suppression in masking.

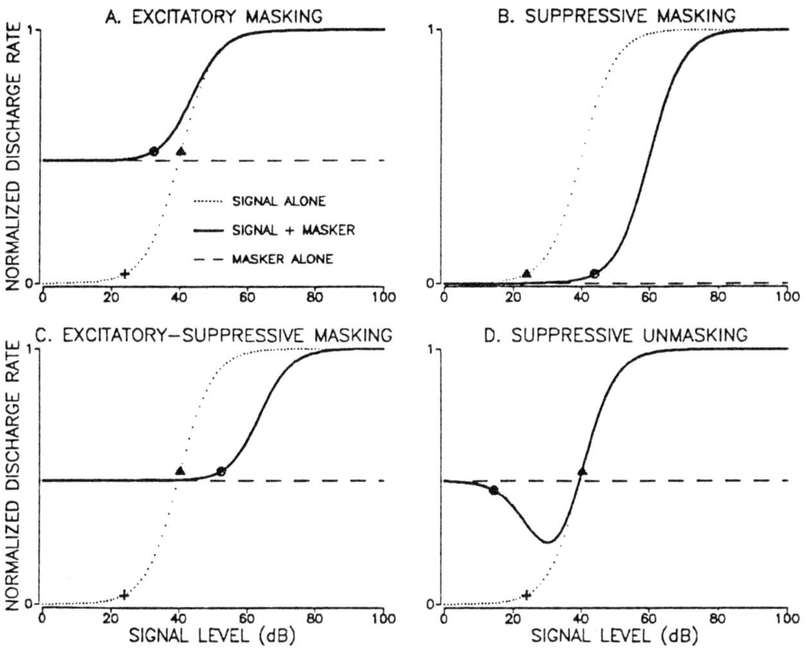

Figure. 1. Schematic discharge rate of an auditory-nerve fiber as a function of the level of a tone signal, both in the presence and in the absence of different maskers. Crosses refer to thresholds in quiet, circles to simultaneous masked thresholds, and triangles to nonsimultaneous thresholds.

masker is never lower than the rate for the signal alone. The physiological masked threshold is the level at which the rate produced by the signal plus the masker exceeds the rate for the masker alone by a certain probabilistic criterion. Masking is said to occur because the masked threshold is higher than the threshold in quiet, which is the level for which the response to the signal alone exceeds spontaneous rate by criterion. In contrast to the excitatory masking of Fig. 1A, Figure 1B illustrates suppressive masking. The masker produces no increment in discharge rage over spontaneous, but shifts the rate-level function for the signal towards high intensities, resulting in a threshold elevation. Excitatory masking and suppressive masking are not mutually exclusive, as shown in Fig. 1C. The masker is excitatory, and suppresses the response to the signal because the rate for the signal plus masker is lower than the rate for the signal alone over a range of signal levels.

One can discriminate between the three forms of masking shown in Fig. 1A-C by measuring three types of thresholds from auditory-nerve fibers for each masker and signal frequency. Two of these thresholds have already been defined: These are the threshold in quiet, and the simultaneous masked threshold. The third threshold is the signal level for which the discharge rate in response to the signal alone exceeds the response to the masker alone by criterion. This "nonsimultaneous" threshold is similar in concept to the pulsation threshold in psychophysics (Houtgast, 1974). Like the pulsation threshold, it is not, strictly speaking, a *masked* threshold because the signal is detectable below threshold. The key point is that the difference between the simultaneous threshold and the nonsimultaneous threshold gives a measure of the contribution of suppression to masking because there is no suppression when the signal and the masker are not simultaneously present. Figure 1A shows that, when masking is excitatory, the simultaneous threshold is slightly lower than the nonsimultaneous threshold, and both masked thresholds exceed the threshold in quiet. In contrast, when masking is suppressive (Fig. 1B), the simultaneous threshold is higher than the nonsimultaneous threshold, and the threshold in quiet coincides with the nonsimultaneous threshold. When masking is both excitatory and suppressive (Fig. 1C), the simultaneous threshold is above the nonsimultaneous threshold, and both masked thresholds exceed the threshold in quiet[2].

Method

Methods for recording from auditory-nerve fibers in anesthetized cats were basically as described by Kiang *et al.* (1965). For each fiber, three threshold measurements were made for a range of signal frequencies centered at the CF. The masker was always a 1-kHz tone at either 60 or 80 dB SPL. Figure 2A shows the method for measuring simultaneous masked thresholds, which mimics the two-tone, two-alternative forced choice paradigm of psychophysics. A pair of stimuli is presented repeatedly in random order. One stimulus is a 50-ms burst of sound consisting of a fixed 1-kHz masker and a variable tone signal, while the other stimulus is the masker alone. The signal level is adjusted by means of a PEST procedure (Taylor and Creeman, 1967) so that the spike count in response the signal plus the masker exceeds the count for the masker alone for 75% of the presentations. Figure 2B shows the method for measuring nonsimultaneous masked thresholds. The stimulus pair now consists of the masker alone and the signal alone, and the signal level is adjusted by PEST so that the spike count for the signal exceeds the count for the masker 75% of the time. Thresholds in quiet were measured by the same method as either masked threshold except that the masker was omitted.

Results

Figure 3A shows the threshold in quiet, the simultaneous masked threshold, and the nonsimultaneous threshold as a function of signal frequency for three auditory-nerve fibers from one cat. The masker was a 1-kHz tone at 60 dB

---

2. More precisely, because the difference between simultaneous and nonsimultaneous thresholds is slightly negative for excitatory masking, this difference might remain negative even when there is a small suppression. However, a positive difference always indicates a contribution of suppression to masking.

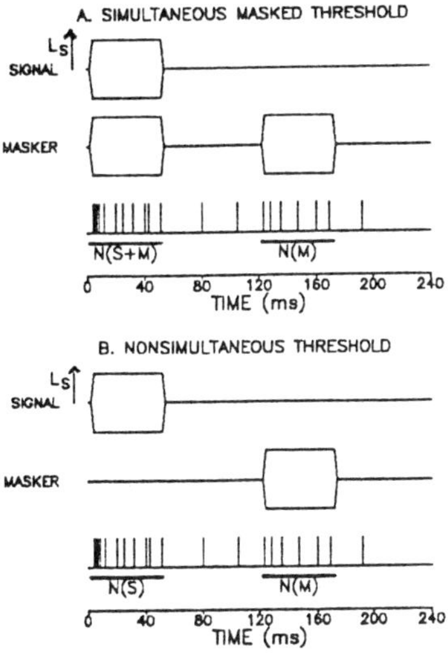

Figure 2. Stimulus paradigms used measuring simultaneous and nonsimultaneous masked thresholds of auditory-nerve fibers.

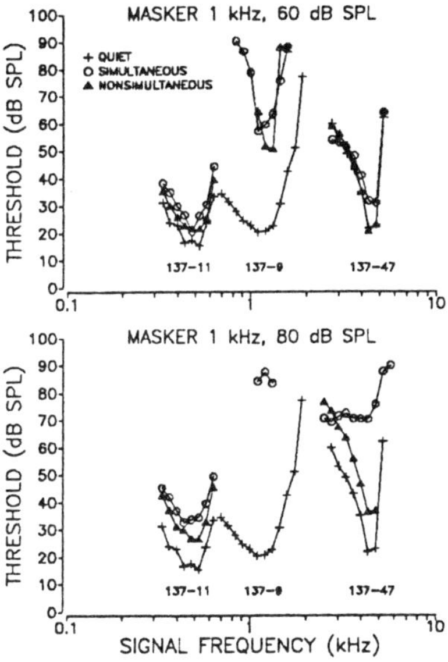

Figure 3. Threshold in quiet, for simultaneous masked threshold, and nonsimultaneous threshold as a function of signal frequency for three auditory-nerve fibers from one cat, and for two intensities of a 1-kHz masker.

SPL. The CF of the center fiber is 1.2 kHz, close to the masker frequency. For this fiber, thresholds in both masking conditions are elevated by about 30 dB over thresholds in quiet. Masking is much smaller for the other two fibers, whose CF's are far from the 1-kHz masker frequency. For both the 0.5-kHz and the 1.2-kHz fibers, masking is largely excitatory because thresholds in the simultaneous and nonsimultaneous conditions are similar. In contrast, masking is suppressive for the 4.6-kHz fiber, because the simultaneous masked thresholds exceed thresholds in quiet by about 10 dB near the CF, while the nonsimultaneous thresholds nearly coincide with thresholds in quiet.

Figure 3B shows masked thresholds for the same fibers as in Fig. 3A when the level of the 1-kHz masker is raised to 80 dB SPL. For the 1.2-kHz fiber, simultaneous masked thresholds were greater than 95 dB SPL, except for 3 signal frequencies near the CF[3]. For the 0.5-kHz fiber, the 20-dB increase in masker level results in only a 12-dB increase in simultaneous masked

3. This fiber was "lost" before nonsimultaneous thresholds could be measured.

thresholds, and even less for nonsimultaneous thresholds. In contrast, for the 4.6-kHz fiber, there is a 40-dB increase in simultaneous masked thresholds for signal frequencies near the CF. Nonsimultaneous thresholds are considerably lower than simultaneous thresholds, suggesting that masking is primarily suppressive for this fiber.

In order to relate these physiological data to psychophysical masking patterns, we need to examine masked thresholds of auditory-nerve fibers as a function of their points of innervation along the cochlea. It seems likely that, for any given signal and masker, it is the fibers with the lowest masked thresholds that provide most information for detecting the signal. Therefore, for each masker level and signal frequency, a V-shaped curve was fit to the patterns of fiber thresholds against CF. The tip of the V defines the "best threshold" for that signal frequency. Figure 4 shows best thresholds as a function of signal frequency, in quiet, and for both a simultaneous and a nonsimultaneous 1-kHz masker at 60 dB SPL. Best thresholds in simultaneous masking are maximum for signal frequencies near the 1-kHz masker, and decay more gradually from maximum for signal frequencies above the masker frequency than for frequencies below the masker, as shown by Sinex and Havey (1986). Best thresholds in the nonsimultaneous condition are below simultaneous thresholds over a broad range of signal frequencies both below and above 1 kHz. Thus, suppression contributes to masking for these frequencies. However, for signal frequencies near the masker, nonsimultaneous thresholds exceed simultaneous threshold, indicating that masking is excitatory in that range. Overall, the nonsimultaneous masking pattern is more sharply tuned than the simultaneous pattern.

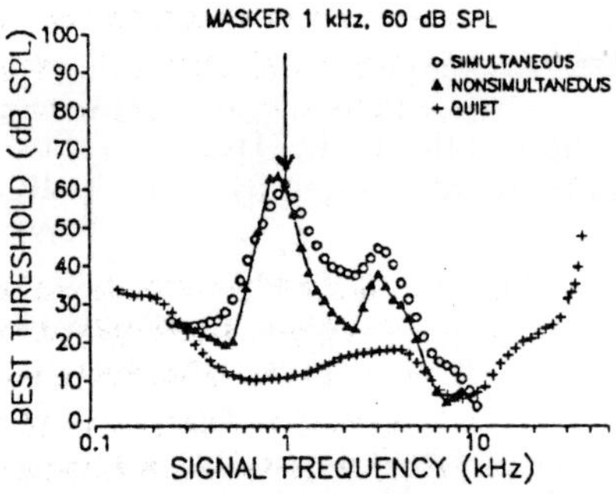

Figure 4. Best thresholds of auditory-nerve fibers as a function of signal frequency, in quiet, and for both simultaneous and nonsimultaneous 1-kHz masker at 60 dB SPL. Each data point is obtained from threshold measurements in at least 10 auditory-nerve fibers.

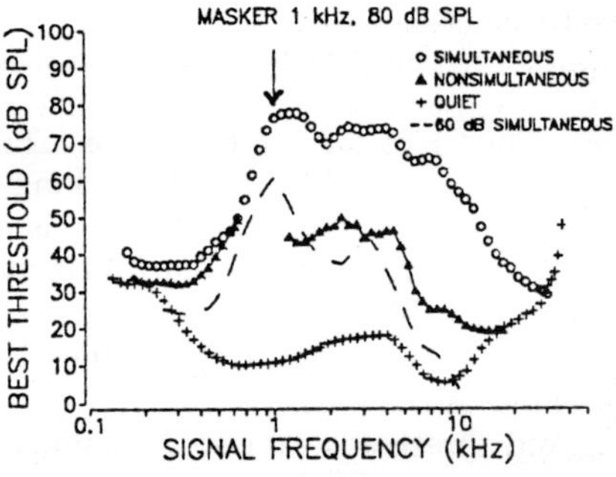

Figure 5. Same as Fig. 4 for an 80-dB masker. The available data did not allow reliable estimates of best nonsimultaneous thresholds for signal frequencies near 1 kHz.

Figure 5 shows best thresholds patterns when the level of the 1-kHz masker is raised to 80 dB. At this level, simultaneous masking extends much farther toward the high frequencies than at the lower level. For signal frequencies near and below 1 kHz, simultaneous masking grows by 15 to 20 dB for the 20 dB increase in masker level. In contrast, for signal frequencies well above 1 kHz, the difference in thresholds between the two levels reaches 40 to 50 dB. This supralinear growth of physiological masking for signal frequencies above the masker has been observed by Sinex and Havey (1986). A key question is whether it is due to an increase in suppression or an increase in excitation. Figure 5 shows that, for the 80 dB masker, nonsimultaneous thresholds are about 40 dB below simultaneous thresholds for signal frequencies well above the masker. This threshold difference, which we attribute to suppression, is only 5 to 10 dB for the 60-dB masker (Fig. 4). Therefore, it seems that the supralinear growth of masking is primarily due to the rapid growth of suppression rather than to the growth of excitation. This result fits well with the fact that the rate of growth of two-tone rate suppression with suppressor level is about 2 dB/dB for suppressors below the CF (Abbas and Sachs, 1976; Delgutte, 1986; Costalupes *et al.*, 1987).

Discussion

The goal of this study was to identify the contributions of suppression and spread of excitation to tone-on-tone masking by comparing the masked thresholds of auditory-nerve fibers measured with simultaneous and nonsimultaneous techniques. For 1-kHz maskers at 60 and 80 dB SPL, simultaneous masked thresholds were above nonsimultaneous thresholds over most of the range of signal frequencies, with the possible exception of the immediate vicinity of the masker frequency (Fig. 4 and 5). This shows that physiological masking is, in general, both excitatory and suppressive. Excitatory masking dominates for signal frequencies near and below the masker frequency, although suppression also contributes somewhat below the masker frequency. Suppressive masking dominates for signal frequencies well above the masker, particularly with the 80-dB masker.

The role of suppression in masking is complicated by the possibility that an off-CF signal might suppress the response to a simultaneous masker, as illustrated in Fig. 1D. The masker produces an increment in rate over spontaneous. When the signal level is raised in the presence of the masker, discharge rate first decreases due to suppression by the signal, then increases when the signal becomes excitatory. The masked threshold is now the level at which the rate for the signal plus masker is *lower* than the rate for the masker by criterion. The masked threshold is below the threshold in quiet, indicating that signals which, by themselves, cannot be detected, become detectable when the masker is introduced. This "unmasking" phenomenon should be taken into account in estimating best thresholds. For about 20 auditory-nerve fibers, we measured "unmasking thresholds" by substituting a probability criterion of 25% for that of 75% in the PEST procedure, and reversing the direction of level changes. With a 1-kHz simultaneous masker at 60 dB SPL, unmasking thresholds were above the best threshold curve of Fig. 4 for all fibers and all signal frequencies. On the basis of these preliminary data, it does not appear likely that taking into account the suppression of the masker response by the signal would greatly change the physiological masking patterns of Fig. 4 and 5. A similar conclusion was reached by Sinex and Havey (1986).

Our conclusions concerning the role of suppression in simultaneous masking differ somewhat from those of Pickles (1984). By comparing the discharge rates of auditory-nerve fibers at masked threshold with the rate at the threshold in quiet, Pickles concluded that masking is excitatory, except for a narrow range of signal frequencies below the masker frequency in which masking is suppressive. However, a greater rate at masked threshold than at the threshold in quiet only implies that masking is *partly* excitatory, and does not rule out a suppressive component (Fig. 1C). Thus Pickles' results are consistent with our conclusion that masking is generally both excitatory and suppressive.

The physiological masking patterns of Fig. 4 and 5 resemble psychophysical masking patterns in many respects (Wegel and Lane, 1924; Houtgast, 1974). Both have a maximum near the masker frequency, and a pronounced skew towards high frequencies. Both physiological and psychophysical masking patterns are more sharply tuned in nonsimultaneous than in simultaneous masking[4]. In simultaneous masking, both physiological and psychophysical masked thresholds grow faster than linearly with masker level for signal frequencies above the masker, a phenomenon called "upward spread of masking". Because nonsimultaneous thresholds (which do not include effects of suppression) do not grow so rapidly with masker level, we concluded that the upward spread of simultaneous masking is due primarily to the supralinear growth of suppression rather than to the growth of excitation. If true, this conclusion has implications for the interpretation of psychophysical experiments. For example, Zwicker (1970) explained the decrease in puretone intensity difference limens (DL) with increasing stimulus level in terms of the nonlinear growth of simultaneous masking patterns. Our results suggest that this interpretation is incorrect because the nonlinear growth in masking is due to suppression, which does not occur for single tones. Florentine and Buus (1981) have provided an alternative explanation for the decrease in DL with intensity which does not require a nonlinear growth in excitation patterns.

In conclusion, both suppression and spread of excitation are important for explaining psychophysical data on simultaneous masking in terms of physiological mechanisms. Specifically, our results suggest that spread of

---

4. Lufti's (1988) recent psychophysical data show roughly the same sharpness of tuning in simultaneous and in forward masking. However, his results are limited to signal frequencies within a half-octave of the masker frequency, whereas we find the largest difference between the two masking conditions for signal frequencies well above the masker.

excitation determines the overall shape of masking patterns, while suppression is largely responsible for the upward spread of simultaneous masking and for differences between simultaneous and nonsimultaneous masking. This implies that psychophysical masking patterns obtained by simultaneous techniques can only provide a crude representation of the pattern of activity produced by the masker at peripheral stages of the auditory system because these masking patterns also reflect suppression of the signal by the masker. This representation will be particularly distorted when the masker includes intense low-frequency components such as the first formant of speech.

Acknowledgement

This research was supported by NIH grant NS13126. I thank L.D. Braida, M.C. Brown, J.L. Goldstein, and N.Y.S. Kiang for their valuable comments.

References

Abbas, P.J., and Sachs, M.B. (**1976**). "Two-tone suppression in auditory-nerve fibers: Extension of a stimulus-response relationship," J.Acoust.Soc. Am. **59**, 112-122.

Costalupes, J.A., Rich, N.C., and Ruggero, M.A. (**1987**). "Effects of excitatory and nonexcitatory suppressor tones on two-tone rate suppression in auditory-nerve fibers," Hearing Res. **26**, 155-164.

Delgutte, B. (**1986**). "Two-tone rate suppression in auditory-nerve fibers: Variations with suppressor level and frequency," Abstr. 9th Midwinter Res. Meet. A.R.O., Clearwater, FL.

Fletcher, H. (**1940**). "Auditory patterns," Rev. Mod. Physics **12**, 47-65.

Florentine, M., and Buus, S. (**1981**). "An excitation-pattern model for intensity discrimination," J.Acoust.Soc.Am. **70**, 1646-1654.

Houtgast, T. (**1974**). *Lateral Suppression in Hearing*. (Academische Pers, Amsterdam).

Javel, E., McGee, J., Walsh, E.J., Farley, G.R., and Gorga, M.P. (**1983**). "Suppression of auditory-nerve responses II. Suppression threshold and growth, isosuppression contours," J.Acoust.Soc.Am. **74**, 801-813.

Kiang, N.Y.S., Watanabe, T., Thomas, E.C., and Clark, L.F. (**1965a**). *Discharge patterns of single fibers in the cat's auditory nerve*. Research Monograph #35 (MIT Press, Cambridge, MA).

Liberman, M.C. (**1978**). "Auditory-nerve response from cats raised in a low-noise chamber," J.Acoust.Soc.Am. **63**, 442-455.

Lufti, R.A. (**1988**). "Interpreting measures of frequency selectivity: Is forward masking special?," J.Acoust.Soc.Am. **83**, 167-177.

Pickles, J.O. (**1984**). "Frequency threshold curves and simultaneous masking functions in single fibres of the guinea pig auditory nerve," Hearing Res. **14**, 245-256.

Sachs, M.B., and Kiang, N.Y.S. (**1968**). "Two-tone inhibition in auditory-nerve fibers," J.Acoust.Soc.Am. **43**, 1120-1128.

Schalk, T.B., and Sachs, M.B. (**1980**). "Nonlinearities in auditory-nerve fiber responses to bandlimited noise," J.Acoust.Soc.Am. **67**, 903-913.

Sinex, D.G., and Havey, D.C. (**1986**). "Neural Mechanisms of tone-on-tone masking: Patterns of discharge rate and discharge synchrony related to rates of spontaneous discharge in the chinchilla auditory nerve," J.Neurophysiol. **56**, 1763-1780.

Taylor, M.M., and Creeman, C.D. (**1967**). "PEST: Efficient estimates of probability functions," J.Acoust.Soc.Am. **41**, 782-787.

Wegel, R.L., and Lane, C.E. (**1924**). "The auditory masking of one pure tone by another and its possible relation to the dynamics of the inner ear," Physics Rev. **23**, 266-285.

Zwicker, E. (**1970**). "Masking and psychological excitation as consequences of the ear's frequency analysis," in *Frequency Analysis and Periodicity in Hearing*, edited by R. Plomp and G.F. Smoorenburg (Sijthoff, Leiden), pp 376-396.

Comments

Moore:

At first sight, there appears to be a discrepancy between your results and the view commonly held by psychophysicists that the effects of suppression are not revealed in simultaneous masking (Houtgast, 1974; for a review see Moore and O'Loughlin, 1986); you suggest that suppression is largely responsible for the upward spread of simultaneous masking. I think that the discrepancy can be resolved if we postulate that the excitation pattern for a pure tone (the masker in this case) can be sharpened by suppression; activity at the peak of the pattern suppresses weaker activity on the skirts, an effect which we can call self-suppression. Your masking patterns determined in 'nonsimultaneous masking' include the effects of this self-suppression. Indeed, when only a single pure tone is presented at a time, physiological estimates of frequency selectivity always include the effects of self-suppression. In simultaneous masking the suppression is applied both to the signal and to the masker. This does not change the signal-to-masker ratio in any channel (relative to what it would be without suppression), but the overall effect is that the signal threshold is higher in simultaneous than in nonsimultaneous masking. In summary, I would interpret your results in this way: Masking patterns are sharply tuned in nonsimultaneous masking since the effects of self-suppression are revealed. Masking patterns in simultaneous masking are less sharply tuned since the suppression affects both the masker and the signal; the simultaneous masking patterns can be thought of as revealing what the excitation pattern of the masker would be like if no suppression were occurring.

Moore, B.C.J. and O'Loughlin, B.J. (1986). "The use of nonsimultaneous masking to measure frequency selectivity and suppression", in: Frequency Selectivity in Hearing, edited by B.C.J. Moore (Academic).

Reply by Delgutte:

Moore postulates the existence of self-supression for single tones in order to resolve the apparent discrepancy between my results and the view that effects of suppression are not revealed in simultaneous masking. I will argue that this notion of self suppression is unnecessary, and inconsistent with the generally-accepted physiological definition of suppression. In physiology, suppression is aid to occur when the response of an auditory-nerve fiber to a tone stimulus (the *excitor*) is decreased by the introduction of a second stimulus (the *suppressor*). According to this definition, suppression does not occur for single-tone stimuli providing that the response increases monotonically with intensity.

My results can be reconciled with psychophysicists' views of masking without postulating the existence of self suppression if we distinguish between the suppression exerted by the masker on the tone signal (*"masker-to-signal suppression"*) and the effects of suppression among different frequency components of a complex masker (*"within-masker suppression"*). Specifically, it is hypothesized that both masker-to-signal and within-masker suppressions occur in simultaneous masking, whereas only within-masker suppression occurs in nonsimultaneous masking. If the masker is a single tone, there is no within-masker suppression. The observation that masking patterns are broader in simultaneous than in nonsimultaneous masking is explained by the fact that simultaneous masking is due to masker-to-signal suppression in addition to spread of excitation, as shown in my paper. A two-tone masker consisting of an excitor and a suppressor produces less nonsimultaneous masking than the excitor alone because the excitation produced by the excitor decreases when the suppressor is introduced. Thus, nonsimultaneous masking reveals the effects of *within-masker* suppression, consistent with physiological data. The observation that effects of *within-masker* suppression are not revealed in simultaneous masking can be explained by assuming that, when the signal is at the excitor frequency, the suppressor attenuates the responses to both the signal and the excitor by *the same amount* (Houtgast, 1974). With this assumption, the simultaneous masked threshold should be about the same in the presence and in the absence of the suppressor, consistent with psychophysical findings. The assumption that the excitor and the same-frequency signal are equally suppressed is consistent with physiological data showing that the suppression (expressed in decibels) produced by a fixed stimulus is approximately constant over of broad range of excitor intensities (Javel *et al.*, 1978).

In summary, the distinction between within-masker suppression and masker-to signal suppression provides a simple explanation for differences between simultaneous and nonsimultaneous masking with holds for single-tone and multiple-component maskers, and is consistent with physiological and psychophysical data. The view that effects of suppression are revealed in nonsimultaneous masking, but not in simultaneous masking, is confirmed, with the restriction that this statement applies to *within-masker* suppression.

Javel, E., Geisler, C.D., and Ravindran, A. (1978). "Two-tone suppression in auditory nerve of the cat: Rate-intensity and temporal analyses," J. Acoust. Soc. Am. 63, 1093-1104.

Rosen:

What is the reason for the second, higher frequency peak apart from the expected peak at 1 kHz in figure 4?

Reply by Delgutte:

I do not know. Perhaps it is related to the "3-kHz notch" often seen in patterns of auditory-nerve fibre thresholds against CF. (Liberman, 1978).

Pickles:

1. The results and analysis presented in my 1984 paper quite clearly support the composite excitatory-suppressive model which you put forward here. The results of that paper showed that the masker suppressed the signal, and masked the suppressed signal with excitation.

2. Is it right to call the curves of the present paper "non-simultaneous thresholds"? Surely, in the configuration shown in Fig. 2b, there is no masking of the signal by the masker (particularly when the signal comes first!). Rather, do not the "nonsimultaneous masked functions" of your figures just correspond to iso-rate tuning curves?

Pickles, J.O. (1984). "Frequency threshold curves and simultaneous masking functions in single fibres of the guinea pig auditory nerve," Hearing Res. 14, 245-256.

Frequency-difference thresholds for tone and noise stimulus combinations in the cat

J. A. Costalupes

Dept. of Otolaryngology, University of Minnesota
Minneapolis, MN 55455 USA

Introduction

Relatively little is known about the properties of frequency resolution in the behaving cat. While behavioral detection thresholds have been described for a number of stimulus conditions, descriptions of the ability of cats to resolve spectral information is a necessary adjunct to physiological studies in using the cat as an animal model of hearing in humans. In this study, frequency-difference thresholds are described for a 1-kHz tone in quiet and in noise over a range of intensities using a detection index analogous to the criterion-free measure used in human studies. Results are compared with human studies and with what is known about the underlying representation of this stimulus complex in the pattern of neural activity.

Method

One healthy cat was trained as a psychophysical observer. The cat was approximately nine months old at the time of testing and had no previous testing experience. External ears were inspected periodically and appeared normal throughout the study. A behavioral audiogram obtained at the end of testing indicated that the cat's hearing range was within normal limits previously reported for the cat using a food-reinforcement behavioral paradigm (Orr *et al.*, 1977; Gerken and Sandlin, 1977; Costalupes, 1983a).

All testing was conducted in a behavioral testing apparatus similar to the one described by Orr *et al.* (1977). The cat was restrained in an upright sitting position by a neckyoke fastened to a pair of sidepanels attached to the floor of the apparatus. An array of three high-intensity "ready" lights, a feeding nozzle, and trough were immediately in front of the cat. Two large mechanical footpedals were located at the cat's forepaws so that it could sit comfortably with one foot on each pedal. The device was enclosed in a wire cage located on a table in the middle of a sound-attenuating chamber. Tone and noise stimuli were delivered by an 8-in dual cone speaker suspended near the cat's head. The sound field was approximately flat up to 8 kHz and harmonic distortion was within acceptable limits. Tone levels are expressed here as dB *re* 20 μPa (i.e., dB SPL) and noise spectrum level is expressed as dB *re* 20 μPa/$\sqrt{}$Hz. All experiments were run under computer control.

Frequency-difference thresholds were obtained using a two-alternative forced choice procedure. The method was a modification of the method described by Orr *et al.* (1977) for obtaining absolute thresholds from cats. The procedure called for the cat to depress both footpedals to begin a trial, to hold both pedals for a silent hold period, and to release one of the pedals to indicate detection of the corresponding stimulus.

A trial consisted of the silent hold period followed by a series of 200-ms tone bursts (rise/fall times=10 ms) delivered at 50-ms intervals. The tone burst sequence ran continuously until one of the pedals was released. Illumination of the ready lights indicated that a trial could be initiated by depressing both footpedals. The duration of the hold period varied from 1-5 s and was randomly selected in 500-ms increments on each trial. If either pedal was released during the initial 500-ms of the hold period, the trial was aborted and recycled without delay. This allowed the cat to make arbitrary movements without initializing a trial. If either pedal was released during the remainder of the hold period, the trial was aborted and recycled after a 4-s timeout, during which the ready lights were extinguished and the footpedals were inoperative. Such a response was scored as an early release.

The hold period was followed by presentation of the tone burst sequence. The standard stimulus was a 1000-Hz tone. Two stimulus conditions were used. On test trials, standard tone bursts alternated with higher frequency comparison tone bursts. The cat indicated detection of the alternating tone sequence by releasing the left footpedal. On control trials, only standard tone bursts were presented. The cat indicated detection of the control sequence by releasing the right footpedal. Responses were counted only when they occured at least 150 ms after the onset of the second tone burst in the series. Shorter response latencies were treated as early releases. A correct response (i.e., releasing the left footpedal for the alternating sequence and the right pedal for the control sequence) was rewarded with 2-3 cc of liquefied cat food. An incorrect response resulted in a 4-s timeout, during which the ready lights were extinguished and the footpedals were inoperative. In the event of an incorrect response on a control trial, the control stimulus was repeated on subsequent trials until a correct response was scored. Control trials were randomly distributed throughout the block of 35-50 trials and accounted for about one-third of the total trials in a block.

The frequency of the comparison tone was varied on each trial by titration. Following a correct response to the alternating stimulus, the frequency separation between standard and comparison tones was reduced by one-half. Following an incorrect response, frequency separation was doubled. Maximum and minimum separations were 256 Hz and 4 Hz for the tone alone condition and 512 Hz and 8 Hz for the tone in noise condition. The cat's performance was evaluated by pooling results at each frequency separation across blocks. Responses on control trials were classified according to the magnitude of the nearest preceeding frequency separation and were similarly pooled across blocks.

Training on the task to a criterion performance level required about ten weeks. Actual testing lasted about four months, during which the cat ran two one-hour sessions a day, seven days a week. Throughout the study the cat maintained excellent health and a gentle, good-natured disposition.

Results

Tone alone

Results are based on data obtained from fifteen individual blocks using a 1000-Hz standard tone at an intensity of 65 dB SPL. Contingencies were set regarding early release rates and tracking behavior. Figure 1 shows correct responses to the alternating stimulus sequence (i.e., hits) as a function of frequency separation (ΔF). Performance results at 256 Hz were contaminated by a ceiling effect and have been excluded. As the arrow indicates, the 50% hit rate extrapolated from the ordinate occurs at a frequency separation of 21 Hz. This is somewhat larger than the range of values reported for the cat by Elliott *et al.* (1960), who obtained a mean value of 8 Hz. Operant response levels were probably strongly influenced by their avoidance conditioning method. Hienz and Sheckler (1987), on the other hand, used a food-reward paradigm and reported thresholds of 35-60 Hz for a 1000-Hz tone in the cat.

Analysis of response latencies supports the reliability of the method. Figure 2 shows response latencies obtained from the hit values in Fig. 1. Maximum mean latency occurs at 16 Hz and decreases monotonically as frequency separation increases. The shift to shorter response latencies at 4 and 8 Hz suggests that the cat did not respond reliably to the stimulus at these frequency separations. Response latencies noted here are consistent with

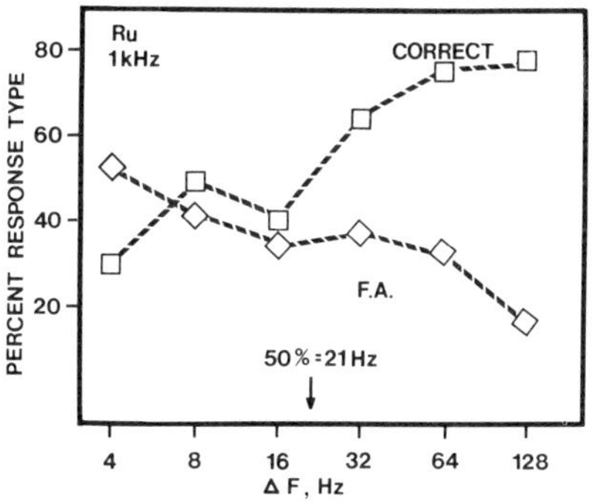

Figure 1. Percent hits (squares) and false alarms (diamonds) as a function of frequency separation. Arrow indicates 50% hit rate.

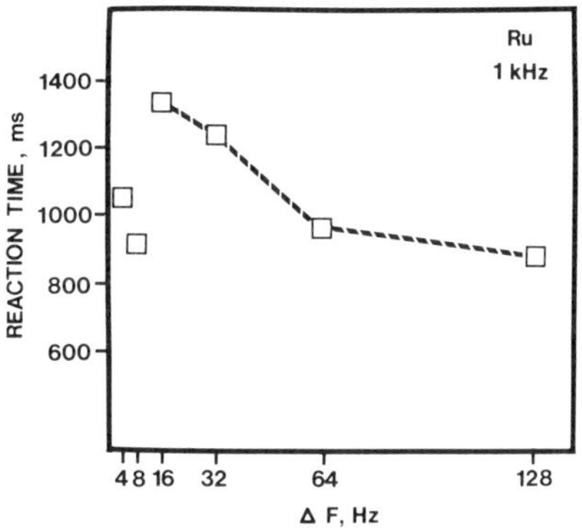

Figure 2. Mean response latencies (ordinate) for hit responses shown in Fig. 1 as a function of frequency separation (abscissa).

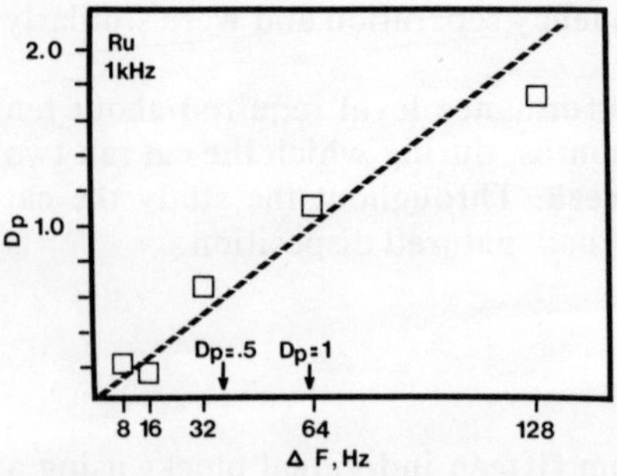

Figure 3. Dp (ordinate) as a function of frequency separation for the tone alone. Straight line is a best fit through the origin. Arrows indicate Dp=0.5 (31 Hz) and Dp=1.0 (63 Hz).

latencies reported previously for the cat (Costalupes, 1983a).

Figure 1 also indicates incorrect responses to the control stimulus (i.e., false alarms) associated with each frequency separation. The figure shows that false alarm rates tend to decrease at successively wider frequency separations. This trend was noted for data similarly obtained from the chinchilla by Nelson and Kiester (1978).

One of the objectives of this study was to obtain a criterion-free response measure of frequency-difference thresholds in the cat. To achieve this, the hit and false alarm rate data were converted to a detectability index comparable to d'. Since the assumptions underlying the use of d' may not apply in the case of the behaving cat, the measure is refered to as Dp. Figure 3 shows Dp as a function of frequency separation for the data in Fig. 1. Note that frequency is represented on linear cordinates for clarity. The straight line has been fit to pass through the origin. The arrows indicate that a Dp of 0.5 corresponds to 31 Hz and a Dp of 1.0 corresponds to 63 Hz. A regression line fit to the data on a log frequency abscissa revealed corresponding Dp's of 26 and 59 Hz, respectively.

Tone in noise

Another objective of the study was to describe frequency-difference thresholds for a 1000-Hz tone in the presence of continuous, wideband noise. It is of interest to determine how noise affects frequency-difference thresholds and, in particular, how detectability will be affected for a given signal-to-noise ratio when overall level is varied. The four noise spectrum levels selected were 10, 20, 30, and 40 dB. Corresponding tone levels of 42, 52, 62, and 72 dB were selected as being approximately 10 dB above the mean behavioral detection threshold for a 1-kHz tone in noise reported for the cat (Costalupes, 1983b).

Figure 4 shows Dp as a function of frequency separation for the 1000-Hz stimulus in the presence of continuous noise at four intensities indicated in the figure. Data are based on five blocks run at each combined noise and tone level. Symbols are indicated only where reliable estimates of Dp could be obtained. The straight line is a regression line fit to the tone alone data and is included for comparison with the noise data. Regression lines were similarly fit to each set of data points for the tone in noise condition and Dp=1 was extrapolated. Although it is not clear whether the slopes of the lines fit to each set of points varied in any systematic way, a comparable overall decrease in the detectability of the alternating stimulus sequence is apparent at each of the stimulus levels. A notable exception occured at a noise spectrum level of 10 dB, where the cat's performance deteriorated markedly. As shown in Fig. 4 (filled squares), reliable estimates of Dp could be determined only at the two widest frequency separations. These data are based on two rather than five blocks of trials due to the cat's intolerance toward working at this stimulus level. This can be attributed to a loss of detectability of the tone signal in the presence of noise at this level. It has been shown that a precipitous rise in the signal-to-noise ratio at the threshold for detection occurs for most cats at noise spectrum levels of 3-13 dB and below (Costalupes, 1983b). Thus, it is likely that the relative level of the tone stimulus was too near detection threshold for the cat to work comfortably.

Figure 5 describes the behavior of frequency-difference thresholds for 1000-Hz tones in noise over a range of intensities at a selected signal-to-noise ratio. Frequency-difference thresholds were determined at Dp=1 from the data shown in Fig. 4. Frequency-separation corresponding to Dp=1 is indicated along the ordinate and noise spectrum level is indicated along the abscissa. Recall that the signal-to-noise ratio of the stimulus combination was approximately 10 dB above mean detection threshold at each of the overall intensities, although there may have been some loss in detectability at the lowest noise level. The data reveal an overall decrease in frequency-difference thresholds as absolute levels rise from moderate to high intensities. There appears to be little improvement, however, at the three highest levels tested.

Discussion

Previous studies have reported similar trends in cat behavioral data and human psychophysical data (Watson, 1963; Pickles, 1975; Costalupes, 1983b), suggesting that the cat is a good animal model of hearing in humans. Results of this study indicate that frequency-difference threshold at 1 kHz is much larger and the psychometric function is shallower than in humans (Jesteadt and Sims, 1975). The psychometric function for the cat is similar to that reported for the chinchilla (Nelson and Kiester, 1978), suggesting similarities in the peripheral apparatus of these species.

Results of the tone in noise experiments, however, reveal properties similar to those observed in human subjects. Dye and Hafter (1980) reported that frequency discriminaton for a 1-kHz tone in noise at a selected signal-to-noise ratio improved as overall level was raised. For a 4-kHz tone, on the other hand, performance declined with intensity. They interpreted this difference as evidence for a temporally-based mechanism for coding spectral information at low frequencies and a rate-based mechanism for high frequencies. Performance could have been impaired, however, at 4 kHz by

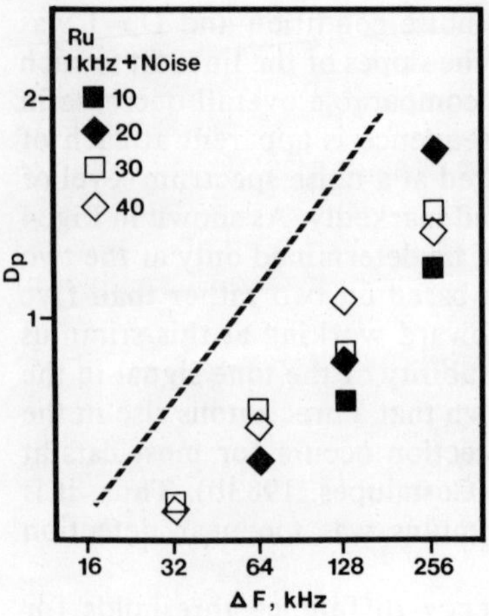

Figure 4. Dp (ordinate) as a function frequency separation for tone in noise. Four noise levels are indicated in the figure. S/N is constant. Straight line is from Fig.1 refit on log coordinate.

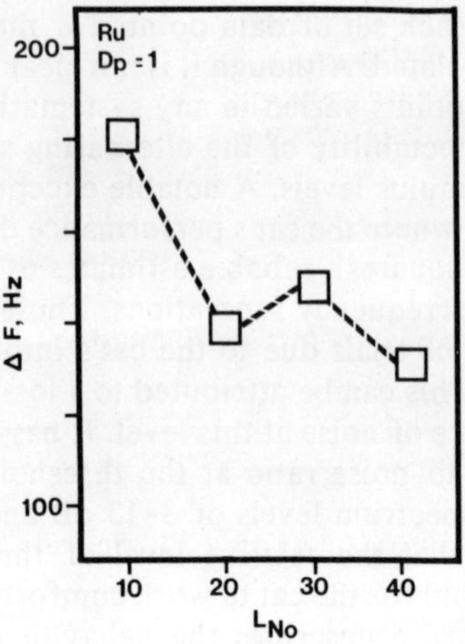

Figure 5. Frequency-difference of threshold at Dp=1 as a function of noise spectrum level.

the level-dependent increase in the relative efficacy of the noise masker specific to high-frequency stimuli (Moore, 1975).

A number of physiological studies have suggested that rate information in the discharge patterns of auditory nerve fibers may be adequate to account for behavioral thresholds over most of the range of audible frequencies (Sachs and Young, 1979; Ehret and Moffatt, 1984; Costalupes, 1985; Shofner and Sachs, 1986; Young and Barta, 1986). Representation of a 1-kHz tone plus noise stimulus in the rate response of large populations of auditory nerve fibers reveals a filter-like distribution of tone-evoked rate activity (Costalupes, 1985). At a signal-to-noise ratio near behavioral detection threshold, tone-evoked rate increases are noted among low and medium spontaneous rate fibers with best frequencies around 1 kHz over a range of best frequencies roughly equivalent to a critical band. The edges of the filter are defined by a sharp transition from a tone-evoked rate increase to a tone-evoked rate decrease, which is a reduction in the steady-state response to the continuous noise due to two-tone suppression. Maximum suppression, particularly on the high-frequency side, occurs at the edge of the filter and decreases in magnitude with distance from the test tone frequency. If overall stimulus level is increased at a constant signal-to-noise ratio, the magnitude of the tone-evoked rate increase within the filter becomes progressively smaller whereas the magnitude of suppression becomes progressively greater with level (Costalupes, 1985).

It remains to be determined whether spatial displacement of the neural representation corresponding to values noted in this study provides adequate rate information to account for frequency-difference thresholds in noise. In addition, the rate representation must maintain its saliency even at high noise levels to be consistent with the behavioral data. Changes in activity in the region of strong suppression at the outer edge of the filter may tend to preserve the salience of the rate representation. A neural critical bandwidth of 417 Hz geometrically centered at 1 kHz (Costalupes, 1985) will have lower and upper limits at 812 Hz and 1230 Hz. If the test tone is changed to 1140 Hz (i.e., say Dp=1 at 140 Hz), fibers with best frequencies near 1140 Hz will not show a large change in tone-evoked rate since these fibers are well within the neural bandwidth for the 1-kHz tone and respond strongly to that tone as well. The upper limit of the neural filter centered at 1140 Hz is 1368 Hz; thus, some fibers that were suppressed by the 1000-Hz tone will exhibit a tone-evoked rate increase in response to the 1140-Hz tone. The effect would depend strongly on the slope of the filter edge, but since the region involved corresponds to about 0.363 mm along the cochlear partition, 200 or more low and medium spontaneous rate fibers could show a response change. Other regions of the neural array could similarly be affected. Thus, off-frequency components of spectrally-complex stimuli may serve important functions in a rate-based coding scheme.

References

Costalupes, J.A. (**1983a**). "Temporal integration of pure tones in the cat," Hearing Res. **9**, 43-54.

Costalupes, J.A. (**1983b**). "Broadband masking noise and behavioral pure tone thresholds in the cat," J.Acoust.Soc.Am. **74**, 758-764.

Costalupes, J.A. (**1985**). "Representation of tones in noise in the responses of auditory nerve fibers in the cat," J.Neurosci. **5**, 3261-3269.

Dye, R. and Hafter, E.R. (**1980**). "Just noticeable differences of frequency for masked tones," J.Acoust.Soc.Am. **67**, 1746-1753.

Ehret, G. and Moffatt, A.J. (**1984**). "Noise masking of tone responses and critical ratios in single units of the mouse," Hearing Res. **14**, 45-57.

Elliott, D.N., Stein, L., and Harrison, M.J. (**1960**). "Determination of absolute intensity thresholds and frequency-difference thresholds in cats," J.Acoust. Soc.Am. **32**, 380-384.

Gerken, G.M. and Sandlin, D. (**1977**). "Auditory reaction times and absolute threshold in the cat, " J.Acoust.Soc.Am. **61**, 602-607.

Hienz, R.J. and Sheckler, D. (**1987**). "A comparison of different methods for determining frequency-difference thresholds in cats," ARO Abstr. **10**, 84.

Jesteadt, W. and Sims, S.L. (**1975**). "Decision processes in frequency discrimination," J.Acoust.Soc.Am. **57**, 1161-1166.

Moore, B.C.J. (**1975**). "Mechanisms of masking," J.Acoust.Soc.Am. **57**, 391-399.

Nelson, D.A. and Kiester, T.E. (**1978**). "Frequency discrimination in the chinchilla," J.Acoust.Soc.Am. **64**, 114-126.

Orr, J.L., Moody, D.B., and Stebbins, W.C. (**1977**). "Behavioral system and apparatus for tone detection and choice reaction times in cat," J.Acoust. Soc.Am. **62**, 1268-1272.

Pickles, J.O. (**1975**). "Normal critical bands in the cat," Acta-Otolaryngol. **80**, 245-254.

Sachs, M.B. and Young, E.D. (**1979**). "Encoding of steady-state vowels in the auditory nerve: representation in terms of average rate," J.Acoust.Soc.Am. **66**, 470-479.

Shofner, W.P. and Sachs, M.B. (**1986**). "Representation of low frequency tone in the discharge rate of populations of auditory nerve fibers," Hearing Res. **21**, 91-95.

Young, E.D. and Barta, P.E. (**1986**). "Rate response of auditory nerve fibers to tones in noise near masked threshold," J.Acoust.Soc.Am. **79**, 426-441.

Watson, C.S. (**1963**). "Masking of tones by noise for the cat," J.Acoust.Soc. Am. **35**, 167-172.

Comments

Hafter:

Dye and Hafter (1980) showed that for constant signal-to-noise ratios the effects of level on frequency discrimination could not be described by a single process. Rather, thresholds declined with higher levels for low frequencies but grew worse for high frequencies. Interestingly, the cross-over point was in the region of your experiment. Thus, I think that you should be cautious about inferring a single-factor model from data collected only at 1 kHz.

Reply by Costalupes:

I agree and I hope to test frequency discrimination at other frequencies. The choice of 1 kHz was predicated on my physiological studies (Costalupes, J.Neurosci. 5, 1985) that showed rate-change information for a 1-kHz tone in noise confined to a specific region in the neural array away over a wide range of stimulus conditions.

Houtsma:

Your data tell us that, for a trained cat, the frequency difference limen (taken at d' = 1) is about a semitone. This is very large compared with frequency DLs measured in humans. Would it be possible to improve the cat's performance further by combining, for instance, positive reinforcement of correct responses with appropriate negative reinforcement of incorrect responses? I think one wants behavioral data from humans and animals to agree within reasonable limits as long as it is assumed that the underlying physiology is not essentially different.

Reply by Costalupes:

Studies in which avoidance conditioning is used often reveal lower thresholds in cats, although one must be careful not to confuse motivation with higher alarm rates. I'm not sure I would expect strong agreement between human and animal data in view of morphological and structural differences, physiological similarities notwithstanding.

Frequency discrimination: evaluation of rate and temporal codes

E. Javel, J.B. Mott, N.L. Rush, and D.W. Smith

Boys Town National Institute
Omaha, Nebraska 68131, U.S.A.

Introduction

A long-standing controversy in the auditory literature involves the neural mechanisms underlying frequency discrimination. What we shall call the "rate-place" argument focuses on the detection of changes in the spatial locus of the cochlear excitation pattern (Winslow, 1985). In its simplest form, this theory presumes that any change in signal frequency causes a concomitant shift in the cochlear position of the traveling wave maximum, thereby possibly altering discharge rates of responsive auditory nerve fibers. The central auditory processor's task is to detect these changes by monitoring the neural population response.

The alternative argument to the rate-place argument is the temporal mechanism. This scheme takes advantage of the well-known phenomenon of synchronization or phase-locking of auditory nerve fiber responses at low and moderate signal frequencies. As applied to the task of frequency discrimination, the temporal theory presumes that changes in signal frequency are detected by monitoring changes in the times of occurrence of discharges, either in single fibers or across groups of fibers. Inputs to this analysis are time intervals between successive neuronal discharges (i.e., inter-spike intervals or ISIs).

Most auditory scientists agree that the rate-place code must operate at high frequencies because neural phase-locking does not exist above 4-5 kHz (Rose *et al.*, 1967). The principal issue is how lower frequencies are discriminated. Siebert (1970), Luce and Green (1974), and Goldstein and Srulovicz (1977) all conducted mathematical analyses of neurophysiological data in an attempt to predict performance on frequency discrimination tasks. These studies concluded that optimum processing of temporally-encoded frequency information leads to perceptual performance which exceeds that observed psychophysically. Goldstein and Srulovicz, in addition, pointed out that processing of inter-spike intervals correctly predicts the duration and intensity dependence of perceptual frequency discrimination as well as the behavior of the Weber fraction across frequency (Moore, 1973; Wier *et al.*,

1977). Of necessity, however, this earlier work used long-term average ISI histograms as inputs to the analysis, and they also assumed that responses of several neurons' activities are summed prior to the decision process.

The goal of the experiments described here was to evaluate the ability of single auditory nerve fibers to utilize rate-based and temporal-based information to detect changes in the frequency of a pure-tone signal. To do this, we employed an adaptive tracking procedure in a two-alternative forced-choice (2AFC) paradigm. By controlling the input to the decision process, namely overall discharge rate versus phase-locked activity, we studied single fibers' frequency difference limens (DLs) as signal frequency, intensity and duration were varied. Our data indicate that temporal-based decision processes produce frequency DLs that are much smaller than those obtained using rate-based measures. However, the actual DLs are not nearly as small as those predicted by the theoretical work, and the ability of temporal-based measures to discriminate frequency declines sharply at higher frequencies. Temporal-based decision processes produced data that behaved in the same general manner as perceptual data for varying signal intensity and duration, whereas rate-based processes did not.

Methods

Techniques to obtain single-fiber recordings from the auditory nerves of healthy adult cats were the same as those used previously in work originating from our laboratory (Javel, 1981). After a fiber was encountered, spontaneous discharge rate was determined and a tuning curve was taken using a computer-automated procedure. Frequency discrimination data were then obtained adaptively using a 2AFC procedure. The frequency of one of the tones in the trial was usually set to the fiber's characteristic frequency (CF), and the frequency of the tone in the other interval was free to vary. All stimuli were synthesized digitally using custom-made hardware. Based on the fiber's responses to each tone, a decision was made as to which interval possessed the higher discharge rate (in rate-based measures) or the higher frequency (in temporal-based measures). If the correct interval was selected, the trial was either repeated or the signal frequencies were spaced more closely, depending on the target probability of a correct response. Percent correct was converged upon by varying the number of trials in a block (Levitt, 1971). Step size was halved after every negative-going response reversal, until a pre-selected minimum step size was attained. Fibers usually tracked a given DL for 150 trials, regardless of the response behavior occurring therein.

The rate-based decision process simply involved selecting the signal interval that had at least one more spike in it. Thus, this procedure tracks differences in discharge rate that depend on signal duration. For example, a duration of 100 ms tracks a rate difference of 10 spikes/s, 50 ms tracks 20 spikes/s, and so on. Similar measures have been used on the single-fiber level by others investigate auditory intensity discrimination, absolute and masked

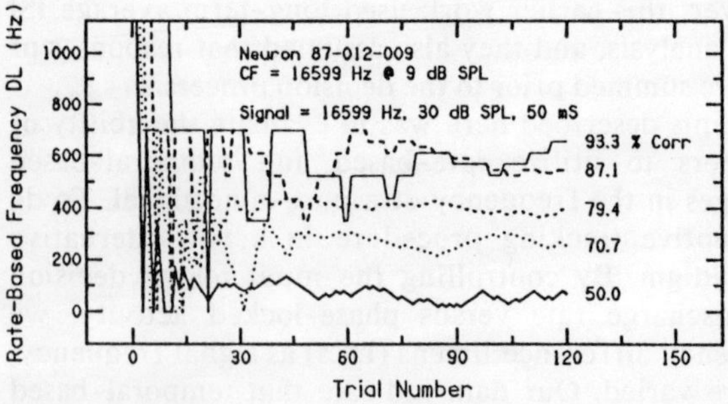

Figure 1. Examples of rate-based 2AFC adaptive tracks. The frequency tested was a CF tone presented at 30 dB SPL. The parameter is target percent correct, obtained by varying the number of trials in a block.

thresholds, and forward masking.

The temporal-based decision process operated differently. We assumed that the fiber "knew" the stimulus frequency whose DL was being examined. With each incoming ISI, the computer determined how many cycles of the stimulus frequency had intervened between the previous spike and the current spike, then assigned the interval to the appropriate mode or peak in an ISI histogram. The deviation between the expected and obtained ISIs was computed for each interval, and these were summed for all ISIs occurring during the tone. After each stimulus had ended, estimated frequency was computed as the inverse of the expected signal period plus the average deviation. Although we could specify the longest ISI length to be used in the analysis, we did not apply any weighting schemes, i.e., all ISIs counted equally. This technique is identical to that described by Luce and Green (1974) in deriving their neural timing model.

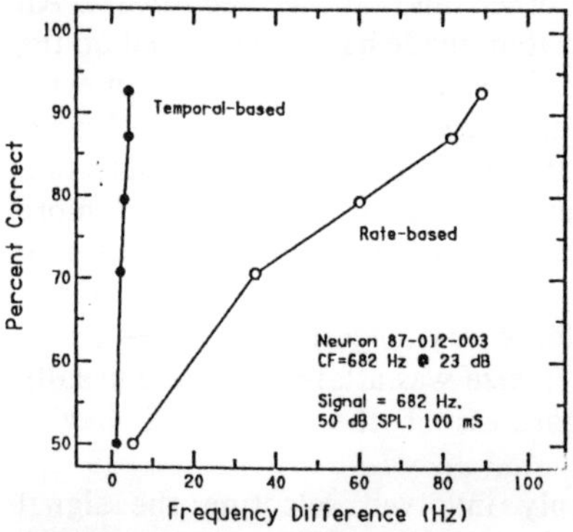

Figure 2. Neurometric functions obtained at CF (682 Hz) from the same fiber using rate- and temporal-based processes.

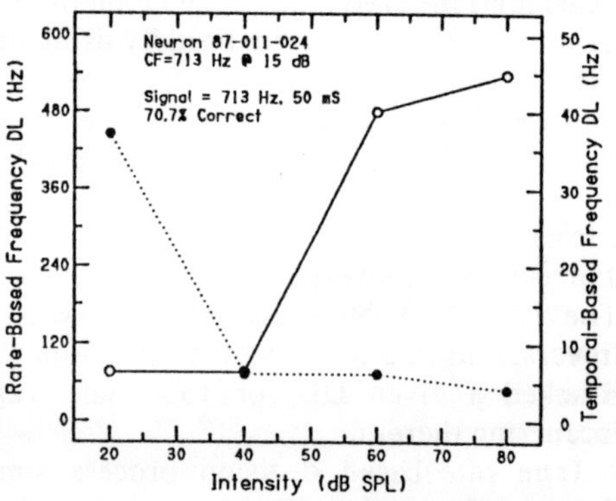

Figure 3. Rate-based (open symbols) and temporal-based (filled symbols) frequency DLs obtained at CF at several intensities.

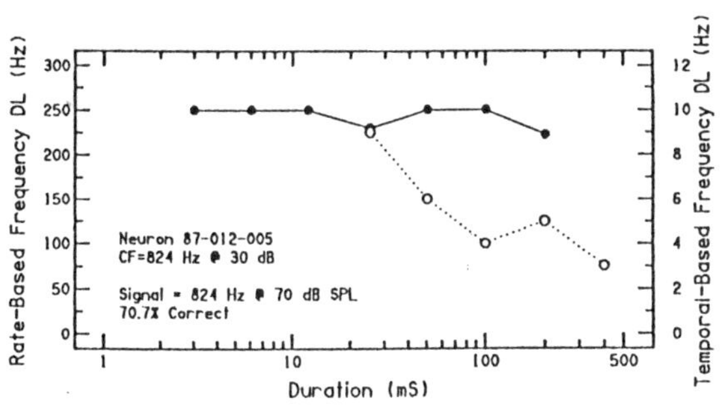

Figure 4. Rate-based (filled symbols) and temporal-based (open symbols) frequency DLs obtained at CF and 70 dB SPL from the same fiber as signal duration was varied.

Results

Examples of adaptive response tracks are shown in Fig. 1. The rate-based DLs shown were obtained from a fiber with a high (16599 Hz) CF. The test frequency was at CF, the intensity was 30 dB SPL, and signal duration was 50 ms. The parameter in Fig. 1 is percent correct, which as stated above was converged upon by varying block size. These data demonstrate the rapidity at which the tracking procedure achieved a DL and its good overall reliability. DLs tracked using the temporal-based decision process were equally fast-settling and reliable.

Psychometric (or, more accurately, neurometric) functions were obtained by forcing fibers to track pre-selected probabilities of correct response, similar to the data shown in Fig. 1. Examples of two neurometric functions, one for rate-based frequency DLs and the other for temporal-based DLs, are shown in Fig. 2. Both functions were obtained from the same low-CF (682 Hz) fiber for tones of 100 ms duration presented at 50 dB SPL. The DLs shown were taken at CF. The temporal-based decision process produced neurometric functions that exhibited much smaller DLs and grew much more rapidly with increasing frequency.

Varying stimulus intensity produced data that differed greatly between rate- and temporal-based decision processes. An example of frequency DLs obtained at CF at various signal intensities is shown in Fig. 3. The percent correct tracked in this case was 70.7%. This value corresponds to a *d'* of almost 1, an index of detectability often equated with "just-detectable" performance. The temporal-based DLs shown in Fig. 3 (filled symbols connected by dashed lines) behaved like perceptual data in that the DLs decreased with intensity. Rate-based DLs (open symbols connected by solid lines), on the other hand, increased with intensity.

In human listeners, decreasing signal duration below 400 ms produces monotonically increasing frequency DLs (Moore, 1973). Comparable data from a cat auditory nerve fiber are shown in Fig. 4. As signal duration was varied from 3 ms to 200 ms, rate-based DLs (filled symbols connected by solid lines) obtained at CF did not change at all. However, temporal-based DLs (open symbols connected by dashed lines) behaved similar to the

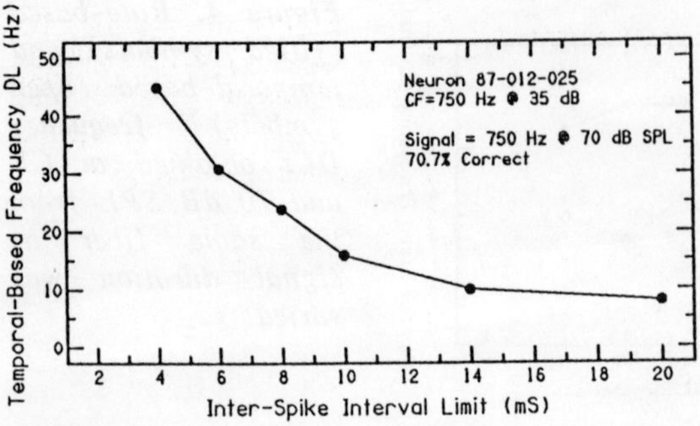

Figure 5. Temporal-based DLs obtained at 70 dB SPL as a function of the length of the longest ISI allowed to enter the decision process.

perceptual data, increasing as signal duration decreased.

An obviously important determinant of temporal-based frequency DLs is the maximum allowable length of the ISIs entering the decision process. All the temporal-based data shown to this point were obtained using ISIs up to 20 ms. We selected this value because it roughly corresponds to the signal period at which musical pitch becomes tonal. As stated earlier, all ISIs received equal weight in the decision process. Goldstein and Srulovicz (1977) have shown that the longer the ISI the listener is allowed to use, the better his frequency discrimination performance will be. This is a simple outgrowth of the increasing time difference between an expected and an obtained ISI as the number of intervening signal periods increases.

We examined the effect of limiting the maximum length of ISIs entering the decision process. Representative data are shown in Fig. 5. These were obtained from a fiber whose CF was 750 Hz, the frequency we tested. As the length of the maximum ISI was decreased, temporal-based DLs likewise suffered, declining over a 5:1 range as the maximum ISI length was reduced from 20 ms to 4 ms. Although we have not tested it as yet, we would expect this effect to be strongly intensity dependent because mean ISI length is a sensitive function of overall discharge rate and hence of intensity.

Representative data on the behavior of temporal-based frequency DLs obtained across frequency at the same sensation level (i.e., suprathreshold intensity) are shown in Fig. 6. DLs obtained from this fiber were uniformly small up to 800 Hz, above which they increased sharply. The highest frequency tested for this fiber was 1 kHz, which lay near the upper edge of the fiber's tuning curve. One can readily compute the Weber fractions from these data and determine that the fraction decreases up to 700 Hz, after which it increases.

We have similar data from other fibers at higher frequencies. These data suggest that the DL (and the Weber fraction) continue to grow above 1 kHz. In no case have we been able on single trials to obtain temporal-based DLs above 2 kHz. This finding is in sharp contrast to the earlier modeling work, Goldstein's and Srulovicz's for example, which employed dense, long-term ISI histograms at their inputs. Our data suggest that limited random samples

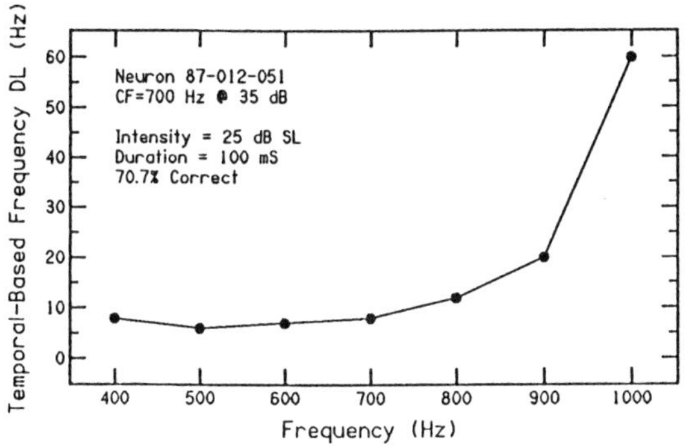

Figure 6. Temporal-based frequency DLs obtained at 25 dB sensation level (SL) at several frequencies.

of ISIs from these distributions do not provide a strong enough input to the temporal-based decision process to effect a reliable estimate of signal frequency.

Because the degree of response synchronization at a given frequency depends only on sensation level and not on CF, one would expect temporal-based DLs obtained across frequency to be essentially the same regardless of the CF of the fiber investigated. On the other hand, spontaneous rate has somewhat of an effect on the magnitude of obtained DLs, with low-spontaneous-rate fibers generally providing smaller temporal-based DLs at a given sensation level than those obtained from high-spontaneous-rate fibers. This is ostensibly due to the tighter distribution of phase-locked discharges within the stimulus period commonly seen in low-spontaneous-rate fibers (Johnson, 1974).

Rate-based DLs across frequency exhibited a completely different behavior than temporal-based DLs. An example is shown in Fig. 7. The CF of the fiber whose responses are shown here was 4210 Hz. DLs at several frequencies were obtained, all at 60 dB SPL, and these are shown as filled symbols. Unlike the temporal-based DLs shown in Fig. 6, the rate-based DLs are a simple, virtually linear function of frequency, up to the edge of the fiber's response area.

The response area of the fiber providing the data for Fig. 7 is shown in Fig. 8. The intensity at which the data for Fig. 7 were obtained, namely 60 dB SPL, produced the iso-intensity line indicated by filled circles in Fig. 8. Given the nature of the rate-based decision process, which as stated earlier simply tracks the frequency at which the elicited discharge rate is some known number of spikes per second lower than that elicited by the test frequency, we can utilize the response area to predict what the rate-based DLs should be. These are shown as open symbols in Fig. 7. The correspondence between obtained and expected rate-based DLs is extremely close.

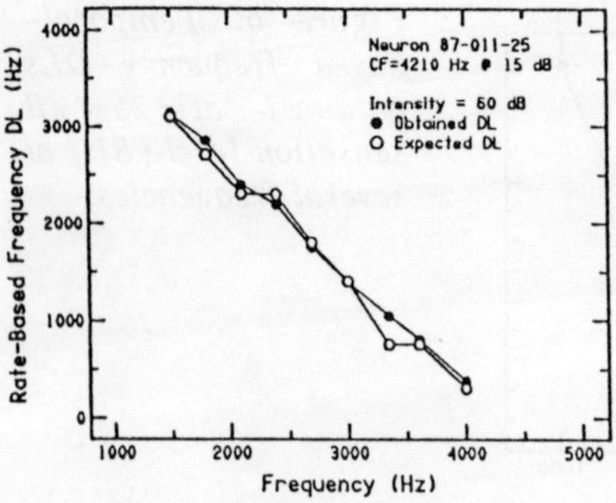

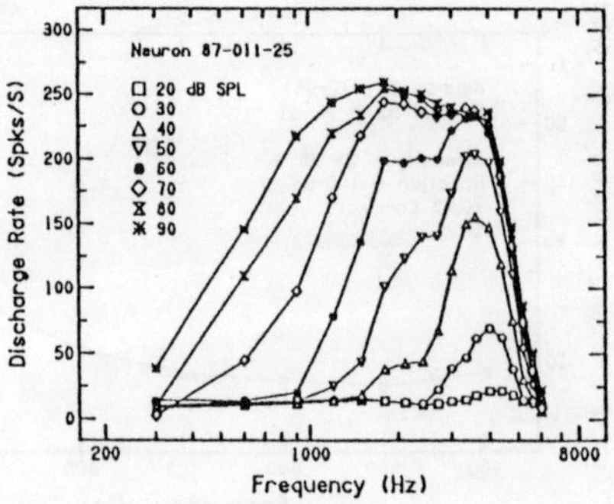

Figure 7. Rate-based DLs obtained from a fiber at 60 dB SPL and several frequencies. Obtained DLs are indicated by filled circles, expected DLs by open circles (see text).

Figure 8. Response area for the fiber whose DLs are shown in Fig. 7.

Discussion

We have shown here that when auditory nerve fibers are allowed to utilize phase-locked frequency information in judging differences in signal frequency, the DLs that result are considerably smaller than those provided by analogous rate-based measures. Moreover, the data obtained using temporal-based decision processes behave in the same manner as perceptual data when signal intensity and duration are varied, but performance improves more rapidly than one might like.

Two findings from our temporal-based data are especially noteworthy. The first is that performance of single fibers declines rapidly above 800 Hz. Although this may reflect limitations of the decision process we employed in this study, it is more likely that performance is particularly sensitive to and determined by the limited numbers of ISIs available per trial. Unlike earlier mathematical studies, which utilized complete, dense ISI histograms as inputs, our technique forced decisions to be made using only small numbers (typically 5-50) of ISIs. We think that limited random samples of ISIs more accurately reflect the input to the decision process, assuming of course that the process actually utilizes the frequency information contained in synchronized discharges.

The second noteworthy finding is that even though temporal-based frequency DLs are sensitive, the human ear is even better. On the average, the temporal-based DLs we obtained were a factor of 4 worse than DLs obtained from human listeners at the same frequencies and comparable sensation levels. Whether this means that human listeners sum temporal information from several fibers and make decisions based on the sum, cannot be determined from these data. The important point, however, is that the actual temporal-based performance of single auditory nerve fibers is not nearly as efficient as optimum processing schemes operating on dense ISI histograms have suggested. On the other hand, temporal-based performance of single fibers matches behavioral data from cats at frequencies below 2 kHz (Elliott *et al.*, 1960).

Finally, a word should be said about our rate-based measures. The technique we employed here does not constitute an adequate test of rate-place theories because those theories base their decisions on the neural population response, which we did not measure. What our data show, however, is that on the single-fiber level rate-based frequency DLs are so large that an enormous amount of response integration must be done to obtain performance which approximates that of the human ear at low and middle frequencies. Whether the auditory system is capable of performing such a large-scale integration at any site, including the cortex, is something that has yet to be demonstrated.

Acknowledgements

This work was supported by research grants awarded by NIH to EJ. JBM and DWS were NINCDS postdoctoral fellows.

References

Elliott, D.N., Stein, L., and Harrison, M.J. (**1960**). "Determination of absolute intensity thresholds and frequency-difference thresholds in cats," J.-Acoust.Soc.Am. **32**, 380-384.

Goldstein, J.L., and Srulovicz, P. (**1977**). "Auditory-nerve spike intervals as an adequate basis for aural frequency measurement," in *Psychophysics and Physiology of Hearing*, edited by E.F.Evans and J.P.Wilson (London, Academic Press), pp. 337-346.

Javel, E. (**1981**). "Suppression of auditory nerve responses. I. Temporal analysis, intensity effects and suppression contours," J.AcoustSoc.Am. **69**, 1735-1745.

Johnson, D.H. (**1974**). *The Response of Single Auditory-Nerve Fibers in the Cat to Single Tones: Synchrony and Average Discharge Rate.* Doctoral thesis, Mass. Inst. Technol.

Levitt, H. (**1971**). "Transformed up-down methods in psychoacoustics," J. Acoust.Soc.Am. **49**, 467-477.

Luce, R.D., and Green, D.M. (**1974**). "Neural coding and psychophysical discrimination data," J.Acoust.Soc.Am. **56**, 1554-1564.

Moore, B.C.J. (**1973**). "Frequency difference limens for short-duration tones," J.Acoust.Soc.Am. **54**, 610-619.

Rose, J.E., Brugge, J.F., Anderson, D.J., and Hind, J.E. (**1967**). "Phase locked response to low frequency tones in single auditory nerve fibers of the squirrel monkey," J.Neurophysiol. **30**, 769-793.

Siebert, W.M. (**1970**). "Frequency discrimination in the auditory system: Place or periodicity mechanisms?," Proc. I.E.E.E. **58**, 723-730.
Wier, C.C., Jesteadt, W., and Green, D.M. (**1977**). "Frequency discimination as a function of frequency and sensation level," J.Acoust.Soc.Am. **61**, 178-184.
Winslow, R.L. (**1985**). *A Quantitative Analysis of Rate-Coding in the Auditory-Nerve*. Doctoral thesis, Johns Hopkins Univ.

Comments

Costalupes:

The argument that the nervous system should be able to detect a change in frequency in the activity of a single fiber strikes me as a bit specious. Would you want to propose then that the nervous system would -- in the case of a rate-place model -- represent *intensity* in terms of the number of active fibers and *frequency* in terms of a rate change in a specific fiber Also, while I agree with your point regarding dense ISI histograms, it might be worth noting that even your method produced temporally-based frequency DLs much smaller than those obtained from behaving cats. The rate-based DLs in Fig. 2 look rather like the behavioral data. Do you suppose this is just fortuitous?

Reply by Javel:

We are not suggesting that frequency is coded by rate at the single fiber, and we are not attempting to differentiate frequency coding from intensity coding! All our data shows that single fibers perform better on a frequency discrimination task when they base decisions on temporaly coded information, relative to performance based solely on changes in discharge rate.

The correspondence of the rate-based performance shown inn Fig. 2 to your behavioral data is purely fortuitous. Had we tested this fiber's ability to discriminate a higher frequency, performance would have been better; likewise, performance would have been worse if we had tested at a lower frequency.

An important consideration in evaluating the temporal code is the growth of performance as a function of frequency separation. As Fig. 2 shows, performance using temporal cues improves much more rapidly than the behavioral performance you measured. Although neural performance will improve less rapidly if we limit the lengths of the ISIs allowed to enter the decision process (Fig. 5), this will not degrade performance to the degree required to approximate your data. Further degradation of performance can be achieved by assuming that temporal jitter is introduced at higher-order synapses. Clearly, temporal-based frequency coding has difficulty accounting for your data.

Moore:

I am surprised that you used fibres with CF close to the signal frequency to evaluate the rate-based process. These are the fibres which would show the smallest change in response to a change in frequency. Have you studied the effectiveness of a rate-based process using fibres tuned somewhat away from CF, particularly below CF?

Reply by Javel:

Magnitudes of rate-based DLs obtained from single fibers depend on the position of the test frequency within the fibers' response area, the shape of the response area, and intensity. Given this, one expects rate-based DLs to be the smallest for frequencies located on the most steeply sloping parts of the response area. For example in Fig. 8 the smallest Dls would be obtained at frequencies above CF and, to a lesser extent, at frequencies well below CF.

We emphasize that rate-based DLs obtained from single fibers do not constitute an appropriate test of the rate-place code's ability to discriminate frequency. We only included them here to provide data analogous to the temporal-based measures that form the focus of this work. A better test of the rate-place code involves analyzing the neural activity in cochlear excitation patterns. Although it is not shown here, we have developed a non-stochastic exitation pattern model specifically for the purpose of predicting relative performance on frequency discrimination tasks. Our model integrates changes in rate elicited by two tones, providing a d'-like measure of detectability. Its outputs match the behavioral data relatively well for frequencies below 2 kHz, but predicts DLs that are too small at higher frequencies. The best -performing fibers (in terms of the amount they contribute to d') invariably are located just apical to the travelling wave peaks. These fibers, of course, are tuned to frequencies slightly below those being tested. Fibers tuned to others frequencies contribute to the model's output, but to a lesser degree.

Duifhuis and Miller:

You mention that temporal models do not predict an increase in $\Delta f/f$ with increasing frequency which models are you referring to? As for serious temporal models, such as these based on Goldstein's optimum processor theory, they do accurately predict the JNDf with frequency as determined psychophysically (e.g. Henning, 1965; Moore, 1973). It is this agreement that has provided the sound underpinning of Goldstein's optimum processor theory.

Reply by Javel:

Temporal-based models accurately predict $\Delta f/f$, as you state, but the goodness of fit is better al low frequencies than at high frequencies. In humans, $\Delta f/f$ rises rather quickly above 2 kHz, just as temporal models predict will happen in the face of declining discharge synchronization. The situation is somewhat different for cats, however. Elliott *et al.* (1960)

measured $\Delta f/f$ to rise rather slowly at frequencies above 2 kHz. I think that the behavioral data from cats are a more appropriate reference, and it is these data to which I was alluding.

In terms of single-fiber performance on the frequency discrimination task, our data suggest that the upper cutoff frequency is around 1.5 kHz, not the 3-4 kHz that the modelling work predicts. The discrepancy is probably due to differences in sample interval, single fiber performance being based on 5-50 ISIs whereas model performance is based on thousands of ISIs. I find it difficult to imagine that the CNS can sum temporarily coded information to the degree required by the temporal models.

Single fiber responses to complex sounds in the pigeon

J. Wiebe Horst, Hero P. Wit and Hans M. Segenhout

Institute of Audiology, University Hospital Groningen
P.O. Box 30.001, 9700RB Groningen, The Netherlands

Introduction

Responses to complex sounds have been studied in single cochlear nerve fibers of mammals for a variety of stimuli. Although several aspects of the stimulus spectra can be processed adequately by the auditory system, it is clear that nonlinear processes play an important role in the transduction of complex sounds and make coding of some aspects of the sounds less translucent. In the case of speech stimuli, Young and Sachs (1979) reported that an interplay of various nonlinear processes results in a relatively linear coding of gross spectral features of the stimuli in the temporal aspects of single fiber responses. Horst *et al.* (1985, 1986a) on the other hand showed that for special choices of stimulus spectra the temporal responses give a distorted impression of the stimulus spectra. In fact, certain aspects of the stimulus spectrum may be enhanced. This phenomenon was also found in the microphonics of guinea pigs and pigeons (Wit *et al.*, 1986), which suggests that the bird cochlea also acts in certain aspects nonlinearly. The latter was investigated in single fiber responses of the pigeon to complex stimuli. The present paper shows some data of a pilot study.

Material and methods

Experiments were carried out in 5 homing pigeons (*Columba livia*), under anaesthesia with a gas mixture of oxygen (1 l/min) and fluothane (1.5 %). Access to the cochlea was obtained by a retro-auricular approach and a small hole was carefully cut in the recessus scalae tympani. Through this hole part of the cochlear nerve was visible. Action potentials were recorded extracellularly from single fibers of this nerve with glass micropipettes (3M KCl; 20 MΩ). Stimuli were delivered to the ear canal of the pigeon by a ½-inch condensor microphone (B&K 4166) in a closed system. Sound pressure was monitored inside this system with a ¼-inch condensor microphone (B&K 4136), as close to the ear canal as possible. At the beginning of each experiment, sound pressure level in the ear canal was recorded as a function

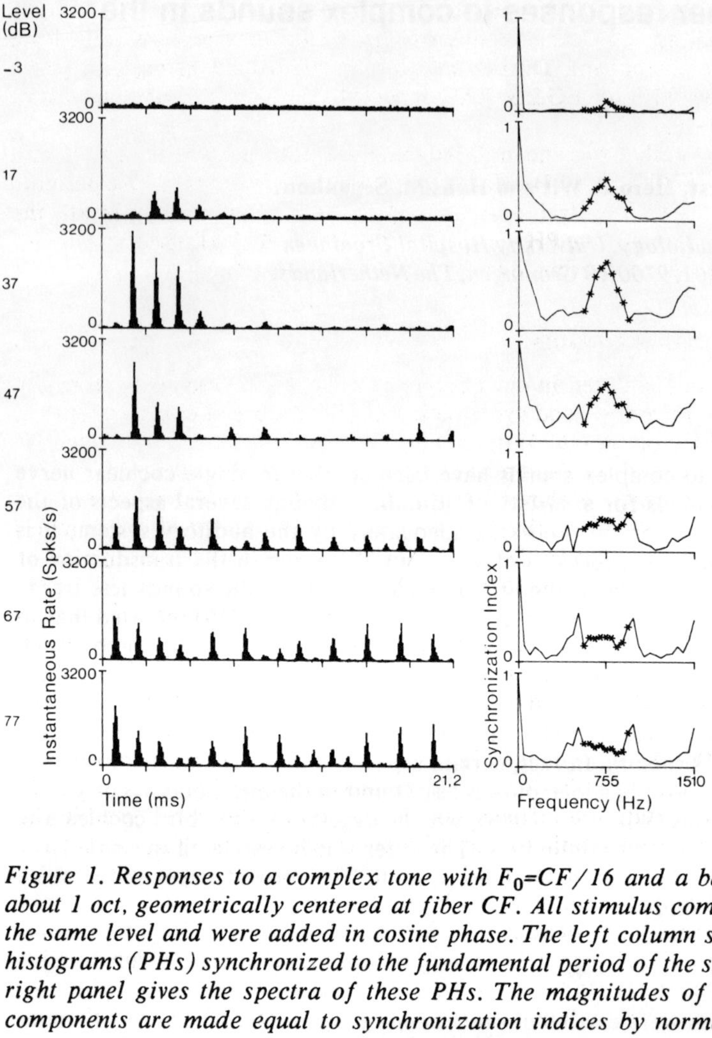

Figure 1. Responses to a complex tone with F_0=CF/16 and a bandwidth of about 1 oct, geometrically centered at fiber CF. All stimulus components had the same level and were added in cosine phase. The left column shows period histograms (PHs) synchronized to the fundamental period of the stimulus. The right panel gives the spectra of these PHs. The magnitudes of the spectral components are made equal to synchronization indices by normalizing with respect to the DC component. The total stimulus level is indicated to the left of each panel in dB SPL.

of frequency. The resulting calibration curve was stored in computer memory and used during the experiments to equalize individual components during synthesis, so that they possessed the desired acoustic levels.

As stimuli we used multi-component sounds defined by a center frequency CF (usually the best frequency of the nerve fiber) and a spectral spacing factor N. Thus the fundamental frequency F_0 was CF/N. The basic stimulus consisted of successive equal-amplitude harmonics of F_0. Spectra were about one octave wide, centered geometrically around CF. Variations of the basic stimulus consisted of a change in phase spectrum and/or a change in the level of the center component. During an experiment, period histograms (PHs) were recorded with an EG&G-PAR model 4203 signal averager and later processed off-line.

After a nerve fiber was encountered the best frequency was estimated with a variation of Møller's (1977) method: In response to a random phase periodic stimulus with flat spectral envelope, a PH was determined. Next, the amplitude spectrum of the PH was determined under ASYST using an Olivetti PC. This resulted in an estimate of the fiber's best frequency.

Results and discussion

The fibers encountered in our experiments ranged in frequency from 250 to 3200 Hz and showed good synchronization for pure and complex tones as reported by Sachs *et al.* (1974) in the same animal. For the complex tones we used mostly flat amplitude and phase spectra (all components in cosine phase).

I. A typical response is shown in Fig.1. CF was 755 Hz, N was 16. The left column shows PHs synchronized to the fundamental period of the stimulus for different stimulus levels. The right column shows the amplitude spectra of the period histograms. At the lowest stimulus level, the PH consisted mainly of spontaneous activity. Locally in the period the spontaneous activity was modulated by the influence of the stimulus. With increasing stimulus level, the response to the stimulus grows and the spontaneous activity is more suppressed. Thus, at intermediate levels the response is fairly limited in time. At the highest stimulus levels the response is spread out through the whole period. Also the envelope of the PH becomes flatter. All this is in agreement with responses measured by Horst *et al.* (1986a) in single fibers of the cat. In the frequency domain the influence of the auditory filter is reflected in the amount of synchronization to the stimulus components. With increasing stimulus level there is an increase of synchronization at low levels and a change in spectrum at intermediate and high levels. At the highest levels the response spectra show dominant peaks near the edges of the stimulus spectrum. These effects can be described by the action of a compressive nonlinearity, which causes enhancement of the low amplitude portions of the PHs (Horst *et al.*, 1986a; Wit *et al.*,1986; Shamma *et al.*,1987). The enhancement of certain spectral aspects of the stimulus is reminiscent of Houtgast's psychophysical data (1974).

II. The influence of a CNL has been studied in several cochlear models (e.g. Duifhuis,1976). In order to check whether a description of certain aspects of the responses in terms of a compressive nonlinearity was adequate, we used some other stimuli where the action of a compressive nonlinearity would show up particularly strongly. This is the case for stimuli with a peaky envelope, where a small part of the stimulus energy is distributed more or less evenly over the low amplitude part of the stimulus. A CNL would boost this part of the stimulus. Since this involves the major part of the stimulus period,

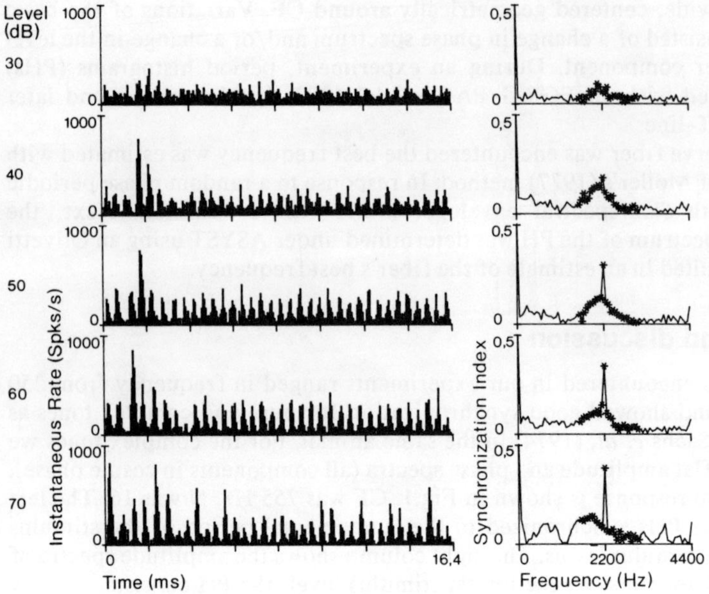

Figure 2. Period histograms and their spectra in response to a stimulus with the CF component inverted in phase. CF/F_0=36.

the effects on the response spectrum can be dramatic. In the case of flat phase spectrum e.g., the low amplitude part of the period contains mainly frequencies near the spectral edges. If one stimulus component is deleted or inverted in phase, the low-amplitude part is mainly tuned to this absent or inverted component. Fig. 2 shows responses for the case with inverted CF (the other case is discussed below). Again we see a gradual change in the PH, where the low amplitude part keeps growing at the cost of the peaked part of the PH. In the frequency domain, the main consequence of these changes is a domination of the spectrum by the CF component.

III. Another check of the adequacy of the description of the responses in terms of a CNL was made by using a random-phase stimulus. Horst *et al.* (1986b) have shown for the cat on stimulation with a random-phase stimulus with equal-amplitude components that the shape of the response spectra is fairly independent of the stimulus level. This shows that any sign of a CNL in the PH does not influence substantially the shape of the response spectra. This can be understood by realizing that one stimulus period can be considered as a (band-pass filtered) noise sample. (One stimulus period of the cosine-phase stimulus can be regarded as a band-pass filtered pulse). The noise sample has a more even envelope than a filtered pulse, since this envelope can be regarded as a low-pass filtered noise. As a consequence, enhancement of low

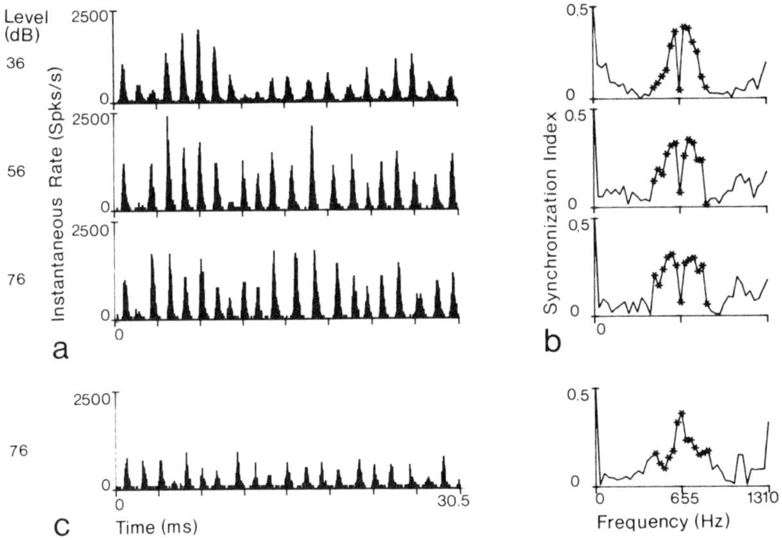

Figure 3. (a) Period histograms in response to a stimulus with random phase spectrum and the CF component deleted. (b) Amplitude spectra of the period histograms of fig.3a. (c) Period histogram and its spectrum in response to a stimulus with the same amplitude spectrum as in fig. 3a and 3b (i.e. the CF component deleted) but flat phase spectrum (all components in cosine phase). $CF/F_0 = 20$. Note the relatively high synchronization at CF.

amplitude portions by a CNL will be relatively small compared to the case of the periodic pulse. Additionally, due to the random-phase spectrum, any influence of a CNL would on the average be the same for every spectral component and not alter the response spectrum. This also implies that removing or adding one component would not cause any nonlinear changes in the response spectrum. Both expectations were borne out by experiment. Here we only show the case of the deleted component. The PHs are plotted in Fig.3a. Clearly, there is a modulation of the PH envelope at the lowest stimulus level, which decreases with increasing stimulus level. This shows the influence of a CNL. In figure 3b the spectra are fairly independent of the stimulus level. As expected, no appreciable response at CF is found. For comparison, we also stimulated this fiber with a cosine-phase complex where the CF was missing. The response at the highest level shown in Fig.3c is clearly dominated by a response to the (missing) CF. Obviously, randomizing the stimulus phase has a linearizing influence on the signal transduction. This problem was discussed theoretically for a general input-output system by Price (1958).

IV. Whereas the major part of the nerve fiber responses was in agreement with a CNL, a considerable minority did not show signs of a CNL. An example is shown in figure 4 with responses to a stimulus with flat phase

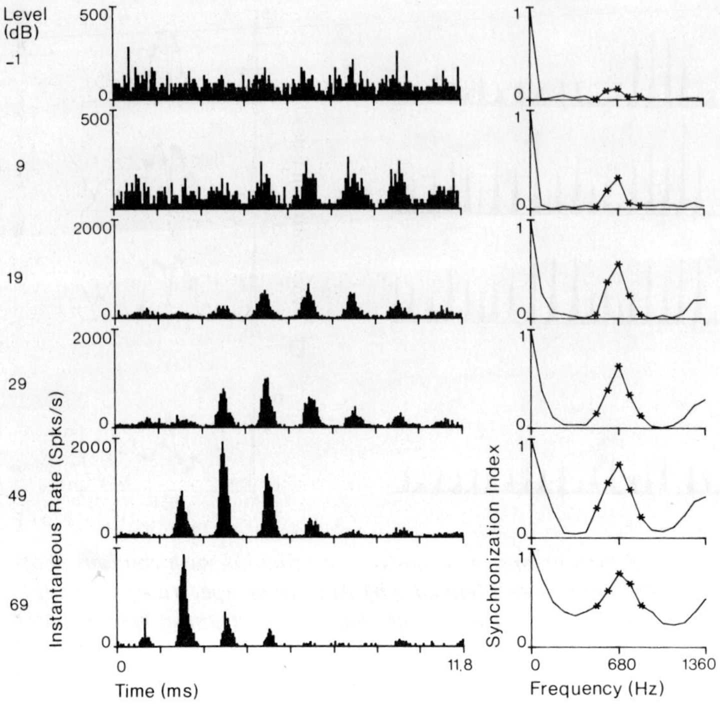

Figure 4. Period histograms and their spectra in response to a stimulus with flat amplitude spectrum and all components in cosine phase. $CF/F_0 = 8$.

spectrum and with N=8. This fiber had a CF of 680 Hz. At all stimulus levels there is a clear modulation of the PH and no indication of a flattening of the envelope. There even is a tendency for a narrowing of the envelope. Additionally, there is a clear advance of the whole PH in time. It is not immediately clear how to reconcile these data with those from mammalian nerve fibers. Indeed, Kiang *et al.*(1965) and Pfeiffer and Kim (1972) found that the response to click stimuli was slightly extended to shorter delay time with increasing stimulus level, but their data do not show an advance of the whole response envelope to shorter delay times, which is clearly the case in the present reponses. The phenomenon of decrease of delay times with level has been explored theoretically by Goldstein *et al.*(1971). They related this effect to a widening of the auditory filter with stimulus level, and also showed that this would result in an advance of the whole response to shorter delay times. Although there is a slight widening of the response spectra, this is not a clear effect. In order to check the relevance of this explanation we would need responses from one and the same fiber to stimuli with a flat phase spectrum and to stimuli with a more stochastic character. This is one of our objects for further research.

A confounding factor is the influence of refractory effects. Gray (1967) and, more recently, Gaumond *et al.* (1983) showed that these effects may have considerable influence on the relation between excitation function and PH. In the case of pulse-like stimuli the PH would underestimate the duration af the excitation function. If this effect also plays a role in the present responses, then the spectra of the excitation functions would have different shapes than the present response spectra. In order to disentangle nonlinear effects in the frequency domain (e.g widening of the auditory filter) and the temporal domain (compressive or expansive nonlinearities, refractory effects) the methods developed by Gray and Gaumond have to be incorporated in our investigation.

Final remark

The spectral contents of period histograms in response to complex tones can seriously change with level. Such nonlinear changes contradict often made suggestions that cochlear responses can to a great extent be described by means of an automatic gain control (AGC). Apparently, those cases where this description holds and the responses behave fairly independently of level, are caused by special choice of the stimulus (e.g. a random-phase stimulus) or by a fortunate interaction of nonlinearities.

References

Duifhuis, H. (**1976**). "Cochlear nonlinearity and second filter: possible mechanisms and implications," J.Acoust.Soc.Am. **48**, 888-893.

Gaumond, R.P., Kim, D.O. and Molnar, C.O. (**1983**). "Response of cochlear nerve fibers to brief acoustic stimuli: Role of discharge-history effect," J. Acoust.Soc.Am. **74**, 1392-1398.

Goldstein, J.L., Baer, T., and Kiang, N.Y.S. (**1971**). "A theoretical treatment of latency, group delay, and tuning characteristics for auditory-nerve responses to clicks and tones," in *Physiology of the auditory system* edited by M.B. Sachs (Nat. Educat. Cons., Baltimore) pp. 133-141.

Gray, P.R. (**1967**). "Conditional probability analysis of the spike activity of single neurons," Biophys.J. 7, 759-777.

Houtgast, T. (**1974**). *Lateral suppression in hearing*. Doctoral dissertation, Free University, Amsterdam.

Horst, J.W., Javel, E., and Farley, G.R. (**1985**). "Extraction and enhancement of spectral structure by the cochlea," J.Acoust.Soc.Am. **78**, 1898-1901.

Horst, J.W., Javel, E., and Farley, G.R. (**1986a**). "Coding of spectral fine structure in the auditory nerve.I. Fourier analysis of period and interspike interval histograms". J.Acoust.Soc.Am. **79**, 398-416.

Horst, J.W., Javel, E. and Farley, G.R. (**1986b**). "New effects of cochlear nonlinearity in temporal patterns of auditory nerve fiber responses to harmonic complexes." In: *Peripheral Auditory Mechanisms*, edited by

J.B.Allen, J.L.Hall, A.Hubbard, S.T.Neely and A.Tubis (Springer-Verlag, Berlin,Heidelberg, New York) pp. 298-305.

Kiang, N.Y.S., Watanabe, T., Thomas, E.C., and Clark, L.F. (**1965**). *Discharge patterns of single fibers in the cat's auditory nerve.* (M.I.T., Cambridge, MA).

Møller, A.R. (**1977**). "Frequency selectivity of single auditory-nerve fibers in response to broadband noise stimuli," J.Acoust.Soc.Am. **62**, 135-142.

Pfeiffer, R.R. and Kim, D.O. (**1972**). "Response patterns of single cochlear nerve fibers to click stimuli:Descriptions for cat," J.Acoust.Soc.Am. **52**, 1669-1677.

Price, R. (**1958**). "A useful theorem for nonlinear devices having Gaussian inputs, IRE Trans.Inform.Theory, **II-4**, 69-72.

Sachs, M.B., Young, E.D., and Lewis, R.H. (**1974**). "Discharge patterns of single fibers in the pigeon auditory nerve," Brain Research **70**, 431-447.

Shamma, S.A. and Morrish, K.A. (**1987**). "Synchrony suppression in complex stimulus responses of a biophysical model of the cochlea," J.Acoust.Soc. Am. **81**, 1486-1498.

Wit, H.P. and Horst, J.W. (**1986**). "Contrast enhancement in frequency spectra of cochlear microphonic responses to complex stimuli," Hearing Res. **21**, 59-65.

Young, E.D. and Sachs, M.B. (**1979**). "Representation of steady-state vowels in the temporal aspects of the discharge patterns of populations of auditory-nerve fibers," J.Acoust.Soc.Am. **66**, 1381-1403.

Comments

Evans:

1. Recent data obtained in our laboratory, from single cochlear nerve fibres in the cat, confirm your results in the pigeon, including, importantly, the illustrated result with a flat phase, one octave wide, spectrum having $CF/f_0=8$. Randomising the phase of the stimulus components had little or no effect. (Because I tend to use autocorrelogram analyzes of the spike discharges, my remarks only apply to the spectral magnitude results.)

2. With a hardware model (Evans, 1980) consisting of a linear front-end filter followed by an Automatic Gain Control (AGC) preceding the non-linear stages of rectification, log compression and probabilistic spike generation the following results were obtained. The model predicts all of the spectral magnitude results shown in the right half of each of the figures in your paper. The crucial point is that the time-constant of integration of the AGC must be short compared with the waveform repetition period of the stimuli having $CF/f_0>20$, and must be of the same order or larger than that of the $CF/f_0=8$ stimulus. In order to model satisfactorily period histograms to low frequency tones, the time constant had been chosen as 10-12 ms, and satisfies these criteria.

3. N.P.Cooper and I (data to be published) have shown that the effects of refractiveness analyzed by Gaumond, Miller and others are virtually insignificant under similar conditions to these, which can be regarded as "steady state" in relation to the tens of msec required for full recovery from the effects of refractoriness (see our comment on Karamanos and Miller, this meeting).

Evans, E. F. (1980). An electronic analogue of single unit recording from the cochlear nerve for teaching and research. J Physiol. 298, 6-7P.

Reply by Horst:

1. I am glad you reconfirmed our data in the cat (Horst *et al.*, 1985, 1986 a,b). Note, however, that fibers where the shape of the response spectrum hardly changed with stimulus level (shown here in Fig.4, for $CF/F_0=8$) formed a minority both in the cat and in the pigeon.

2. I made my remark on AGC because our data clearly contradict the existence of an AGC that would serve to maintain the envelope of the period histogram at all stimulus levels. Obviously, mechanisms such as compression or limitation are needed in order to describe the data. An AGC with a time constant short compared to the fundamental period, would have similar effects on the temporal envelope. There is ample evidence that compression or saturation can be found in (I) BM mechanics and (II) hair cell transduction as well as in (III) the hair-cell nerve-fiber synapse and it is becoming clear that the stages I and II are coupled. Therefore, a separate linear front-end filter is not likely. A separate compressive nonlinearity (CNL) before the spike generator would influence the shape of individual peaks in the period histogram into the direction of blocks. So, we have to be careful about using separate CNLs in models of the cochlea. A CNL coupled with a bandpass filter, or an AGC would not have this drawback. More research is needed to determine to what extent CNLs and/or AGCs determine the fiber's response.

3. I am looking forward to see those data. However, our peak instantaneous discharge rates both in the cat and the pigeon show a dependence on CF (and as a consequence on the fundamental period) indicating that refractory effects do influence the shape of the response.

The representation of concurrent vowels in the temporal discharge patterns of auditory nerve fibers

A. R. Palmer

Institute of Hearing Research, University of Nottingham, University Park, Nottingham NG7 2RD, England.

Introduction

In the real world, sounds are rarely heard in quiet without any interference from background noises. While the frequency selectivity of the cochlea provides a means of rejecting some unwanted signals, purely place-based schemes for the encoding of even relatively simple speech sounds, such as steady-state voiced vowels, appear to break down at high sound levels and in the presence of wideband noise (Sachs & Young, 1979; Sachs *et al.*, 1983). On the other hand, in the presence of such wideband noise there is still a good representation of the vowel spectra in terms of the temporal aspects of the cochlear nerve fiber activity (Delgutte, 1980; Sachs *et al.*, 1983; Delgutte & Kiang, 1984).

The voice of a competing speaker represents a particularly difficult interfering noise in speech perception, since both the target voice and the the background have similar spectral and temporal characteristics. Nevertheless, listeners can perform well above chance in identifying pairs of vowels, even when both have the same fundamental frequency (F0) or when they are unvoiced (Scheffers, 1983). In these cases, the identification, whether place-based or using temporal cues, must depend upon some kind of profile analysis or template matching (Klatt, 1980a; Scheffers, 1983). When a difference in F0 is introduced between members of a pair of voiced vowels, listeners hear two voices rather than one and their identification performance improves. This improved performance presumably results from extra information present in the neural representation, which aids the process of template matching by enabling segregation of components from the two sources with different F0. A difference in F0 has little effect on template matching based on place alone (Scheffers, 1983).

In the present study I have investigated the representation of concurrent voiced vowels on different F0s in the temporal aspects of the discharge of cochlear nerve fibers. Two different ways of signalling the F0s were assessed: modulation of the discharge of single fibers and the distribution of responses synchronized to harmonics of F0. Across the population of fibers there are regions where individual harmonics are not resolved, but the discharge is modulated at one or other of the two F0s. However, even for single vowels this modulation is virtually eliminated by wideband noise masking (Miller & Sachs, 1983). The second measure which should be resistant to noise (Sachs *et al.*, 1983) uses the distribution of the activity synchronized to the harmonics of the double vowel to estimate the two F0s. Using these F0 estimates a good separation of the spectra of the two constituent vowels can be achieved.

Methods

Details of the methods used for nerve-fiber recording and for the generation and presentation of the stimuli may be found in Palmer *et al.* (1986).

Pigmented guinea-pigs (200-450g) were anesthetized with a neuroleptic technique (0.06 mg atropine sulphate; 30 mg/kg sodium pentobarbitone; 4 mg/kg droperidol; 1 mg/kg phenoperidine; see Evans, 1979). The trachea was cannulated and the core temperature was maintained at 37 °C.

Glass micropipettes filled with 2.7 M KCl (impedance 10-30 MΩ) were then introduced under direct vision into the auditory nerve via a posterior craniotomy, after retraction of the cerebellum and brainstem. The bulla pressure was equalized with a small-bore nylon tube and the cochlear action-potential threshold to tone pips was monitored periodically via a wire on the round window. Nerve-fiber discharges were amplified, filtered, discriminated from baseline noise and then fed to a laboratory computer which recorded their time of occurrence with respect to the stimulus with 10 μs accuracy.

Bursts of wideband noise were used as search stimuli and the best frequency, minimum threshold and spontaneous rate of each fiber were routinely determined.

The speech sounds were produced using a software cascade synthesizer (Klatt, 1980b). Three steady-state approximations to the single vowels /i/ /a/ and /)/ were used with either four (to match our earlier studies) or five formants (producing a more natural spectrum). The formant frequencies (F1-F3), the fundamental frequency of voicing (F0) and the formant bandwidths are shown in Table 1. The spectrum of the four-formant vowel /a/ may be

Table 1. Voicing fundamental frequency (F0) and frequency and bandwidth in Hz of the first three formants F1-F3 of the synthetic vowels /i/ /a/ /)/.

Vowel	F0 Freq.	F1 Freq.	BW	F2 Freq.	BW	F3 Freq.	BW
/i/	125	270	90	2290	110	3010	170
/a/	100	730	90	1090	110	2440	170
/)/	100	450	90	750	110	2850	170

found in Fig.1 of Palmer *et al.* (1986). The sampling rate was 10 kHz in all cases. The double vowels were produced by combination of the /i/ with either the /a/ or the /)/.

The times of occurrence of the cochlear nerve spikes were used to construct period histograms locked to the 40 ms period of the double vowels. 40 ms gives four complete pitch periods of the vowel on 100 Hz and five of the vowel on 125 Hz. The choice of F0s which bear an integer relationship (4:5) to one another reduces the computational overhead in the analyses, but has the unfortunate consequence that harmonics at exact multiples of 500 Hz are shared by the two vowels of the concurrent pair. The contribution, to the overall discharge, made by spikes synchronized to the individual harmonics of the stimulus was quantified by taking the Fourier transform of the period histogram. Results were pooled from different animals.

Results

When several equal amplitude components pass through a single neural filter, beating occurs which results in modulation of the neural discharge at the common F0 (Smoorenburg & Linschooten, 1977; Delgutte, 1980; Miller & Sachs, 1983, 1984). As a result of rectifier distortion a peak appears in the Fourier transform of the period histogram at the F0 frequency. This can be used as an indicator of the degree of modulation of the discharge and its distribution across the fiber array is shown in Fig.1 for the double vowel /i/+ /a/. The large synchronization indices at low frequencies indicate responses

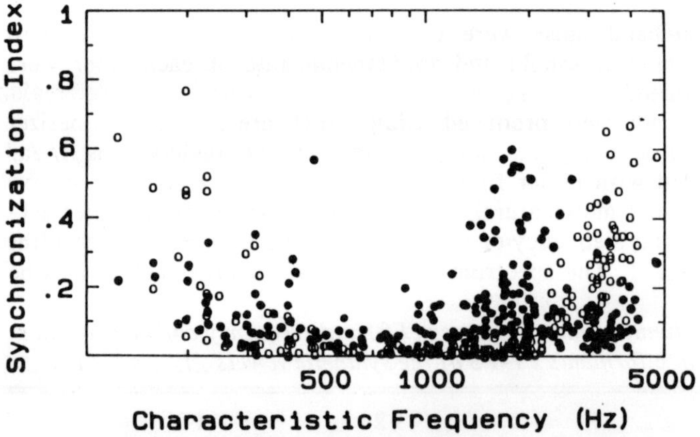

Figure 1. Degree of modulation of period histograms to /i/ + /a/ at 85 dB SPL as a function of fiber CF as indicated by the synchronization index (magnitude of the component in the Fourier spectrum divided by the value at zero frequency). Open symbols show modulation at 125 Hz, closed symbols at 100 Hz.

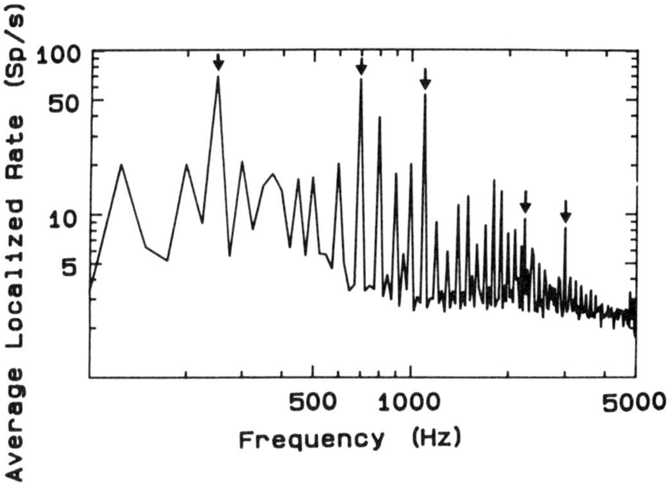

Figure 2. ALSR function for the double vowel /i/ + /a/ at 85 dB SPL. Sampling interval 25 Hz, window ±0.5 octs., N=231.

to the two F0s in fibers with best frequencies at or near the two F0s. Even though the degree of modulation decreases with intensity there are still neurons at this sound level which are modulated at frequencies corresponding to the two F0s; between the F2 of /a/ and the F2 of /i/ the modulations are at 100 Hz and above the F2 of /i/ they are at 125 Hz. The usefulness of these modulations for identifying the F0s is questionable, however, since Miller and Sachs (1983,1984) have shown that such modulations for single vowels are virtually eliminated by wideband noise, as they occur in spectral regions where the vowel components are weakest.

Figure 2 shows the distribution across the fiber array of responses synchronized to the components of the double vowel /i/ + /a/. Shown here is the average localized synchronized rate function (the ALSR after Young & Sachs, 1979) which is computed as the average synchronized discharge (from the FFT) to each frequency in turn in the firing of those neurons whose CF was within ±0.5 octaves of that frequency. It should be stressed that other analyses, not using matched filtering, have yielded similar results. In this figure peaks of synchronized activity can be seen at the frequency positions of the formants of both the /i/ and the /a/ (arrows). It is also evident that synchronized activity occurs only at frequencies corresponding to the harmonics of 100 and 125 Hz and that within this function there is a considerable amount of information as to the F0s of the constituent harmonic series. Three very different analyses have been applied to the data of Fig.2 each of which successfully identified 100 and 125 Hz as the F0s of the two vowels present. The first was an harmonic selection technique after Parsons (1976) in which the center frequencies of harmonics in the ALSR function are

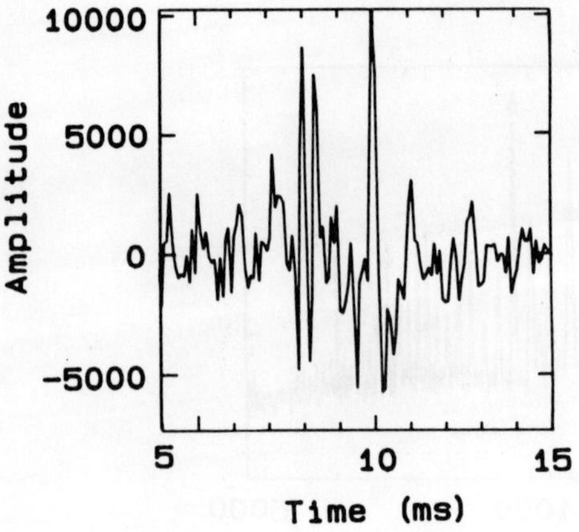

Figure 3. Cepstrum derived from the data shown in Fig.2

used to determine the F0s. The second technique consisted of application of a series of harmonic sieves and summing the components which passed through; sieves with spacings corresponding to the two F0s produced the largest values of the sum. The third analysis is shown in Fig.3 which illustrates the cepstrum obtained from the data of Fig.2 (a cepstrum is a form of non-linear autocorrelation obtained by taking the inverse FFT of the logarithmic power spectrum). Note the two largest peaks in the cepstrum at 8 and 10 ms corresponding to the 125 and 100 Hz F0s.

By using the estimates of the F0s obtained from the population response, a type of harmonic sieve process can be applied to the data of Fig.2 by resampling only at the harmonics of either 125 or 100 Hz. The result of this analysis is shown in Fig.4 by the solid lines (top part shows sampling at 100 Hz, bottom at 125 Hz). The filled symbols have been excluded since these represent responses to the shared harmonics at multiples of 500 Hz; the values used at these frequencies were extrapolated from the adjacent harmonics. The points excluded reflect responses to harmonics of /a/ at 500, 1000 and 1500 Hz and of /i/ at 3000 Hz. The dashed lines show the ALSR functions with 100 Hz or 125 Hz resolution for the responses to /a/ (top) and /i/ (bottom) presented alone and are exactly like previously published data for the guinea-pig (Palmer *et al.*, 1986).

The data for the five-formant vowels were similar in all important respects. The vowel /)/ was included in the stimulus set as its first formant at 450 Hz was much closer to that of the /i/ (at 270 Hz) than was that of the /a/ (at 730 Hz). Even with this closer spacing of the F1s the ALSR to the /i/ + /)/ yielded good estimates of both F0s and good reconstructions of the /i/ and /)/ component spectra. Notice in particular that in the reconstructed spectra the first two formants of both vowels are very prominent as they are in the responses to the vowels alone.

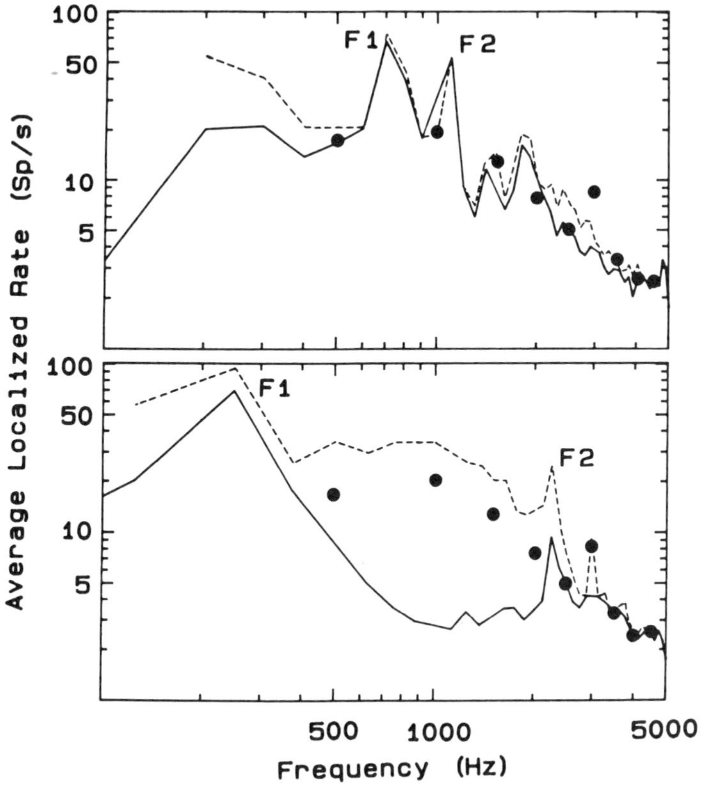

Figure 4. Top: Dashed line, ALSR function for /a/ at 84 dB SPL, N=140, sampled at 100 Hz. Solid line, ALSR function derived by sampling the data of Fig.2 at 100 Hz. Bottom: Dashed line, ALSR function for /i/ at 77 dB SPL, N=147, sampled at 125 Hz. Solid line, ALSR derived by sampling the data of Fig.2 at 125 Hz. Filled symbols indicated shared harmonics (see text).

Discussion

Entirely place-based models for the encoding of voiced speech sounds appear to suffer a number of drawbacks. While at low sound levels, formant-related peaks are evident in the distribution of mean discharge rate across the fiber array, at high levels such peaks are evident only amongst the higher threshold, low spontaneous rate, fibers (Sachs & Young, 1979; Sachs *et al.*, 1983) or during formant transitions (Miller & Sachs, 1984). At high presentation levels in background noise even the low spontaneous rate fibers are unable to show peaks in activity at the formant-related frequencies, nor does the wider dynamic range at the onset of sounds appear to be useful under these conditions (Sachs *et al.*, 1983). Nevertheless, we cannot exclude the possibility that place of activity alone might yet afford a good internal representation of voiced speech sounds, even at high level and in background noise, by taking into account dynamic aspects such as moving formants and wider onset dynamic ranges, higher thresholds for low spontaneous rate fibers, and possible actions of the middle-ear muscles and the descending efferents to the cochlea.

When two vowels are present at once even a perfect place-based code would require some kind of template matching as seems to be the case for many pitch judgements (e.g. Goldstein, 1973). A difference in the F0 of the two vowels has minimal effect on the vowel identification performance by template matching on the basis of place information (Scheffers, 1983). Since performance does improve markedly, probably as a result of segregation into different sound sources, we should look to temporal features for the cues enabling the improved performance. The present study has demonstrated that information is readily available in the distribution of synchronized activity across the fiber array which would allow identification of the two F0s in a concurrent vowel pair. Using this information, good reconstructions of the component vowel spectra are possible from the population response to the concurrent vowels. Thus it would seem likely that the improvement in performance in the psychophysical experiments when a difference in F0 is present between two vowels reflects use of temporal aspects of the nerve fiber activity.

Acknowledgements

I thank Padma Moorjani for technical assistance Dr. R. Stubbs for implementing the harmonic selection and Drs. A. Rees, Q. Summerfield and P. Assmann for reading early drafts of this paper.

References

Delgutte, B., (**1980**). "Representation of Speech-like Sounds in the Discharge Patterns of Auditory-nerve Fibers," J.Acoust.Soc.Am. **68**, 843-857.

Delgutte, B., and Kiang, N. Y. S. (**1984**). "Speech Coding in the Auditory Nerve: V. Vowels in background noise," J.Acoust.Soc.Am. **75**, 908-918.

Evans, E. F. (**1979**). "Neuroleptanesthesia for the Guinea-pig," Arch. Otolaryngol. 105, 185-186.

Goldstein, J. L. (**1973**). "An Optimum Processor Theory for the Central Formation of the Pitch of Complex Tones," J.Acoust.Soc.Am. **54**, 1496-1516.

Klatt, D. H. (**1980a**). "Speech Perception: a Model of Acoustic-phonetic Analysis and Lexical Access," in *Perception and Production of Fluent Speech*, edited by R. Cole (Laurence Erlbaum, Hillsdale, New York), pp. 243-288.

Klatt, D. H. (**1980b**). "Software for a Cascade/Parallel Formant Synthesizer,"

J.Acoust.Soc.Am. **67**, 971-995.

Miller, M. I., and Sachs, M. B. (**1983**). "Auditory-nerve Respresentation of Voice Pitch," in *Hearing - Physiological Bases and Psychophysics*, edited by R. Klinke and R. Hartmann (Springer, Berlin), pp. 344-351.

Miller, M. I., and Sachs, M. B. (**1984**). "Representation of Voice Pitch in Discharge Patterns of Auditory-nerve Fibers," Hear. Res. **14**, 257-279.

Palmer, A. R., Winter, I. M., and Darwin, C. J. (**1986**). "The Representation of Steady-state Vowel Sounds in the Temporal Discharge Patterns of the Guinea Pig Cochlear Nerve and Primarylike Cochlear Nucleus Neurons," J. Acoust.Soc.Am. **79**, 100-113.

Parsons, T. W. (**1976**). "Separation of Speech from Interfering Noise by Harmonic Selection," J.Acoust.Soc.Am. **60**, 911-918.

Sachs, M. B., and Young, E. D. (**1979**). "Encoding of Steady-state Vowels in the Auditory Nerve: Representation in Terms of Discharge Rate," J. Acoust.Soc.Am. **66**, 470-479.

Sachs, M. B., Voigt, H. F., and Young, E. D. (**1983**). "Auditory Nerve Representation of Vowels in Background Noise," J.Neurophysiol. **50**, 27-45.

Scheffers, M. T. M. (**1983**). *Sifting Vowels: Auditory Pitch Analysis and Sound Segregation*, Doctoral Thesis, University of Groningen.

Smoorenburg, G. F., and Linschoten, D. H. (**1977**). "A Neurophysiological Study on Auditory Frequency Analysis of Complex Tones," in *Psychophysics and Physiology of Hearing*, edited by E.F. Evans and J.P. Wilson (Academic Press, London), pp.175-183.

Young, E. D., and Sachs, M. B. (**1979**). "Representation of Steady-state Vowels in the Temporal Aspects of the Discharge Patterns of Populations of Auditory Nerve Fibers, " J. Acoust. Soc. Am. 66, 1381-1403.

Comments

Schroeder:

This is an exciting contribution to monoural speech perception (and separation) on the neurophysiological level. Interestingly the separation of two (or more) voices picked up by the same microphone has been a long-time goal of *artificial* intelligence (AI). As a first signal-processing step, one usually measures the different pitches and splits the received signal by appropriate comb-filters "tuned" to the different fundamental frequencies. (Subsequent steps invoke formant track continuity etc.) In the pitch measurement step, I have found that the (inverse) Fourier transform of the *amplitude* spectrum (the *square-root* of the power spectrum) can cope better with multiple pitches than the (justly famous) *cepstrum*, which is based on the *logarithm* of the power spectrum. Both logarithm and square root are of course compressive ("convex") functions but, for some reason, the square root seems to work better in AI.

Pitch-period following response of cat cochlear nucleus neurons to speech sounds

D.O. Kim and G. Leonard

Div. of Otolaryngology/Surgery; Neuroscience Program
University of Connecticut Health Center
Farmington, CT 06032

Introduction

Several studies conducted in the 1970's investigated the response of cochlear nucleus neurons to speech stimuli (e.g., Moore and Cashin, 1974, Caspary *et al.*, 1977). In more recent years, the response of the primary auditory nerve fibers to certain speech stimuli have been relatively well characterized (e.g., Sachs and Young, 1979; Miller and Sachs, 1984; see Carlson and Grandstrom, 1982). This has led to a renewed interest in further studies of the cochlear nucleus which can compare the input to and the output from the cochlear nucleus thereby helping to elucidate how the cochlear nucleus neurons transform the signals established in the primary auditory nerve fibers in response to speech (e.g., Palmer *et al.*, 1986; Blackburn *et al.*, 1986; Kim *et al.*, 1986).

One of the most striking examples of a specialized signal processing of the cochlear nucleus, which was observed in our recent study (Kim *et al.*, 1986), is a phenomenon that we called the "pitch-period following response" (PFR). The PFR corresponds to spike discharges of a neuron which are phase-locked to the fundamental period (i.e., the pitch period) of a complex periodic stimulus such as voiced speech sounds.

In this study, we have conducted single unit recordings of responses from neurons in the dorsal and posteroventral cochlear nucleus (DCN and PVCN) of decerebrate cats using speech sounds as stimuli. We found that different neurons exhibited a widely varying temporal precision of the PFR. We present in this paper an analysis of the PFR of various types of neurons in the DCN and PVCN.

Methods

This paper is based on data from 12 healthy adult cats. The cats were initially anesthetized by an intraperitoneal injection of sodium pento-barbital (30 mg/kg). The left pinna was resected and an acoustic coupler, incorporating a calibrated probe tube and a Beyer DT48 earphone, was attached to the bone around the eardrum. The bulla was left intact except for installation of a ventilation tube (0.86 mm I.D.). The dorsal surface of left cochlear nucleus was exposed by opening the cranium and aspirating a section of the cerebellum. The cats were rendered decerebrate by a total transection of the brainstem at the level of the superior colliculus. Subsequent to the decerebration, each of the cats was maintained over a period up to four days in an unanesthetized condition. Attempts were made to maximize the number of neurons recorded from individual animals by limiting the number of stimuli applied to each neuron and by conducting the recordings around the clock for several days in a manner analogous to the population study of primary auditory nerve fibers (Pfeiffer and Kim, 1975).

The recording electrodes were glass microelectrodes which were filled with 3M KCl (typically 50 MΩ) or with 4% Chicago Sky Blue (typically 70 to 100 MΩ after beveling). The DCN surface was visualized through an operating microscope when placing the recording electrode. The electrode penetrations were oriented parallel to both sagital and transverse planes. In some cats, the electrode tip locations were marked by iontophoretically injecting small amounts of the dye (Lee *et al.*, 1969). We were able to visualize blue dye spots in histological sections and confirmed that the electrode penetrations advanced from the DCN molecular layer through the deep DCN and into the PVCN.

A system including a DEC Micro-PDP11 computer, a University-of-Wisconsin Digital Stimulus System and a Unit Event Timer was used to control the stimulus and to process the spike data. We used vowels synthesized with "KLTEXC", which is the Klatt (1980) algorithm implemented by the D. Pisoni group of University of Indiana. One of the stimuli was a synthetic vowel [ϵ] whose parameters were: F0 = 128 Hz, F1 = 512 Hz, F2 = 1792 Hz, F3 = 2432 Hz, B1 = 60 Hz, B2 = 90 Hz, B3 = 200 Hz. (The Fi and Bi are the frequency and the bandwidth of the the i-th formant, respectively.) We also used a synthetic vowel [a] (whose parameters are shown in Kim *et al.* 1986) and natural human speech signals [la] and [ra] spoken by a male and a female speaker.

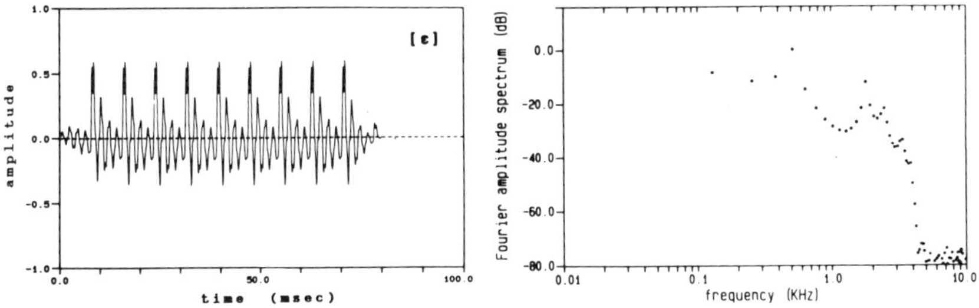

Figure 1. Waveform and amplitude spectrum of a synthetic vowel [ϵ] as a voltage applied to the earphone. F0=128Hz, F1=512Hz, F2=1792Hz, F3=2432Hz, B1=60Hz, B2=90Hz, B3=200 Hz.

Figure 1 shows the waveform and amplitude spectrum of [ε]. The vowel stimulus, whose duration was 80 ms, was presented with an 8-ms rise-fall time and repeated every 400 ms with an intervening silent time. Spike discharges in response to [ε] at a particular stimulus level were collected from each neuron for 40 seconds. A similar procedure was used with [a]. In the case of [la] and [ra], the stimulus duration was 250 ms and the stimulus was repeated every 1250 ms. Spike discharges in response to these syllables were collected from each neuron for 50 seconds. In all cases, the occurrence time of each spike was stored with a 20 μs resolution.

Results

Figure 2 shows four examples of poststimulus time (PST) histograms obtained from four different cochlear nucleus neurons using the stimulus [ε] at 55 dB SPL. (The dB SPL in this paper represents an rms level re 20 μPa.) The four responses are chosen to illustrate a wide range in the temporal precision of the PFR. As a means of quantifying the temporal precision of the PFR, we introduce a measure to be called "periodicity strength". The periodicity strength is a special case of the vector strength (Goldberg and Brown, 1969). We define the periodicity strength, PS, to be equal to the vector strength of the spike discharges of a neuron being stimulated with a complex periodic signal where the entire fundamental period is equated to 2π radians:

$PS = ((\Sigma x_i)^2+(\Sigma y_i)^2)^{\frac{1}{2}} / N$, where

$x_i = \cos(2\pi t_i/T_0)$; $y_i = \sin(2\pi t_i/T_0)$;
t_i = time of occurrence of the i-th spike relative to the stimulus onset;
T_0 = fundamental period of the complex periodic stimulus signal,
N = total number of spikes observed in the computation window.

The top PST histogram of Fig. 2 is an example of a very high (0.999) periodicity strength. This neuron (#P21-11) had a CF of 1157 Hz and is an "onset" type in its response to a pure tone at CF (Pfeiffer, 1966). The second neuron is a "chopper" type with CF of 1358 Hz. The lower periodicity strength of this response represents the fact that the spike discharges are more broadly distributed over each fundamental period.

The third neuron in Fig. 2 is a "primarylike" type with CF of 1157 Hz. It is interesting to note that the first neuron and the third neuron have the same CF but are quite different in their periodicity strength characteristics. The third and top histograms may be considered as the input and output, respectively, of a time-domain contrast-enhancement processing. Such a contrast enhancement could be accomplished through a coincidence detection mechanism (Kim *et al.*, 1986).

The fourth neuron is a "primarylike" type with CF of 762 Hz. This neuron's CF is close to the first formant of [ε], 512 Hz, and the neuron's response is dominated by the first formant frequency component.

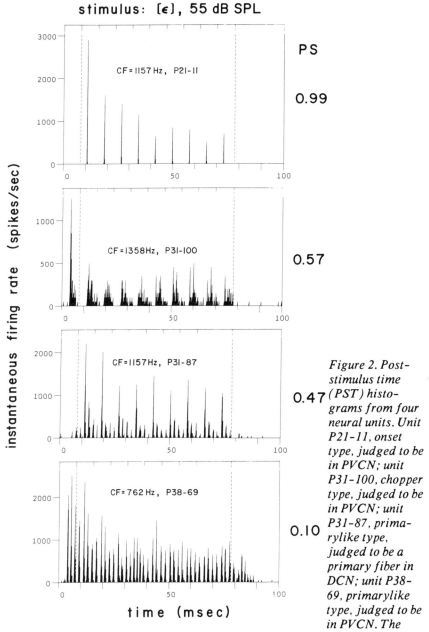

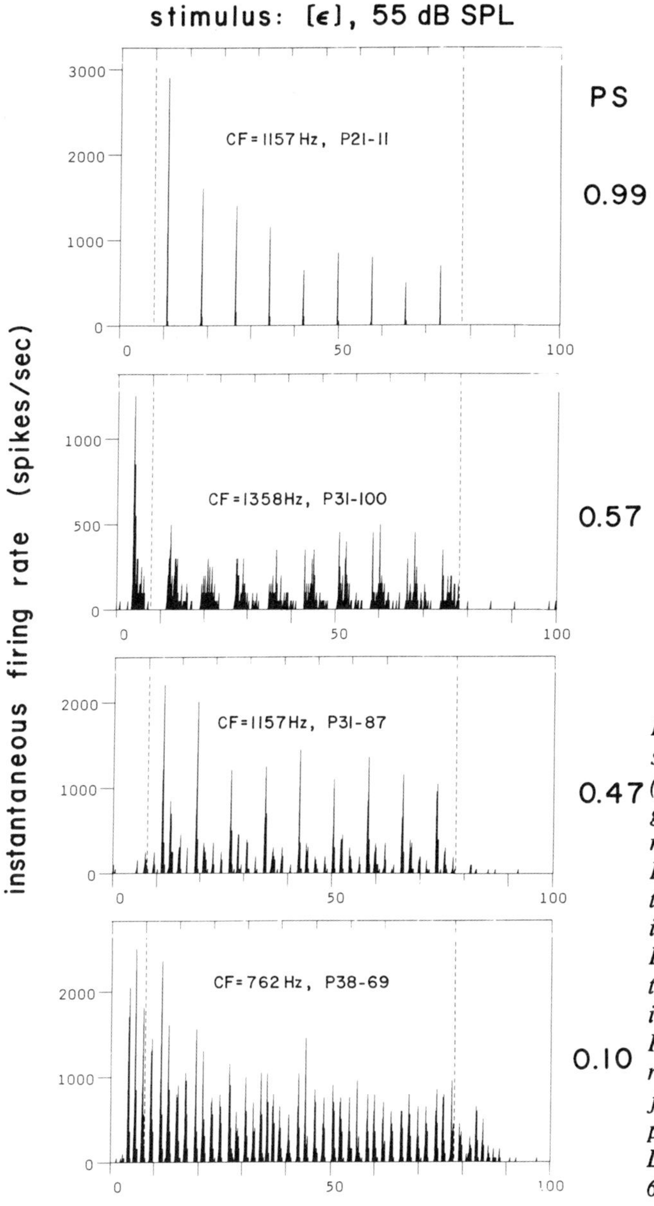

Figure 2. Post-stimulus time (PST) histograms from four neural units. Unit P21-11, onset type, judged to be in PVCN; unit P31-100, chopper type, judged to be in PVCN; unit P31-87, primarylike type, judged to be a primary fiber in DCN; unit P38-69, primarylike type, judged to be in PVCN. The periodicity strength (PS) was computed over a time window indicated by two vertical dashed lines in each histogram. Stimulus: [ϵ], 55 dB SPL.

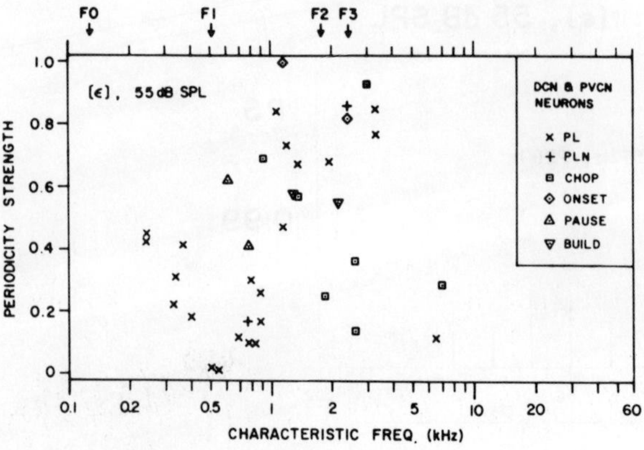

Figure 3. Periodicity strength versus CF for a number of neural units recorded in DCN and PVCN of 5 cats. Stimulus: [ϵ], 55 dB SPL.

Figure 3 shows a plot of periodicity strength versus a neuron's CF for a number of neurons recorded in the DCN and PVCN with [ϵ] at 55 dB SPL. The sample of neurons represent all of the neurons recorded from a set of 5 cats whose spike discharges exhibited a significant excitatory response to the stimulus. Thus, not shown in Fig. 3 are a number of neurons recorded in these cats whose spike discharges were inhibited or little affected by the stimulus. The neurons are classified, as indicated by different symbols in Fig. 3, on the basis of the type of the PST histogram obtained with a pure tone at CF. Data of Fig. 3 indicate that the periodicity strength is strongly influenced by the CF of each neuron. The neurons with CF near the first formant of [ϵ], 512 Hz, show small values of the periodicity strength. Similarly, the periodicity strength values tend to decrease as the CF approaches the second formant of the vowel, 1792 Hz. In the two regions of CF between the first and second formants and just above the third formant, 2432 Hz, the periodicity strength values are the largest. The data obtained with [a] are qualitatively similar to the above results.

Although the neurons exhibiting the largest periodicity strengths near 1.0 were of the "onset" type, there is a large variability in the periodicity strength in each of the different types of neurons. The data that we presently have do not permit us to determine clearly whether there is a systematic difference in the periodicity strength for different types of neurons having same CF.

Figure 4 illustrates examples of a precise PFR (from neuron #P21-11) in response to natural human speech sounds [la] sampled from a male and a female speaker. The pitch period (averaged over the signal) of the male voice was 7.93 ms (corresponding to 126 Hz) and that for the female voice was 5.02 ms (199 Hz). The data of Fig. 4 demonstrates that the neuron was capable of accurately following the voice pitch period over a range encompassing male and female voices.

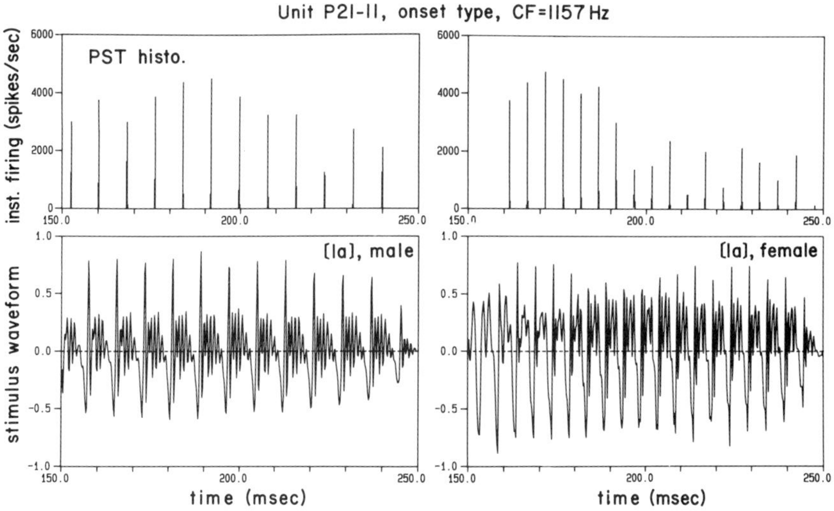

Figure 4. Upper panels: pitch-period following response of a neuron judged to be in PVCN to [la] spoken by a male and a female speaker. Lower panels: stimulus waveforms as voltages applied to the earphone. Stimulus level, 55 dB SPL. The total duration of [la] was 250 ms and the time window displayed in each PST histogram corresponds to the vowel portion of the syllable.

Discussion

Previous single unit recordings from the cochlear nucleus using speech stimuli reported examples of responses which show some degree of synchronization to the pitch period (Moore and Cashin, 1974; Caspary *et al.*, 1977; Palmer *et al.*, 1986). However, data reported in our present paper and in Kim *et al.* (1986) document more clearly the existence of a highly precise pitch-period following response.

Data from the previous studies and the present study both show that there is a large diversity in responses to speech stimuli among various types of cochlear nucleus neurons having similar CF. We suggest that the periodicity strength would be a useful measure in distinguishing each neuron's pitch-period encoding behavior.

Miller and Sachs (1984) investigated representations of voice pitch in discharge patterns of the primary auditory nerve fibers in terms of the "synchronization index" at the fundamental frequency. We believe that the synchronization index at the fundamental frequency and the periodicity strength are mathematically equivalent but their definitions emphasize different aspects. The periodicity strength definition conveys more directly the concept that the histograms of Fig. 2 (top) and Fig. 4 should have a near-perfect score. Both their data on the primary fibers and our data on the cochlear nucleus neurons show that the response of the neural units having CF near formant frequencies are dominated by a formant frequency component (Fig. 2, bottom) leading to low periodicity scores and that the neural units having CF just above the third formant show higher periodicity scores. A major difference between the two sets of data is that the cochlear nucleus neurons exhibit higher periodicity scores than the primary fibers in the CF regions between the first two formants and just above the third formant. In other words, the precise PFR illustrated in Fig. 2 (top) and Fig. 4 (also Fig. 2 of Kim *et al.*, 1986) are observed in the cochlear nucleus but not in the primary auditory nerve fibers.

The ability to follow the time-varying pitch (i.e., intonation) of the speaker's voice is a significant aspect of speech recognition. Some theories and models for the pitch of complex signals attempt to represent response properties of the primary auditory nerve fibers (see e.g., de Boer, 1976; Evans, 1978). At the present time, there is much less information about the discharge patterns of the cochlear nucleus neurons in response to complex periodic signals than about the response of the primary auditory nerve fibers. Thus, neurophysiological data such as presented in this paper should be useful in further developments of models of pitch perception.

Acknowledgements

This study was supported by a grant (No. NS23693) from US-NIH and grants from the University of Connecticut Health Center. We thank K.L. Jones, H.H. Nguyen and J.G. Sirianni for their general assistance, and D.L. Oliver and D.K. Morest for their help in histological processing.

References

Blackburn, C.C., Shofner, W.P. and Sachs, M.B.(**1986**). "The representation of the steady-state vowel sound /ϵ/ in the temporal discharge patterns of cat anteroventral cochlear nucleus neurons," Assoc.Res.Otolaryngol. 9th Meeting Abs., p130.

de Boer, E.(**1976**). "On the "residue" and auditory pitch perception," in Handbook of Sensory Physiology, Vol. V, Part 3, pp 479-583.

Carlson, R. and Grandstrom, B.(**1982**). The Representation of Speech in the peripheral auditory system, Symposium Proc. (Elsevier, New York), p1-291.

Caspary, D.M., Rupert, A.L. and Moushegian, G.(**1977**). "Neuronal coding of vowel sounds in the cochlear nuclei," Exper.Neurol. **54**, 414-431.

Evans, E.F.(**1978**). "Place and time coding of frequency in the peripheral auditory system: Some physiological pros and cons," Audiology **17**, 369-420.

Goldberg, J.M. and Brown, P.B.(**1969**). "Response of binaural neurons of dog superior olivary complex to dichotic tonal stimuli: Some physiological mechanisms of sound localization," J.Neurophysiol. **32**, 613-636.

Kim, D.O., Rhode, W.S. and Greenberg, S.R.(**1986**). "Responses of cochlear nucleus neurons to speech signals: Neural encoding of pitch, intensity and other parameters," in Auditory Frequency Selectivity, edited by B.C.J. Moore and R.D. Patterson (Plenum, New York), pp281-288.

Klatt, D.H.(**1980**). "Software for a cascade/parallel formant synthesizer," J. Acoust.Soc.Am. **67**, 971-994.

Lee, B.B., Mandl, G. and Stean, J.P.B.(**1969**). "Microelectrode tip position marking in nervous tissue: A new dye method" Electroenceph. Clin. Neurophysiol. **27**, 610-613.

Miller, M.I. and Sachs, M.B.(**1984**). "Representation of voice pitch in discharge patterns of auditory-nerve fibers," Hearing Res. **14**, 257-279.

Moore, T.J. and Cashin, J.L.(**1974**). "Response patterns of cochlear nucleus neurons to excerpts from sustained vowels," J.Acoust.Soc.Am. **56**, 1565-1576.

Palmer, A.R., Winter, I.M. and Darwin, C.J.(**1986**). "The representation of steady-state vowel sounds in the temporal discharge patterns of the guinea pig cochlear nerve and primarylike cochlear nucleus neurons," J.Acoust. Soc.Am. **79**, 100-113.

Pfeiffer, R.R.(**1966**). "Classification of response patterns of spike discharges for units in the cochlear nucleus: Tone-burst stimulation," Exp.rain Res. **1**, 220-235.

Pfeiffer, R.R. and Kim, D.O.(**1975**). "Cochlear nerve fiber responses: Distribution along the cochlear partition," J.Acoust.Soc.Am. **58**, 867-869.

Sachs, M.B. and Young, E.D.(**1979**). "Encoding of steady-state vowels in the auditory nerve: Respresentation in terms of discharge rate," J.Acoust.Soc. Am. **66**, 470-479.

Comments

Van Stokkum:

Can adaptation explain your findings, especially of your unit P21-11? In the grassfrog I found indications for a relation between a following response to pulses or clicks and adaptation (van Stokkum, 1987).

Van Stokkum, I.H.M. (1987). "Sensitivity of neurons in the dorsal medullary nucleus of the grassfrog to spectral and temporal characteristics of sound." Hearing Res. 29, 223-235.

Reply by Kim:

We may consider that adaptation is a possible process that gives rise to the pitch-period following response of cat cochlear nucleus neurons, as you suggest. An alternative type of model, which I prefer now, is a coincidence-detection model where an output spike of a cochlear nucleus neuron requires simultaneous arrival of a sufficient number of input spikes of primary auditory nerve fibers that converge on a common cochlear nucleus neuron (Kim *et al.*, 1986). Regardless of which type of model one uses, it is interesting to note that your study showed that spike discharges of certain neurons in the frog dorsal medullary nucleus were time-locked to pulses of the mating call analogues to our cat cochlear nucleus data.

Rosen:

One thing which most psychoacousticians agree on is that the perception of pitch is determined primarily by the lowest harmonics. However, your Fig. 3 shows that fundamental periodicity is most strongly represented in neurons with relatively high characteristic frequencies, so it seems highly unlikely that the performance of human listeners could be based on the outputs of such neurons. Presumably, these pitch-following neurons are responding to a number of interacting harmonic components, so that randomizing the phase of the components, which has little or no effect on the perception of pitch by human listeners, will be likely to cause large changes in the corresponding periodicity strength.

Reply by Kim:

We will determine answers to these and related questions by direct experiments.

Houtsma:

Your physiological results are important for our general understanding of pitch perception in at least two respects. Firstly, you have found synchronisation to F_0 in a nucleus which is sufficiently central to have efferent contralateral connections. This may, at least in principle, account for virtual pitch of dichotic partials (Houtsma and Goldstein, 1972). Secondly, one may consider the shapened tuning for F_0, exhibited by some cochlear nucleus units, as represented by the variance reduction between the noisy frequency respresentations of partials and the best estimate of the fundamental in the Optimum Processor Theory (Goldstein, 1973). I think it would be very interesting to see whether the sharpened tuning effect in your experiment is maintained when some of the harmonics from your stimulus are moved to the other ear.

Houtsma, A.J.M. and Goldstein, J.L. (1972). "The central origin of the pitch of complex tones: evidence from musical interval recognition". J. Acoust. Soc. Am. 51, 520-529.

Goldstein, J.L. (1973). "An optimum processor theory for the central formation of the pitch of complex tones", J. Acoust. Soc. Am. 54, 1496-1516.

Miller:

If, in fact, the neurons you have studied are encoding the pitch cue via the envelope modulations seen in primary auditory nerve fibers, then it seems to me that this is a major piece of evidence in support at the residue pitch theory of Schouten. Do you agree?

Reply by Kim: Yes.

The influence of noise on the neuronal responses to pure and amplitude-modulated tones in the guinea-pig inferior colliculus

A. Rees

MRC Institute of Hearing Research
University Park, Nottingham NG7 2RD, England.

Introduction

Neurons in the central nucleus of the mammalian inferior colliculus (IC) respond to amplitude-modulated tones with a discharge modulated at the same frequency as the stimulus. The shape of the modulation transfer function (MTF), which describes a neuron's sensitivity to modulation as a function of stimulus modulation frequency, is influenced by changes in the mean intensity of the modulated tone, and by the addition of continuous broadband noise (Rees and Møller, 1987). When the mean stimulus level is raised, the MTFs become more bandpass-like as a result of a reduction in the depth of the modulated response at low modulation frequencies. However, this effect can be reversed by the addition of progressively higher levels of continuous broadband noise. The observed change in sensitivity to low modulation frequencies when noise is added to a modulated tone at a constant level is similar to that obtained when the intensity of the modulated tone is reduced.

Another well-documented effect of noise is the shift which it induces in the intensity dynamic range of cochlear-nerve fibers (Evans, 1974; Costalupes *et al.*, 1984), and of neurons in the cochlear nuclei (Gibson *et al.*, 1985) and auditory cortex (Phillips and Cynader, 1985; Phillips and Hall, 1986). In noise, such shifts would reduce the effective level of a modulated tone with respect to the neuron's dynamic range. A correlation should exist between the effects of noise on the dynamic range and the MTF, if such changes are manifestations of the same mechanism.

The present study tested this hypothesis by recording the responses of neurons in the central nucleus of the guinea-pig inferior colliculus to pure and amplitude-modulated tones, presented both in quiet, and in the presence of different levels of broadband noise.

Methods

Recordings were made from single neurons in the central nucleus of the inferior colliculus of pigmented guinea-pigs (250-450 g). The animals were anesthetised with a neuroleptic technique (sodium pentobarbitone 30 mg/kg, I.P.; 4mg/kg droperidol,I.P.; 1mg/kg phenoperidine I.M. and 0.06mg atropine sulphate, S.C.). They were tracheotomized and their core temperature maintained at 37°C.

Sound stimuli were presented monaurally to the contralateral ear, via a calibrated, closed acoustic system. Recordings were made with stereo-taxically-placed tungsten microelectrodes. Electrolytic lesions were made in each track to enable subsequent histological verification of the recording sites.

Characteristic frequency (CF) and threshold were determined for each unit along with its frequency/intensity response area for 50 ms tone bursts. Rate-intensity functions (RIFs) were generated from the responses to 50ms (5ms rise/fall time) CF tone bursts pseudo-randomly varied in level over a 90dB range in 5 dB steps. Each point on the RIF was calculated from the responses to 20 presentations of the stimulus.

Period histograms locked to the modulation waveform were constructed from the discharges in response to a sinusoidally amplitude-modulated CF tone (depth 50%). The vector strength (Goldberg and Brown, 1969) for each histogram was measured, enabling the gain of the response modulation to be calculated with respect to that of the stimulus as a function of modulation frequency; this gives the MTF. A measure of significance was calculated for each point using the factor $2nR^2$ (where n is the number of discharges and R is the vector strength of the histogram). A criterion value of 9.21 for this factor gives a probability of $p < 0.01$ that a non-uniform distribution of firing has occurred by chance (Mardia, 1972; Buunen and Rhode, 1978). Values

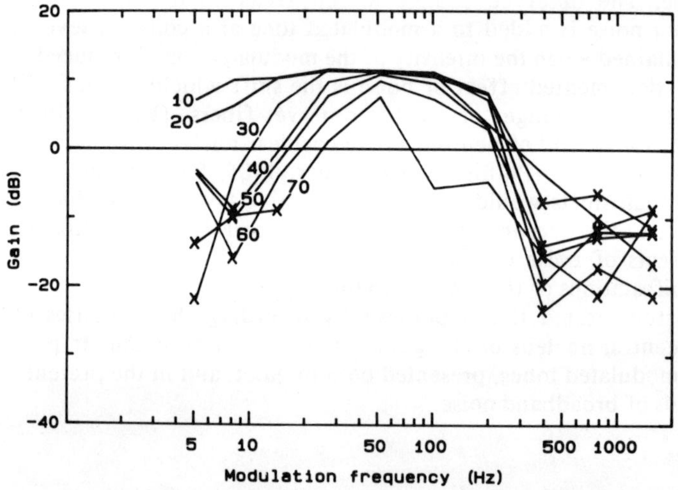

Figure 1. MTFs for an IC neuron at different carrier levels (parameter, dB re threshold). CF= 5.5 kHz.

which fall below this criterion are denoted by a cross in Figures 1 and 4. In addition, the neuron's mean discharge rate as a function of modulation frequency was calculated from the total number of spikes collected in each period histogram. The continuous broadband noise had a bandwidth of 0-20 kHz and its spectrum level is expressed in dB re 20 μPA/Hz$^{\frac{1}{2}}$.

Results

The results are based on recordings made from 124 single neurons in the central nucleus of the inferior colliculus with CFs between 0.6 and 20kHz.

Comparison of responses to pure and amplitude modulated tones in quiet

Figure 1 shows a series of MTFs calculated from the responses of a single neuron to a modulated CF tone at a range of different mean carrier levels. As the mean carrier level of the stimulus is increased there is a reduction in the gain of the neuron's response to the lowest modulation frequencies, with relatively little effect at higher modulation frequencies. The net effect is an increase in the slope of the low-frequency segment of the MTF with stimulus intensity making the MTF more bandpass.

For the same neuron, the change in mean firing rate as a function of the level of tone at CF (in 10 dB intervals) is shown by the RIF (filled circles) in Fig. 2a. For this neuron there is an initial steep rise in discharge rate as the level of the stimulus is raised to approximately 20 dB above the unit's threshold, with a more gradual increase for higher sound levels.

The slope of the low-frequency limb of each MTF was estimated by fitting a regression line through the points below the peak frequency, and is shown by the squares in Fig. 2a as a function of the mean carrier level of the

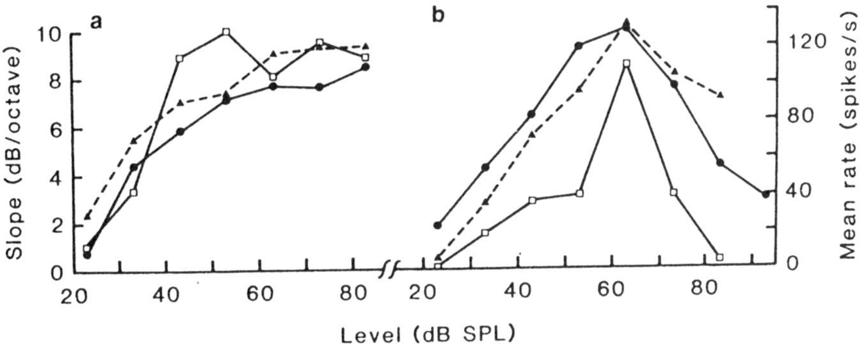

Figure 2. Mean discharge rate to a pure (filled circles) and modulated (triangles) CF tone and the slope of the low-frequency segment of the MTF (squares), as a function of stimulus intensity. Mean-rate reponses to modulated tones (triangles) have been multiplied by 4 to facilitate scaling. Data for two units a) CF =5.5kHz, b) CF =9kHz.

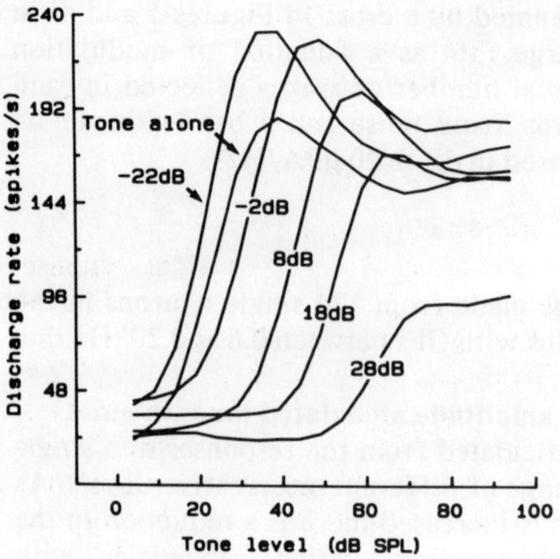

Figure 3. RIFs for an IC neuron to a CF tone (4.8 kHz) presented in quiet and in different levels of broadband noise (parameter, noise spectrum level).

modulated stimulus. The changes in the MTF slope as a function of mean level parallel those in the neuron's mean firing rate, although the slope of the MTF does not show the same gradual increase above 40 dB SPL seen in the mean discharge rate values.

The third curve on the graph shows the mean discharge rate during the response to the modulated tone at low modulation frequency. The two mean-rate functions are similar in form, but differ in absolute values due to the different stimulation paradigms.

Figure 2b shows a similar plot for a second neuron, which had a nonmonotonic RIF, with a reduction in response when the stimulus level exceeded 63 dB SPL. The low-frequency slope of the MTF is similarly a nonmonotonic function of level with a peak at 63 dB SPL. As in Fig. 2a, the mean discharge rate calculated from the response to modulation takes the same form as the RIF.

Effects of noise on rate-intensity functions

Figure 3 shows a series of RIFs from an IC neuron to CF tone stimuli presented in quiet and in increasing levels of broadband noise. Increasing the spectrum level of the noise shifts the RIF to a higher tone level, and also changes the maximum firing rate of the neuron. The maximum firing rate in response to the tone in low levels of noise is greater than the corresponding response to the tone in quiet, but at higher noise levels the maximum firing rate falls below that obtained in the tone-alone condition.

To measure the horizontal shift induced by noise, the RIFs were normalised after first subtracting the spontaneous activity and any direct response to the continuous noise. The shift at each noise level was measured, relative to the tone-alone condition, at 50% of the maximum firing rate. Above a threshold noise level, there is a linear relationship between the spectrum level of the noise and the magnitude of the shift, with a mean slope of 0.97 (S.D. ± 0.24; n=66). Neurons with monotonic and nonmonotonic RIFs showed shifts in the presence of noise, with many units showing shifts as large as 60dB. Similar shifts in the RIFs were measured when the noise was gated on and off with the tone. However, the shift was much smaller for inversely gated noise (noise off while tone on).

The effects of noise on the response to amplitude modulation

The MTFs in Fig. 4 illustrate the changes induced in the neuronal response to a modulated tone by the addition of continuous broadband noise. For a modulated tone presented in quiet at 9dB above threshold (filled circles) the MTF is lowpass, while at 39 dB above threshold the function is bandpass (open squares). The remainder of the curves represent the responses to a modulated tone at 39dB above threshold to which progressively higher levels of broadband noise have been added. As the level of the noise is raised the modulation gain at the low modulation frequencies increases and the slope of the low-frequency limb of the transfer function decreases.

For some units the changes in MTF slope with noise level were more complex as might be expected from their nonmonotonic responses with intensity.

Comparison of noise effects on rate-intensity and modulation transfer functions

From Fig. 2 it is clear that, in quiet, the modulation gain at low modulation frequencies is not related to the stimulus level, but to the mean discharge rate evoked by that level, even in nonmonotonic units. This relationship does not generally hold, however, between the response to low modulation frequencies

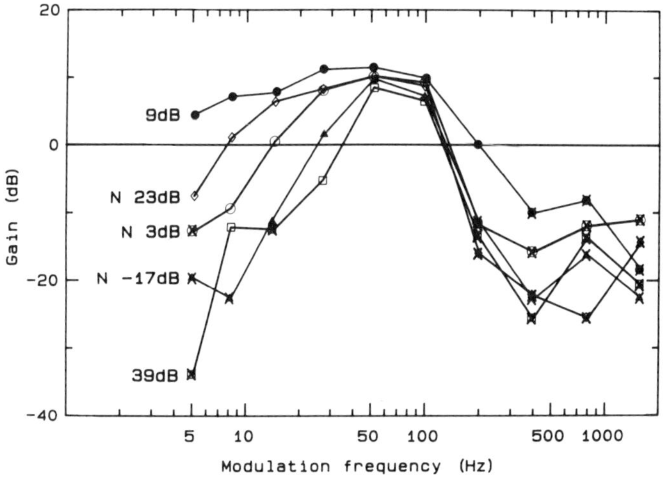

Figure 4. MTFs for an IC neuron at two mean carrier levels in quiet (9 and 39 dB re threshold) and at 39dB carrier level in the presence of different levels of broadband noise ('N' parameter, noise spectrum level). CF = 4.25 kHz.

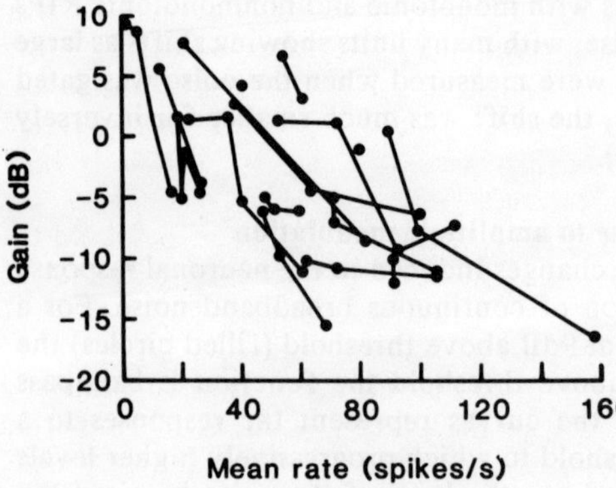

Figure 5. Modulation gain at low modulation frequency (5.1 or 8.2 Hz) plotted as a function of the neuron's mean discharge rate in response to modulated tones presented in broadband noise. Data for 14 units.

and the discharge rate estimated from the RIF, when both are measured in the same level of noise. For a few units there was an inverse relationship between the response to modulation at low frequencies and the mean rate estimated from the RIF, but for the majority no manipulation of this mean-rate estimate (subtraction of spontaneous rate or normalisation) produced any consistent relationship.

A correspondence was obtained, however, when the modulation gain at low modulation frequency (5.1 or 8.2 Hz) was compared with the neuron's mean firing rate in response to the same modulation rate, as shown in Fig. 5. Across this sample of neurons there is a clear trend for a decline in the gain at low modulation frequency with increasing mean discharge rate.

Discussion

The shifts in the dynamic range of IC neurons which occur in broadband noise are similar to those reported at other levels in the auditory pathway (Evans, 1974; Costalupes *et al.*, 1984; Gibson *et al.*, 1985; Phillips and Cynader, 1985; Phillips and Hall, 1986). The slope of the function relating the RIF shift to the noise level for neurons in the IC (i.e. 0.97) is higher than that reported for fibers in the cochlear nerve (Costalupes *et al.*, 1984) and neurons in the ventral cochlear nucleus (Gibson *et al.*, 1985). It is, however, similar to that measured for neurons in the dorsal cochlear nucleus (DCN, Gibson *et al.*, 1985). The increase in slope seen here may reflect the activity of the direct input from the DCN to the IC, or alternatively, it could be generated within the IC itself via inputs from the other pathways. The requirement that the noise occur simultaneously with the tone in order to produce a shift of the rate-intensity function is consistent with data obtained at more peripheral levels which suggest that most of the shift in the saturation point arises as a result of suppression within the cochlea rather than from adaptation (Geisler and Sinex, 1980; Costalupes *et al.*, 1984), possibly supplemented in more central nuclei by lateral inhibition.

The main finding of this study is that the sensitivity of neurons in the IC to low frequencies of modulation is greatest under conditions where the neuron has a relatively low mean discharge rate, and decreases when the mean discharge rate increases. This is true for modulated signals both in quiet and in noise, but the initial hypothesis that the effects of noise on the RIFs and MTFs should be correlated is not confirmed. The reason for this lack of correlation is that while, in quiet, the RIF provides a good estimate of the mean discharge rate for modulated stimuli, this is not the case when both the RIF and MTF are measured in broadband noise. This finding suggests that, in the IC, there are some differences in the way modulated stimuli and pure tones are processed when broadband noise is present.

As a possible explanation for the relationship between mean firing rate and the response to modulation, one might speculate that at low modulation frequencies, the strength of the afferent input determining the neuron's mean firing rate increases in proportion to the stimulus level up to saturation, but the strength of a separate, time-varying component remains constant or is reduced. Thus there is a large percentage modulation at low levels which decreases with increasing intensity. At higher modulation frequencies, the modulated excitatory input to the neuron increases in proportion to the mean stimulus level.

Acknowledgements

I am grateful to Alan Palmer for his collaboration in this study, and to Mark Haggard and Quentin Summerfield for their comments on the manuscript.

References

Buunen, T.J.F. and Rhode, W.S. (**1978**). "Responses of fibers in the cat's auditory nerve to the cubic difference tone," J.Acoust.Soc.Am. **64**, 772-781.

Costalupes, J.A., Young, E.D. and Gibson, D.J. (**1984**). "Effects of continuous noise backgrounds on rate response of auditory nerve fibers in cat," J.Neurophysiol. **51**, 1326-1344.

Evans, E.F. (**1974**). "Auditory frequency selectivity and the cochlear nerve," In *Facts and Models in Hearing*, edited by E. Zwicker and E. Terhardt (Springer-Verlag Berlin).

Geisler, C.D. and Sinex, D.G. (**1980**). "Responses of primary auditory fibers to combined noise and tonal stimuli," Hearing Res. 3, 317-334.

Gibson, D.J., Young E.D. and Costalupes J.A. (**1985**). "Similarity of dynamic range adjustment in auditory nerve and cochlear nuclei," J.Neurophysiol. **53**, 940-958.

Goldberg, J.M. and Brown, P.B. (**1969**). "Responses of binaural neurons of dog superior olivary complex to dichotic tonal stimulation: Some physiological mechanisms of sound localization," J.Neurophysiol. **32**, 940-958.

Mardia, K.V. (**1972**). *Statistics of Directional Data*, (Academic Press,

London).
Phillips D.P., and Cynader, M.S. (**1985**). "Some neural mechanisms in the cat's auditory cortex underlying sensitivity to combined tone and wide-spectrum noise stimuli," Hearing Res. **18**, 87-102.
Phillips D.P. and Hall S.E. (**1986**). "Spike-rate intensity functions of cat cortical neurons studied with combined tone-noise stimuli," J.Acoust.Soc. Am. **80**, 177-187.
Rees, A. and Møller, A.R. (**1987**). "Stimulus properties influencing the responses of inferior colliculus neurons to amplitude-modulated sounds," Hearing Res. **27**, 129-143.

Comments

Costalupes:

You mentioned that the rate of horizontal shift for IC cells is similar to that reported for DCN cells. The rate functions in Fig. 3 bring to mind other similarities that might further suggest ascending input from the DCN: these include the increase in peak rate in the presence of noise, the change from nonmonotonic to monotonic rate functions, and the similar slopes of the dynamic portions of the rate functions over a range of noise levels. Gibson, Young and I also found that substantial horizontal shift could be effected by a BF tone background. Have you looked at tone-evoked shifts among the IC-cells?

Reply by Rees

I agree, the effects of noise on the responses of IC neurons are similar in many respects to those reported by Gibson et al. for DCN units. Alan Palmer and I have discussed this in detail elsewhere (Rees and Palmer, 1988, J. Acoust.Soc.Am. 83, 1488-1498). Our findings suggest that the elevation of peak firing rate in the presence of noise at low spectrum levels is enhanced in the IC. Of course similarity does not necessarily imply causality, and one cannot rule out the possibility that some of these effects may be generated within the IC itself from afferent inputs other than those from the DCN. We have only studied one or two units with two tone stimuli, always with the second tone set at a frequency in the region of side-band suppression. Horizontal shifts did occur but they were not as dramatic as those generated by noise.

Patterson:

In your paper you concentrate on the low frequency slopes of your MTFs, which are level dependent and relatively shallow. In contrast, the high frequency slopes are largely independent of level and rather steep. They fall 20 dB in the octave 200-400 Hz in the absence of noise, and 20 dB in the octave 100-200 Hz with noise (even when the noise is very low level). If these effects are consistent across units and CFs they could help explain psychophysical data on monoural phase perception. In the absence of noise, in the region below 200 Hz, phase changes can produce strong timbre changes, but they fade away quickly in the octave above 200 Hz (Patterson, 1987). Furthermore, one class of these timbre discriminations is particularly sensitive to disruption by noise, (Patterson, 1988, this volume) as are your data in the region above 100 Hz. The psychophysical (MTF has a much shallower high frequency slope which is less compatible with timbre discrimination data.

Patterson, R.D. (1987). "A pulse ribbon model of monaural phase perception", J. Acoust. Soc. Am. 82, 1560-1586.

Reply by Rees:

The most likely determinant of the high-frequency slope of the MTF is the ability of the neuron to synchronise its firing to the modulation waveform of the stimulus. There is a progressive reduction in the value of this cut-off from peripheral to more central nuclei which probably occurs as additional synapses in the pathway reduce the accuracy with which rapid, temporally varying information is transmitted from one nucleus to the next (see Rees and Møller, 1987, Hearing Res. 27, 129-143 for discussion). I would hesitate to draw parallels between human psychophysical studies and responses of single neurons in other species. The MTF cut-off for cells in the inferior colliculus may be similar to the frequency at which changes occur in the perception of monaural phase, but this may be coincidental. The high-frequency cut-offs of the MTFs for cells at other levels are quite different, in the auditory cortex for example they occur at much lower frequencies (Schreiner and Urbas, 1986, Hearing Res. 21, 227-241).

On the interpretation of neural interaction in the auditory nervous system

Jos J. Eggermont

Department of Psychology, The University of Calgary
Calgary, Alberta, Canada

Introduction

The study of neural interaction requires the simultaneous recording from at least two neural units. Such recordings can be done using independent electrodes and obtaining single unit records from each of them, or by recording with a single electrode and using spike-separation techniques. Both methods have their advantage and disadvantage. Using independent electrodes it is often hard to record from neighboring units, using a single electrode one usually has problems in separating superimposed waveforms but one can be reasonably sure that the units recorded from will originate from a limited space. Both methods have been used to probe for interaction in the auditory nervous system. The goal of such studies is often to identify underlying connectivity of the neurons in order to arrive at a wiring diagram. Occasionally one aims to study the difference in coding of stimuli by a single-unit measure such as rate or synchrony and that in small neuronal groups using the additional information about the correlations in neural firing between the units (Epping and Eggermont, 1987). In this paper I will first review all the studies that pertain to neural interaction in the auditory nervous system. From this review two aspects will emerge, the first one is that, except in one study, it has not been possible to obtain correlations that point to inhibitory interactions, secondly neural correlation appears to be dependent on the type of stimulus used. In the second part of the paper I will present studies on a very simple neuronal network that elucidates these points and will be useful in the interpretation of neural interaction studies.

Correlation studies in the auditory nervous system

Johnson and Kiang (1976) tested the independence of spontaneous activity in **auditory nerve** fibers by using two independent electrodes. As the test statistic they used the comparison of forward and backward recurrence times of order one. In 21 fiber pairs with spontaneous activity ranging from 7.5-131.5 spikes per second these recurrence times were the same within statistical limits, indicating that a spike in unit 2 was as likely to follow a spike in unit 1 as vice versa. This implies that there was no causal relationship between the firings, this was found for fiber-pairs with identical CF and with different CF. Their results suggest that transmitter release at various synaptic terminals- even those on the same haircell- is independent.

The principal cells in the Dorsal Cochlear Nucleus (DCN) receive direct input from auditory nerve (AN) fibers as well as from interneurons. Electrophysiologically on distinguishes so-called type II/III cells with a V-shaped tuning curve and an excitatory area flanked by inhibitory side bands, from type IV cells with broad tuning curves which are mainly inhibitory. Voigt and Young (1980) studied 41 unit pairs in the DCN of decerebrated, unanesthetized cats both with dual and single electrodes. Best frequencies (BF) of the fibers in the pair were the same when recorded on one electrode, in case two electrodes were used and separation was less than 400 μm BFs were less than one half octave apart. In 25 out of the 41 pairs a clear correlation was observed, 17 of these 25 pairs consisted of a type II/III unit and a type IV unit. In 12 out of these 17 pairs the correlogram showed an inhibitory trough consistent with a monosynaptic inhibition of a type IV unit by a type II/III unit. It was concluded that a type IV unit- most likely a principal cell- is subjected to both an excitatory drive from the auditory nerve and an inhibitory drive from a low spontaneous type II/III cell- most likely a granule cell or small cell. No sign of common input on the type II/III and type IV units could be demonstrated, suggesting that the type II/III interneurons do not receive direct input from the auditory nerve.

Correlation studies in the auditory midbrain of mammals are currently not available. However, a comprehensive study has been conducted in the **torus semicircularis** (TS) of the paralyzed and locally anesthetized grassfrog (Epping and Eggermont,1987). A total of 264 pairs was studied using both single and dual electrodes. Since spontaneous activity was usually less than one spike per second the study was carried out under stimulus conditions. After the necessary correction for correlation between the neuronal firings through stimulus-locking neural correlations were observed in 37 out of the 264 pairs. No difference was found in the results for the one and two electrode recordings, except that no neural correlation was observed for interelectrode distances of more than 300 μm. Common input accounted for correlations observed in 31 out of these 37 pairs while 6 pairs showed evidence for a unidirectional,excitatory interaction. No signs of inhibitory interactions were found. About half of the neural correlations, both in shape of the correlogram and in the correlation strength, were found to be stimulus (type) dependent.

The **Medial Geniculate Body** (MGB) in the paralyzed, weakly anesthetized, cat was extensively studied by Heierli *et al.* (1987), who recorded from a total of 950 nerve cell pairs. About 40% of the neuron pairs fired independently, 20% showed a correlogram indicative of common input, in 15% evidence was found for an excitatory synaptic interaction, and in only 2% of the pairs an inhibitory synaptic interaction could be demonstrated. The remaining neuron pairs were reported to show a weak or ambiguous interaction (23%). All these results were obtained for spontaneous activity. Under stimulus conditions indications were obtained for change in the type and strength of the interaction. From the 92 pairs that were evaluated for stimulus effects in 53% a qualitative change in the form of the correlogram was observed, 16% showed a quantitative change and 3% showed no effect, the remaining cases were ambiguous. Interaction type distribution did not differ in the various parts of the MGB.

Dickson and Gerstein (1974) studied 61 neuron pairs in the auditory cortex of paralyzed cats under spontaneous activity, and 107 pairs under stimulus conditions. In 51 out of these 107 pairs both neurons had a phasic response to tone bursts, in 32 of the 107 cases only one neuron was affected by the stimulus, in the remaining cases both neurons were unresponsive to the stimuli used. From the total of 168 pairs investigated, 54 pairs showed a strong neural correlation but only 5 of these were other than common input, 31 pairs showed a weak neural interaction, and the remaining pairs did not show any signs of neural interaction. Of the 48 pairs with neural interaction that were tested for stimulus dependence this was found in 15 cases. Most of this dependence could be attributed to a change in firing rate of both neurons giving a better opportunity to detect any correlation. Only in 5 cases a change in the peak of the correlogram was observed while the neurons' firing rates stayed the same. Thus there appears to be little direct stimulus dependence of neural correlation in the auditory cortex. The majority of the observed correlation was due to common input, probably due to incoming neurons from the thalamus. Frostig *et al.* (1983) corroborated most of these findings in a study comprising 117 neuron pairs sampled with the single electrode, multi unit, spike separation technique. In 14% of the cases a flat correlogram was obtained, in 12% evidence for a direct excitatory interaction was found, in 74% there was either common input (66%) or reciprocal input (8%). The inability to detect inhibitory interactions was addressed to low background firing rates and inhibition being rare within local groups as sampled with one electrode.

The major conclusions to be drawn from this survey is that, with the exception of the DCN example, inhibition cannot be demonstrated using cross correlation between the firings of two nerve cells, and that in nearly all cases the outcome of the correlation procedure is dependent on the type of stimulus used.

Correlation in a simulated neural network

In order to study the effects of neural firing rate on both the detectability of inhibitory connections and the form and strength of the correlation, a simple neural network was simulated. The network, shown as an insert in Figure 1, represents four neurons that receive common input from a driver-neuron, and that are mutually inhibiting each other. The matrix of connection strengths is shown in Table I. We assume that the driver unit is not accessible to the recording electrode and that all four output neurons can be monitored

Table I: Connection strength of neural network

output \ input:	1	2	3	4	driver
1	*	-16	-2	-64	0.5
2	-1	*	-4	-8	4
3	-2	-64	*	-256	16
4	-4	-128	-16	*	32

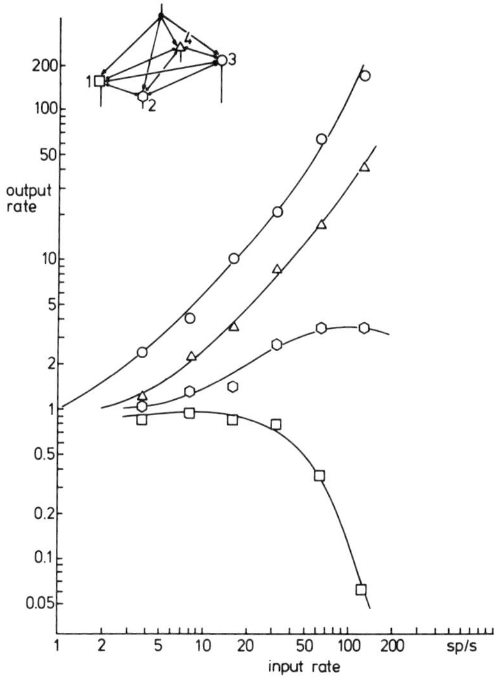

Figure 1. Input-output functions for the four observable neurons in the network. The insert shows the wiring diagram of the neural network.

Over:
Figure 2. Cross-correlation functions between all pair combinations of the *four output neurons of the network for input rates of 8, 32, and 128 spikes per second. All correlograms are scaled on their own maxima, the number of bins is 101.*

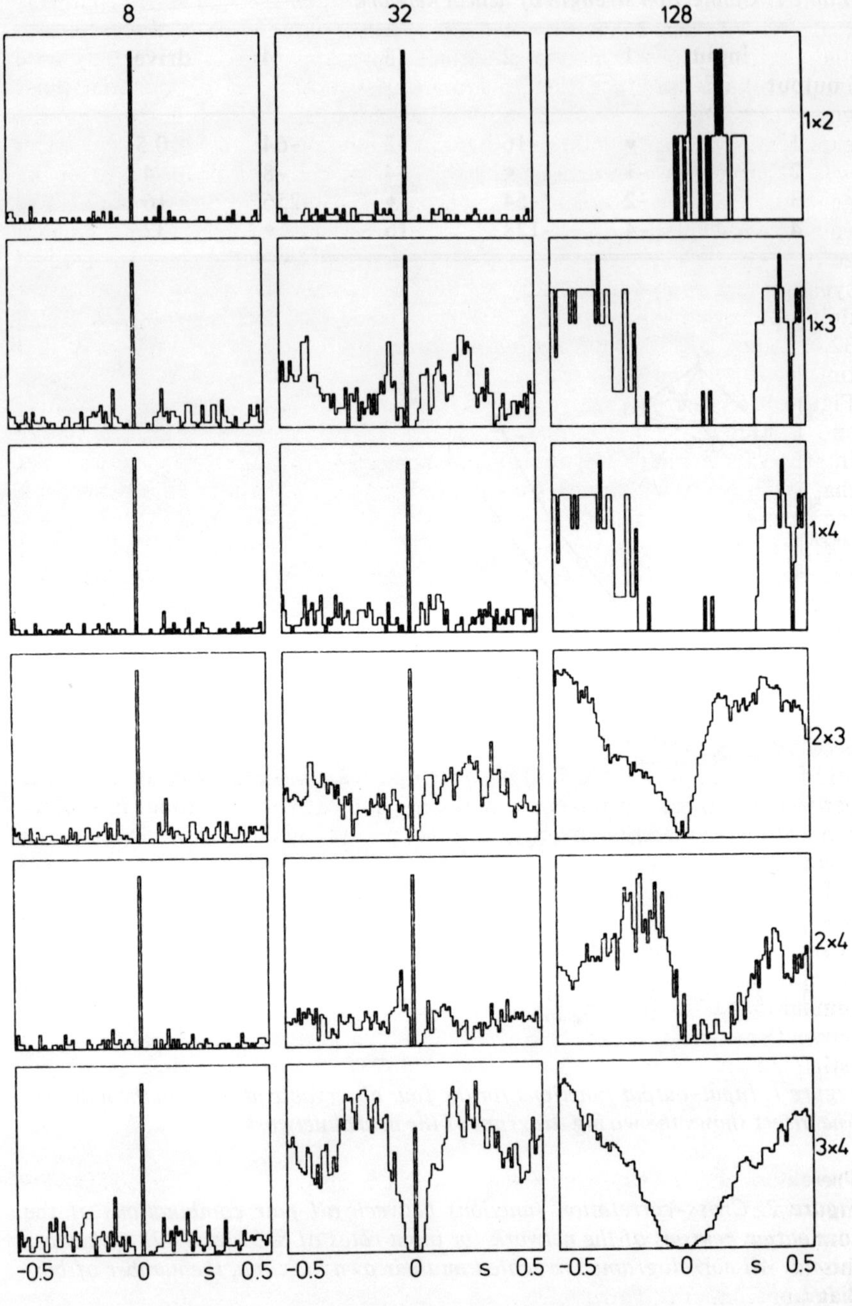
8
32
128
1×2
1×3
1×4
2×3
2×4
3×4
-0.5
0
s
0.5
-0.5
0
s
0.5
-0.5
0
s
0.5

simultaneously and separately. The model neurons used have the following features (Van den Boogaard *et al.*, 1986): linear summation of the excitatory and inhibitory post synaptic potentials (epsp and ipsp) produced by each input spike to produce the "membrane potential", and exponential pulse generation whereby the probability of an output spike is proportional to the exponential of the "membrane potential". The shape of the epsp's and ipsp's was a simple decaying exponential with a time constant of 10 ms. After the generation of a spike the "membrane potential was reset at a large negative value from which it recovered with a time constant of 1 ms. The spontaneous activity of the neurons was set at one spike per second. There was a fixed synaptic and conduction delay of one ms between the neurons. The driver unit produced a Poisson-distributed spike train with average rate of 4, 8, 16, 32, 64, and 128 spikes per second, the simulations covered 33 seconds of real time activity. The input-output behavior of the four neurons is shown in Figure 1. It is observed that neuron 1 never fires above its spontaneous level and is suppressed for input rates above 16 per second. Neuron 2 slowly increases its firing rate to about 3 times the spontaneous rate and saturates at that level. Neurons 3 and 4 show a monotonous increase in firing rate with increasing driver rate.

Correlograms were computed between all six pairs of the four output neurons for a time frame of -500 to 500 ms, the number of bins was 101. Because the delays from the driver unit to each of the four units were identical common input will result in a peak in the central bin. This aspect of the interaction can be observed clearly in the case of the 8 spikes per second input rate (Figure 2). When the input rate is increased to 32 per second the central peaks stay present but for the correlation between neurons 3 and 4 becomes lower than the activity at lags of about 200 ms, clear evidence of an inhibitory trough is now found as well (Figure 2). At input rates of 128 spikes per second most correlations now are indicative of strong inhibitory connections, extending over long time periods and in most cases being asymmetric (Figure 2).

From the values in the central bin we calculated the pair wise connection strengths between the four neurons. The first step is to determine the value (V) in the central bin as well as the expectation (E) in case of independent firing of the two neurons. For a neural model as used here, with a linear summation of input activity and an exponential pulse generator, it has been shown (Van den Boogaard *et al.*,1986) that the connection strength, w, can be estimated as:

$$w = \ln V - \ln E.$$

The values obtained were between -5 and 5 and are shown in Table II for the input rates of 8, 32, and 128 spikes per second. It can be seen that the connection matrix that is obtained is critically dependent on the input rate, this as we will see is of considerable assistance in recreating the wiring diagram from cross correlation studies. On basis of the correlogram shape we can obtain additional information about the direction of the inhibition and about symmetries in the interconnections. Taking all this into account we arrived at the wiring diagrams for the three input rates considered in detail, they are shown in Figure 3.The connection matrices derived from the cross-correlation study are symmetric, further elaboration could be done by estimating values at say + and - 50 ms to estimate unidirectional values.

Table II: Connection strengths as derived from the correlograms

input rate	8			32			128		
neuron	1	2	3	1	2	3	1	2	3
2	4.34			3.58			4.61		
3	3.19	3.20		1.57	1.19		-5.00	-1.02	
4	3.81	3.60	2.46	2.30	1.93	0.07	-5.00	0.01	-3.51

While at low input rates the common input character is the only obvious finding, at higher input rates we also observe more of the inhibitory connections but loose some of the evidence for common input. This common input character of the network at the input rate of 128 spikes per second remains only for the correlation between units 1 and 2. From an analysis of the relation between w and E it became clear that negative w values, signifying inhibitory connections, occur only for E values larger than 10-50. This means that the number of coincidences in the background per 10 ms bin should be in that range, this corresponds to product rates of 1000-5000 per second. Assuming that both neurons have about the same firing rate it would mean that inhibition can only be detected when the neurons' firing rates are higher than 33-70 spikes per second.

For the DCN such firing rates are quite common and the cross correlation studies reveal the underlying inhibitory interaction. For the TS, MGB, and auditory cortex firing rates are considerably lower and it becomes more difficult if not impossible to show any of the inhibitory connections. Using stimulation to increase the neurons' activity is not always the solution, since this requires a stimulus correction procedure to account for correlation through stimulus-locking. This correction is not model free and does not work if the stimulus is too strong and causes all the firings to be very rigidly synchronized to the stimulus (Epping and Eggermont, 1987).

Conclusions

From the review about neural interaction in the auditory nervous system and the analysis of a neural network designed to show some of the features that were found in this survey we can come to some general statements and suggestions for neural interaction studies. First of all the spontaneous and

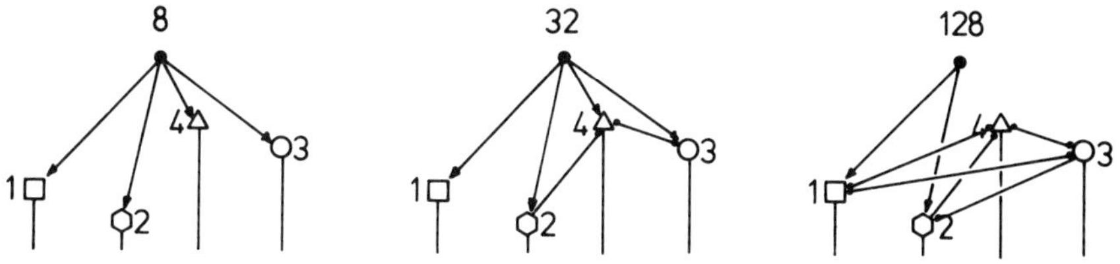

Figure 3. Wiring diagrams as estimated from the three input-rate conditions.

stimulus driven firing rates of the neurons in a particular neural structure determine completely the detectability of neural inhibitory interactions. For firing rates below 33 spikes per second it is much more likely to detect common input and unilateral excitatory interactions than inhibitory interactions. Secondly at higher firing rates the presence and detection of inhibitory interactions may interfere with the detectability of common input in the network. It is suggested therefore that an analysis of a neural network is to be performed with a large class of stimuli and stimulus levels in order to cover an as wide range of firing rates as possible, and to allow for the detection of all types of neural interaction. Finally it is suggested that it is not the stimulus type that causes changes in the neural interaction but rather the firing rates in the network. This study has shown that stimulus dependent neural interaction can occur in a network with fixed connections. Thus changing correlation strengths in itself are not sufficient evidence to conclude changing connection strengths between neurons.

Acknowledgements

This investigation was supported by the Alberta Heritage Foundation for Medical Research, and the Natural Sciences and Engineering Research Council of Canada.

References

Boogaard, H. van den, Hesselmans, G., and Johannesma, P. (**1986**). "System identification based on point processes and correlation densities. I. The nonrefractory neuron model". Math. Biosciences **80**, 143-171.

Dickson, J.W., and Gerstein, G.L.(**1974**)."Interaction between neurons in auditory cortex of the cat".J.Neurophysiol. **37**, 1239-1261.

Epping, W.J.M., and Eggermont, J.J.(**1987**)."Coherent neural activity in the auditory midbrain of the grassfrog." J.Neurophysiol. **57**, 1464-1483.

Frostig, R.D., Gottlieb, Y., Vaadia, E., and Abeles, M.(**1983**). "The effects of stimuli on the activity and functional connectivity of local neuronal groups in the cat auditory cortex". Brain Res. **272**, 211-221.

Heierli, P., Ribaupierre, F. de, and Ribaupierre, Y. de (**1987**)."Functional properties and interactions of neuron pairs simultaneously recorded in the medial geniculate body of the cat". Hearing Res. **25**, 209-225.

Johnson, D.H., and Kiang, N.Y.S.(**1976**)."Analysis of discharges recorded simultaneously from pairs of auditory nerve fibers". Biophysical J. **16**, 719-734.

Voigt, H.F., and Young, E.D.(**1980**). "Evidence of inhibitory interactions between neurons in the dorsal cochlear nucleus". J.Neurophysiol. **44**, 76-96.

Comments

Lewis:

Yours is a message that should be repeated often. With its many bidirectionally interacting processes (both within neurons and among them), any neural network is inherently irreducible (e.g., in the formal sense of the theory of marking processes). Our problem, as biologists, will be to bring our reductionist instincts into harmony with the irreducible world we face.

Selectivity for interaural time-difference and amplitude-modulation frequency in the auditory midbrain of the grassfrog

Willem J. Melssen and Ivo H.M. van Stokkum

Department of Medical Physics & Biophysics, University of Nijmegen, P.O. Box 9101, 6500 HB Nijmegen, the Netherlands

Introduction

Anurans are able to localize species-specific sounds (e.g. Walkowiak and Brzoska, 1982). The basis for this localization capability lies in their acoustic periphery. Variation of sound source position gives rise to sound intensity differences less than 2 dB outside the eardrums, but to amplitude differences of tympanic membrane movement upto 9 dB (Michelsen *et al.*, 1986). The directionality of the frog's acoustic periphery is affected if the relatively large Eustachian tubes are partially obstructed (Rheinländer *et al.*, 1981). On basis of Laser Doppler Velocity measurements Aertsen *et al.* (1986) proposed a model for the acoustic periphery of the grassfrog. In this model both eardrums and the mouth-cavity are considered as three coupled oscillators. Simulations of this model showed that the frog's periphery acts as a combined pressure-pressure gradient receiver. The azimuthal angle of sound incidence is transformed into a frequency-dependent interaural intensity difference at the level of both inner ears. Because of the intensity-latency characteristics of auditory nerve fibers, interaural intensity differences are transformed into interaural time differences (ITDs) in the millisecond range (Feng, 1982).

Grassfrog calls consist of regular trains of identical pulses (e.g. Brzoska *et al.*, 1977). In dorsal medullary nucleus units strong time-locking to these pulses is found, whereas in the torus semicircularis (TS) only a minority of units exhibits time-locking (Van Stokkum, 1987; Epping and Eggermont, 1986a). In the dorsal medullary nucleus and superior olivary nucleus the first binaural interaction takes place (Feng and Capranica, 1976, 1978).

In most experiments, based on the ITD paradigm, rather simple stimulus ensembles were used: clicks, tonepips and broadband noise. In this report results are presented, obtained from experiments where a temporally structured stimulus was used: amplitude modulated tonebursts (AMF).

Previous studies (Rose and Capranica, 1985, Epping and Eggermont, 1986b) reported several neural response types to monaurally presented amplitude modulated tonebursts in the torus semicircularis. The objective of this study is to investigate the relation between selectivity for amplitude modulation frequency and interaural time-difference.

Materials and methods

Animal preparation and recording procedure are descibed extensively in Epping and Eggermont (1986a).

Stimuli were presented to the animal by two electrodynamic microphones (Sennheiser MD211N) coupled to the frog's tympanic membranes. The frog's mouth was kept open in order to decouple the tympanic membranes. Sound pressure level was measured in situ with half inch microphones (Brüel and Kjær 4143) connected to each coupler. Amplitude and phase characteristics of the couplers were almost equal in the range of interest. Stimulus intensity generally was 90 dB peak SPL. For units with low thresholds, which could experience acoustic crosstalk (Feng and Capranica, 1976) the stimulus was presented at 70 dB peak SPL.

The amplitude of a toneburst was modulated by a sinusoid, multiplied by an exponential function, with a modulation depth of 100% (Epping *et al.*, 1986b). Carrier phase was set to zero at the beginning of each sinusoid. In general, the stimulus was presented at the unit's best excitatory frequency (BEF), as determined with monaurally presented tonepips. AMFs were 9, 18, 36, 72 and 144 Hz. In addition an unmodulated toneburst with rise- and falltimes of 5 ms was presented. Each toneburst had a duration of 680 ms and was presented binaurally at onset intervals of 3 s. The following ITDs were applied: -5, -3, -1, 0, 1, 3, 5 ms. A negative ITD indicates a leading ipsilaterally presented toneburst. Each combination of AMF and ITD was presented 5 times. Total stimulus duration was 630 s.

Neural responses to the stimulus are represented as eventdisplays, reordered according to the parameters AMF and ITD. Counting of the number of neural events per AM-ITD toneburst resulted in an average rate histogram (ARH). The degree of time-locking to each pulse train was expressed in a synchronization index (SI). A SI of one indicates perfect time-locking to the stimulus envelope as expressed in the period histogram, whereas a SI of zero indicates no synchronization.

Results

Recordings of 50 units were made in 9 grassfrogs. The response of one unit was totally suppressed. In some cases, depending on recording stability, the stimulus was repeated with a different carrier frequency or a different overall sound intensity. Figure 1 shows neural response types of five representative TS units. Unit 322,0,2 (Fig.1a) exhibits strong time-locking to all AMFs. At low AMFs, timelock to the stimulus can be recognized as regular, vertically aligned, dot patterns. The synchronization index varied between 0.5 and 1 and did not change as function of ITD. A small, ITD dependent, change in firing rate is present for an AMF of 72 Hz. Unit 322,3,0 (Fig.1b) shows a sustained response to all AM tonebursts. This unit responds with 1 or 2 spikes

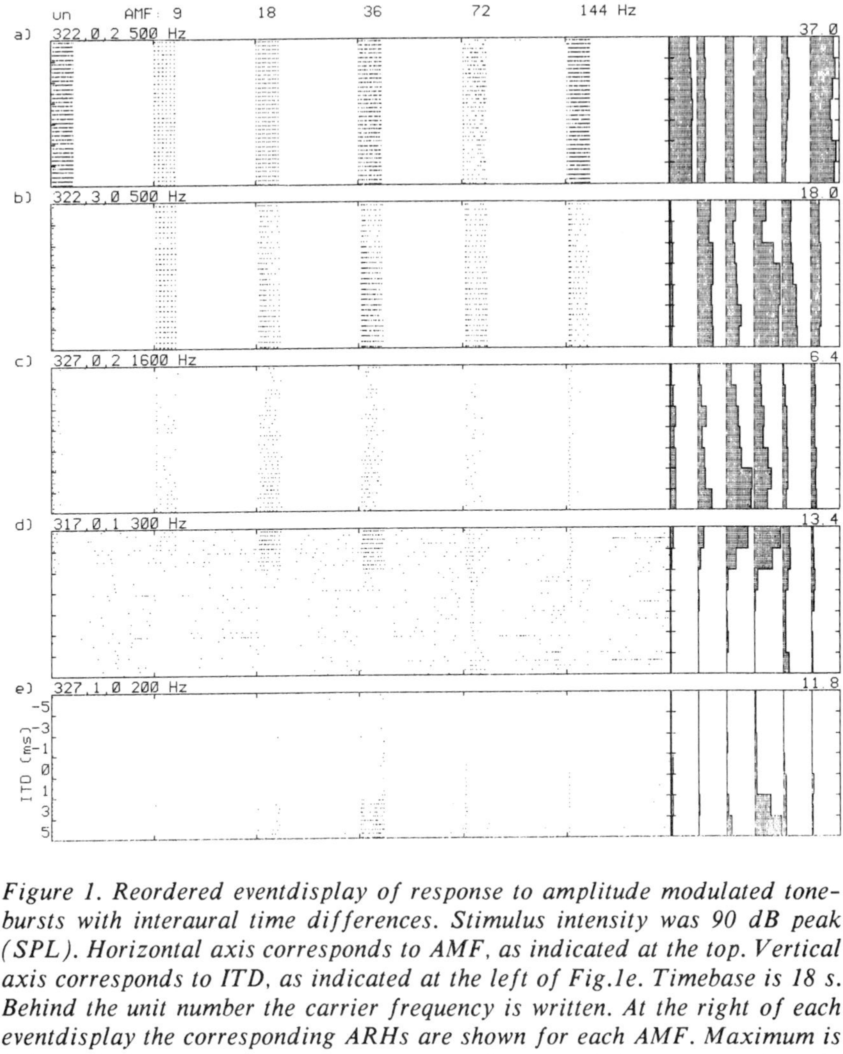

Figure 1. Reordered eventdisplay of response to amplitude modulated tonebursts with interaural time differences. Stimulus intensity was 90 dB peak (SPL). Horizontal axis corresponds to AMF, as indicated at the top. Vertical axis corresponds to ITD, as indicated at the left of Fig.1e. Timebase is 18 s. Behind the unit number the carrier frequency is written. At the right of each eventdisplay the corresponding ARHs are shown for each AMF. Maximum is indicated above each block of histograms. Because of strong adaptation the first stimulus sequence was discarded from the response analysis of unit 322,3,0. Number of events: a) N = 3956; b) N = 1327; c) N = 385; d) N = 833; e) N = 185

at the onset of the unmodulated tonebursts. Time-locking is present for AMFs of 9 and 18 Hz (SI = 0.85, 0.7). The ARHs show a dip at an ITD of 3 ms for AMFs from 9 to 36 Hz. This ITD dependence is strongest for the 36 Hz AMF. Unit 327,0,2 (Fig.1c) exhibits a bandpass response to AM tonebursts;

high rates are present for 18 and 36 Hz modulators. In this particular range of AMF the neural response varies strongly with ITD. Here, the synchronization index is less than 0.5. This unit's best excitatory frequency was 1600 Hz. So far, ipsilaterally leading tonebursts excerted an inhibitory influence on neural firings. Figure 1d (unit 317,0,1) shows a spontaneously firing neuron with a BEF of 200 Hz. For negative ITDs a sharp bandpass response is visible.

Table I: Selectivities for AMF and ITD.

ITD\ AMF	+	?	-	Σ
+	16	13	0	29
?	4	3	0	7
-	5	4	4	13
Σ	25	20	4	49

Contralaterally leading tonebursts with low AMFs cause total suppression of the unit's spontaneous activity. The response of unit 327,1,0 (Fig.1e) varies strongly with ITD and AMF. For negative ITD this unit responds maximally with one offset spike at an AMF of 36 Hz. For positive ITD phasic responses are present for AMFs of 0, 72 and 144 Hz. A strong sustained response is present only for an AMF of 36 Hz.

General results are summarized in Table I. A unit was termed ITD selective if a clear trend was observed in the ARH for one or more AMFs. All units of Fig.1 satisfied this criterion. A unit was termed AMF selective when there was no response to one or more AMFs. Examples thereof are the units of Figs.1d,e. Moderately selective units are indicated by a question mark in Table I. Approximately 60% of the units showed a selectivity for ITD. The degree of selectivity could vary from relatively small changes in firing rate upto total suppression of the neural activity. Units nonselective for AMF were also nonselective for ITD. There was a trend ($P < 0.05$, χ^2-test) that non-selectivity for AMF was correlated with non-selectivity for ITD.

Eight out of ten units remained ITD selective at a 20 dB lower overall sound intensity. But the degree of ITD selectivity turned out to be intensity dependent. Of three units tested, two were ITD selective at two carrier frequencies.

Discussion

It has been demonstrated that a large number of neurons in the torus semicircularis is involved in the processing of both temporal and directional features of sound. In many cases neural responses to AMF and ITD were not separable: selectivity for AMF depends on ITD and vice versa. These data suggest that the tuning to AMF and ITD is based on the same underlying neural mechanism: interaction of excitatory and inhibitory influences, originating from both contralateral and ipsilateral neural pathways. Timecourse, strength and the temporal relation between excitatory and inhibitory post synaptic potentials determine a unit's selectivity for AMF and ITD. The strongest ITD effects were observed with AMFs of 36 and 72 Hz. The period of the 36 Hz modulator is approximately equal to the interpulse interval of the original mating call of the grassfrog. The risetime of the 72 Hz envelope matches rather well the risetime of a single mating call pulse. This suggests tuning for species-specific sounds.

Often a unit's response was qualitatively invariant with respect to overall sound intensity and carrier frequency. Most ITD-rate histograms were flat or sigmoidally shaped. None of the ITD-rate histograms showed a dominant peak or trough, indicating a preferred ITD. If we hypothesize that ITD corresponds to sound source laterality, these findings indicate that an accurate determination thereof can be achieved by ensemble coding.

Summarizing, identification and localization of sound are not two independent processes: probably both tasks are performed simultaneously in the auditory midbrain of the grassfrog.

Acknowledgements

This investigation was supported by the Netherlands Organization for the Advancement of Pure Research (ZWO). The authors thank Koos Braks for animal preparation. Willem Epping is thanked for helpful discussions and critical reading of the text.

References

Aertsen A.M.H.J., Vlaming M.S.M.G., Eggermont J.J., Johannesma P.I.M. (**1986**). "Directional hearing in the grassfrog (*Rana temporaria* L.). II. Acoustics and modelling of the auditory periphery," Hearing Res. **21**, 17-40.

Brzoska, J., Walkowiak, W., Schneider, H. (**1977**). "Acoustic communication in the grassfrog (*Rana t. temporaria* L.): calls, auditory thresholds and behavioral responses," J.Comp.Physiol. **118**, 173-186.

Epping, W.J.M., Eggermont, J.J. (**1986a**). "Sensitivity of neurons in the auditory midbrain of the grassfrog to temporal characteristics of sound. I. Stimulation with acoustic clicks,". Hearing Res. **24**, 37-54.

Epping, W.J.M., Eggermont, J.J. (**1986b**). "Sensitivity of neurons in the auditory midbrain of the grassfrog to temporal characteristics of sound. II. Stimulation with amplitude modulated sound," Hearing Res. **23**, 55-72.

Feng A.S., Capranica R.R. (**1976**). "Sound localization in anurans. I. Evidence of binaural interaction in dorsal medullary nucleus of bullfrogs (*Rana catesbeiana*)," J.Neurophysiol. **39**, 871-881.

Feng A.S., Capranica R.R. (**1978**). "Sound localization in anurans. II. Binaural interaction in superior olivary nucleus of the green treefrog (*Hyla cinerea*)," J.Neurophysiol. **41**, 43-54.

Feng A.S. (**1982**). "Quantitative analysis of intensity-rate and intensity-latency functions in peripheral auditory nerve fibers of northern leopard frogs (*Rana p. pipiens*)," Hearing Res. **6**, 241-246.

Michelsen A., Jørgensen M., Christensen-Dalsgaard J., Capranica R.R. (**1986**). "Directional hearing of awake, unrestrained treefrogs," Naturwissenschaften **73**, 682-683.

Rheinländer J., Walkowiak W., Gerhardt H.C. (**1981**). "Directional hearing in the green treefrog: A variable mechanism?" Naturwissenschaften **67**, 430-431

Rose G.J., Capranica R.R. (**1985**). "Sensitivity to amplitude modulated sounds in the anuran auditory nervous system," J.Neurophysiol. **53**, 446-465.

Van Stokkum, I.H.M. (**1987**). "Sensitivity of neurons in the dorsal medullary nucleus of the grassfrog to spectral and temporal characteristics of sound," Hearing Res. **29**, 223-235.

Walkowiak, W. and Brzoska, J. (**1982**). "Significance of spectral and temporal parameters in the auditory communication of male grassfrogs," Behav. Ecol.Sociobiol. **11**, 247-252.

Simultaneous processing of sound pressure and particle motion enables spatial hearing in fish

Nico A.M. Schellart and Rob J.A. Buwalda

Laboratory of Medical Physics, University of Amsterdam, Amsterdam, the Netherlands

Introduction

The auditory system of bony fishes is a unique development in hearing. Without a cochlea, but with the swimbladder as a middle-ear analogon, fish hearing rivals that of many higher vertebrates in sensitivity, frequency selectivity and wave form resolution (cf. Popper and Fay, 1984). The gas-filled swimbladder transforms sound pressure into pulsations that reach the nearby labyrinths, thus displacing the hair cells relative to the inert otoliths. In addition to sound pressure (p), a fish detects the particle motion vector (**v**) because the acoustically transparent fish is carried along with the incident wave and thus oscillates about its otoliths. Both inputs are depicted in Fig. 1. The temporal and amplitude relationships between p and **v**, in combination with **v** direction, characterize the source position. This dual sensitivity might provide fish with superior spatial hearing in their 3-D environment, without need for the binaural intensity or timing difference cues available to terrestrial vertebrates. Accordingly, fish have been shown to discriminate acutely between sound sources differing in distance, azimuth, and/or elevation (cf. Schuijf and Buwalda, 1980; Schuijf and Hawkins, 1983).

That fish can analyze the p-**v** relations to some extent is borne out by the results of Schuijf and Buwalda (1975) and Buwalda et al. (1983). They demonstrated that the directional responses of fish err by 180° if in the field emitted by an underwater sound source the pressure phase is inverted, the p-**v** phase relation then mimicking that of an oppositely positioned source. In

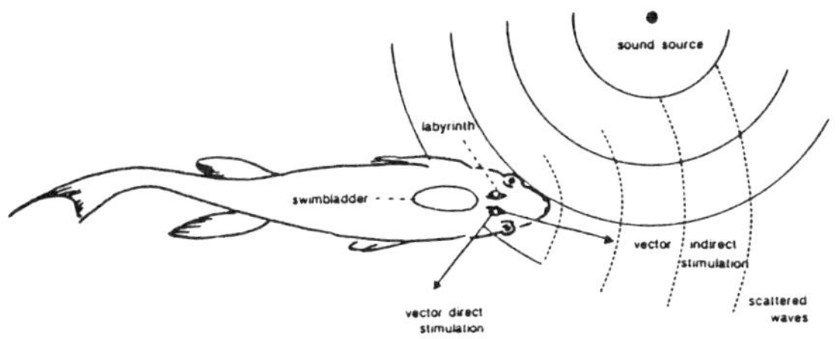

Figure 1. Schematic representation of the direct and indirect stimulation of the fish otolith organs. (The wave fronts and vectors are not drawn to scale.)

these and other experiments featuring real or simulated source directions in horizontal or vertical planes, the fish's directional responses appeared to be governed by **v** direction and p-**v** phase relations in the incident wave.

These results support the hypothesis that the fish's spatial hearing abilities, like the vestibular orientation abilities mediated by the same organ system, depend on the detection of vector input, but with coherent (pressure) input added to remove the ambiguity produced by the alternating direction of the acoustic vector input. The exact physiological basis, however, remains to be elucidated. Both the "direct" incident particle motions (in line with the source) and the p-induced swimbladder pulsations (the "indirect" input, with body-fixed orientation) stimulate the ears. Superposition of direct and indirect input results in a rotatory movement ("orbit") of the hair cells with respect to the otoliths (Schuijf, 1981; De Munck and Schellart, 1987).

There are two strategies to realize a mechanism for extracting the positional information encoded in this stimulus. One is the segregation of the p and **v** information from the rotatory stimulation of the hair cells. One implementation of this strategy is peripheral segregation through local specificity for either input, based e.g. on structural adaptations ("acoustic windows") locally promoting or impeding the reception of swimbladder pulsations, or based on hair cells being oriented parallel or orthogonal to the indirect input vector (Buwalda, 1981). Peripheral segregation may be supplemented or even replaced by central binaural subtraction processes resulting e.g. in the removal or segregation of the (bilaterally symmetrical) indirect input components. Such schemes allow a separate central processing of **v**-input (e.g. for binaural "vector weighing", i.e. determining the **v**-direction from the output ratio of binaurally symmetrically oriented otolith organs) and of p-correlated input, and of the relations between p and **v** (Buwalda, 1981). So far, peripheral segregation has only been demonstrated in the goldfish with its specialized swimbladder-ear link (cf. Popper and Fay, 1984).

The other strategy is to analyze the hair cell orbits themselves, i.e. to extract monaurally the orbit parameters uniquely defining the source position: an approach called the orbit model (Schellart and de Munck, 1987). The basic concept of this model is that the stimulus is mapped out on the sensory macula, thus providing a basis for a central mapping of the orbit parameters.

The aim of this chapter is to present a theoretical framework for the orbit model, to discuss some physiological implications, and to evaluate its merits in the light of new and existing behavioural data on cod and trout.

The indirect displacement wave

In order to find the orbits of the hair cells with respect to the otoliths, the direct displacement wave and the wave scattered by the swimbladder have to be calculated. De Munck and Schellart (1987) derived an expression for the nearfield of the scattered wave as a function of frequency and hydrostatic pressure for an elongate, spheroidal air bubble. Such a bubble, an ellipse of revolution, approximates the shape of the swimbladder. The bubble-water system can be described as a damped mass spring system with system constants m, A and K. The displacement $\mathbf{r}_{sc}$ is:

$$\mathbf{r}_{sc}(x,t) = p_f[8\pi a(-m\omega^2 + iA\omega + K)]^{-1}.\nabla \ln[(a+S)/(-a+S)]$$

with a the spheroid's half interfocal distance and $S=-x+[(a-x)^2+y^2+z^2]^{\frac{1}{2}}$. The sound pressure p_f emitted by the source is $(U/R).\exp\{i(-\omega Rc^{-1}+\omega t)\}$, with U the strength of the source, R its distance to the bladder and c the sound velocity in water. The resonance frequency of a bubble in water is $(K/m)^{\frac{1}{2}}$. K and m can be calculated from the bladder's geometry, the hydrostatic pressure and system constants of water and air (De Munck and Schellart, 1987).

For any point on a particular isopressure surface - all spheroids with half interfocal distance a centered around the bubble - the displacement amplitude is proportional to the distance between that point and the centre of the spheroid. So, near the apex of the bubble the scattered displacement field is strongest whereas it is weakest in the middle. At the apex the strength strongly decreases for increasing distance.

To compute the total displacement, first $\mathbf{r}_f$, the contribution of the incident sound wave arriving from the source, has to be calculated. $\mathbf{r}_f$ is:

$$\mathbf{r}_f = Ur_0^{-1}\omega^{-2}R^{-1}(-i\omega c^{-1} - R^{-1}).\exp\{i(-\omega Rc^{-1} + \omega t)\},$$

with r_0 the density of water. Since both displacements are not in phase, the orbits will, in general, be elliptical. However, very close to the bladder surface the displacement orbits are linear and perpendicular to the bubble surface owing to the dominance of $\mathbf{r}_{sc}$. At large distances from the bubble the orbits are practically linear again and point to the source owing to the dominance of $\mathbf{r}_f$. At the apex strong changes of orbit size, shape and orientation occur for slight changes of position. This means that the precise macular position is crucial for its displacement orbit. For any given posi-tion, the macular displacement orbits can be calculated when it is assumed that the tissues surrounding the bladder and lying in between swimbladder and otolith organs behave like water except for their experimentally determined damping A (yielding a quality Q between 1 and 2). Moreover, the fish should lack special sound transmitting structures, such as the goldfish's Weberian ossicles coupling the swimbladder to the otolith systems. A final condition, justified for frequencies > 50 Hz by De Vries' (1950) measurements, is that the otoliths do not oscillate (with respect to the source).

The calculations have been made for the otolith systems of the cod and trout as a function of depth, of sound frequency, and of distance and direction of a (monopole) source in the same horizontal plane as the fish.

The displacement orbits of the otolith systems: the orbit model

Figure 2 gives the orbits of both utricular maculae of a 30 cm cod for

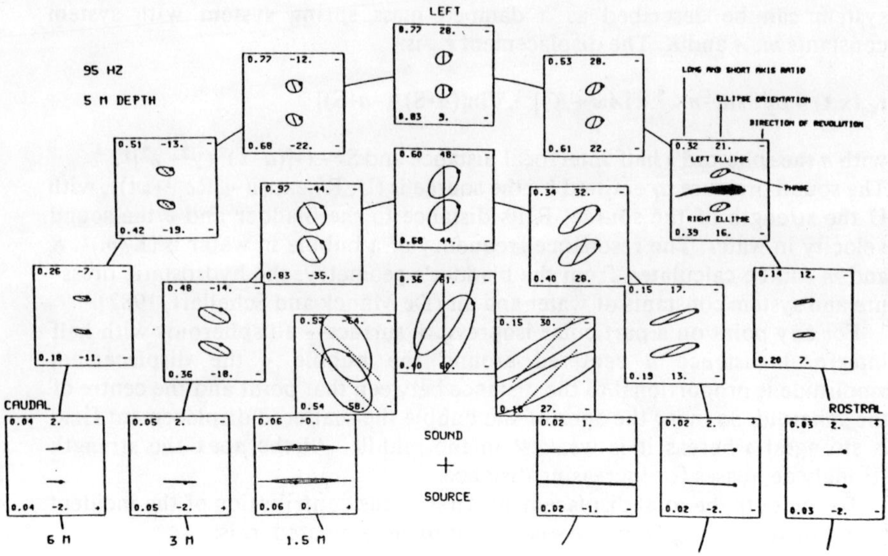

Figure 2. Orbits of the utricular macula of a 30-cm cod.

conditions that are typical for many behavioural field experiments (95 Hz and 5 m depth). Each box gives the bladder relative to the source for fish positions at the left. Mirrored fish positions give, of course, the same results. The values of the orbit parameters indicated in each box are 1) the ratio of the short versus the long axis (called the axis ratio) at the left; 2) the orientation of the length axis (the ellipse orientation, in degrees) in the middle; and 3) the direction of revolution indicated by a plus or minus sign at the right. Values and orbit at the top hold for the left utriculus. The dashed line within each orbit represents the direct input. Owing to the generally nonzero axis ratios the direction of revolution will be distinguished easily (except near 0° and 180°). Figure 2 shows that the axis ratios and ellipse orientations change considerably as a function of source position for distances within the nearfield (< 3 m). Each orbit is completely described by the axis ratio, the orientation, the direction of revolution and its phase. There is hardly any phase difference between the orbits of the left and right utriculi, and neither is there much difference between the orbit length axes.

Computation of the displacement orbits for the sacculus and lagena yielded roughly similar results, although their orbit parameters change less as a function of source position, owing to the shorter distance of these otolith systems to the swimbladder. In Fig.3, for a 28 cm trout the range of change of the orbit parameters is depicted when the source rotates over 180° around the fish. For the utriculus, the ranges are generally largest. This holds for the cod utriculus as well. The range of change depends not only on the relative distance of macula to swimbladder, but also on source position and frequency.

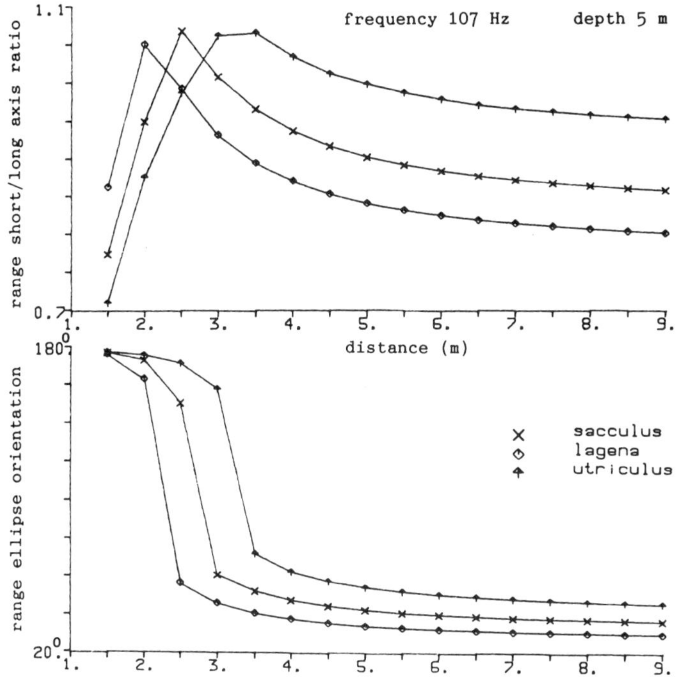

Figure 3. Range ofchange of the orbit parameters of the three trout maculae when the source angle varies between 0° and 180° for distances from 1.5 to 9 m. Along the ordinate, the difference between the highest and lowest value found has been depicted.

At 5 m depth, the optimal source distance is 3 m and the optimal frequency approx. 107 Hz. Smaller fish have higher optimal frequencies and smaller optimal distances.

Physiological implementation of the orbit model

The sensitivity of the utriculus, the detector best positioned according to the orbit model, is roughly restricted to the horizontal plane, in contrast to the other two otolithic maculae. Consequently, the utriculus is most effectively stimulated by sound waves that propagate in the horizontal plane. The fan-like orientation of the utricular hair-cell sensitivity axes gives the functional basis to supply the neuronal signals representing the orbit parameters. At any instant during an orbit cycle, there is a group of hair cells that are stimulated more than other ones at the same instant. The axis of sensitivity of the former group coincides with the instantaneous excursion at the orbit. Owing to the fan-like configuration, during each sound cycle a wave of excitation travels over the macula utriculi either clockwise or counterclockwise. The direction of revolution can be extracted by unidirectional forward excitation or inhibition in a tangential chain of neurons. In this way the 180° ambiguity can be solved in the macula itself or in a central projection of it. The fan sector of maximal excitation within a sine wave period, corresponding to the point of maximal excursion, gives the ellipse orientation. The response strengths of the (perpendicularly oriented) fan sectors of maximal excitation and of minimal excitation determine the axis ratio. So, the fan-like pattern of the directionality of the hair cells enables an analysis of the orbit parameters, even within a single utriculus. The orbit model can be extended to the vertical planes by employing the information from the sacculus and/or lagena, where hair cell directionality is mainly restricted to vertical directions.

No single parameter is a reliable indicator of source position. In combination, however, the orbit parameters can unambiguously encode the source's position. If the orbit parameters have a topological central representation, and if in addition some logical operations between the parameters are performed by neuronal interaction, directional and distance hearing can well be achieved by central mapping. Such a central reconstruction of auditory space from several parameters is also the basis of acoustic localization in most terrestrial vertebrates. Unlike these, however, fish might, according to the orbit model, localize in an essentially monaural manner, since the inputs to both utriculi (or other otolith organs) are nearly identical (Fig. 2).

Behavioural evidence for the orbit model

It should be stressed that many properties of the orbit model ultimately depend on the validity of the assumptions made for calculating the orbits. Consequently, some experiments aiming at testing the model may actually have more bearing on the assumptions and estimates of physical parameters than on the concept of the orbit model itself.

A property of the orbit model leaning heavily upon the assumption of linea recta transmission of swimbladder pulsations is that the left and right utricular orbits are nearly identical, making localization essentially a monaural process. It has been found that unilateral cutting of saccular and lagenar nerves eliminates localization, but not hearing itself (Schuijf, 1975). This would seem to indicate that directional hearing, at least in cod, is a binaural process needing these otolith systems, but, on the other hand, it does not exclude involvement of the utriculus. This should properly be tested in the reverse experiment, i.e. functionally eliminating one or both utriculi, and observing the fish's localizing abilities remaining unimpaired. However, utricular dysfunctioning affects the fish's equilibrium and is thus likely to produce stress leading to unreliable performance in behavioural tests. Clarifying the auditory role of the utriculus requires as yet untried methods that allow a temporary and reversible blocking of the utriculus, and/or a restraining of the fish during testing to minimize the effects of unbalance.

From the point of view of the orbit model proper, it is doubtful whether cod or trout can distinguish between 0° and 180° since the orbits are linear. However, in the experiments of Schuijf and Buwalda (1975) cod were perfectly capable of discriminating these two situations. One possible explanation is that the expected poor performance at 0° and 180° did not show up because the source direction did not coincide precisely with the longitudinal axis of the fish. When the fish moves its head or body through some 5 to 10°, the change in direction of revolution of both orbits solves the 180° ambiguity, since this change uniquely depends on the direction of the turn and the position of the source. For situations other than 0° and 180° this argument does not hold, but in that case the direction of revolution is easily detected.

Another explanation is revealed in Fig. 2. It can be seen that, for equal input strength, the orbit lengths for 0° and 180° differ markedly: the cod may have used the resulting intensity cue without any directional sensation coming into play. This pronounced difference is a manifestation of a more general phenomenon that may be termed the "anisotropy" of the orbit model. The effects of this anisotropy can be tested in psychophysical experiments relating the detectability or discriminatability of the stimulus to the source direction or position. Such tests have been carried out on cod and trout, employing the methods described by Buwalda (1981), viz. sound field synthesis by standing wave superpositioning for stimulus control, and heart rate conditioning for response measurement. The specific situations studied include determining: a) the just noticeable change in source azimuth or elevation; b) the signal detection threshold as a function of source direction; c) the (masked) detection threshold for a pure displacement signal ("direct input") in a pressure noise masker as a function of the displacement vector direction: this "directional masking" paradigm was designed to reveal the effective direction of the swimbladder-oriented "indirect input". The experiments were repeated at different pressure/displacement ratios in order to vary the relative strength of direct and indirect inputs, thus to emphasize any anisotropic effects. The results can be summarized succinctly: no anisotropy whatsoever was revealed in any of the conditions tested. Directional acuity and hearing sensitivity appear to be uniformly distributed over space.

This surprising outcome is clearly at odds with the predictions of the orbit model in its simple monaural form. It does, however, not invalidate the concept of the orbit parameters being used for reconstructing auditory space. A model featuring orbit analysis on a binaural basis, or a monaural analysis followed by binaural interaction to restore bilateral symmetry and smooth any inherent monaural anisotropy, is well conceivable. It would be attractive in that it combines the physiologically plausible aspects of the orbit model with the advantages of binaural processing, a mechanism that is plausible both from an evolutionary and from a functional point of view.

Acknowledgement

We thank Dr. Alfons B.A. Kroese for critically reading the manuscript.

References

Buwalda, R.J.A. (**1981**). "Segregation of directional and nondirectional acoustic information in the cod," in *Hearing and Sound Communication in Fishes*, edited by W.N. Tavolga, A.N. Popper, and R.R. Fay (Springer, New York), pp. 139-171.

Buwalda, R.J.A., Schuijf, A., and Hawkins, A.D. (**1983**). "Discrimination by the cod of sounds from opposing directions," J.Comp.Physiol. **150**, 175-184.

Munck, J.C. de, and Schellart, N.A.M. (**1987**). "A model for the nearfield acoustics of the fish swimbladder," J.Acoust.Soc.Am. **81**, 556-560.

Popper, A.N., and Fay, R.R. (**1984**). "Sound detection and processing by teleost fish: a critical review," in *Comparative Physiology of Sensory Systems*, edited by L. Bolis, R.D. Keynes, and S.H.P. Maddrell (Cambridge University Press, Cambridge), pp. 67-101.

Schellart, N.A.M., and Munck, J.C. de (**1987**). "A model for directional and distance hearing in swimbladder-bearing fish based on the displacement orbits of the hair cells," J.Acoustic.Soc.Amer. **82**, 822-829.

Schuijf, A. (**1981**). "Models of acoustic localization," in *Hearing and Sound Communication in Fishes*, edited by W.N. Tavolga, A.N. Popper, and R.R. Fay (Springer, New York), pp. 267-310.

Schuijf, A. (**1975**). "Directional hearing of cod (Gadus morhua) under approximate free field conditions," J.Comp.Physiol. **98**, 307-332.

Schuijf, A., and Buwalda, R.J.A. (**1980**). "Underwater localization: a major problem in fish acoustics," in *Comparative Studies of Hearing in Vertebrates*, edited by A.N. Popper and R.R. Fay (Springer, New York), pp. 43-77.

Schuijf, A., and Buwalda, R.J.A. (**1975**). "On the mechanism of directional hearing in cod (*Gadus morhua* L.)," J.Comp.Physiol. **98**, 333-343.

Schuijf, A., and Hawkins, A.D. (**1983**). "Acoustic distance discrimination by the cod," Nature **302**: 143-144.

Vries, H.L. de (**1950**). "The mechanics of the labyrinth otoliths," Acta Otolaryngologica **38**: 208-230.

Comments

Narins:

Does the swimbladder in your model provide differential input to the two ears? I ask in light of new evidence from laser doppler vibrometry studies which have suggested the existence of an "indirect" input to the auditory system of the frog. Anurans (frogs and toads) have large, permanently open Eustachian tubes which serve to couple, via the buccal cavity, the inner surfaces of the tympanic membranes. Sound impinging on the outer surface of one eardrum interacts with sound arriving at the inner surface of that eardrum, resulting in a pressure-gradient receiver. Input to the inner surface of the eardrum comes from the contralateral ear. We (Narins, Ehret and Tautz, 1988) have recently identified a second input to the tympanic membrane inner surface in the treefrog, namely via the lungs, larynx, buccal cavity and Eustachian tubes. The vibrational velocity of the lateral body wall overlying the lung cavity is on the order of 10 dB below that of the ipsilateral eardrum. Perhaps the complex interactions between the direct and indirect inputs to the amphibian ear have their evolutionary origins in the fishes and therefore your model for spatial hearing may have rather broad implications.

Section 5

Psychophysics of pure and complex tones

Nonlinear level effects, and across-frequency processing for simple tones is in issue in the first three papers. The next five deal with perceptual properties of complex signals, focussing on temporal, spectral and phase information. Two papers deal with pitch perception. The last two concern binaural hearing.

Irregularities in the masked threshold of brief tones and filtered clicks

J.M. Festen and W.A. Dreschler[2]

Experimental Audiology, ENT department, Free University Hospital, Amsterdam, The Netherlands
[2]Clinical Audiology, Academic Medical Center, Amsterdam, The Netherlands

Introduction

In studies on the spectro-temporal properties of the auditory system often detection thresholds for brief signals are measured. In the interpretation of results frequently the implicit assumption is made that we are dealing with a linear system; i.e. we assume that detection of the signal as a function of masker level is determined solely by the signal-to-noise ratio. No direct justification of this premise is available from the literature. In a classical paper Hawkins and Stevens (1950) presented only masked thresholds for long tones of various frequencies showing a constant S/N ratio at threshold as a function of the level of a white-noise masker. Notably, subjects were instructed to adjust the level of the tone such that a definite pitch could just be recognized rather than some increment in the noise. Among others, Plomp and Bouman (1959) studied the masked threshold for tones of various frequencies as a function of the signal duration, but only for a fixed masker level. They described their data with a model in which at some stage in the auditory system the activity asymptotically reaches a final value proportional to signal intensity with a time constant between 150 and 375 ms. For the detection of short signals they obtained masking curves with a slope of 3 dB for each doubling in signal duration. Only for very short signals steeper slopes were found and it was concluded that for the detection of short signals the energy within a critical band centered at the signal frequency is integrated.

A closely related topic is the detection of just-noticeable signal increments. This intensity resolution is in a first approximation described as a constant fraction of the signal intensity, known as Weber's law, but many data appeared to deviate from this rule (cf. Rabinowitz *et al.*, 1976). However, for signal detection in the presence of a masker that is spectrally different from the signal, very few deviations from the simple rules introduced above have been reported. Campbell (1964) measured the detection threshold for narrow bands of noise of various frequencies in a wide-band masking noise and found that "the threshold S/N ratios were not constant once the masker was well above threshold". Campbell and Lasky (1967) also found irregular threshold curves as a function of masker level for 20, 400, and 1000-ms tones in a single- or multi-tone masker, with the larger effects for the brief tones. The effects in both studies were attributed to the existence of different neural detection mechanisms operating at different levels. Carlyon and Moore (1986) suggested a similar explanation for intermediate-level deteriorations in the threshold of 20-ms tones of 4000 and 6500 Hz in narrow-band noise of the same duration. But in the latter study the nonconstant S/N ratio at threshold occurred only when the masker was gated together with the signal. In general we can conclude, that deviations from the simple rules outlined above show up in particular for brief signals.

Masking functions for filtered clicks

Recently, when investigating differences in the masking of clicks by wide and narrow-band maskers we obtained an unexpected result. The masked threshold for octave-filtered clicks (f_c = 1000 Hz) was measured in a 2AFC adaptive procedure both for a white-noise masker low-pass filtered at 4 kHz and for an octave-filtered noise masker coinciding in frequency with the click. The presentation of the click was temporally centered in the masker burst with a duration of 400 ms. Further details of the measurement procedure are given in the next section. Results as a function of masker level are shown in Fig.1 for one listener. For other listeners similar results were obtained. The straight-line fit to the data in Panel (a) has been redrawn in Panel (b); this line clearly shows an approximately 6-dB deterioration of the threshold at intermediate levels in the wide-band masking condition. In the present paper conditions for which this phenomenon exists, are traced to some extend and a possible explanation is given.

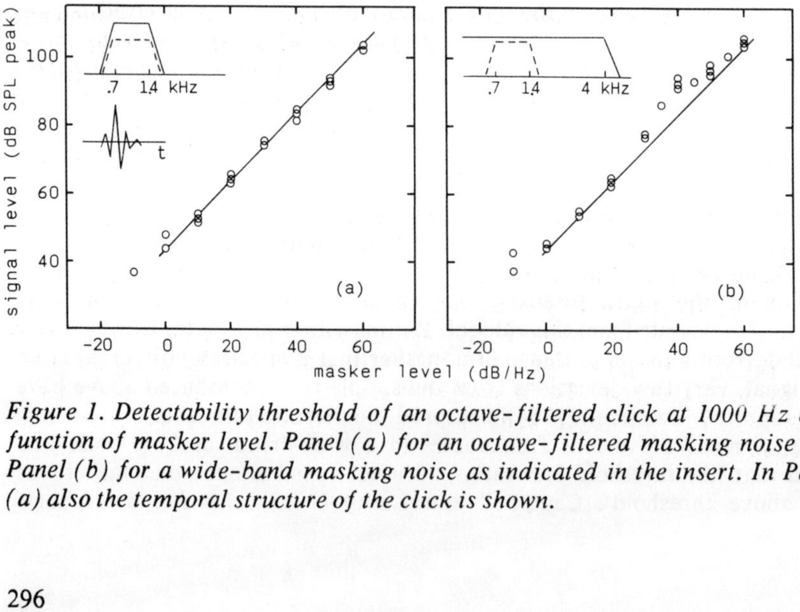

Figure 1. Detectability threshold of an octave-filtered click at 1000 Hz as a function of masker level. Panel (a) for an octave-filtered masking noise and Panel (b) for a wide-band masking noise as indicated in the insert. In Panel (a) also the temporal structure of the click is shown.

Experiments

Throughout this study a fixed 2AFC adaptive procedure was used with minor differences in masker and signal timing among the experiments. In the experiments with filtered clicks the masker was presented in two 400-ms bursts with an inter-burst interval of 800 ms. The click was presented at random in either the first or the second masker burst with a delay of 200 ms relative to the masker onset. For each threshold determination the adaptive procedure started above threshold and in the first phase the click level was lowered after each correct response. After the first incorrect response the procedure changed to "2 up, one down" estimating a signal level with on the average 71% correct responses (cf. Levitt, 1971). This procedure was continued for a period of three reversals in the signal level. Following this two-stage starting procedure requiring typically about 30 trials the actual measurement was carried out, and contained a fixed number of 20 trials (3 up, one down, 79% correct). The step size was 2 dB throughout the whole run and after each response the listener obtained visual feedback (correct/incorrect). For the experiments in which Gaussian-shaped tones were applied the masker bursts were 500 ms with 300-ms inter-burst interval and the signal was for each signal duration centered in the masker burst.

Effects of click and masker bandwidth

In order to study the onset of the threshold deterioration shown in Fig.1, thresholds for filtered clicks were measured as a function of masker bandwidth and at three levels (20, 40, and 60 dB/Hz). The results are shown in Fig.2a. For a large masker bandwidth threshold differences between 20 and 40 dB/Hz masker level are substantially larger than 20 dB; between 40 and 60 dB/Hz substantially smaller differences are found as can be seen also in Fig.1b. When narrowing the masker bandwidth signal thresholds for high and low masker levels are unaffected until the masker width equals the signal width (700 Hz). However, at the intermediate masker level (40 dB/Hz) the threshold already starts to drop for frequencies below about 2500 Hz and when signal and masker have the same width the irregularity has disappeared. For even narrower maskers part of the signal energy is outside the masker frequency band and the threshold sharply drops.

From informal listening it appeared that for very wide-band clicks no irregular masking curves were found. Therefore also the click threshold in wide-band noise was measured as a function of the click bandwidth for the same three masker levels. Results are shown in Fig.2b. Again for narrow-band clicks irregular masking functions are found, but for increasing signal bandwidth, the irregularities gradually diminish and beyond about 2500 Hz they have disappeared. For a click bandwidth of 700 Hz the results are comparable with the wide-band data from Panel (a) as is indicated with dashed lines.

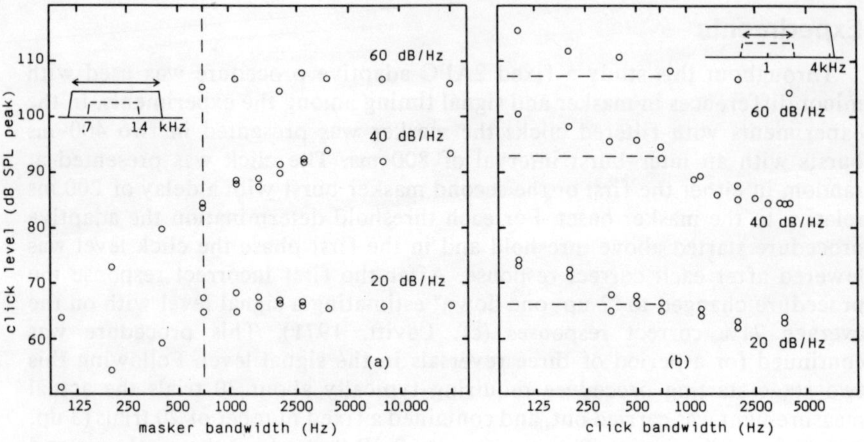

Figure 2. Click threshold as a function of masker bandwidth (Panel a) and as a function of click bandwidth (Panel b) for three masker levels (20, 40, and 60 dB/Hz). Stimulus spectra are shown schematically in the two panels.

Effect of signal duration/bandwidth in Gaussian-shaped tones

The data in Fig.2b show a nonlinear growth of masking for a narrow spectral width of the click. Further narrowing of the signal spectrum will ultimately result in a pure tone for which no nonlinearities were reported (Hawkins and Stevens, 1950). We expect, therefore, that the nonlinearity will disappear if we extend the measurements from the previous section to signals with a smaller bandwidth. To investigate this we used short tonal signals with a Gaussian envelope. The carrier phase was locked to the envelope in such a way that the top of the envelope always coincides with the top of the carrier. So the peak amplitude was constant irrespective of the signal duration. For very short duration we have an impulse signal and for longer duration we have an oscillating signal. The Gaussian envelope was truncated at 0.76% of its peak amplitude. The spectrum of the signal is approximately also Gaussian and its spectral width varies inversely with its duration.

Masked thresholds for signals with a 1000-Hz carrier were measured as a function of signal duration. The masker was low-pass noise filtered at 8000 Hz with a spectrum level of 20, 40, or 60 dB/Hz. Results are shown in Fig.3. For the high and the low noise levels the signal threshold gradually increases for decreasing signal duration with 10 dB per decade. Again at 40 dB/Hz higher thresholds were found than expected on the basis of a constant S/N ratio. This effect disappears both for very brief signals (equivalent rectangular duration < 0.5 ms) as was found in the previous sections and for long signals (> 5 ms).

The data in Fig.3 show still an other unexpected effect. Apart from the irregularity, thresholds increase with 10 dB per decade even for very short

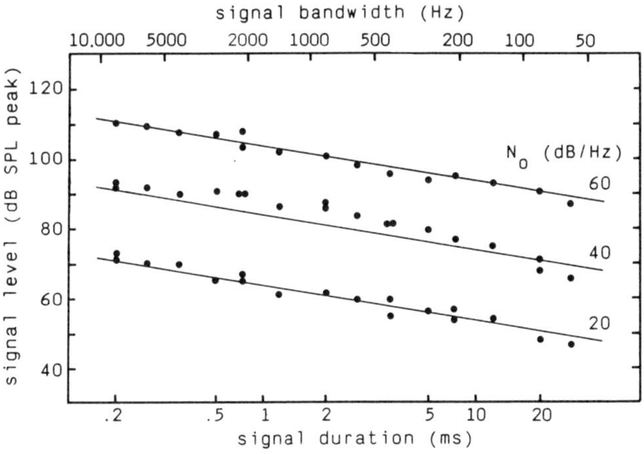

Figure 3. Detection threshold for Gaussian-shaped tone pulses with a 1000-Hz carrier as a function of the equivalent rectangular duration. The masker is white noise low-pass filtered at 8 kHz with a spectrum level of 20, 40, or 60 dB/Hz. Equivalent rectangular signal bandwidth is shown above the figure.

signals with a bandwidth much wider than the critical band at 1000 Hz. This implies an integration of energy over a much wider range than the critical band. At 1000 Hz signals shorter than about 10 ms are spectrally wider than the critical band, thus for the larger part of the data in Fig.3 the current hearing theory predicts a steeper slope. For very short durations, however, there is a small artifact. Between an equivalent rectangular duration of about 0.8 and 0.2 ms the signal changes from a very brief oscillating signal to a single impulse. As a consequence the total signal energy drops with only 3 dB instead of 6 dB over this range of durations.

Effect of signal frequency

In this section we present the results of an experiment on the frequency dependence of the threshold deteriorations found sofar for band-limited brief signals over a restricted range of intensities. With a Gaussian-shaped tone pulse of fixed duration and bandwidth (2 ms and 800 Hz) thresholds were measured as a function of masker level for various central frequencies. The results of this experiment for two listeners are shown in separate panels of Fig.4. The data in Panel (b) are from the same listener as shown in the other figures. For 1000 Hz the data are similar to those in Fig.1b. For other central frequencies comparable irregular masking curves are found, but the thresholds corresponding to a high S/N ratio occur at different masker levels. For f_c = 4000 Hz only minor irregularities are present. Also for different listeners the irregularities in the masking curves for the same central frequency are found for different masker levels.

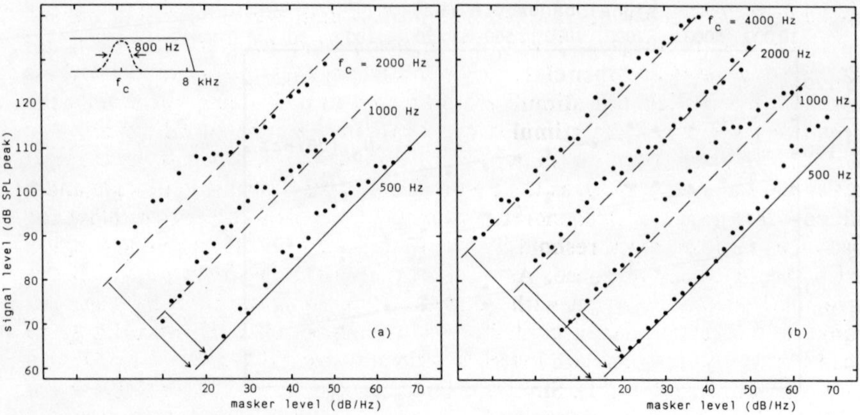

Figure 4. Detectability thresholds as a function of masker level for a Gaussian-shaped tone pulse with an equivalent rectangular bandwidth of 800 Hz. The two panels show data for different listeners. The axes refer to the 500-Hz data. The data for the other central frequencies and the straight line representing a constant S/N ratio have been shifted for each octave over 10 dB along both axes. The spectral configuration of the stimulus is shown in the insert.

Discussion

The results presented in Fig.2a show that a broad-band masker is more effective than a masker of the same spectral width as the signal, at least for specific intensities. The most obvious conclusion from this finding is that the broad-band noise masks off-frequency energy in the signal. However, two problems remain. Firstly, if we raise the level, off-frequency energy will come above threshold and may contribute to the detection and thus to the masking difference between octave and broad-band noise. But why would this difference disappear for even higher levels as is shown in Fig.1b? Secondly, the irregular masking curves were obtained for the broad-band masking condition for which it is assumed that the off-frequency energy in the signal is masked. To check this, part of the experiments was repeated with an extra notched noise with a spectrum level 20 dB higher than the broad-band noise. As expected the additional notched noise did not significantly change the results.

A possible explanation for the data presented here can be given, when we assume that for click-like stimuli with a restricted bandwidth the threshold as a function of masker level is essentially nonlinear and thus is not reached for a constant S/N ratio. For instance, in a simple model the detection of a click in noise would require the neural activity to increase with a certain amount. In this view the existence of classes of neurons with different thresholds as has been found among others by Liberman (1978) may easily cause such a level dependent S/N ratio at the masked threshold. A high S/N ratio will be needed to reach the threshold at levels where many neurons from one class are saturated while in an other class for only relatively few units the threshold is reached. When click-like stimuli are presented in wide-band noise, only the frequency region of the stimulus can contribute to the threshold and the irregularities are found as shown in Fig.1b. However, when the masker is given the same bandwidth as the signal, the exitation patterns coincide and a much wider range of freqencies may contribute to the detection. Now for each masker level the threshold will be determined by the frequency region with the optimum response. As is shown in Fig.4 the level at which the irregularities occur changes with frequency, thus for stimuli in which a broad range of frequencies may contribute to the detection it is more likely to incorporate also regions with low S/N ratio at threshold and the irregularities will disappear (see Fig.1a). Similar effects occur if in a wide-band noise the stimulus bandwidth is widened. For a more wide-band stimulus a broader range of frequencies may contribute to the detection threshold and again no irregularities will be found (see Fig.3).

The explanation given above does not hold for the other extreme in Fig.3; for long-duration Gaussian-shaped tones again a normal increase of the detection threshold with masker level is found. However, these stimuli are perceived as having a distinct pitch and for their detection other mechanisms may play a role. In Fig.2b click-like stimuli with a bandwidth of about 100 Hz show an irregular growth of masking while a tonal stimulus of comparable bandwidth in Fig.3 does not. Also the absence of an irregular growth of masking for f_c = 4000 Hz in Fig.4 may be due to these other detection mechanisms.

References

Campbell, R.A. (**1964**). "Masker level and noise-signal detection," J.Acoust. Soc.Am. **36**, 570-575.

Campbell, R.A. and Lasky, E.Z. (**1967**). "Masker level and sinusoidal-signal detection," J.Acoust.Soc.Am. **42**, 972-976.

Carlyon, R.P. and Moore, B.C.J. (**1986**). "Detection of tones in noise and the "severe departure" from Weber's law," J.Acoust.Soc.Am. **79**, 461-464.

Hawkins, J.E. and Stevens, S.S. (**1950**). "The masking of pure tones and of speech by white noise," J.Acoust.Soc.Am. **22**, 6-13.

Levitt, H. (**1971**). "Transformed up-down methods in psychoacoustics," J.Acoust.Soc.Am. **49**, 467-477.

Liberman, M.C. (**1978**). "Auditory-nerve response from cats raised in a low-noise chamber," J.Acoust.Soc.Am. **63**, 442-455.

Plomp, R. and Bouman, M.A. (**1959**). "Relation between hearing threshold and duration for tone pulses," J.Acoust.Soc.Am. **31**, 749-758.

Rabinowitz, W.M., Lim, J.S., Braida, L.D., and Durlach, N.I. (**1976**). "Intensity perception. VI. Summary of recent data on deviations from Weber's law for 1000-Hz tone pulses," J.Acoust.Soc.Am. **59**, 1506-1509.

Across-frequency integration in signal detection

W. van den Brink and T. Houtgast

TNO Institute for Perception
Soesterberg, The Netherlands

Introduction

In a previous experiment (Houtgast, 1987) it was found that the detection threshold of a signal may decrease considerably with increasing signal bandwidth: when a broadband signal is labelled by the number (n) of the 1/3-octave-band elements included, its masked threshold can be 10log(n) dB lower than the masked threshold of each individual 1/3-octave-band element presented alone. This was observed for a brief signal (10 ms) in which the 1/3-octave-band elements were well synchronized and their relative levels were adjusted with respect to their individual masked thresholds. The 10log(n) rule, i.e., a 3 dB decrease for each doubling of signal bandwidth, implies a very efficient across-frequency integration process, as efficient as the across-time integration underlying the classical data on the masked threshold of a pure tone (a 3 dB decrease for each doubling of tone duration, within certain limits) (Plomp & Bouman, 1959). The 10log(n) rule for across-frequency integration is not in line with current theories on the effect of signal bandwidth on signal detection. Basically, two types of theories are prevailing. The first type is essentially based on the idea that detection is governed by "the best" critical band (Gässler, 1954; Zwicker and Feldtkeller, 1967) involved (the band with the highest individual d' or S/N ratio), which would predict no effect of bandwidth on signal detection for our stimuli. The second type (Green, 1958, 1960), the optimum detector model with adjustable frequency and time window and various statistical multi-channel combination rules, would predict typically a 5log(n) rule, which is less effective than the one observed in the experiment mentioned above. This paper reports on a series of detection experiments which is carried out on the role of various stimulus parameters on across-frequency integration.

Signal definition

In experiments I & III the signals consisted of Gaussian tone pulses, being defined by the following mathematical expression:

$$f(t) = C \sin\{2\pi f_0(t - t_0)\} \exp[-\{a f_0(t - t_0)\}^2] \qquad (1)$$

The value of a determines the signals effective duration and its effective bandwidth. We used a=0.2, for which the effective bandwidth is just within one third of an octave. The value of f_0 determines the signals central frequency. Broadband signals were obtained by summation of Gausssian tone pulses with appropriate f_0-values.

In experiment II the signals were bandpass impulse responses. They were defined in the frequency domain using 2048 samples. Bandpass regions were calculated and spectral filtering was applied according to what spectral slope was needed (1/f, 1/1f). The signals were then Fourier transformed using a FFT-algorithm producing time signals consisting of 2048 samples.

Level definition

The levels of the present brief signals were defined on the basis of the signal energy E within 1/3-octave bands. For the individual Gaussian tone pulses, this corresponds to their actual energy. For the broad-band stimuli in experiment II, the energy was determined after 1/3-octave-band filtering, and specified for each relevant 1/3-octave band. The energy E within a 1/3-octave band is always related to the spectral density N_0 of the noise within the same 1/3-octave-band. N_0 is the noise intensity in a 1-Hz interval and consequently, the mean noise energy within a frequency-time window for which the product bandwidth and duration equals one. The ratio E/N_0 plays an essential role in detection theory.

Measuring procedure

A 2-IFC method with feedback was used in all the experiments, with an adaptive-level procedure. The masker consisted of continuous white or pink noise and the intervals were marked by warning lights. Four subject are used in the series of experiments; some tentative data will be presented here. Each data point is based on typically 500 trials.

Experiment I

This experiment is concerned with the masked threshold of individual Gaussian tone pulses for various central frequencies as described by Eq.1, each covering essentially only one 1/3-octave band. The masker was continuous pink noise. The thresholds in terms of E/N_0 for five subjects typically correspond to a constant value of about 9 to 10 dB for the four central frequencies considered, which agrees well with data from literature (Green, 1958).

The broad-band signals considered in the next experiment were defined such that E/N_0 was the same for each 1/3-octave band within the signal bandwidth, thus ensuring that all frequency regions within the signals

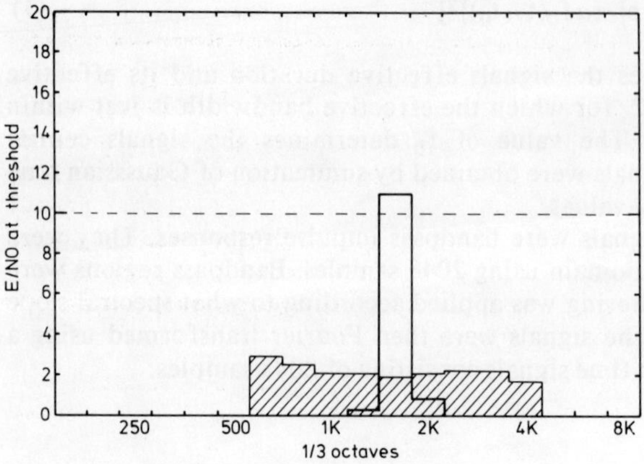

Figure 1. E/N_0-spectra at masked threshold for two signals: one covering a single 1/3-octave band, and one covering nine adjacent 1/3-octave bands (Example for one subject).

bandwidth equally contribute to signal detection.

Experiment II

In this experiment the signal bandwidth was varied, expressed by the number of 1/3-octave bands involved. The masker was either white or pink noise. The central frequency of the signal was fixed at 1.6 kHz, and the number of 1/3-octave bands covered was 1, 3, 5, 9 or 13. Additionally, for the pink-noise masker, a step-function was included as one of the signals; this signal produces E-values within 1/3-octave bands which decrease by 3 dB per octave, thus ensuring a constant E/N_0 value over a wide frequency range. As an example, Fig.1 presents the E/N_0 spectra for two signals at masked threshold: one covering a single 1/3-octave band as in Exp I, and one covering nine 1/3-octave bands (one subject, masker white noise).

The data show that, at masked threshold, the E/N_0 for the signal covering nine 1/3-octave bands is about 9 dB lower than for the signal covering only a single 1/3-octave band. Figure 2 presents the E/N_0 at masked threshold for two subjects as a function of the number (n) of the 1/3 octave bands covered by the signal. This refers to the pink-noise masker; for the white-noise masker identical results were obtained. The relation corresponding to 10log(n) is indicated by the dotted line. Essentially, the data follow this relation, leveling off at a bandwidth covering about nine 1/3-octave bands. Thus, the across-frequency integration underlying the 10log(n) rule appears to operate over a bandwidth of typically three octaves.

Experiment III

This experiment is concerned with signals exciting a number of non-adjacent 1/3-octave bands, with a total bandwidth not exceeding three octaves. One series of signals consists of three signal-excited 1/3-octave bands, with a spacing of either 0, 1, 2 or 3 1/3-octave bands (thus, the latter signal covering nine 1/3-octave bands). A second type consists of five signal-excited 1/3-octave bands, with a spacing of either zero or one 1/3-octave bands (thus, the latter signal also covering nine 1/3-octave bands). As in experiment II, all spectra were centered symmetrically around 1.6 kHz on a log-f scale.

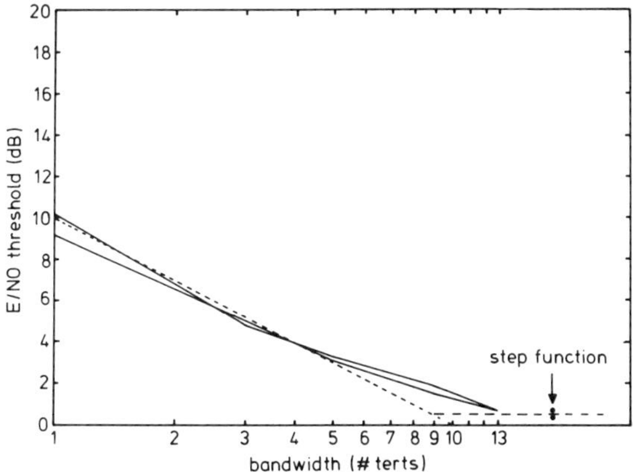

Figure 2. E/N_0 per 1/3-octave band at masked threshold as a function of the number of 1/3-octave bands excited by the signal. Two subjects, pink-noise masker.

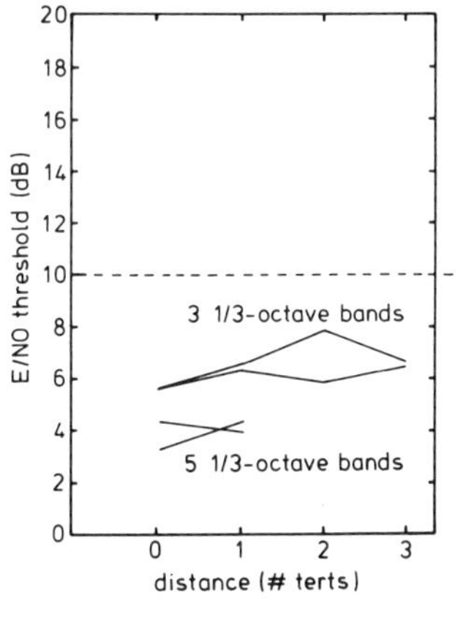

Figure 3. Masked threshold as a function of the seperation between the signal-excited 1/3-octave bands. The horizontal axis represents the number of 1/3-octave bands separating the excited 1/3-octave bands. One set refers to three signal-excited bands, another set to five signal excited bands. Two subjects, pink noise masker.

Across-frequency integration

The data, which are presented in Fig.3, suggest that the 10log(n) rule, n being the number of signal-excited 1/3-octave bands, essentially also applies in case of non-adjacent signal bands, although there is a slight tendency towards a little higher thresholds for increasing seperation.

Conclusions

For brief signals, exciting a number (n) of 1/3-octave bands with equal E/N_0, the masked threshold appears to decrease with 10log(n). The present tentative data suggest this efficient across-frequency integration to extend over about three octaves. Further experiments are in progress on the effects of, for instance, signal duration, over-all stimulus level or the degree of synchronization of the signal envelopes within the various 1/3-octave bands excited by the signal.

Acknowledgement

This investigation was supported by the Netherlands Organization for tge Advancement of Pure Research (Z.W.O.).

References

Buus, S., Schorer, E., Florentine. M. and Zwicker, E. (**1986**). "Decision rules in Detection of Simple and Complex Tones," J.Acoust.Soc.Am. **80**, 1646-1657.

Dallos, P.J. and Olsen, W.J. (**1964**). "Integration of Energy at Threshold with Gradual Rise-Fall Tone Pips," J.Acoust.Soc.Am. **36**, 743-751.

Gässler, G. (**1954**). "Über die Hörschwelle für Schallereignisse mit verschieden breitem Frequenzspektrum," Acustica **4**, 408-414.

Green, D.M. (**1958**). "Detection of Multiple Component Signals in Noise," J.Acoust.Soc.Am. **30**, 904-911.

Green, D.M. (**1960**). "Auditory Detection of a Noise Signal," J.Acoust.Soc. Am. **32**, 121-131.

Houtgast, T. (**1987**). "On the Significance of Spectral Synchrony for Signal Detection," in *Auditory Processing of Complex Sounds*, edited by W.Yost an C.Watson, (LEA London) pp. 118-125.

Plomp, R. and Bouman, M.A. (**1959**). "Relation between Hearing Thresholds and Duration for Tone pulses,"J.Acoust.Soc.Am. **31**, 749-758.

Zwicker, E. and Feldtkeller, R. (**1956**). *Das Ohr als Nachrichtenempfänger*, (Hirzel, Stuttgard).

Comments

Scharf:

The finding that threshold, expressed as overall signal level, remains constant as signal bandwidth increases up to several octaves is at variance with many data in the literature (e.g., Buus *et al.*, JASA, 1986; Gässler, Acustica, 1954). The difference may be related to the very brief signal duration used in the present studies. However, another problem is the inconsistency with data on loudness summation near threshold in the quiet (Scharf, JASA, 1962; Scharf & Hellman, JASA, 1966). Loudness **decreases** with bandwidth, beyond the critical band, below 10 or 15 dB SL. If threshold is constant with bandwidth, then the loudness of a narrow band signal must grow more rapidly from threshold than that of a wide-band signal. Data reveal just the opposite, i.e. more rapid growth for a wide-band signal (see: Scharf, in: *Hearing*, Carterette and Friedman, eds., 1978). And the same rules apply to the loudness of very brief signals as to longer duration signals. It is difficult to understand the basis for a radical change in functional relations when a sound goes from threshold to slightly above threshold.

Across-frequency processing in temporal gap detection

John H. Grose and Joseph W. Hall III

The University of North Carolina at Chapel Hill
Division of Otolaryngology
Chapel Hill, North Carolina

Introduction

One psychophysical measure of the temporal acuity of the auditory system is temporal gap detection. This refers to the ability of a listener to discriminate between a stimulus having a temporal discontinuity (or gap) and a continuous stimulus. For a wideband noise stimulus, the gap detection threshold is approximately 1-2 ms (Plomp, 1964; Shailer and Moore, 1983). Perhaps the aspect of gap detection that has received the most attention is the effect of the frequency composition of the noise stimulus on the gap threshold. In studies where the bandwidth of the noise at the different frequency regions was constant in relative, rather than absolute, frequency (e.g., Fitzgibbons and Wightman, 1982), there was a substantial improvement in gap detection with increasing stimulus frequency. Because the noise bandwidth changes as a function of the stimulus frequency in such studies, it is not possible to attribute this effect solely to noise frequency region. Indeed, the change in noise bandwidth could affect temporal resolution, since random amplitude fluctuations become increasingly prominent as a function of decreasing noise bandwidth. It is likely that such amplitude fluctuations in the low-frequency, narrowband noise stimulus might be confused by the listener with an experimentally imposed gap. This would reduce the sensitivity of the listener to the stimulus interruption, resulting in relatively large gap thresholds (see discussion by Shailer and Moore, 1985). However, even when the absolute noise bandwidth is held constant, there is evidence that somewhat superior performance still occurs for higher-frequency noise stimuli (Shailer and Moore, 1983). Therefore, in general, gap detection for noise stimuli appears to be superior at high frequencies. One interpretation of the improvement of gap detection with increasing stimulus frequency is in terms of the filter analogy often used to characterize the frequency selectivity of the ear: a wide high-frequency filter, associated with a relatively short time constant, would allow better processing of the transient temporal aspects of the waveform (Duifhuis, 1973).

A second issue concerning temporal resolution, also related to the frequency selectivity of the ear, is the question of whether the auditory system processes information across different critical bands (CBs) in gap detection, or whether the auditory system simply bases detection on the CB providing the best temporal information. The results of experiments using wideband noise stimuli are consistent with the idea that gap detection is based upon the highest frequency information available (e.g., Buus and Florentine, 1982; Fitzgibbons and Wightman, 1982; Shailer and Moore, 1983). This would agree with the interpretation that the auditory system uses the CB having the widest bandwidth, and therefore, best temporal resolution. There may be some exceptions to this rule, however. For instance, Shailer and Moore (1985) reported that under some circumstances the auditory system appears to be able to combine information over more than one CB in order to improve temporal resolution. For low-frequency, band-pass noise stimuli, they found that extending the low-frequency cut-off beyond the bandwidth of the CB resulted in improved gap detection. A general interpretation of this result is as follows. For low-frequency noise stimuli the output from any particular CB is characterized by the relatively large amplitude fluctuations inherent in narrowband noise. An experimentally-introduced gap in such a noise is difficult to discriminate from the randomly occurring ongoing fluctuations. However, if noise is present in more than one CB a new cue becomes available which might help the auditory system discriminate a "real" gap from a random noise fluctuation. Whereas the random fluctuations of noise are uncorrelated between the two bands, the experimentally-imposed gap will be correlated between the bands. If the auditory system is able to use this information to reduce uncertainty about the presence of a "real" gap, then gap detection would improve when information is present in more than on CB. The following experiment was performed to test further the hypothesis that the auditory system is able to analyze information across CBs or different auditory channels in order to improve temporal resolution.

Method

Gap detection was measured on four normal-hearing subjects using noise stimuli composed of one, two, or three 50-Hz wide narrow bands of noise. When the noise stimulus was composed of more than one noise band, the noise bands either had envelopes that were random with respect to each other, or had identical (comodulated) envelopes. It was hypothesized that when the envelopes of the noise bands had identical envelopes, performance would not be different from performance for one band alone: in other words, because the fluctuation and gap information in the multiple bands would be identical, the additional bands would not provide any further information over one band.

Each 50-Hz wide noise band was derived by low-pass filtering a wideband noise at 25 Hz and then multiplying the filter output by a pure tone of the desired center frequency. The center frequencies used were 800, 1000 and

1200 Hz. For the stimuli composed of two 50-Hz wide bands having uncorrelated envelopes, two bands having independent envelopes (centered on 800 and 1000 Hz, 800 and 1200 Hz, or 1000 and 1200 Hz), were presented. For the stimulus composed of three 50-Hz wide bands having uncorrelated envelopes, all three noise bands were presented. For the stimuli composed of two 50-Hz wide bands having identical envelopes, a two-tone complex (800+1000, 800+1200, or 1000+1200 Hz) was multiplied by a noise low-passed at 25 Hz. Similarly, for the stimulus composed of three 50-Hz wide bands having identical envelopes, a three-tone complex (800+1000+1200 Hz) was multiplied by a noise low-passed at 25 Hz. Thus eleven monaural conditions were presented: each of the three center frequencies alone; each of the three possible pairs of center frequencies (both comodulated and non-comodulated); and the three center frequencies together (both comodulated and non-comodulated).

Four binaural conditions employing 50-Hz wide noise bands were also run. Three of the conditions were dichotic. In the first, two uncorrelated bands centered on 1000 Hz were presented to the two ears. In the second condition three bands (centered on 800, 1000, and 1200 Hz) were presented to each ear; the bands within each ear were comodulated, but the envelopes between the two ears were uncorrelated. In the third condition, bands at 800, 1000, and 1200 Hz were again presented to both ears; however in this condition not only were the noise envelopes not correlated between the ears, but they were also not correlated within each ear. The final binaural condition was diotic. The diotic stimulus consisted of three comodulated 50-Hz wide noise bands centered on 800, 1000, and 1200 Hz.

Gap detection thresholds were determined using a three-alternative forced-choice procedure, using an adaptive three-down one-up strategy to estimate 79.4% detection (Levitt, 1971). In two intervals a 1-s stimulus was presented without a gap, whereas in the third (at random) the stimulus containing the gap was presented. The gap was initiated 500 ms after stimulus onset. The gap interval was subtracted from the remainder of the stimulus to keep the total duration of the stimulus 1 s. The gap was defined in terms of the 3 dB down point. The initial gap-size was 80 ms. The gap size was decreased by a factor of 1.4 after three consecutive correct responses, and was increased by a factor of 1.4 after one incorrect response. A threshold run was stopped after 12 reversals, and the average of the final eight reversals was taken as the threshold for a run. Four threshold runs were made, and the threshold for a condition was estimated as the average of the four runs. The intervals were marked by a 0.5-s warning light, followed by three 1-s interval lights. The inter-stimulus interval was 400 ms. Visual feedback was provided after each trial.

Detection of spectral splatter was controlled in two ways. One was presentation of stimuli at a low level of 15 dB SL . The other was the use of a relatively long cosinusoidal rise/fall time (15 ms) for gap on-set and off-set.

Results

The results of the monaural conditions are shown in Fig. 1. As can be seen, the gap detection thresholds for the individual 50-Hz bands were approximately 50 ms. This value is high when contrasted with the minimum value reported for wideband stimuli at high sensation level (approximately 1-2 ms), but agrees with past experiments where stimuli of similar bandwidth and level were used (e.g., Shailer and Moore, 1985). When two-component comodulated bands were presented, gap detection did not improve appreciably with respect to that for single 50-Hz wide components. Similarly, there was no apparent advantage for the comodulated three-component stimulus.

In contrast, there was a substantial advantage for the uncomodulated noise bands. For the two and three-component uncomodulated noise bands gap detection was approximately 30-35 ms. There was no apparent advantage for the three-component stimulus over the two-component stimulus.

The binaural conditions exhibited similar effects, as shown in Fig. 2. The diotic condition (consisting of three comodulated bands to each ear) showed a gap detection threshold that was similar to that for a single 50-Hz wide band presented to a single ear. However, the three dichotic conditions showed superior performance. The conditions employing a single band to each ear, and three bands which were comodulated within an ear, but not between ears,

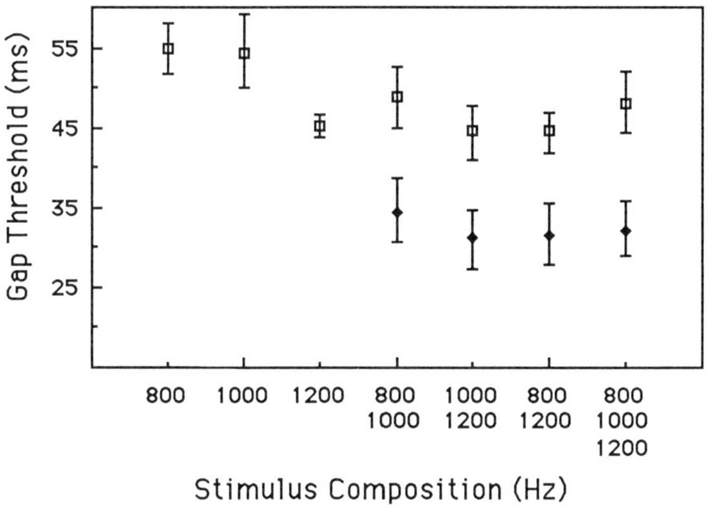

Figure 1. Average gap detection thresholds for single bands at 800, 1000, or 1200 Hz; two-component bands at 800+1000 Hz, 1000+1200 Hz, or 800+1200 Hz; and a three-component band at 800+1000+1200 Hz. Single and comodulated bands are represented by open squares, and uncomodulated bands by solid diamonds.

each resulted in gap detection of about 30 ms. The condition where the envelopes of the three bands were not only uncorrelated within an ear, but also uncorrelated between the ears, resulted in the best detection (approximately 20 ms).

Discussion

The present results suggest that the auditory system is able to combine information across critical bands (or between the two ears) in order to improve temporal acuity. The apparent ability of the auditory system to perform across-frequency comparisons of modulation pattern has also been demonstrated recently in other phenomena, particularly Comodulation Masking Release (CMR) and Comodulation Difference Detection (CDD). In CMR, the masked threshold of a signal is reduced when the components of the masker are made to comodulate rather than modulate independently (Hall *et al*., 1984). In CDD, where the signal is a band, or bands, of noise interspersed with other bands of noise, performance is poor when the signal and the background are comodulating, but performance improves markedly when the signal modulates independently with respect to the comodulating background, (McFadden, 1987; Cohen and Schubert, 1987). Thus in CMR, CDD and the present study of gap detection, it is evident that auditory performance can be based upon an across-frequency comparison of envelope

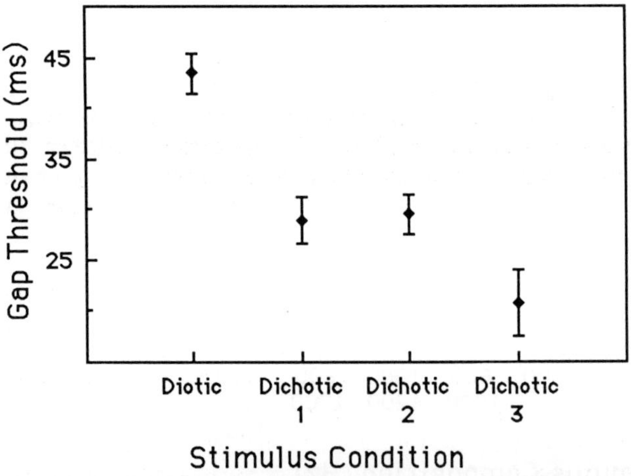

Figure 2. Average gap detection thresholds for the binaural conditions. In "Dichotic 1" a single band is presented to each ear; in "Dichotic 2" a three-component band is presented to each ear such that the bands are comodulated within an ear, but not comodulated between ears; in "Dichotic 3" a three-component band is presented to each ear such that the bands are not comodulated within or between ears.

information, rather than upon an analysis of the output of a single CB or auditory channel. The present results also appear to be closely related to those of Richards (1987). Richards showed that listeners could detect a difference in the correlation of the envelopes of frequency-separated narrow noise bands. In our conditions where a common gap occurs among several uncorrelated bands, a cue of change in across-frequency envelope correlation is available. In light of the results of Richards, it seems likely that this cue was used by our listeners.

The improvement in temporal acuity found in the present study of gap detection is associated with conditions where the modulation patterns across frequency are otherwise *uncorrelated*, save for the common interruption. Superficially this conclusion may appear to be at odds with the results of CMR which indicate that an improvement in performance is associated with conditions where the modulation patterns across frequency are *correlated*, save for the channel in which the signal is presented. However, closer examination reveals the two demonstrations to be entirely complementary. In CMR, when a complex of separate components is comodulating and a signal is added to one of the components, the modulation pattern in the signal channel ceases to be entirely coherent with the remaining channels and the resulting across-frequency difference may cue the signal's presence. In the present study, when a temporal interruption is added synchronously to a complex of independently modulating components, an across-frequency similarity now cues the presence of the gap. In both cases, as well as in CDD, it appears that the cue is associated with the ability to distinguish between common temporal events or modulations and independent events or modulations. Inasmuch as commonality of amplitude modulation pattern is an important grouping factor in attributing components to a common source (Darwin, 1983; McAdams, 1984), such a cueing mechanism might act to facilitate a segregation between a target event (signal or gap) and the background pattern. In other words, the across-channel comparisons thought to underlie the present results on gap detection, as well as CMR and CDD, suggest that the system might use such comparisons to differentiate between different stimulus sources which are present simultaneously.

Following on from this argument, it is of interest to consider the possible relevance of this auditory property to naturally encountered sounds, in particular speech. Consider first a speech signal in quiet. In this case there may be no significant benefit to analyzing the temporal fluctuations across frequency, as they will be comodulated and, therefore, largely redundant. Analyzing the temporal information from a single CB would be nearly as informative about the modulation pattern as analyzing information across many CBs. This is somewhat analogous to the conditions in the present experiments where no benefit of presenting additional comodulated noise bands was found. If a primary function of across-frequency comparisons is to aid in the grouping of components into common sources, then such a process would be of no benefit to speech in quiet since only a single source is present.

However, speech often occurs in a noise background which, as often as not, is other speech sounds. In such conditions, a within band analysis of envelope information may be of limited benefit. The comodulation of speech components from a single source is degraded by the addition of other fluctuations. The resulting problem for the auditory system is somewhat analogous to trying to detect a "real" gap in the fluctuating noise stimuli used in the present experiments. Therefore, from a standpoint of a within-band analysis, the noise background would have the effect of increasing uncertainty about the locations of the temporal peaks and gaps in the signal. Under this circumstance an across-frequency analysis of temporal envelope may be beneficial. Whereas all frequency regions of the speech signal would be associated with similar problems for within-band analyses, a comparison across bands might aid the auditory system to identify the "real" gaps (associated with the signal), as apparently occurred for the uncomodulated stimuli in the present experiments: a gap would be more likely to be accepted as "real" (and processed as part of the desired sound) when occurring at more than one frequency region. Obviously there are many characteristics of a speech sound that could provide cues which would help a listener to track a desired source in a noise environment; the across-frequency processing of temporal fluctuations is one such factor which may underlie perceptual grouping at unfavorable signal-to-noise ratios.

In summary, the present study demonstrated that gap detection for a narrow band of noise can be improved by the addition of another independent band (or bands) containing the gap. This result supports the notion that the auditory system is able to combine information across channels in order to improve temporal acuity.

Acknowledgements

Research supported by Air Force Office of Scientific Research.

References

Buus, S. and Florentine, M. (**1982**). "Detection of a temporal gap as a function of level and frequency," J.Acoust.Soc.Am. **72**, S89.

Cohen, M.F. and Schubert, E.D. (**1987**). "The effect of cross-spectrum correlation on the detectability of a noise band," J.Acoust.Soc.Am. **81**, 721-723.

Darwin, C.J. (**1983**). "Auditory processing and speech perception," in *Attention and Performance X*, edited by H. Bouma and H. Bouwhuis (Erlbaum, Hillside, NJ).

Duifhuis, H. (**1973**). "Consequences of peripheral frequency selectivity for nonsimultaneous masking," J.Acoust.Soc.Am. 54, 1471-1488.

Fitzgibbons, P.J. and Wightman, F.L. (**1982**). "Gap detection in normal and hearing-impaired listeners," J.Acoust.Soc.Am. **72**, 761-765.

Hall, J.W., Haggard, M.P. and Fernandes, M.A. (**1984**). "Detection in noise by spectro-temporal pattern analysis," J.Acoust.Soc.Am. **76**, 50-56.

Levitt, H. (**1971**). "Transformed up-down methods in psychoacoustics,"

J.Acoust.Soc.Am. **49**, 467-477.
McAdams, S. (**1984**). "The auditory image," in *Cognitive Processes in the Perception of Art*, edited by W.R. Crozier and A.J. Chapman (Amsterdam, North Holland).
McFadden, D. (**1987**). "Comodulation detection differences using noise-band signals," J.Acoust.Soc.Am. **81**, 1519-1527.
Plomp, R. (**1964**). "Rate of decay of auditory sensation," J.Acoust.Soc.Am. **36**, 277-282.
Richards, V.M. (**1987**). "Monaural envelope correlation perception," J.-Acoust.Soc.Am. **82**, 1621-1630.
Shailer, M. and Moore, B.C.J. (**1983**). "Gap detection as a function of frequency, bandwidth and level," J.Acoust.Soc.Am. **74**, 467-473.
Shailer, M. and Moore, B.C.J. (**1985**). "Detection of temporal gaps in band-limited noise: effects of variations in bandwidth and signal-to-masker ratio," J.Acoust.Soc.Am. 77, 635-639.

Comments

Tyler:

I am a bit unclear how "across-band" modulation relates to speech perception. In speech, the formants will change rapidly as a function of time, and therefore there may not be sufficient time for "across-band" modulation to be of any benefit. What duration is required of the stimulus for the "across-band" modulation to be utilized?

It may be that "across-band" modulation helps the brain follow formant transitions. As formants move into adjacent frequency regions, identifying the pattern of regions with changing, correlated envelopes could be used to determine where the formant has moved. For example, there could be a constant frequency first formant and a changing second formant. The frequency regions that have correlated envelopes could serve as a cue to follow the second formant transition.

Reply by Grose:

Our point is simply that the phenomenon of perceptual grouping due to common amplitude trajectories, which our results support, may be of benefit in tracking a single speaker in a noisy background. As for the dependence of CMR on stimulus duration, we have observed a masking release for a train of three 50-ms tone bursts.

Hafter:

It seems that your gap effects with multiple bands are considerably smaller than those which you have reported in comodulation masking. Could this be because the two tasks use quite different mechanisms? If gaps are detected by some kind of energy detector as proposed by Green in the last paper, then one should expect a change in performance proportional to the number of independent bands. Your data in Fig.2 for one, two and six such bands are of the right order. Thus, unlike the case with CMR, one need not propose that the listener tracks commonality across bands, just that they make independent computations of the likelihood.

Reply by Grose:

We agree that the "multiple look" hypothesis is compatible with the improved performance observed for the dichotic multiple non-comodulated bands. However, there are two considerations which might favor our across-frequency difference hypothesis. The first is that it is not totally clear why the "multiple look" mechanism would be of benefit for the non-comodulated case, assuming some internal noise in each case. The second is that the across-frequency envelope correlation cue associated with the synchronous gap which is available in the non-comodulated case is very much like that available in the work of Richards on across-frequency detection of envelope correlation. It seems likely that if such a cue is available in our stimuli, then it will be used by the listener.

Aspects of monaural synchrony detection

Virginia M. Richards

Psychoacoustics Lab, Department of Psychology, University of Florida, Gainesville Florida 32611, USA

Introduction

Recent experiments investigating comodulation masking release, or CMR (Hall, Haggard and Fernandes, 1984) have established that the detectability of a tone in a narrow band of noise is improved when a second band, identical to the first save for a frequency translation, is also present. The presumed reason for the reduction in masking is that the temporal pattern of the second band in some way 'cues' the listener to the presence of the signal. The present paper examines one possible mechanism, an across-frequency envelope comparator. When the signal is not present, the two bands of noise are synchronous. The addition of a tone to one of the bands acts to reduce synchrony; i.e., the envelope correlations are reduced.

In several recently completed experiments, we have examined this hypothesis. The experiments were designed to determine: (a) whether envelope synchrony was detectable and (b) whether the just noticeable change in envelope correlation was sufficient to account for the CMR effect (Richards, 1987). In the first experiment we asked listeners to discriminate between simultaneously presented bands of noise that had either identical or statistically independent envelopes. The bands of noise were 100 Hz wide and were presented diotically. The center frequencies, f_L and $f_L+\Delta f$ Hz, were varied systematically. For frequency separations less than an octave, $\Delta f<f_L$, discriminations were best for f_L=2500 and 4000 Hz, somewhat poorer for f_L=1000 Hz, and impossible for f_L=350 Hz. As the frequency of separation approached an octave, discriminations dropped to chance levels. Thus, the initial question of inquiry has been answered: envelope synchrony is detectable (see also Goldstein, 1966).

To determine whether changes in envelope synchrony are sufficient to account for thresholds obtained using the CMR paradigm, we determined the change in envelope correlation needed to discriminate between sounds composed of two bands of noise whose envelopes were either fully or partially correlated. Psychometric functions relating percent correct and the change in envelope correlation were obtained for three subjects. Next, a computer simulation was run to determine the reduction in envelope correlation concomitant with the addition of a tone to one of the otherwise identical bands. The results of these experiments, one psychophysical and one computational, are presented in Table 1. The first column shows the level of the signal relative to the level of the band of noise, E/N_0 in dB. The second column shows the average envelope correlation obtained for the relative signal level indicated in column 1. The third column presents the expected percent correct discriminations based on values derived from the psychometric functions. Based on changes in envelope correlation, we expect an E/N_0 of between 0 and 5 dB to be needed in order to detect the presence of a tone. In contrast, the data of Green, McKey and Licklider (1964) suggest than an E/N_0 of about 12 dB would be needed for the detection of a tone in noise. Thus, when synchrony cues are available, we would expect signal detection thresholds to drop some 5 to 10 dB below those obtained using a single bands of noise. Such values are in line with the data of Cohen and Schubert (1987), who used similar stimulus parameters.

Examination of the envelope synchrony hypothesis

The current experiment was initiated in order to determine whether envelope comparisons *per se* were the basis of the synchrony detection. The experiments described above concentrated on envelope correlations alone. However, in those experiments envelope similarity, power spectrum similarity and phase function similarity (the phase angle of the carrier

Table 1: A tone is added to one of two otherwise identical bands of noise. The resulting envelope correlation is indicated, along with the expected percent correct discrimination based on psychometric data.

E/N_0	r	E(% Correct)
15	0.34	94
10	0.54	92
5	0.77	80
0	0.90	65
-5	0.95	58

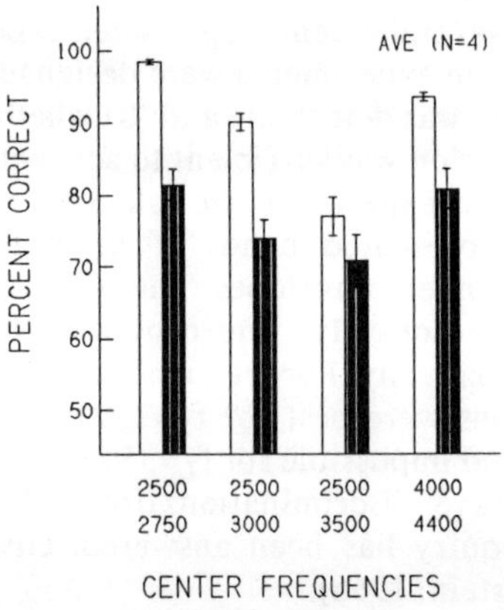

Figure 1. Average percent correct discriminations for the 'shifted' (open) and 'envelope only' (closed) conditions as a function of center frequency.

frequency as a function of time) co-varied; the synchronous bands of noise had identical envelopes, identical power spectra (save for a shift in center frequency) and identical phase functions. Similarly, the bands with statistically independent envelopes had different power spectra and different phase functions. At high frequencies the confounding of envelope and phase is not likely to be serious; it is unlikely that the auditory system is able to incorporate information concerning phase. The potential use of a power spectrum cue is more viable. Either a 'mini-profile analyzer' or a gross energy comparator could have been used to discriminate between synchronous and independent bands. Thus, in this experiment we separated the envelope and power spectrum cues in a factorial manner, and determined the relative contribution of those cues. Due to space limitations, only a portion of the factorial design will be considered here.

In each interval of the 2IFC paradigm, each sound was composed of two bands of noise. Three conditions were run, and in each condition listeners discriminated between sounds composed of bands that shared at least one aspect and bands that were independent. In the first condition, which will be referred to as the 'shifted' condition, one interval contained bands of noise that were the same save for a frequency translation and the second interval contained independent bands of noise. Thus, both envelope and power spectrum cues were available; the envelopes and power spectra were either identical or different. In the second, 'envelope only' condition, only envelope changes reliably cued the listener. One interval contained bands of noise that had identical envelopes but different power spectra and the other interval contained independent bands. The third, 'spectrum only' condition employed only power spectrum cues. In that condition, one interval contained bands of noise with identical power spectra (save for a frequency translation), and the other interval contained independent bands of noise. The idea was to evaluate the combined effects of envelope and power spectrum similarities, and then to determine the relative strength of each cue. Four different center frequency pairs were tested; (2500,2750), (2500,3000), (2500,3500), and (4000,4400) Hz.

The bands of noise were computed digitally, each being the sum of 11 tones spaced 10 Hz apart in frequency. In the 'shifted' condition, amplitudes and phases were chosen randomly for each of the lower noise-band components, and the same amplitudes and phases were used for the higher band. To prevent subjects from learning the noise bursts (each signal was 100 ms long), 32 such pairs were computed and stored. The 'spectrum only' bands were generated in a similar manner, except that the phases used in the high- and low-frequency bands were chosen independently. Thus the two bands had identical spectra but different envelopes. To generate the 'envelope only' pairs, a low-frequency band was generated using randomly chosen amplitudes and phases. Then a high-frequency band was generated such that it was the mirror image of the low-frequency band; the amplitudes were rotated about the center frequency, and the phases were both rotated and negated. This manipulation lead to two bands of noise with identical envelopes but with different relative spectra. Note that these 'envelope only' bands are physically realizable, the same would result if a narrow band of noise was multiplied by a high frequency tone. Finally, the independent bands were chosen from the pool of 64 available bands of noise, with the restriction that the low- and high-frequency bands had not been generated as a pair.

Figure 1 presents the averaged data for the 'shifted' (open bars) and 'envelope only' (closed bars) conditions. The averages are based on the data of four normal hearing listeners. The abscissa shows the center frequencies of the bands employed, and the ordinate presents the percent correct discriminations. The error bars indicate the standard errors of the mean. Synchrony was detectable for all stimulus conditions tested. In both the 'shifted' and 'envelope only' conditions increases in frequency separation lead to reduced discriminability. Performance levels were slightly poorer in the 'envelope only' condition than in the 'shifted' condition. The average difference was a 13 % advantage to the 'shifted' condition, but the magnitude of the difference was subject dependent.

No listener was able to perform above chance in the 'spectrum alone' condition, even though three of the four subjects completed in excess of 1000 trials in the (2500,2750) Hz condition. This indicates that spectral comparisons were not available.

Summary

The experiments described here examined synchrony detection. The extent to which across-frequency synchrony shapes the characterization of our auditory world may be worth speculation, but the experiments described here are not sufficient to approach that question. In general, though, it appears that synchrony detection is quite robust, and that 'envelope synchrony detection' is a reasonable term; changes in envelopes synchrony were detectable even in the absence of spectral cues.

Acknowledgements

This research was supported in part by the Air Force office of Scientific Research and in part by an NIH post-doctoral fellowship. I thank Drs. Leslie Bernstein, Craig Formby, Timothy Forrest and David M. Green for their comments on earlier versions of this paper.

References

Cohen, M. F., and Schubert, E. D. (**1987**). "Influence of place synchrony on detection of sinusoids," J.Acoust.Soc.Am. **76**, 50-56.

Goldstein, J. L. (**1966**). "An investigation of monaural phase perception," Doctoral dissertation, The University of Rochester.

Green, D. M., McKey, M. J., and Licklider, J. C. R. (**1964**). "Detection of a pulsed sinusoid as a function of frequency," in *Signal Detection and*

Recognition by Human Observers, edited by J. Swets (J. Wiley and Sons, New York), pp 508-522.
Hall, J. W. III., Haggard, M. P., and Fernandes, M. A. (**1984**). "Detection in noise by spectro-spatial pattern analysis," J.Acoust.Soc.Am. **81**, 452-458.
Richards, V. M. (**1987**). "Monaural envelope correlation perception," J. Acoust.Soc.Am. **82**, 1621-1630.

Comments

Moore and Schooneveldt:

To perform your task based on 'spectrum only', subjects would have had to detect changes in spectral structure occurring *within* each band of noise; only then could they have detected the similarity of structure across bands. Since both the spacing of the components and the overall bandwidth of each band of noise was much less than the auditory filter bandwidth at 2500 Hz (about 300 Hz), it is not surprising that subjects were unable to perform the task on the basis of 'spectrum only'. What at first sight does appear surprising is that subjects performed slightly less well for the 'envelope only' condition than for the 'shifted condition'. We believe that this can be explained in terms of a within-channel cue similar to that described by Schooneveldt and Moore (1987). Trace (B) below shows a sample of the waveform of two 100-Hz wide bands separated by 250 Hz in the 'shifted' condition. The waveform shows regular envelope fluctuations (a form of beats), occurring 250 times per second and superimposed on the irregular slower fluctuations inherent to the noise bands. When the noise bands are independent, the regular fluctuations and use them to perform the task. Trace (A) also shows a sample of the waveform of two 100-Hz wide bands separated by 250 Hz, but for the 'envelope only' condition. Now the envelope fluctuations are less regular, and occur at a slightly higher average rate (the expected number of envelope

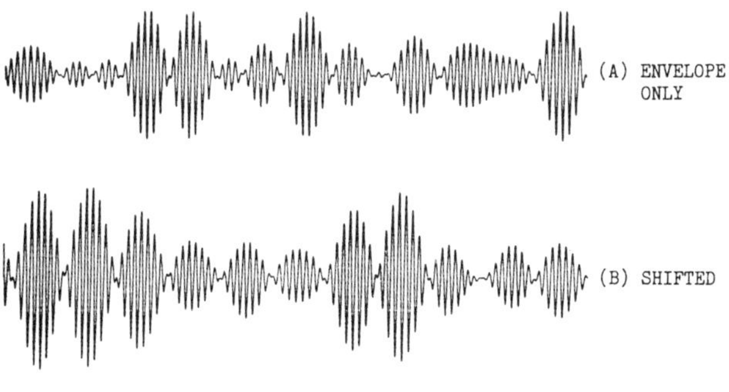

Figure C1

minima per second is about 257). Thus, this stimulus would be somewhat harder to distinguish from two independent bands. In summary, the results may be at least partly explained in terms of a within-channel cue, rather than in terms of the detection of envelope synchrony across channels.

Schooneveldt, G.P. and Moore, B.C.J. (1987). "Comodulation masking release (CMR): Effects of signal frequency, flanking-band frequency, masker bandwidth, flanking-band level, and monotic versus dichotic presentation of the flanking band," J.Acoust.Soc.Am. 82, 1944-1956.

Reply by Richards:

As Moore and Schooneveldt indicate, the "beats" of the two carriers are regular for the "shifted" condition, and irregular for the "envelope only" condition. Two bands of noise that have the same envelope, A(t), that are centered at frequencies f_1 and f_2, when summed have an envelope that is given by

$$A(t)\cdot\sqrt{\{2 + 2\cos[2\pi(f_2-f_1)t + \Phi_2(t)-\Phi_1(t)]\}} \quad (1)$$

where $\Phi_i(t)$ is the phase function of band i.

In the "shifted" condition, $\Phi_1(t)=\Phi_2(t)$, and so equation (1) reduces to $A(t)\sqrt{\{2 + 2\cos(2\pi(f_2-f_1)t)\}}$: The envelope of the summed bands and the envelope of the beating carriers. In the "envelope only" condition, $\Phi_1(t)\neq\Phi_2(t)$, and so the "beating" carriers have a phase modulation component.

The difference in the regularity of the summed envelopes is indicated below. The drawing presents the envelopes of the "shifted" (solid) and "envelope only" (dashed) waveforms. The duration is 100 ms and the center frequencies differ by 250 Hz.

The role of the change in regularity, however, remains to be determined. For the conditions described in the current chapter, the "beat" rates range from 250 to 1000 Hz; detection of regularity would require exquisite temporal resolution (by comparison, temporal modulation transfer functions show considerable attenuation at such high rates). Second, the extend to which bands centered at 2500 and 3500 Hz are "summed" requires consideration.

Finally we have found that listeners are able to discriminate between "shifted" and "envelope only" waveforms on an average of 85% of the trials. This result is consistent with the mechanism proposed by Moore and Schooneveldt.

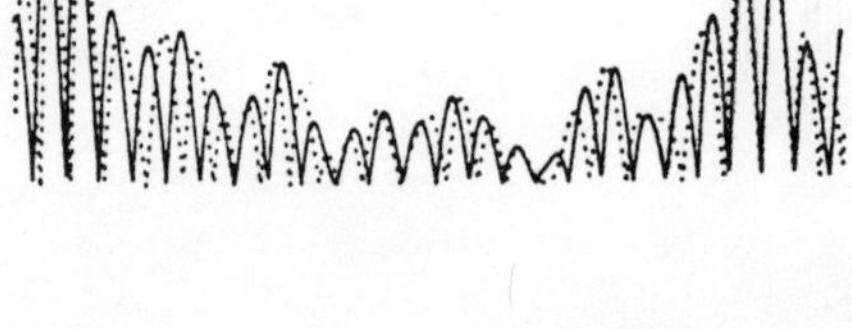

Detection of amplitude modulation and gaps in noise

David M. Green and Timothy G. Forrest

Psychoacoustics Laboratory, Department of Psychology, University of Florida, Gainesville, Florida, 32611, USA

Introduction

Nearly ten years ago, Viemeister (1979) proposed a model to explain how human observers detect amplitude modulation of a noise signal. In this paper, we modify that model slightly and extend its application to the detection of brief temporal gaps in noise. Measuring gap detection has become an increasingly popular way of assessing temporal properties of the auditory system (Penner, 1977; Fitzgibbons, 1983; Green, 1985). Simulation using a modified model provides excellent predictions of the thresholds obtained with partially filled gaps as well as their psychometric functions. Despite this success, the computer simulations indicate that the gap threshold is not strongly influenced by the two major variables of the model, namely, filter bandwidth and integration time. Thus, the applicability of this model to the understanding of hearing impairment remains unclear.

The paper begins with a brief description of the detection tasks and Viemeister's original model. Next, modifications of the original model are described and our reasons for their adoption are explained. The applicability of this modified model to partially filled noise gaps is then described. Finally, we explore the model's predictions about how gap threshold should change as a function of the two major parameters of the model. We begin with a description of the task.

Detection task

All the detection data we will discuss were based on a choice between two stimulus alternatives. One stimulus alternative was an uninterrupted or continuous noise which we refer to as the standard. The other stimulus alternative was noise which was interrupted or altered in amplitude in some fashion. One such alteration was a temporal gap in the noise process, illustrated at the top left (see Fig. 1). The second alteration was amplitude modulation of the noise waveform, illustrated in the bottom left of Fig. 1. These two alterations define two detection tasks called gap detection and

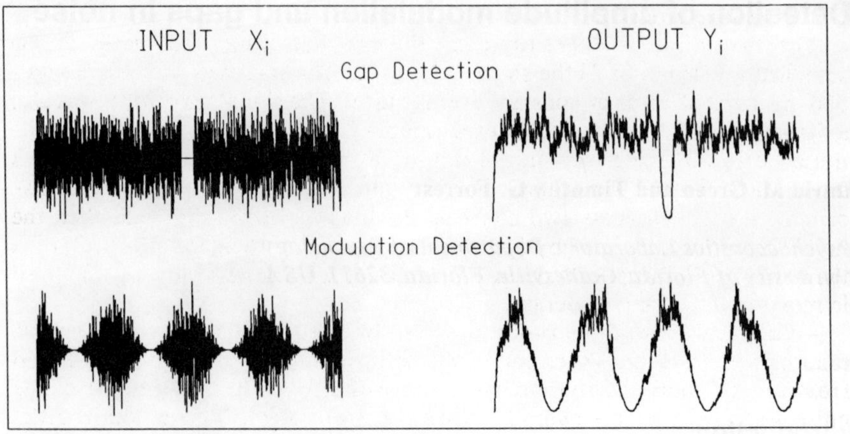

Figure 1. Input and output waveforms for broadband noises with a gap (top) or sinusoidally-amplitude modulated noise (bottom).

modulation detection. Disregard the right column of Fig. 1, it represents the output of a model that we will discuss shortly. All the data reported in this paper were obtained from one of these two detection tasks. The following is a brief summary of the details of the stimulus.

Two-alternative forced-choice procedures were used to estimate all thresholds. The standard was either continuously present or was presented for 500 ms and occurred in one of the two stimulus intervals. The signal was presented in the other interval of the forced-choice task. A two-down one-up adaptive procedure was used to estimate threshold. We generally report the mean of three listeners' thresholds.

Broadband noise was computer generated and presented over 12-bit D to A converters at a rate of 25,000 points per second, and lowpass filtered at 10,000 Hz. More details of the stimulus procedure can be found in Forrest and Green (1987).

The simulations reported in this paper were obtained by programming the model to act as a human observer. The input to the model was the digital version of the signals heard by the observers. The model analyzed two sound buffers corresponding to the two intervals of the forced-choice procedure (standard and signal) and made a choice between the two. The signal level was adjusted adaptively to estimate a threshold for the model, just as it had been for the human observers. All computations were carried out on a microcomputer (IBM AT or equivalent). The human observers took about 5 minutes to run 50 trials and to obtain a threshold estimate with about 10 to 15 reversals. The model took about 3 to 10 times longer.

Gap detection procedure

The two stimulus alternatives of the gap detection task were: 1) the standard waveform or 2) the signal waveform. The standard waveform was a 500-ms burst of noise of constant average level. The signal waveform was also a 500-ms burst of noise, except each sample from the temporal center of the noise burst was scaled by an amount equal to (1-k). The duration of this attenuated segment was called the noise gap. The task problem was to discriminate between these two alternatives. If the value of $k = 0.5$, then the noise was reduced in level by 6 dB for the duration of the gap. If $k = 1.0$, then the noise was fully cancelled during the gap, a condition typical of that used in most studies of gap detection.

An atypical part of the procedure used in these experiments was that we randomized the level of each sound as it was presented. The level was selected from a rectangular distribution with a range of 10 dB. The median level of the noise was about 65 dB overall, 25 dB spectrum level. We randomized the presentation level because the introduction of the gap reduces the total energy in the noise waveform by an amount that depends on the size of the gap and the amount of the attenuation. Randomization discourages observers from trying to use overall level as a detection cue, and makes the primary detection cue one of temporal variation of noise level present within the half-second sample.

Modulation detection procedure

The two stimulus alternatives of the modulation detection procedure were: 1) the standard waveform or 2) a signal waveform. The standard waveform was a continuous noise presented throughout the 50 trials of the two-alternative forced-choice task. The signal waveform, 500 ms in duration, was a set of noise sample multiplied by a sinusoid. Thus, the signal waveform may be described as

$$s(t) = [1 + m \cos(2\pi f_m t)] \cdot n(t) \qquad (1)$$

where n(t) is the unmodulated or standard noise waveform, f_m is the rate of modulation in Hertz, and m is the degree of modulation.

A somewhat atypical part of the procedure used in these experiments was that the signal waveform was adjusted in power, so that the average power of the signal and standard waveforms were equated. When noise is amplitude modulated, the modulated waveform is increased in average power by an amount that depends on the degree of modulation. The expected, or average, power of s(t), $\langle S \rangle$, is given by

$$\langle S \rangle = (1+m^2/2) \cdot \langle N \rangle \qquad (2)$$

where $\langle N \rangle$ is the expected power of the standard noise. Thus, unless $m = 0$, a potential cue for detecting the presence of modulation is the increase in overall power caused by amplitude modulating the noise. This potential

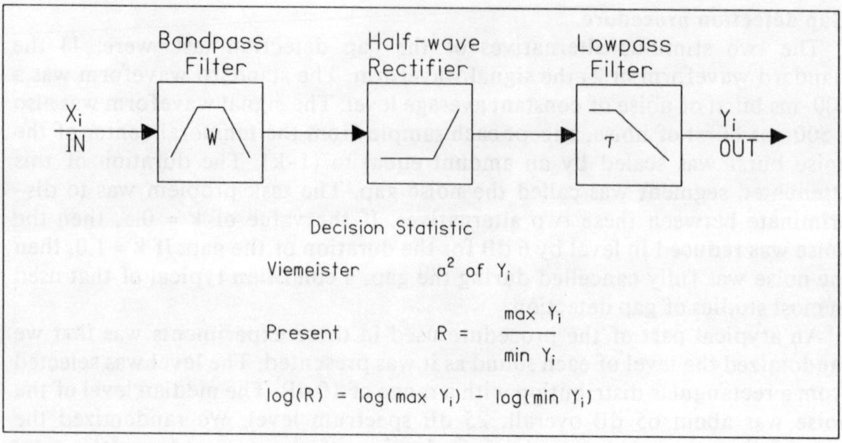

Figure 2. Viemeister's three stage model. Samples of the input waveforms (X_i) pass through an initial bandpass filter with bandwidth (W), then through a half-wave rectifier and a simple lowpass filter. A decision statistic (bottom) is computed from samples of the output waveform (Y_i).

artifact was appreciated by Viemeister (1979) and is responsible for the asymptotic value of the threshold for high modulation frequencies, where m is large (see Fig. 7 of Viemeister, 1979). In all our experiments, we scaled the signal waveform, so that the expected power of the signal was exactly $<N>$, independent of the value of m.

Viemeister's MTF model

The three stages of Viemeister's MTF model are shown in Fig. 2. The incoming signal is first bandpass filtered, with a filter of bandwidth, W. Next the signal is half-wave rectified. Finally, the output of the rectifier is smoothed with a simple one-stage (6 dB per octave) lowpass filter. The output of the model, Y_i, provides the input to a decision stage that selects which of the two stimulus alternatives is correct. In Viemeister's original work, he used the variance of the Y values. Such a decision statistic will be larger, on average, when the noise has been amplitude modulated, as shown in Fig. 1. The figure shows the output of the model to either a gap (top) or amplitude modulated (bottom) input.

Our modification of the original model consisted of changing the decision statistic. Instead of using the variance of the output number, Y_i, we used the ratio, R, of the maximum of Y_i to the minimum of Y_i observed during the bulk of the observation interval. Specifically, we considered all values of Y_i that occurred after the initial three time-constants of the 500-ms observation interval. After determining the maximum and minimum values of Y_i that occurred during that interval, we computed the ratio, R. The decision rule

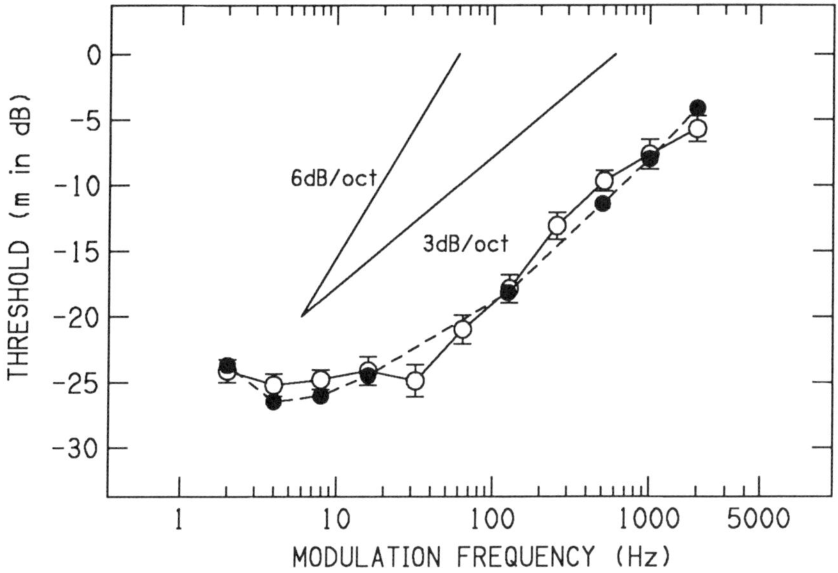

Figure 3. Temporal modulation transfer function for human subjects (solid symbols) and a three-stage model simulation (open symbols). Model parameters are $W = 4000$ Hz and $\tau = 3$ ms.

assumed that the stimulus with the larger value of R was the signal. Such a decision rule is somewhat inefficient compared to the calculation of the variance of Y_i because it is based on only two of the many samples of Y_i present during an observation interval. We adopted this rule for several reasons.

First, we wanted a decision statistic that would function sensibly even with changes in overall level of the sound, as was true in our gap detection experiment. The variance statistic would change systematically with overall level, whereas the expected value of R is independent of the overall sound level. Second, the R statistic produces the 3-dB-per-octave slope observed in psychophysical data for large modulation rates, as we shall now demonstrate.

Modulation detection data

Figure 3 shows the average data of our observers, solid symbols, as well as the data from our simulation, open points. For these simulations, the first stage bandwidth was 4000 Hz and the time constant of the lowpass filter was 3 ms. As can be seen, the data appear to fall along a 3 dB per octave line at high frequencies. This is somewhat unexpected, since the final lowpass filter has an attenuation skirt of 6 dB per octave. We believe that this shallow slope arises because, as the frequency of modulation increases, a greater number of

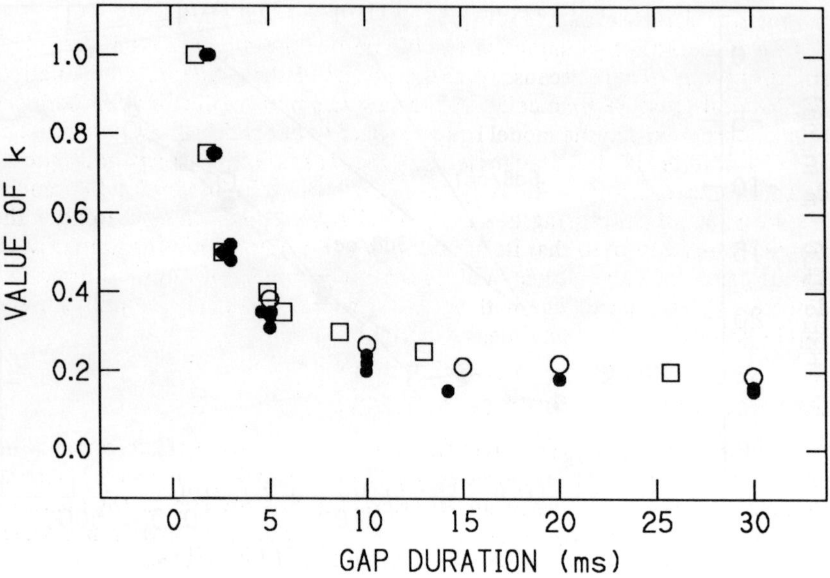

Figure 4. Gap detection data for partially filled gaps in noise for human subjects (solid symbols) and the three-stage model (open points). Model parameters are W = 4000 Hz and τ = 3 ms.

potential maxima and minima are produced. This increase in the number of extrema increases the number of potential signals observed in any observation interval and ameliorates the rapid fall in sensitivity that one would expect from the attenuation produced by the lowpass filter. A problem with this explanation is that sensitivity below the cut off frequency is constant and independent of modulation rate (Fig. 3). Viemeister's model, which uses the variance as the decision statistic, will produce a 6 dB per octave decline at high frequencies, if the noise samples are equalized in overall power, as we have shown elsewhere (Forrest and Green, 1987). Viemeister's original data do not show the 6 dB per octave slope because the noise was not equalized in power (ibid, see Fig. 9). We are now in a position to compare the computer simulations and data obtained from human observers in the gap experiments.

Gap detection data

Figure 4 shows the data for the detection of partially filled gaps in noise. The figure presents data obtained from human observers, solid points, and computer simulations for corresponding conditions, open symbols; again, the parameters of the simulation were W = 4000 Hz and τ = 3 ms. As can be seen, the fit of the model to the data is very satisfactory. Thus, a single model produces reasonably good predictions of both the gap (Fig. 4) and the modulation detection data (Fig. 3).

One of the striking characteristics of gap thresholds is their stability. This stability arises in part because of the steepness of the psychometric function. For k = 1.0 (complete cancellation) the psychometric function for both the human observers and the model has a range of only 1 ms! For smaller values of k (0.50 and 0.35) the psychometric functions are less steep and human detection performance is actually superior to that obtained with the model. We are presently exploring a variety of different ideas on how to alter the computer simulation so that its predictions will better mimic the human data. The urgency of this project will be apparent when we consider how gap detection thresholds change with the other parameters of the model, namely, bandwidth and integration time.

Gap detection as a function of W and τ

Because estimates of gap thresholds are stable, they are often touted as an excellent way to assess temporal parameters of hearing-impaired listeners. Clinical investigators have often reported that gap thresholds for hearing-impaired listeners are appreciably greater than those obtained from normal listeners. Gap thresholds for the hearing-impaired may be in the 10- to 20-ms range when measured with k = 1.0 in broadband noise (Formby, personal communication). Other experiments show that gap thresholds increase systematically, for both normal and hearing-impaired listeners, as the bandwidth of the noise is decreased (Fitzgibbons and Wightman, 1982; Fitzgibbons, 1983; Shailer and Moore, 1983; Buus and Florentine, 1985). The gap thresholds found in these experiments are factors of 3 to 5 larger than the typical gap threshold value of 2-3 ms found with most normal observers in broadband noise. We naturally wondered if we could alter the parameters of the computer model to produce data that would simulate such large gap thresholds. The following table shows how the simulated gap threshold changes as the two major parameters of the model are altered. The columns

Table 1. Effect of bandwidth (W) and tau (τ) on simulated gap detection thresholds. Entry is the mean value of a silent gap needed to achieve about 70% correct in an adaptive task. The standard deviation of these estimates is about 17% of the mean.

	Bandwidth (Hz)			
	400	800	1600	3200
Tau(ms)				
1.5	6.20	3.92	2.01	1.31
3.0	6.16	3.76	2.28	1.40
6.0	7.57	4.67	2.73	1.95
12.0	7.62	5.21	3.17	2.55

show the variation in bandwidth and the rows are different time-constant values.

The first thing to note about the table are the relatively small changes in gap threshold caused by alteration of the time-constant value. A change of nearly an order of magnitude in the value of the time-constant increases the gap threshold by only a factor of two, and then only at the largest bandwidth. For the smaller values of bandwidths, which are needed to produce any significant increase in gap threshold, the changes with τ are minuscule. To achieve gap thresholds approaching the measured values of 10 to 20 ms, we would need to assume totally unreasonable parameter values for the model.

We are now exploring how the introduction of internal noise at different stages of the model will alter this situation. At present, we can only say that the model gives reasonably good predictions for normal hearing listeners, but is not particularly useful in interpreting the results obtained from listeners with abnormally large gap thresholds. Indeed, changes in the major temporal parameter of the model, τ, produce surprisingly little variation in the size of the gap threshold.

Acknowledgments

This research was partially supported by grants from the National Science Foundation and the Air Force Office of Scientific Research. We thank Dr. Craig Formby and Dr. Virginia Richards for their comments on earlier versions of this article.

References

Buus, S. and Florentine M. (**1985**). "Gap detection in normal and impaired listeners: the effect of level and frequency," in *Time Resolution in Auditory Systems*, edited by Axel Michelsen (Springer, Berlin), pp. 159-179.

Fitzgibbons, P. J. (**1983**). "Temporal gap detection in noise as a function of frequency, bandwidth, and level," J.Acoust.Soc.Am. **74**, 67-72.

Fitzgibbons, P. J., and Wightman, F. L. (**1983**). "Gap detection in normal and hearing-impaired listeners," J.Acoust.Soc.Am. **72**, 761-765.

Forrest, T. G., and Green, D. M. (**1987**). "Detection of partially filled gaps in noise and the temporal modulation transfer function," J.Acoust.Soc.Am. **82**, 1933-1943.

Green, D. M. (**1985**). "Temporal factors in psychoacoustics," in *Time Resolution in Auditory Systems*, edited by Axel Michelsen (Springer, Berlin), pp. 122-140.

Penner, M. J. (**1977**). "Detection of temporal gaps in noise as a measure of the decay of auditory sensation," J.Acoust.Soc.Am. **61**, 552-557.

Shailer, M. J., and Moore, B. C. J. (**1983**). "Gap detection as a function of frequency, bandwidth, and level," J.Acoust.Soc.Am. **74**, 467-473.

Viemeister, N. F. (**1979**). "Temporal modulation transfer functions based upon modulation thresholds," J.Acoust.Soc.Am. **66**, 1364-1380.

Comments

Patterson:

It is difficult to understand the motivation behind a model of hearing that ignores cochlear filtering and assumes that a wideband signal is passed directly through to the broad lowpass process that determines the MTF. Would it not be better to assume that bandwidth effects are the result of combining the outputs of sets of adjacent auditory filters, and thereby make the model a lot more realistic?

Reply by Green:

I have always believed that the primary test of a theory was its ability to predict the data, not whether the assumed processes mimicked our **current** understanding of how the system functions on a more molecular level. Indeed, it seems to me that the theory or model must be simpler than the process it hopes to explain at least in some respects, otherwise, it achieves no economy of understanding. The present model has only two free parameters (bandwidth and integration time) and predicts with fair accuracy the results of normal-hearing listeners in two experimental situations, see Fig.3 and Fig.4. But, as Table 1 indicates, it does not provide much understanding of hearing-impaired listeners.

For that reason we have been exploring a model much like that described in your comment. That model, a series of parallel, narrow-band channel, raises the issue of how the output of these several independent channels are combined. This is not an issue where more molecular investigations provide much insight. We are presently exploring a number of different decision rules but, as yet, have nothing to report.

Some observations on monaural phase sensitivity

G.B. Henning

Department of Experimental Psychology
Oxford, OX1 3UD, U.K.

Introduction and Discussion

Ronken (1970) measured Observers' ability to discriminate stimuli differing only in their phase spectra; phase discrimination failed when the duration of his signals was less than about 2 ms. Similar experiments have subsequently been reported (Henning and Gaskell, 1981) in which Observers were able to discriminate between stimuli of equal energy but different phase spectra when the signals were less than 200 μs in duration.

In the latter experiment, Observers were required to discriminate between two stimuli, one of which, a(t), consisted of a 20-μs pulse of unit amplitude (the standard pulse), followed, after a delay of D seconds, by a second pulse of amplitude k. The other stimulus, b(t), comprised the same pair of pulses in reverse order (Fig. 1).

The waveforms to be discriminated, Ronken's stimuli, differ only in their phase spectra:

$$\phi_a(t) = \arctan\,[-k \sin \omega D/(1 + k \cos \omega D)], \qquad (1a)$$

$$\phi_b(t) = \arctan\,[-\sin \omega D/(k + \cos \omega D)]. \qquad (1b)$$

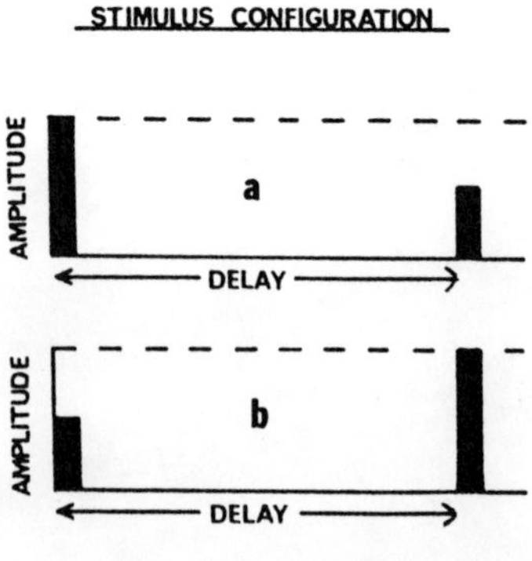

Figures 1a and 1b show the stimuli between which the Observers were required to discriminate in a 2-AFC task. Amplitude is plotted as a function of time in both figures and the vertical black bars represent the 20-μs clicks.

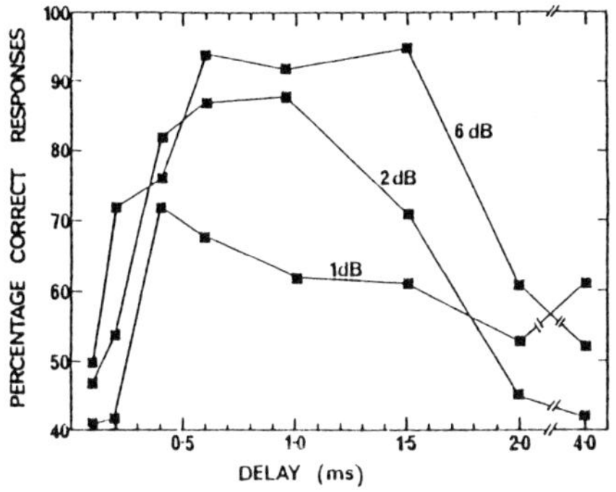

Figure 2. The percentage of "correct" discriminations as a function of the delay, D, between the onsets of the pulses. The parameter is the amplitude of the attenuated pulse relative to that of the standard pulse. Each data point is based on 100 observations from Observer GBH.

The common power spectrum $S(\omega)$ is given by,

$$S(\omega) = (1 + k^2 + 2k \cos \omega D). \tag{2}$$

The results for one of the three Observers in that experiment are shown in Fig. 2. The percentage of "correct" responses from a standard two- alternative forced-choice discrimination experiment is shown as a function of the delay D in milliseconds. Since the cue (or cues) used by the Observers was chosen arbitrarily by them, deviations of more than 10 percentage points from 50% "correct" responses were arbitrarily plotted as greater than 50% correct.

Three different relative amplitudes of the pulses were used: 6 dB, 2 dB and 1 dB below the 30 dB Sensation Level of the standard pulse. In the 6-dB condition the range of delays for reliable discrimination was 200 μs to 2.0 ms, for the 2-dB case 400 μs to 1.5 ms, and for the 1-dB case also from 400 μs to 1.5 ms. In the middle range of delays the results are as might be expected in that performance is better the greater the amplitude difference between the pulses.

The cue that the Observers reported using when the delays were large was "doubleness"; the signal in which the second pulse was larger was frequently reported to sound more "double" than that in which the larger pulse occurred first. With moderate delays, the Observers reported that one stimulus sounded like "tick" and the other like "tock". There was no agreement, however, on which stimulus produced which sensation. At short delays, the stimuli sounded like different allophones of the consonant /t/.

There appear to be three possible explanations based on the properties of the stimuli; only one of them relies explicitly on the extraction of phase info rmation.

A. Running spectrum

The running spectrum, $S_t(\omega)$, of a stimulus, s(t), is defined as

$$S_t(\omega) = \int_{-\infty}^{t} s(\tau) \exp(-j\omega\tau)\, d\tau \,. \tag{3}$$

If the Fourier transform of the stimulus is denoted by $S(\omega)$ then the spectrum and the running spectrum are conveniently related by

$$S_t(\omega) = (2\pi)^{-\frac{1}{2}} S(\omega) * [(\pi\ \delta(\omega) - 1/j\omega) \exp(j\omega t)], \tag{4}$$

where the asterisk represents convolution (Papoulis, 1962). With Ronken's stimuli, the spectrum, $S(\omega)$, and the running spectrum, $S_t(\omega)$, are identical when t is less than zero or greater than the delay, D, plus the duration of the earphone response to the second pulse, denoted T. Since the amplitude spectra of the waveforms to be discriminated are identical, it follows that discrimination on the basis of a running amplitude spectrum is only possible if the spectrum is measured (sampled) some time after the onset of the stimuli but before they end; that is when t is greater than zero but less than D+T.

It is easiest to use Eq. (3) to calculate the running spectra of the stimuli. For stimulus a, then, the running spectrum is given by

$$S_{at}(\omega) = \begin{cases} 0, & t<0, \\ \int_0^t p(t)e^{-j\omega t}dt, & 0 \le t < T, \\ A(\omega)\exp[j\phi(\omega)], & T \le t < D, \end{cases} \tag{5}$$

where $A(\omega)$ and $\phi(\omega)$ are the magnitude and phase of the impulse response of the earphones, respectively. When $D+T \le t$ the running spectra are given by Eqs. (1) and (2). For the three ranges of t in Eq. (5), the running spectrum of the stimuli are identical except for the real attention constant k. Thus any device capable of calculating a running spectrum and of terminating its calculation before D seconds elapse is capable of making the discrimination on the basis of amplitude differences alone: indeed, such a device operating with $t<D$ must use amplitude differences since they are the only differences in the running spectra of the stimulus in that range of t.

B. Duration discrimination

A second class of explanation requires that the Observer calculate some moment of the stimuli to be discriminated and to base his decision on that. The second moment about some suitably chosen point is proportional to the rms duration, Du, and is given by

$$Du^2 = \int_{-\infty}^{\infty} t^2\, |f^2(t)|\, dt. \tag{6}$$

Papoulis (1962) has shown that Du is related to the amplitude spectrum, $A(\omega)$, and the phase spectrum, $\phi(\omega)$, of f(t) by

$$Du^2 = (2\pi)^{-\frac{1}{2}} \int_{-\infty}^{\infty} ([dA(\omega)/d\omega]^2 + A^2(\omega)[d\phi(\omega)/d\omega]^2)\, d\omega. \qquad (7)$$

From Eq. (7), it is readily seen that waveforms with identical amplitude spectra but which differ in their phase spectra may also differ in their duration. Further, the differences in duration are not very different from those that are known to be discriminable from simple duration discrimination experiments (Small and Campbell, 1962; Creelman, 1962).

Inspection of Eq.7. reveals a simple way of testing the notion that Observers use differences in duration to make the discrimination; duration, Du, depends on the magnitude but not the sign of the slope of the phase spectrum, $d\phi(\omega)/d\omega$. Thus waveforms with identical amplitude spectra that have changes in their phase spectra of the same size but different sign have the same duration. Such stimuli were constructed in order to determine whether discrimination between stimili with identical power spectra *and* identical duration, Du, were still possible.

Method

The stimili consisted of the impulse responses of three different digital filters. All three had the same power spectrum - a flat band 180-Hz wide centred on 1-kHz. The phase response of two of the filters was adjusted to produce fixed phase change for 120 Hertz centred on 1000 Hertz. For one of the filters a phase advance was used and for the other, a phase delay. The Observer was required first to discriminate between the impulse response of the phase-delayed filter and the standard impulse, then in a separate experiment between that equal duration impulse responses of the phase-advanced and the phase-delayed filters. A standard two-alternative forced-choice discrimination experiment was used with a 600-ms delay between the first and second observation intervals.

Either 1024 or 2048 point signals were digitally generated and windowed using techniques described in Henning (1983). The signals were read out simultaneously through 16 bit digital-to-analogue converters at a rate of 50 kHertz (Hafter and Lones, 1981) and delivered over TDH-39 earphones (driven in phase). Trials were run in blocks of 50 and each data point is based on 100 observation from one Observer (the author). A continous background of broad-band white Gaussian noise of O-dB Spectrum Level was used.

Discrimination performance was measured as a function of the ratio-signal energy to noise-power density (E_s/N_0) for four different phase shifts.

Results

Figures 3a - 3d show the percentage correct discrimination as a function of the ratio (dB) of signal energy to noise-power density for phase changes of four different sizes. The crucial comparision is shown by the filled circles.

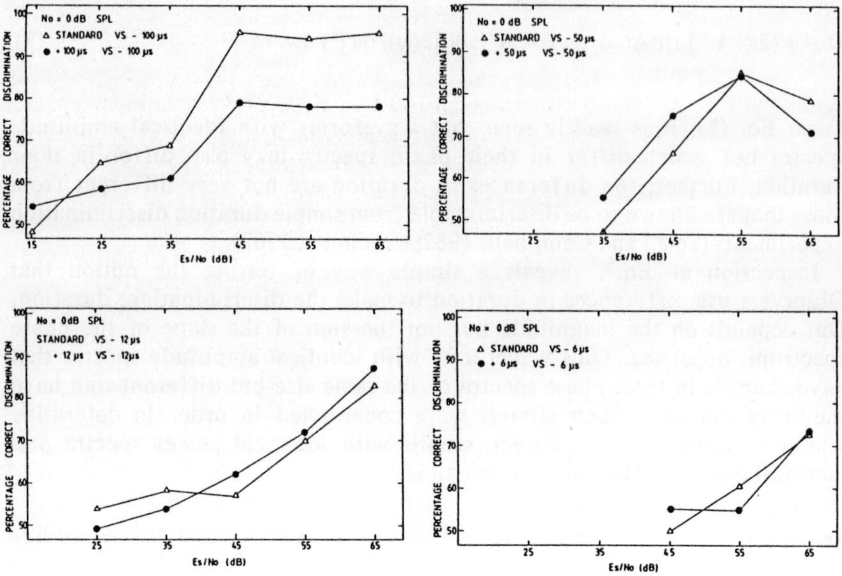

Figures 3a–3d show the percentage of correct discrimination as a function of the ratio of signal energy to noise-power density. The open triangles in each Fig show discrimination between the impulse response of the standard 180-Hz wide filter centered on 1000 Hz and the impulse response of the same filter having a 120-Hz central region with a fixed phase delay. The filled circles show discrimination between the impulse response produced by the 120-Hz wide phase delay and an advance of the same size. The temporal change corresponding to the phase shift at the 1-kHz centre frequency was 100 µs in Fig 3a; 50 µs in Fig 3b; 12 µs in Fig 3c and 6 µs in Fig 3d.

Because the waveforms being discriminated in this case have phase changes of the same size but different sign, they have identical durations, Du, as well as identical power spectra. Since discrimination is still possible in these cases, it is clear that there in some basis for the discrimination of Ronken's stimuli beyond mere differences in duration.

Discussion (cont'd)

It seems unlikely that Observers should be able to create observation intervals as short as 200 microseconds. The resultant critical bandwidths would be very much larger than the largest estimates so far obtained. Further, any such extensive widening should produce an order of magnitude loss in detectability. It is in fact the case that a signal level at least 20 dB above masked thresholds is required before discrimination is measurably different from chance, but the signals are clearly heard, even when they can't be discriminated. If signals from the critical bands were subsequently combined, however, the very short power-specturm measurement could not be excluded because wide band information needed for the discrimination would produce about the amount of noise masking measured.

On the other hand, the fact that the Observer can discriminate between signals of equal duration precludes differences in duration between the stimuli being the cue they use

C. True phase sensitivity

The two mechanisms considered so far allow Observers to discriminate the waveforms but, although both depend on phase differences, neither relies specifically on the determination of phase difference; that is, neither mechanism is directly sensitive to the differences in the time at which energy arrives in different (probably adjacent) frequency bands, and it is entirely possible that Observers are indeed sensitive to these differences as Patterson and Green (1970) and Green (1971) have suggested. If so, we are very sensitive to these monaural phase cues - almost as sensitive as we are to the interaural phase differences that lead to changes in the apparent location of sound sources.

This is apparent in Fig.4 which allows monaural and binaural phase sensitivity to be compared.

Monaural phase discrimination was measured for the impulse responses of three different filters at 65 dB E_s/N_0. The method was exactly as in the previous experiments. For comparison (the dashed line), a 2-AFC lateralization experiment was performed using the impulse response from the phase advanced filter for one ear and the phase delayed impulse response for the other. Waveforms were interchanged between observation interval and the Observer reported which interval contained the leftmost sound.

Lateralization performance based on binaural differences is only a factor of two better than monaural discrimination.

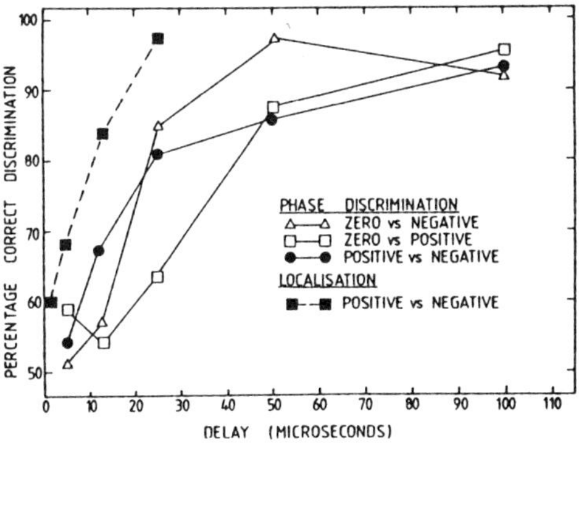

Figure 4 shows percentage correct discrimination as a function of the phase shift (measured as the equivalent delay at the 1-kHz centre frequency) obtained at 65 dB E_s/N_0. The solid lines connect data for monaural discrimination, the dashed line shows 2-AFC lateralization results.

Whatever the underlying explanation of monaural phase sensitivity, the fact that Observers are sensitive to manipulations of phase within such short time periods suggests that we should not neglect to look for cues Observers use in processing complex signals in the potentially important short term phase spectra of the signals.

References

Creelman, C.D. (**1962**). "Human discriminations of auditory duration," J. Acoust.Soc.Am. **34**, 582-593.

Feth, L.L. and O'Malley, H. (**1977**). "Influences of temporal masking on click-pair discriminability," Perc.Psychophys. **22**, 497-505.

Green, D.M. (**1971**). "Temporal auditory acuity," Psychol.Rev. **78**, 540-551.

Hafter, E.R. and Lones, S. (**1981**). Their design.

Henning, G.B. and Gaskell, H. (**1981**). "Monaural phase sensitivity with Ronken's paradigm," J.Acoust.Soc.Am. **70**, 1669-1673.

Henning, G.B. (**1983**). "Lateralization of low-frequency transients," Hearing Res. **9**, 153-172.

Papoulis, A. (**1962**). *The Fourier Integral and its Applications*. (McGraw Hill, New York).

Patterson, J.H. and Green, D.M. (**1970**). "Discrimination of transient signals having identical energy spectra," J.Acoust.Soc.Am. **48**, 894-905.

Ronken, D. (**1970**). "Monaural detection of a phase difference between clicks," J.Acoust.Soc.Am. **47**, 1091-1099.

Small, A.M., Jr. and Campbell, R.A. (**1962**). "Temporal differential sensitivity for auditory stimuli," Am.J.Psychol. **75**, 401-410.

Masking patterns of harmonic complex tone maskers and the role of the inner ear transfer function

Armin Kohlrausch

Drittes Physikalisches Institut, Universität Göttingen, Bürgerstr. 42-44, D-3400 Göttingen, Federal Republic of Germany

Introduction

Masking experiments are a common psychoacoustic technique to investigate signal processing in the human hearing system. On the basis of such experiments the concept of an internal filter evolved within the last 40 years. The shape of this internal filter reflects the interaction between spectral components of the masking signal and the test stimulus. Masker components close in frequency to the test-signal frequency have a stronger impact on the detection threshold than those further away. A primary source for this spectral interaction is found in the excitation pattern generated by the traveling wave propagation on the basilar membrane. It is expressed quantitatively by an attenuation characteristic, the "auditory filter" (e.g., Patterson, 1976).

As long as noise maskers are used, only the amplitude characteristic of the auditory filter can be estimated from the measured detection thresholds. To study the influence of the frequency-specific phase chracteristic, it is necessary to employ maskers with well defined phase spectra. A possible way is the use of harmonic complex tones. By varying the component phases of a harmonic complex, it is possible to generate very different time signals even for constant amplitude spectra. In a recent publication (Smith *et al.*, 1986), we describe thresholds for stationary test signals masked by harmonic complex maskers. We found threshold differences of up to 20 dB for maskers with identical amplitude spectra and identical temporal envelopes. These threshold differences could be explained by calculating the masker's envelope on the basilar membrane using a one-dimensional, linear basilar membrane model (Strube, 1985). Owing to the model's phase-dispersive properties, the maskers have very different envelopes at the output of the inner ear filter.

The experiments of the present study were performed in order to get additional evidence for the role of the (complex) transfer function of the inner ear in masking experiments. We applied the same type of masker as in our previous study and measured, for three different phase choices, the masked thresholds of stationary test signals (experiment 1) and masking period patterns of a 5 ms test signal pulse, added with variable delay to the masker (experiment 2). The experimental data are compared with calculated temporal envelopes of the maskers on the basilar membrane.

Signal generation

The masking signals used in the experiments consisted of equal amplitude sinusoids of common fundamental f_0:

$$m(t) = \sum_{n=n1}^{n2} \sin(2\pi n f_0 t + \theta_n). \tag{1}$$

n1 and n2 were chosen to restrict the spectrum to the range 200 to 2000 Hz. The starting phases θ_n of the masker components were either set to zero, resulting in a periodic pulse sequence (called "sine phase" in the following) or according to a formula given by Schroeder (1970):

$$\theta_n = -\pi n(n+1)/N \tag{2}$$

where N=n2-n1+1 (called "Schroeder phases"). This formula was developed to reduce the peak factor of the resulting time signal and can be used with both a "-" sign (as in Eq. (2)) and a "+" sign. In Fig.1, we have depicted the time

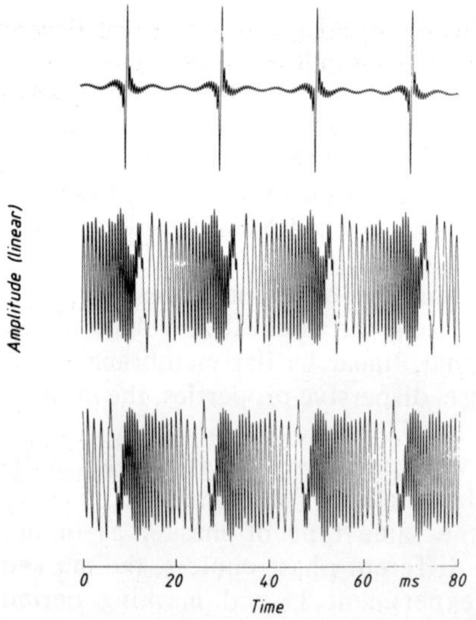

Figure 1. Time functions of harmonic complex signals for three different choices of the component starting phases. Top: $\theta_n=0$ (sine-phase signal), middle: $\theta_n=-\pi n(n+1)/N$ (up chirp), bottom: $\theta_n=+\pi n(n+1)/N$ (down chirp). All signals are composed of the equal amplitude harmonics 4 to 40 of the fundamental frequency 50 Hz. The amplitude of the sine-phase signal is scaled down by 10 dB in comparison to the two Schroeder-phase signals.

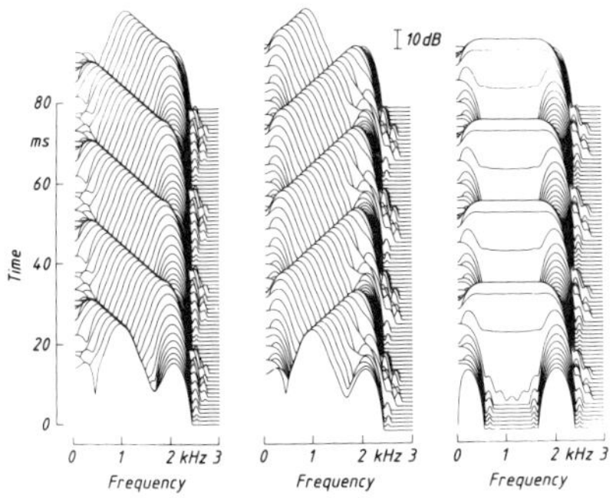

Figure 2. Short-time spectral analysis using 5-ms Hanning windows for the three signals shown in Fig.1. Left: down chirp, middle: up chirp, right: sine-phase signal.

signals for the three different sets of starting phases. In this figure the amplitudes for the sine-phase signal are reduced by 10 dB in comparison to the Schroeder-phase signals. The middle panel in Fig.1 shows the signal according to the "-" sign in Eq. (2) (called "up chirp" due to the increase of the instantaneous frequency within each period) and the lower panel represents the Schroeder-phase signal with a "+" sign ("down chirp"). In Fig.2 we demonstrate the course of the instantaneous frequency by means of short-time spectra. The chirp characteristic is more pronounced in this presentation. In addition, the short-time spectra of the sine-phase signal emphasize that the spectral edges of the complex continue during the minima of the envelope of the time signal! These edge frequencies give rise to a pitch sensation which can be heard for fundamental frequencies up to about 200 Hz. This pitch is not apparent for the Schroeder-phase signals.

Threshold estimation procedure

Masked thresholds were determined using an adaptive 3-Interval Forced Choice procedure. The 320-ms masker was presented in three successive intervals separated by 200-ms breaks. In one randomly chosen interval, the test signal (1100-Hz center frequency) was added to the masker. In experiment 1, the test signal was centered with respect to the masker interval and had a duration of 260 ms including 30-ms raised cosine ramps. In experiment 2, the test-signal pulse (5-ms Hanning envelope) was added with a specific onset time difference t_v to the masker. In both experiments, the subject had to specify the interval containing the test signal. The test-signal level was varied adaptively during the experiment according to a two-down-one-up procedure. After two successive correct responses, the signal level was decreased by 1 dB, after each incorrect response it was increased by the same amount. During the starting period of each measurement, a greater step size was used that was progressively reduced to 1 dB. The threshold value was determined by taking the median probe level of the 20 trials that followed the starting phase (Kollmeier *et al.*, 1988).

For each subject this procedure was repeated at least four times and the median was taken for further calculations. The experiments were controlled

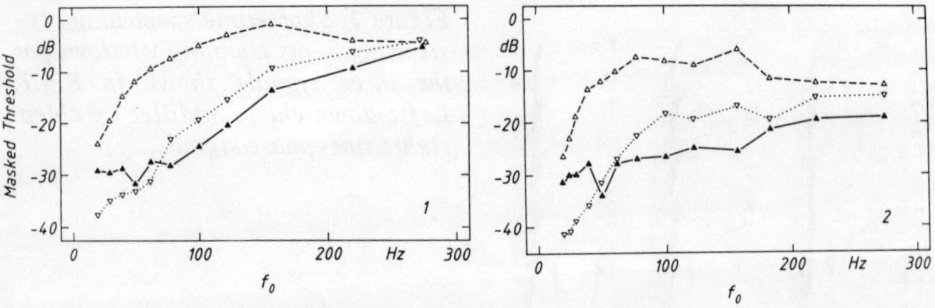

Figure 3. Simultaneous masked thresholds of a 260-ms, 1100-Hz signal in dependence on the fundamental frequency of the harmonic complex masker. Threshold levels are expressed relative to the level of a single masker component. Open triangles: up-chirp masker, filled triangles: down-chirp masker, inverted triangles: sine-phase masker. Results for subject 1 and 2.

by computer (Gould Concept 32/9705) which also generated the stimuli. They were converted to analog signals by means of a 12-bit D/A-converter (sampling rate 20 kHz), low pass filtered at 5 kHz and presented diotically to the listener via headphone (Beyer DT880 monitor with diffuse field equalizer). Three normal hearing subjects aged between 25 and 33 years participated in the experiments.

Experimental results

Experiment 1: Stationary test signal

In the first experiment we measured the simultaneous masked threshold of a stationary (260 ms) test signal, which was always added in phase to the 1100-Hz component of the masker. Experimental parameters were the different phase choices and the fundamental frequency of the masker. The latter was varied between 20 and 275 Hz, giving a masker period between 3.6 and 50 ms.

The results for two subjects are presented in Fig.3. Masked threshold values are expressed relative to the level of the 1100-Hz masker component. As the overall level of the masker was held constant at about 75 dB SPL for all values of f_0, the level of a single masker component decreases by 3 dB (due to the increase of harmonics in the complex) as f_0 decreases by an octave. The three different symbols correspond to the different phase choices, open and closed (upright) triangles denote the two Schroeder-phase maskers and the inverted triangles the sine-phase masker.

As already known from our previous study (Smith *et al.*, 1986), the threshold values for the two Schroeder-phase maskers differ by more than 20 dB in the medium range of f_0. This difference reveals the fact that the linear-FM characteristics of the two maskers (cf. Fig.2) interact in an opposite way with the phase characteristic of the basilar-membrane filter. The down-chirp masker is transformed into a pulse-like signal with an energy concentration within a short epoch and a long part with low envelope values. In contrast, the up-chirp masker retains its flat temporal envelope even on the basilar membrane. With the assumption that the minima of the masker envelope determine the masked thresholds of the stationary test signal, the differences between the two maskers can be explained qualitatively (cf. Smith *et al.*, 1986). This interpretation is supported by the results for the sine-phase masker (inverted triangles in Fig.3). The phases of this masker are adjusted to give a maximal modulation of the temporal envelope of the acoustic input. Therefore, without further phase changes, this masker should have the lowest masked thresholds according to our assumption. The comparison with the thresholds for the down-chirp masker reveals that this is only true in the lowest range of fundamental frequencies. In the medium range of f_0, the thresholds for the sine-phase masker are higher by up to 6 dB compared to the down chirp. In this region of fundamental frequencies and sweep rates, the quadratic phase choice of the down-chirp masker components appears to be cancelled in a near optimal way by the phase transformation of the basilar membrane filter.

Experiment 2: Masking period patterns of a short test-signal pulse

In the second experiment, we used a 5-ms pulse with center frequency 1100 Hz as test signal. The pulse always was added in phase to the 1100-Hz masker component and was presented at different moments within the masker period in order to measure the temporal course of the masker excitation in the spectral region of 1100 Hz. Masked thresholds were measured for three different fundamental frequencies of the masker (25, 100 and 220 Hz) and the three phase choices used in experiment 1. The data points in Figs.4-6 are the median values of 12 threshold extimates (four repetitions for each of the three observers). Typical interquartile values are in the order 2 to 3 dB. The time axis in the figures always covers one period of the masker and denotes the probe onset time relative to the masker onset.

At the highest fundamental frequency (Fig.4), the masking period patterns are very even. This is a consequence of the short masker period (4.5 ms) which is of the same magnitude as the test signal duration (5 ms). Due to the large frequency separation between adjacent masker components (220 Hz), only very few components are effective at the test-signal frequency. Therefore, the relative phases of these components are of minor importance and the different maskers lead to similar threshold values.

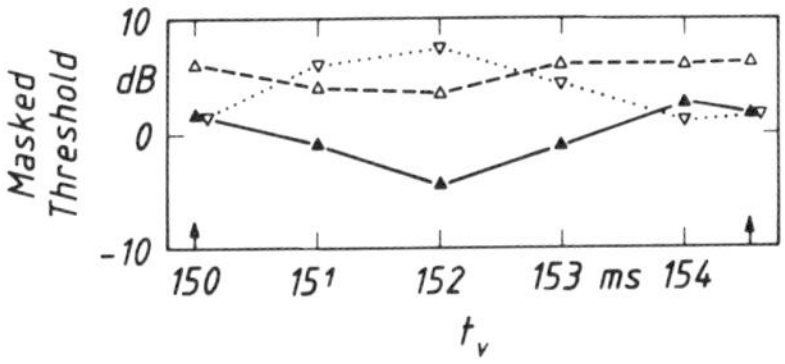

Figure 4. Masked thresholds of a 5-ms test signal (relative to the level of a single masker component) as a function of the onset time difference t_v between masker and test signal. Same symbols as in Fig.3. The arrows mark the duration of the masker's period. Fundamental frequency 220 Hz.

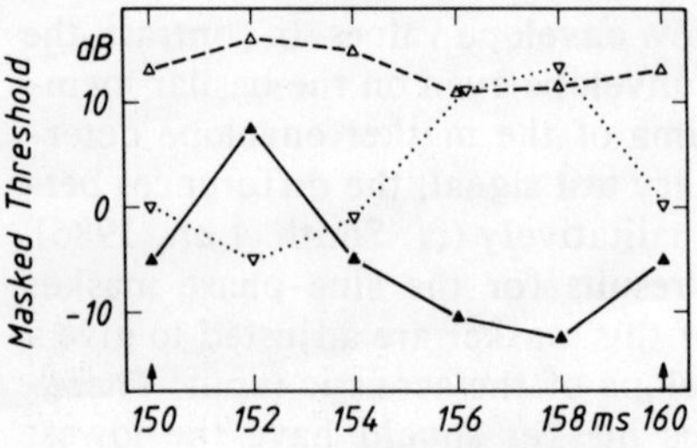

Figure 5. As Fig.4 for a fundamental frequency of 100 Hz.

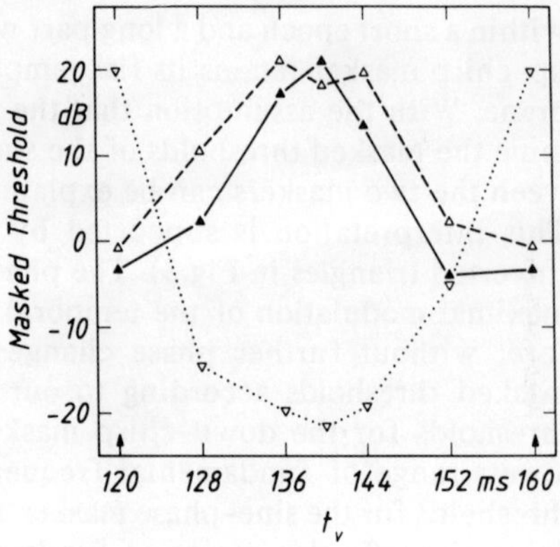

Figure 6. As Fig.4 for a fundamental frequency of 25 Hz.

The differences between the three maskers become more pronounced at 100-Hz fundamental frequency (Fig.5). Comparison of up and down chirps (open and closed triangles) reveals a difference of 20 dB for the minimum of the masking period pattern. This difference has the same amount as the threshold differences found for a stationary test signal (Fig.3) and confirms the correlation between masked thresholds for stationary signals and the minima of masking period patterns. In addition, Fig.5 reveals that the minimum of the

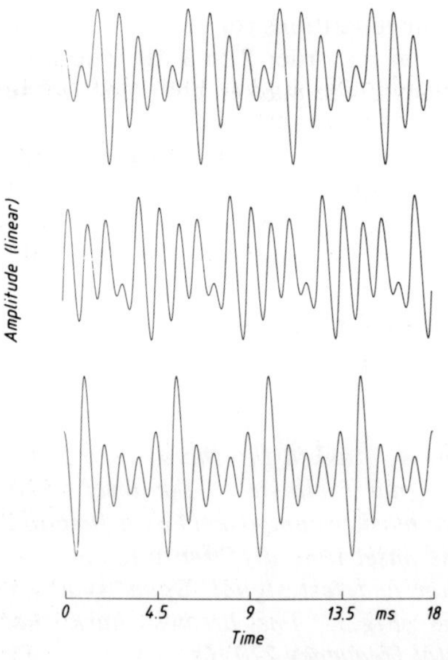

Figure 7. Responses of the basilar-membrane model at resonance frequency 1100 Hz to the sine-phase masker (above), up chirp (middle) and down chirp (bottom). All output functions are shown on the same linear scale. Fundamental frequency 220 Hz.

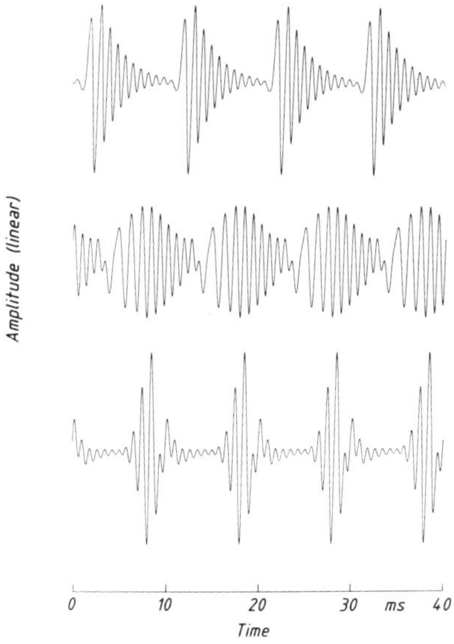

Figure 8. As Fig.7 for a fundamental frequency of 100 Hz.

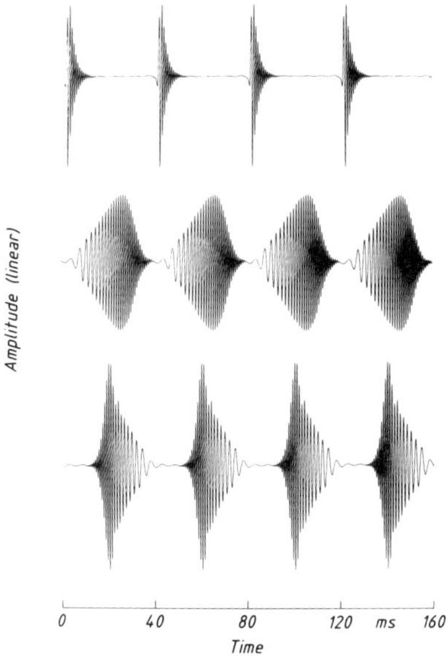

Figure 9. As Fig.7 for a fundamental frequency of 25 Hz, but the output function for the sine-phase masker (upper panel) scaled down by a factor two relative to the Schroeder-phase signals.

pattern for the sine phase masker is considerably higher than that for the down chirp, as we expected from the results of experiment 1.

At the lowest fundamental frequency (Fig.6), the patterns for all maskers are highly modulated. The patterns of the two Schroeder-phase signals are similar in shape and overall value, indicating that sweep direction becomes less important at this fundamental frequency. The sine phase masker produces threshold variations of up to 40 dB for onset-time changes of only 20 ms and resembles very much the envelope of the input signal (cf. Fig.1).

Model calculations

For our model calculations, we used a digitally realized linear cochlea model (Strube, 1985). In this model, the cochlea is treated as a one-dimensional nonuniform transmission line, composed of 120 segments. The filter output is proportional to the model basilar-membrane velocity.

We first gauged the model by determining the segment most sensitive to our 1100-Hz test signal pulse. Subsequently we calculated the output of this segment for the various maskers used in experiment 2. In the following figures, the upper panel always represents the sine-phase masker, below we show the up and the down chirp. Within each figure, the same linear scale is used for the three maskers.

Figure 7 reveals that the output functions for the highest fundamental frequency (220 Hz) are weakly modulated and very similar. This corresponds well to the result of the experiments. At 100 Hz fundamental frequency (Fig.8) the differences between the two Schroeder-phase signals are more pronounced. The valley in the envelope of the down-chirp masker (lower panel) is even more distinct than the valley in the sine-phase signal. This indicates that due to the phase dispersion of the basilar-membrane model the envelope of the down-chirp signal becomes very modulated in the inner ear. For the up chirp, the effect is opposite and the envelope remains nearly constant, resulting in the high masked thresholds for this masker. The functions calculated for the lowest fundamental frequency (Fig.9) show large envelope variations within each period for all maskers corresponding to the experimental results. The duration of the envelope minimum, however, is considerably smaller for the Schroeder-phase signals than for the sine-phase signal. Therefore the detection of a signal presented at the minimum of the masker's excitation is more difficult for the two chirp maskers. This comparison of calculated masker envelopes and masking period patterns shows a close correspondance. We take this result as a confirmation of the phase and amplitude characteristics of the linear basilar-membrane model, at least for the relatively high sensation levels of our experiments. Therefore, in detailed models of temporal aspects in hearing as masking period patterns and forward masking, the basilar-membrane filtered time function of the masking signal should be taken as input for further calculation in order to test the role of higher stages in our hearing system.

References

Kollmeier, B., Gilkey, R.H., and Sieben, U. (**1988**). "Adaptive staircase techniques in psychoacoustics: A comparison of human data and a mathematical model," J.Acoust.Soc.Am. (in press).

Patterson, R.D. (**1976**). "Auditory filter shapes derived with noise stimuli," J. Acoust.Soc.Am. **59**, 640-654.

Schroeder, M.R. (**1970**). "Synthesis of low-peak-factor signals and binary sequences with low autocorrelation," IEEE Trans Inf. Theory **16**, 85-89.

Smith, B.K., Sieben, U.K., Kohlrausch, A., and Schroeder, M.R. (**1986**). "Phase effects in masking related to dispersion in the inner ear," J.Acoust Soc.Am. **80**, 1631-1637.

Strube, H.W. (**1985**). "A computationally efficient basilar-membrane model," Acustica **58**, 207-214.

Comments

Moore:

Your model of the cochlea shows less frequency selectivity than observed psychophysically. For example, your figure 7 shows responses of the model for a resonance frequency corresponding to the fifth harmonic of 220 Hz. The complex waveforms indicate a high degree of interaction between harmonics. However, the auditory filter bandwidth at 1100 Hz is considerably less than 220 Hz (about 140 Hz), so the fifth harmonic should be quite well resolved.

Reply by Kohlrausch:

The observation of Moore is correct that the transfer function of the basilar-membrane filter is wider than the corresponding filter shapes derived from psychoacoustic masking experiments. This can be seen directly in Fig. 5 of the original paper by Strube (1985), where log-amplitude and phase resonance curves for the velocity at a fixed point of the basilar membrane are shown. The implicit conclusion of the comment, however, that there would be no modulation at the output of an appropriate auditory filter is not correct. Using the attenuation characteristic of the rounded-exponential filter (Patterson *et al.*, 1982) for a center frequency of 1100 Hz, I calculated the filter output for the masker with fundamental frequency 220 Hz by adding the 5 most prominent masker components (660, 880, 1100, 1320 and 1540 Hz) with relative amplitudes of -33, -14, 0, -14 and -33 dB in zero phase. The left figure shows two periods (9.1 ms) of the calculated time function. It is obvious that there is some interaction between the masker components even for this auditory filter. An even higher degree of modulation can be seen, if the center frequency of the filter is shifted to 990 Hz, just in between two harmonics of the masker. This is shown in the right figure, where the components 660, 880, 1100 and 1320 Hz are added with relative amplitudes -23.3, -5.4, -5.4 and -23.3 dB. Additional evidence for an interaction between the masker components comes from the psychoacoustic experiments. As well for the stationary test signal (Fig. 3) as for the pulsed test signal (Fig. 4) there is an influence of the relative phases of the masker components on the masked

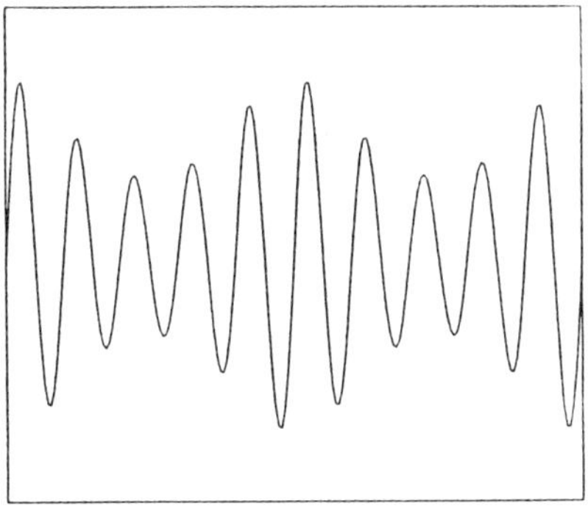

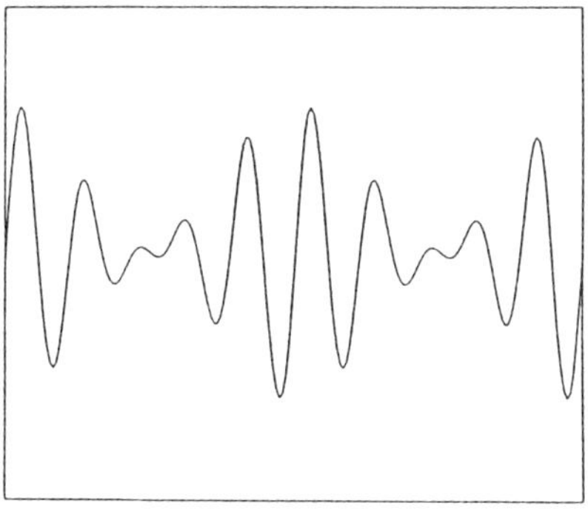

thresholds for f_0 = 220 Hz. In addition, the dependence of the threshold on the temporal position of the pulsed test signal indicates some changes in the masker's envelope during each period, because the test signal is always added in phase to the 1100-Hz component of the masker. Due to large separation of the masker components, however, this interaction is much smaller than at the other fundamental frequencies used in the experiments.

Patterson, R.D., Nimmo-Smith, I., Weber, D.L. and Milroy, R. (1982). "The deterioration of hearing with age: Frequency selectivity, the critical ratio, the audiogram, and speech threshold", J.Acoust.Soc.Am. 72, 1788-1803.

Rebuttal by Moore:

I did not mean to imply that there would be *no* modulation at the output of an auditory filter centered at the filter harmonic, only that there would be less modulation than shown in your Fig.7. The quantitative predictions of your model will obviously depend on the degree of frequency selectivity assumed, and it seems to me that you have assumed frequency selectivity poorer than observed in man.

Moore:

If discrimination of the fundamental frequency of complex tones depends partly on temporal processing, then differences might be expected between up chirps and down chirps of the type described in your paper. We have compared the DLs for fundamental frequency of our subjects for up chirps and down chirps. Fundamental frequencies of 100 and 200 Hz were used. For both the normal and impaired ears there were only small differences between the two types of signals. For the normal ears this is not suprising, since, for them, discrimination of the fundamental frequency of complex tones probably depends primarily on information from the lower harmonics, where interaction of the components would be weak. However, the lack of a difference is somewhat surprising for the impaired subjects, since, for them even the lower harmonics would interact strongly in the peripheral auditory system. It is possible that the phase characteristics of the basilar membrane in impaired ears is different from normal. This could lead to waveforms on the basilar membrane with peak factors which are not consistently greater for down chirps than for up chirps.

Zwicker:

Assuming that somebody produces a 2-ms, 1500 Hz tone burst with rise/fall time of 1 ms and repeats it every 10 seconds, listeners call that a sequence of single tone pips in silence. Somebody else changes the frequency of a tone generator within 10 seconds from 1000 to 2000 Hz; listeners call that a tone with rising pitch. A third person turns on a digital noise generator attached to an octave filter with a passband from 1000 to 2000 Hz; listeners call this a continuous noise. No one of the listeners would call one of the three sounds a harmonic complex tone, although all three sounds can be produced by 10.000 lines of almost equal level (with a frequency separation of 0.1 Hz between 1 and 2 kHz) and different, but proper phase. The description of the stimuli by the listeners indicates how the ear analyses the stimuli. The expression "harmonic complex tones" describes the way of production in the computer and can therefore, be misleading in hearing research if ear-characteristics have to be encovered.

A sinusoidally frequency modulated 1500-Hz tone ($\Delta f = \pm$ 700 Hz; f_{mod} = 32 Hz) produces a spectrum not very different from that of an upward saw-tooth frequency modulation (see Fig.C2). Using such frequencies of modulation sensations correlated to the temporal as well as to spectral resolution are produced.

Therefore, masking-period patterns as described elsewhere (Zwicker, 1974a,b; Kemp, 1982) may be an adequate description of the masking effects illustrating the transition from pure temporal resolution at low, to pure spectral resolution at high modulation frequencies. Such masking-period patterns produced by sinusoidally frequency modulated tones show very clearly the different masking effect of rising in contrast to decreasing frequency movements of the masker. This effect may be produced not only by the frequency selectivity of the cochlear partition but also by the difference of pre- and post-stimulus masking.

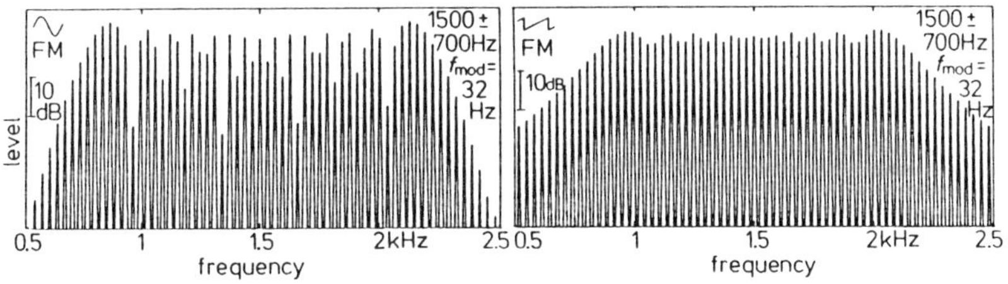

Figure C2. Spectra of sinusoidal and saw-tooth like frequency modulated 1500-Hz tones

Kemp, S. (1982). "Masking period patterns of frequency modulated tones of different frequency deviations", Acustica *50*, 63-69.

Zwicker, E. (1974a). "Loudness and excitation patterns of strongly frequency modulated tones", In: Sensation and Measurement, papers in honor of S.S. Stevens, D. Reidel Publishing Comp., Dordrecht, Holland, 325-335.

Zwicker, E. (1974b). "Mithörschwellen und Erregungsmuster stark frequenzmodulierter Töne", Acustica *31*, 243-256.

Reply by Kohlrausch:

I think there is no doubt among psychoacousticians that the three sound examples described (and produced) by Zwicker should be described as separated tone pulses, as a tone with a rising pitch or as broadband noise rather than by a line spectrum with spacing 0.1 Hz. However, for periodic signals within the range of fundamental frequencies I used it is not a priori clear which perceptual attribute is most important in the experiment (and it possibly changes with the task) and therefore, one should give to the reader as much information about the signals as possible such as exact mathematical definition, time function and short time spectra.

The references given by Zwicker may be looked upon as a good example for a limited view on the signal's properties. In all three papers the asymmetry between upward and downward frequency modulation (FM) was observed for sinusoidally FM maskers. However, none of the papers discusses the possible influence of phase dispersion in the inner ear in these experiments, just because phase spectra are usually not described for sinusoidally frequency modulated signals.

The "explanation" for the asymmetry given in the last sentence of the comment was already mentioned by Zwicker (1974a). S. Kemp (1982), a later coworker of Zwicker in this field, ended his discussion of the effect with the statement: "...it is difficult to see how differences as large as 15 dB between the two peaks in the masking period patterns .... could arise from such considerations" (i.e., forward and backward masking). Therefore, a different view on old unresolved problems may at least sometimes lead to a better explanation for the outcome of the experiments.

Schroeder:

The question is not, I submit, what to *call* Kohlrausch's stimuli but whether they can teach us something about hearing.

Timbre cues in monaural phase perception: distinguishing within-channel cues and between-channel cues

Roy D. Patterson

MRC Applied Psychology Unit
15 Chaucer Road, Cambridge, England

Introduction

Recently, Patterson (1987a) proposed a model of peripheral auditory processing which suggested that global changes in the phase spectrum of a sound would cause timbre changes, in certain circumstances. Global phase changes shift the output of one auditory filter relative to another in time, and previously these shifts were not thought to be audible (de Boer, 1976). To test the hypothesis, Patterson (1987b) presented listeners with a filtered pulse train containing 31 equal-amplitude harmonics, all in cosine phase. Then he introduced a global phase change and increased its magnitude while checking for timbre changes. The experiments revealed that sensitivity to global phase changes existed over a wide range of stimulus conditions.

In fact, it is not actually possible to generate a global phase change without introducing at least a small, local phase change. Local phase changes alter the envelope of the output of the auditory filter in which they occur, and they are known to cause timbre changes when sufficiently large (Mathes and Miller, 1947). The current paper presents a pair of experiments designed to distinguish local and global phase sensitivity, and in so doing, to provide further evidence for global phase sensitivity.

The role of phase in timbre perception

The timbre experiments reported by Patterson (1987b) were performed with local as well as global phase changes. The operation of the model is illustrated in Fig. 1 using a sound (Fig. 1a) with local phase changes that are just audible when the fundamental is 125 Hz and the stimulus level is about 40 dB/component (dB/c). In this case, the odd harmonics are all in cosine phase and the even harmonics are all shifted 40 degrees from cosine phase. This is referred to as an alternating-phase, or APH, wave and the filtered pulse train is referred to as a cosine-phase, or CPH, wave.

In the first stage of the model, an auditory filterbank is used to simulate the frequency analysis performed by the cochlea. The filterbank converts the sound wave into a set of driving waves (Fig. 1b); in the latest version, the transfer function for the auditory filter is the gammatone suggested by Johannesma (1972). In the second stage, a bank of pulse generators converts the driving waves into streams of pulses that, in essence, record the times of the driving-wave peaks; the pulse generators are based on a hair cell simulation suggested by Meddis (1986). Together, the pulse streams form a pulse ribbon (Fig. 1c) which provides a representation of the overall neural firing pattern that the sound might be expected to produce in the auditory nerve. The vertical dimension of the ribbon is filter centre frequency on an ERB-rate scale (Moore and Glasberg, 1983). For a periodic sound like the APH wave, the pattern repeats on the ribbon and the repetition rate corresponds to the pitch of the sound. Timbre is assumed to correspond to the shape of the pulse pattern within a cycle. Thus, the pulse ribbon provides a

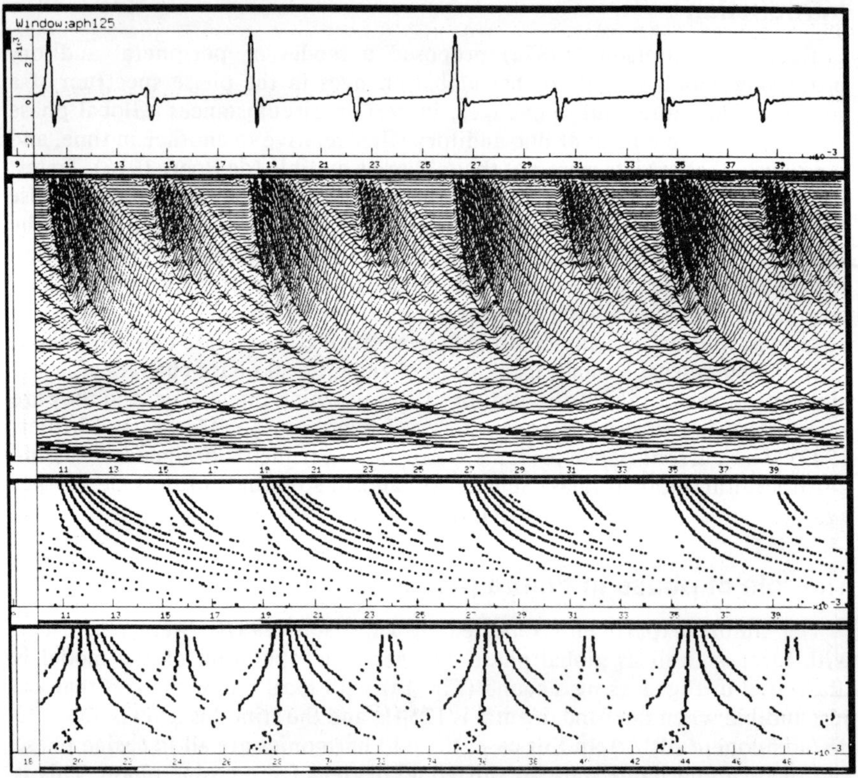

Figure 1. The processing of an APH wave by the pulse ribbon model (D = 40 degrees). The filterbank converts the wave (a) into driving waves (b) which the pulse generators convert into a pulse ribbon, either without (c) or with (d) phase compensation.

convenient means of separating pitch and timbre information, and relating phase manipulations to timbre perceptions in complex sounds.

Timbre cues within filter channels

The APH sound causes secondary maxima to appear in the envelopes of the higher-frequency driving waves midway through the cycle (Fig. 1b) -- maxima that do not occur in the CPH driving waves. Envelope changes of this sort are known to produce timbre changes when they are sufficiently large (Mathes and Miller, 1947). The secondary maxima of the APH driving waves generate a secondary column of pulses midway through the cycle of the pattern that appears on the pulse ribbon (Fig. 1c). In the model, it is these pulses that are assumed to mediate the timbre change. Since it is the interaction of adjacent harmonics within an auditory filter that causes the envelope change, the perceptual feature that accompanies the change is referred to as a within-channel timbre cue. Patterson used the data from the APH experiments to estimate sensitivity to envelope changes within filter channels.

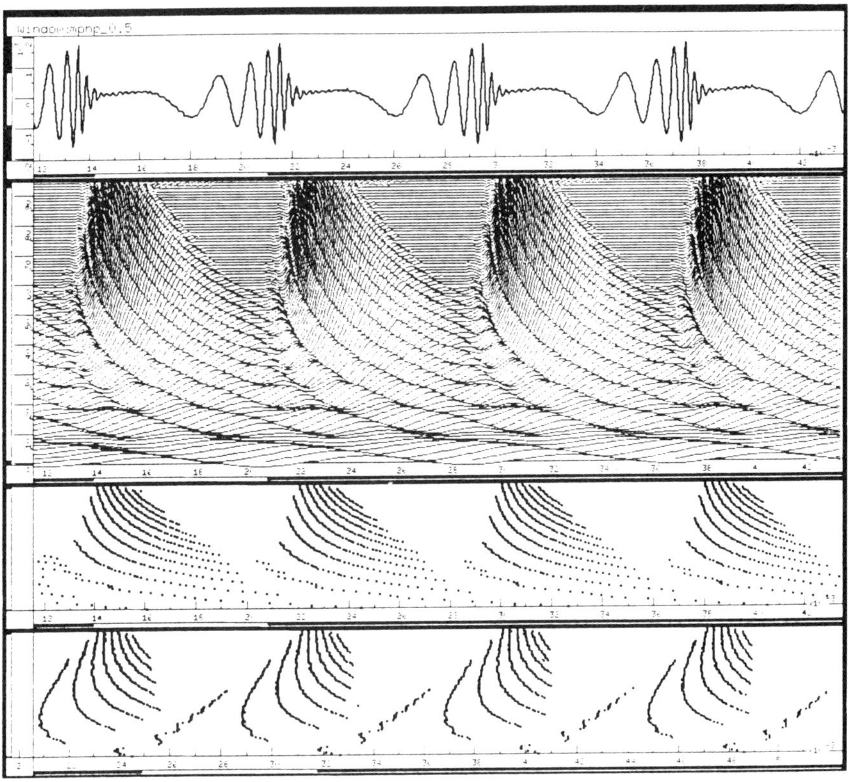

Figure 2. As in Fig. 1, but for an MPH wave (S = 1/2).

Note that the phase lag of the low-frequency channels in Figs. 1b and 1c is not produced by the APH stimulus. It is a property of the filterbank; the low-frequency filters have narrower bandwidths and greater phase lags. Figure 1d presents a version of the pulse ribbon in which the phase lag of the filterbank has been removed and it shows that the envelope maxima of APH driving waves are aligned across channels when measured relative to the phase lag of the filterbank.

Timbre cues between filter channels

Global phase changes were introduced into the CPH wave by applying an acceleration to the phase spectrum. Patterson (1987b) used decelerations as well as accelerations and so the stimuli are referred to as monotonic- phase, or MPH, waves. A decelerating MPH wave is shown in Fig. 2a. Some of the low- and high-frequency energy that would be concentrated in the single pulse of a CPH wave has been separated out in the MPH wave, with the low-frequency energy appearing just before the main pulse and the high-frequency energy appearing just after the main pulse. Figure 2b presents the driving waves of the MPH stimulus, and it shows that they have simple envelopes with no secondary maxima anywhere in the cycle. There is still a phase lag in the low-frequency channels, but a comparison of the magnitude of the time differences in Figs. 1b and 2b reveals that the global phase lag is reduced by the MPH wave. It had generally been assumed that global phase manipulations of this sort would not produce timbre changes (de Boer, 1976; Buunen, 1976).

The primary characteristics of the MPH manipulation are preserved in the initial pulse ribbon (Fig. 2c); there are no pulses midway through the cycle of the pattern and the global phase lag is reduced with respect to that in Fig. 1c. Figure 2d shows the MPH pulse ribbon after compensation for the global phase lag of the filterbank. It shows that the MPH manipulation results in a progressive shift of the envelope maxima relative to filterbank phase. Patterson (1987b) found that, contrary to previous expectations, MPH stimuli do produce timbre changes when compared with CPH stimuli. The MPH stimuli produce only minimal envelope changes, and so he argued that the timbre cue was probably the progressive delay of channels across the pulse ribbon. Since the cue involves a comparison across channels, it is referred to as a between-channel timbre cue.

Differential masking of timbre cues

In the model, the MPH and APH timbre cues differ in terms of the stability of the pulses on which they are based: The MPH cue is based on the most stable pulses in the ribbon - those arising from the largest driving-wave peaks. The cue is assumed to involve a comparison of the most stable pulses in different channels. The APH cue is based on some of the less stable pulses arising from secondary envelope maxima. The cue is assumed to involve a comparison of more and less stable pulses within individual channels. If these assumptions are correct, then we might expect to find that a rising background noise would disrupt the APH/CPH discrimination sooner than the MPH/CPH discrimination, because it would obscure the less stable pulses of the APH/CPH discrimination sooner than the more stable pulses of the MPH/CPH discrimination. A pair of experiments was performed to test this hypothesis.

Method

Four listeners with normal hearing were required to discriminate APH and CPH stimuli, or MPH and CPH stimuli, in the presence of a background noise. The signal level and the magnitude of the phase manipulation were both fixed during a run. The noise level was varied adaptively to determine the level at which the discrimination was just possible; that is, the point where performance was reduced to 71% correct in a two-alternative, forced-choice experiment. Between runs, the magnitude of the phase manipulation was varied to determine whether the MPH/CPH discrimination was, indeed, more resistant to noise masking than the APH/CPH discrimination.

There were two versions of the experiment: To begin with, since the peak factor of the stimulus decreases as the magnitude of the phase manipulation increases, it was important to demonstrate that the individual APH and MPH signals were all equally detectable in the masking noise. The noise masker had a bandwidth in excess of 3.0 kHz, and so in the first experiment, to keep the noise from becoming too loud, the signal level was set at 40 dB/c. The experiment revealed significant differences in the expected direction, but since it did not employ the full range of the phase effect, it did not provide the most sensitive measure of the differences. Accordingly, a second experiment was performed in which the signal level was raised 10 dB. In this case, it was not possible to measure masked threshold for the signals. Aside from the level difference, the two experiments were quite similar.

Stimuli

The signals were flat-spectrum periodic sounds containing 31 harmonics. The fundamental, fo, was 62.5 or 125 Hz in the first experiment and 62.5 Hz in the second. The signals were lowpass filtered at the 25th harmonic and bands of noise with steep cutoffs were used to restrict the listening region to a set of harmonics extending from the 4th to the 24th. A detailed description of the stimuli and the procedure is presented in Patterson (1987b).

The APH manipulation involved shifting every other harmonic away from cosine phase by a fixed number of degrees. The phase difference, D, was varied from 20 degrees -- where it is just large enough to support discrimination in the absence of the masking noise -- up to 80 degrees -- where the secondary maxima in the driving waves are almost as large as the primary maxima. The MPH manipulation involved shifting successive harmonics an ever decreasing amount to produce a phase spectrum in which greater shifts occur between lower harmonics and smaller shifts between higher harmonics. The aim was to produce between-channel phase lags that were roughly con-

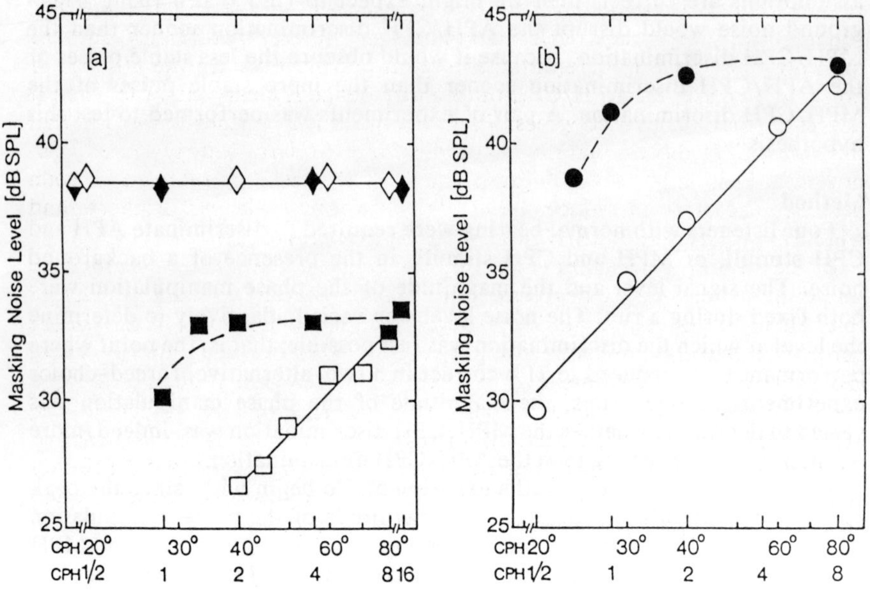

Figure 3. The noise spectrum level required to disrupt timbre discriminations for signals of 40 dB/c (squares) or 50 dB/c (circles); filled and open symbols are for MPH and APH conditions, respectively. The diamonds show masked threshold for 40 dB/c signals.

stant from channel to channel. The initial phase spectrum was created by calculating the number of auditory-filter bandwidths between adjacent harmonics and shifting the phase of the upper harmonic by 180 degrees per bandwidth. Then a scalar, with value S, was applied to the phase spectrum as a whole to produce the MPH manipulation.

The pattern of results was the same for the two fundamentals in the first experiment and so the data were combined. Furthermore, the pattern was quite similar for all four listeners, in both experiments, and so their results were averaged in each case. Each of the means presented in the next section includes the data from at least 32 individual runs.

Results

The average data for experiments one and two are presented in Fig. 3. The detection data (diamonds) in the upper part of Fig. 3a show that the APH and MPH stimuli were equally detectable, and that threshold does not vary with the magnitude of the phase manipulation in either case. In the absence of the noise masker, the MPH/CPH timbre difference is clearly audible provided S is greater than about unity. When the noise is introduced, we find that the discrimination requires a signal-to-noise (S/N) ratio of about 6 dB in the region where S is greater than unity - independent of the value of S (filled squares). Only when the discrimination becomes inherently difficult, does the masking noise have a differential effect on performance. In the absence of noise, at 40 dB/c, the APH/CPH timbre difference is clearly audible when D is greater than about 35 degrees. When the noise is introduced, we find that the APH/CPH discrimination is audible for a S/N ratio of just over 6 dB, provided D is large, say 80° (open squares). But as D is reduced, it soon becomes necessary to reduce the noise level to maintain performance, and when D is 40 degrees, the S/N ratio has to be in excess of 12 dB.

In the second experiment (Fig. 3b), the range of the APH measurements was extended down to 20 degrees by increasing the signal level and restricting fo to 62.5 Hz. The results for D = 20 degrees show that an aspect of the timbre perception that is capable of supporting APH/CPH discrimination in silence, is obscured by a noise whose level is almost 20 dB below that required to mask the presence of the sounds. There is no corresponding effect in the MPH/CPH data. The overall pattern of results is very similar to that found in the first experiment. Indeed, the curves drawn through the MPH/CPH data and the lines drawn through the APH/CPH data are the same in Figs. 3a and 3b, except that they have been shifted up 10 dB in Fig. 3b.

Discussion and Conclusions

The fact that the MPH/CPH discrimination is more resistant to noise masking than the APH/CPH discrimination supports Patterson's (1987a, 1987b) contention that the MPH and APH timbre cues are derived from different parts of the pulse ribbon. In the case of the APH sounds, it is argued that the timbre cue is the column of pulses that appears in the pulse ribbon midway through the cycle of the pattern -- pulses associated with secondary maxima in the envelopes of the driving waves. These maxima are relatively small and this accounts for the fact that the discrimination is disrupted by the introduction of a relatively low-level noise. The MPH cue is assumed to be the slant of the pulse ribbon, derived from pulses associated with the primary maxima in the driving waves. These maxima contain the largest driving-wave peaks and this accounts for the fact that it takes a relatively higher-level noise to disrupt this discrimination.

The contrast between the form of the MPH data and the APH data would appear to rule out the possibility that the MPH timbre cue might be based on small envelope changes occurring in the troughs of the driving waves. The current data do not mean that the MPH timbre cue is necessarily a between-channel cue; it is logically possible for the cue to be a change in the shape of the maximum of the driving-wave envelope. However, as Patterson has pointed out, the timbre cue is available when the shape change is very small, and so it seems more likely that it depends on a between-channel comparison.

Acknowledgements

The author would like to thank Robert Milroy for running the experiments and analysing the results.

References

de Boer, E. (**1976**). "On the residue and auditory pitch perception," in *Handbook of Sensory Physiology, Vol. V*, edited by W.D. Keidel & W.D. Neff (Springer-Verlag, Berlin), pp. 479-583.

Buunen, T.J.F. (**1976**). *On the perception of phase differences in acoustic signals.* Doctoral dissertation. University of Delft, Delft, The Netherlands.

Johannesma, P.I.M. (**1972**). "The pre-response stimulus ensemble of neurons in the cochlear nucleus," in: *Proceedings Symposium on Hearing Theory,* pp. 58-69. IPO, Eindhoven, The Netherlands.

Mathes, R.C. and Miller, R.L. (**1947**). "Phase effects in monaural perception," J.Acoust.Soc.Am. **18**, 780-797.

Meddis, R. (**1986**). "Simulation of mechanical to neural transduction in the auditory receptor," J.Acoust.Soc.Am. **79**, 702-711.

Moore, B.C.J. and Glasberg, B.R. (**1983**). "Suggested formulae for calculating auditory-filter bandwidths and excitation patterns", J.Acoust.Soc.Am. **74**, 750-753.

Patterson, R.D. (**1987a**). "A pulse ribbon model of peripheral auditory processing," in *Auditory Processing of Complex Sounds*, edited by W.A. Yost and C.S. Watson (Erlbaum, New Jersey), pp.167-179.

Patterson, R.D. (**1987b**). "A pulse ribbon model of monaural phase perception," J.Acoust.Soc.Am., **82**, 1560-1586.

The role of FM-induced AM in dynamic spectral profile analysis

Stephen McAdams & Xavier Rodet

Institut de Recherche et Coordination Acoustique/Musique (IRCAM) 31, rue Saint-Merri F-75004 Paris, France

Introduction

Recent work by Green and colleagues (cf. Green, 1983) has begun to demonstrate with psychophysical methods that the human auditory system is capable of extracting a global representation of the spectral envelope of a signal. This may serve to identify the resonance structure characteristics of a sound source. However, this previous work has been exclusively confined to relatively dense steady-state, inharmonic stimuli of simple spectral forms (a single bump in the spectral profile). Dynamic stimuli, those with frequency jitter or vibrato, might be helpful in reducing perceptual ambiguity in cases where there are not enough partials present in a sound to clearly define a spectral envelope. They may do this by tracing out the spectral envelope through time, thus increasing information about the resonance structure.

While this seems intuitively obvious, previous work on high-pitched vowel identification in the presence of frequency vibrato has yielded ambiguous results (Sundberg, 1977). These researchers claim that intonation contours or vibrato had slight, or even detrimental, effects on vowel identification. The present study demonstrates, to the contrary, that if the amplitude behavior of a given partial is coupled with its frequency behavior according to a given spectral envelope, this information can be used by the auditory system to discriminate and identify the vowel quality or timbre of complex harmonic sounds.

Experiment 1: Spectral envelope discrimination

Stimuli

The experiment was conducted with both harmonic complex and sinusoidal stimuli. All tones had a duration of 1 sec and an amplitude envelope with raised cosine attacks (150 ms) and decays (200 ms). Complex tones consisted of the first 8 harmonics of a 675 Hz fundamental. Sine tones were at 1350 Hz, equivalent to the second harmonic of the complex. This high F_0 gives wide harmonic spacing and thus a poor spectral envelope definition in the absence

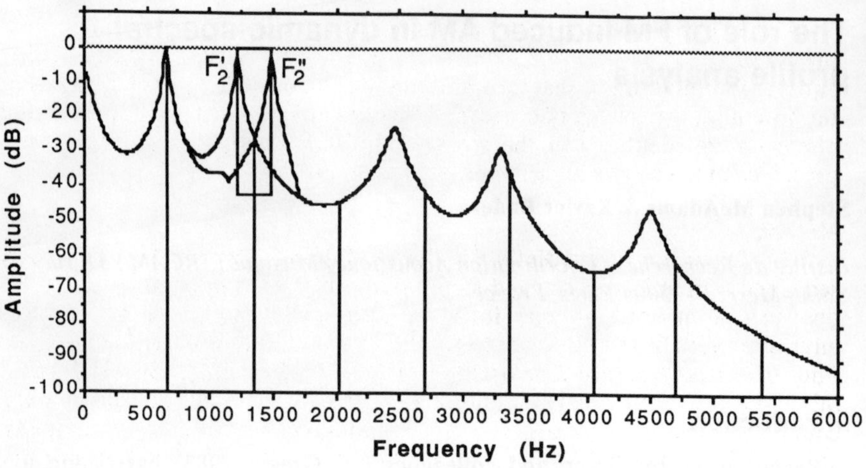

Figure 1. The two spectral envelopes used in the experiment.

of frequency modulation.

Eight peak-to-peak widths were used throughout: 0, 1, 2, 3, 4, 6, 8, 10% of the partials' frequencies. A psychometric function was determined based on this dimension. The vibrato was a sinusoidal frequency modulation with a frequency of 6.5 Hz. The starting phase of the vibrato was randomly selected from 0, $\pi/2$, π, $3\pi/2$. This was necessary to avoid discrimination judgments based on counting the number of peaks in the amplitude envelope for the modulated pure tone condition, since with sine phase vibrato the amplitude would always increase at the beginning for one spectral envelope, and decrease for the other.

The two table-lookup spectral envelopes applied to the components, SE1 & SE2, are illustrated in Figure 1. They are like allophones of /ʌ/ with SE1 being closer to /o/ and SE2 being closer to /æ/. The envelopes were stored in a table which returned the instantaneous amplitude corresponding to the instantaneous frequency of each partial. In this way, the vibrato was coupled to an amplitude modulation defined by the spectral envelope function. The spectral envelopes consisted of 5 formants, 4 of which were identical in the two cases. The only difference was the center frequency of the second formant (F'_2=1215 Hz for SE1, F''_2=1485 Hz for SE2). The skirts of these 2 formants intersect at the center frequency of the second harmonic, and the main difference between them in the region just around this harmonic (at small vibrato widths) is a change in the sign of the spectral slope. The part of the slopes in the boxed area in Fig. 1 covers the range for a 20% peak-to-peak vibrato, and was constructed over this range such that the two envelopes are mirror images (in linear frequency) of one another about the 2nd harmonic frequency. The envelopes were also constructed so that the frequency-amplitude coupling for all other harmonics was identical in the 2 cases.

In the non-roving global amplitude condition, complex tones were presented at 75 dBA and sine tones were presented at 58 dBA, this latter being equal to the intensity of that tone within the complex. The rms amplitudes of the stimuli at a given vibrato width (2 spectral envelopes at 4 vibrato starting phases) were identical. In the roving amplitude condition the tones were presented at the above intensities or at that value ± 5 dB.

Method

Stimuli were presented diotically over headphones. Each trial consisted of a sequence of four tones arranged in two pairs, with each pair constituting one observation interval. In one interval, both tones had the same spectral envelope (SE). In the other interval, they had different spectral envelopes. Four trial structures are thus possible: (SE1 SE1 / SE1 SE2), (SE1 SE2 / SE1 SE1), (SE2 SE2 / SE2 SE1), and (SE2 SE1 / SE2 SE2). These structures were counterbalanced across trials. The starting phase of the vibrato was randomly selected for each of the 4 tones. In the roving condition the amplitude of each tone was randomly selected from the 3 possible values.

The subject's task was to identify the interval containing the "different" pair by pressing a corresponding button. Feedback indicating the correct response was given.

Trials were presented in blocks of 80 with ten repetitions of each of the 8 vibrato widths in random order.

Subjects completed several training blocks until their psychometric functions appeared to stabilize. The number of training blocks varied considerably between subjects (5-35). Then ten blocks were collected, giving a total of 100 2IFC judgments for a data point at each vibrato width. The % correct measures at each vibrato width were averaged across the 10 blocks in order to obtain the mean and standard deviation. This latter statistic was then used to evaluate the reliability of the 75% threshold on the psychometric function as described in the next section.

Four subjects completed the non-roving conditions for complex and sine tones in that order. Afterward, two of these subjects completed the roving conditions for complex and sine tones.

Results

A spline curve was fitted to the 8 data points for each subject in each condition and the 75% point was determined as a measure of threshold performance. In order to have a measure of the variability of this threshold, spline curves were also fitted to points 1 standard deviation above and below the means from which the 75% points were also determined. One notes that these outer points are asymmetric with respect to the mean. Therefore, as a rough measure of the overall variation in the threshold the mean distance between the center point and the outer 75% points was calculated. This measure was used as an estimate of the standard deviation along the stimulus dimension. It is probably an over-estimation of the standard deviation, making the statistical test very conservative.

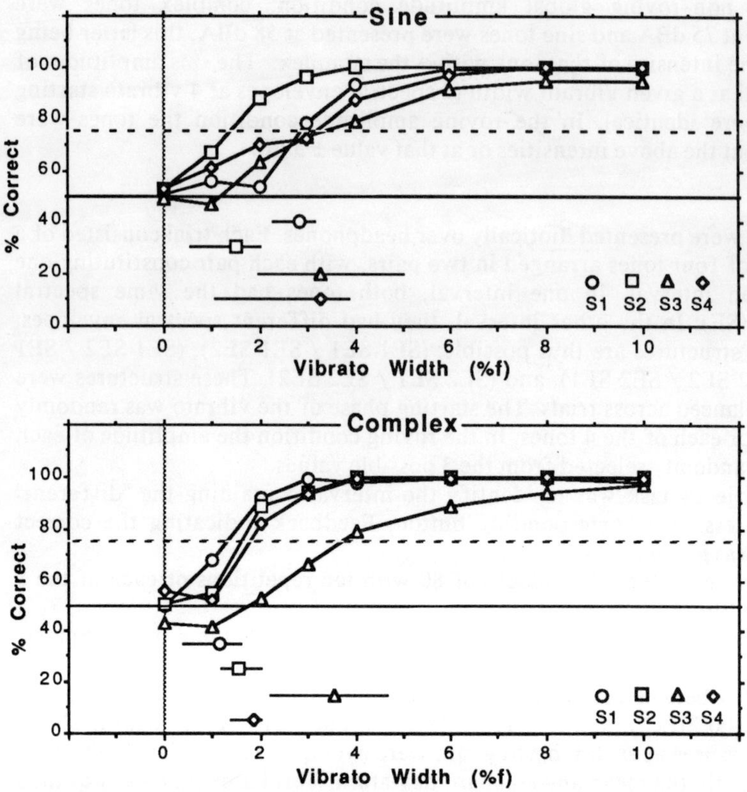

Figure 2. Psychometric functions for 4 subjects (non-roving condition) showing % correct discrimination as a function of vibrato width in %f. The points with horizontal bars in the lower portion of the plot indicate the 75% point of the mean curve and the estimated range of standard error for each subject.

The mean data for 4 subjects are shown for the non-roving condition for both complex and sine tones in Fig. 2. All Ss attain near-perfect performance in the range of vibrato widths used indicating that the stimulus difference is easily discriminable. All psychometric functions are monotone increasing indicating that the perceptual factor upon which discrimination is based varies with vibrato width. The range of threshold vibrato widths for the 4 Ss was 1.2-3.8% (16-51 Hz at the 2nd harmonic). For S1 & S4, complex thresholds are significantly lower than sine thresholds ($p<.01$; t-test). They are approximately equal for S2 & S3. This may indicate differences in decision strategies among the Ss. If complex thresholds were always less than sine

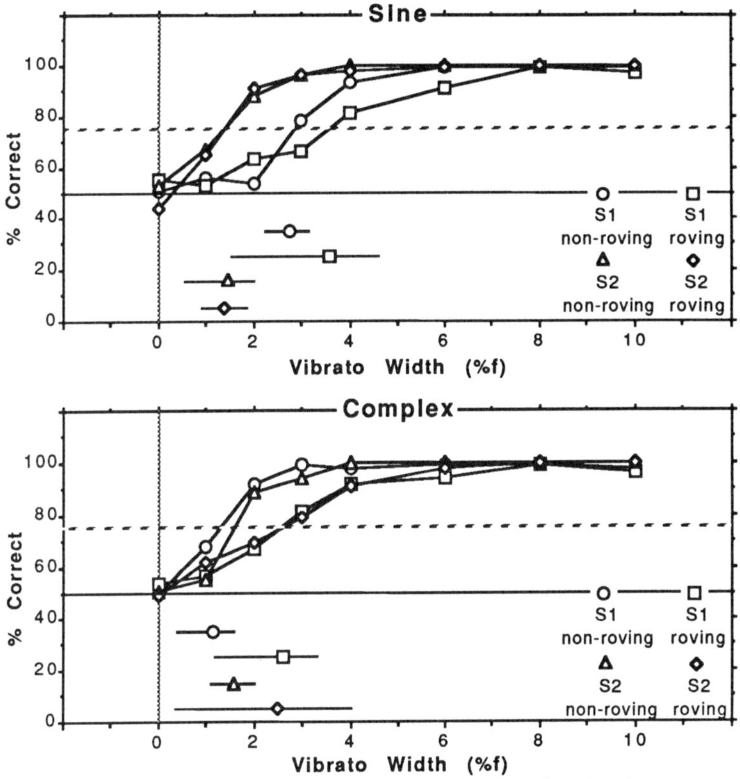

Figure 3. Psychometric functions for 2 subjects showing % correct discrimination as a function of vibrato width. Points with horizontal bars as in Fig. 2.

thresholds, one might hypothesize that the same dynamic frequency-amplitude slope information was more easily interpreted in the global context given by the behavior of the other harmonics. Such may be the case for S1 & S4.

The mean data comparing roving and non-roving conditions for Ss 1 & 2 are shown in Figure 3. Both subjects attain near-perfect performance by 6% peak vibrato width in both of these conditions. For complex tones, the thresholds for roving amplitude stimuli appear to be greater than those without roving for both Ss. Only the difference for S1 is statistically significant ($p<.01$), though it is relatively small. For sine tones, neither S shows an effect of amplitude roving. Comparing sine with complex tones within the roving condition, S1 shows no difference while S2 does, complex tones having a higher threshold ($p>.05$).

We might conclude from these data that the difference in spectral envelope following for minimally different envelopes is indeed possible at relatively low vibrato widths (1.2-3.8%). This discrimination is easier for some Ss in the presence of a vowel-like spectral envelope on flanking harmonics than it is with a single sinusoid. While roving the global amplitude causes some deterioration in performance, its effect is quite small indicating that Ss are not using a within-frequency channel intensity discrimination strategy, but are extracting the spectral profile and storing it in short-term memory.

Experiment 2 : Spectral envelope identification

Stimuli

The stimuli are identical to those used in Experiment 1.

Method

At the beginning of each block the subject was presented with a series of tones alternating between SE1 and SE2, starting from 10% vibrato width and descending progressively through the other values to 0%, each being associated with a differently colored light and button in order to avoid verbal labeling of the sounds. The initial presentation series could be replayed as many times as necessary for the subject to become accustomed to the differences. All 4 Ss had already participated in the previous experiment and were thus quite familiar with the stimuli.

Ss were to identify the single tone presented on each trial. The tone had a randomly selected vibrato starting phase as in Experiment 1. No feedback was given. Trials were presented in blocks of 80 with ten repetitions of each of the vibrato widths. An equal number of SE1's and SE2's was presented in each block. Four Ss performed the experiment for complex tones and then sine tones in the non-roving condition. Two of these Ss then performed the roving condition.

Subjects completed training blocks until their psychometric functions (% correct identification as a function of vibrato width) stabilized. Ten blocks were then collected from which were determined the mean % correct and standard deviation across the 10 blocks. From these values the 75% threshold and range of its standard error were calculated from fitted spline curves as in Experiment 1.

Results

The mean data for 4 Ss are plotted for the non-roving condition for both types of tone in Figure 4. Three of the Ss attain near-perfect performance at a vibrato width of 8% for both sines and complex tones. The range of threshold vibrato widths is 0.6-3.6% (8-49 Hz at the 2nd harmonic). S3 attains threshold for sine tones at 6.2%, but never achieves better than chance performance for complex tones even at the largest vibrato width. This subject claimed to have tried several criteria for identification, but could not latch onto anything that allowed positive identification. With that one exception, all curves are monotone increasing indicating that the perceptual factor permitting identification varies with vibrato width.

Reversing the trend in Experiment 1, Ss 2 & 3 have different thresholds for complex and sines in this identification task ($p<.05$ for S2; threshold for

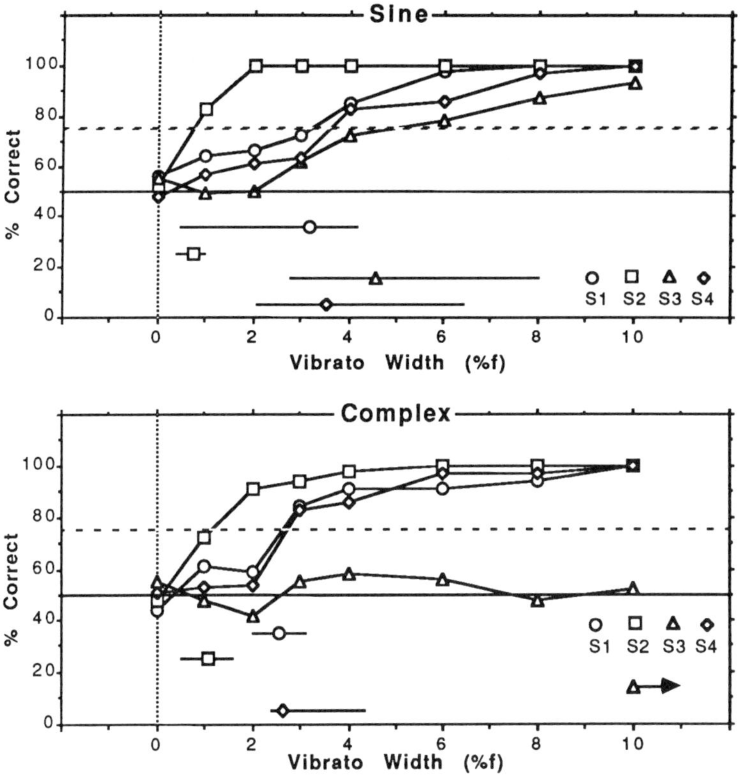

Figure 4. Psychometric functions for identification (non-roving condition). Points with horizontal bars as in Fig. 2.

complex well beyond stimulus range for S3), while Ss 1 & 4 show no difference. The difference shown by S2 is from 0.6% for sines compared to 1.2% for complex tones. The threshold for sines may well be lower since more data would be needed between 0 and 1% to accurately estimate the threshold.

The psychometric functions for roving amplitudes (Ss 1 & 2) showed no differences between sine and complex tones nor between roving and non-roving conditions.

These data suggest that even very similar spectral envelopes can be successfully identified in the presence of vibrato (and with a severely restricted set of choices), when the fundamental frequency is fairly high and the spectral envelope is not well defined by the relative amplitudes of the frequency components in the absence of vibrato.

A possible criticism of this experiment may be that the stimulus set was too small, making the "identification" experiment one of "discrimination across trials". All Ss remarked during the experiment that when the vibrato width was small for several trials, they tended to shift their criterion toward the less bright of the 2 SE's. Subsequently, a large vibrato stimulus would be judged (sometimes erroneously) as SE2. These errors would raise the measured thresholds.

Three of the four Ss (1,3,4) showed a tendency for discrimination thresholds to be lower than identification thresholds in the non-roving condition for both sine and complex tones. The general tendency seems to be for identification to require greater perceptual difference than discrimination. It seems intuitively obvious that sounds must be easily distinguishable in order to be correctly categorized and identified, but given the limited number of stimuli to be identified, these results must be interpreted with caution.

Discussion

The main result of these experiments is that small differences in complex spectral envelopes that are poorly filled with only a few frequency components can be discriminated and identified in the presence of a small amount of sinusoidal vibrato. This performance is relatively unaffected by roving the global amplitude of the stimuli. The range of threshold vibrato widths across subjects and conditions is approximately 0.6-3.8% peak-to-peak (excepting the 6.2% sine identification threshold of S3). At the frequency of the 2nd harmonic, these values are above sinusoidal frequency modulation detection threshold (0.1-0.3% in Hartmann & Klein, 1980). They also correspond to peak-to-peak amplitude variations on the 2nd harmonic of 0.6-4 dB (6.7 dB for S3 sine identification), which are also either at or above detection threshold (0.8 dB at 1000 Hz and 60 dB; cf. Riesz, 1928). One might conclude that the modulation must be detectable along both dimensions in order for its combined effect to be extracted as a spectral envelope tracing.

The apparently small difference in performance introduced by the presence of other harmonics around the 1350 Hz 2nd harmonic (whose frequency-amplitude coupling defines other regions of the spectral envelope) bears some consideration. For the 2 Ss who show this trend (Ss 1 & 4), the average increase in threshold when the flanking harmonics are removed is only on the order of 1% of the component frequency. This corresponds to an average increase of about 1 dB in the peak-to-peak amplitude fluctuation on the 2nd harmonic. What this may suggest is that the information already present in the modulated sine tone is sufficient to explain performance with the complex tones. The reports from Ss about what they listened to in order to make the judgments on sine tones varied. Ss 1 & 4 felt that they were listening for a tone color difference in the two sines. Ss 2 & 3 felt that they were listening to a pitch difference. This latter criterion is easily understood since the amplitude of the sine is greater at lower frequencies for SE1 and greater at higher frequencies for SE2. A strategy that consisted of accumulating a weighted pitch representation of the tone and deciding whether it was the higher or lower would be successful since the discrimination thresholds are above frequency discrimination threshold if one were to measure the distance between the lower excursion of SE1 and the upper excursion of SE2. All Ss, however claimed to use tone color or vowel quality as the cue with the complex tones. It is entirely possible that Ss 2 & 3 used different strategies in the two cases.

Whatever the mechanism responsible for this performance, it is clear that one must take into account the dynamic nature of the stimuli. The basilar membrane activity pattern proposed by Green (1983) as the stimulus structure used to make the profile comparison is never present at any given moment in these stimuli. It is thus necessary for the auditory system to accumulate it through time.

Acknowledgments

The idea for this research arose from discussions with William Hartmann and Yves Potard.

References

Green, D.M. (**1983**). "Profile analysis: A different view of auditory intensity discrimination," American Psychologist **38**, 133-142.

Hartmann, W.M. & Klein, M.A. (**1980**). "Theory of frequency modulation detection for low modulation frequencies," J.Acous.Soc.Am. **67**, 935-946.

Riesz, R.R. (**1928**). "Differential sensitivity of the ear for pure tones," Phys.Rev. **31**, 867-875.

Sundberg, J. (**1977**). "Vibrato and vowel identification," Archives of Acoustics, Polish Academy of Sciences **2**(2), 257-266.

Comments

Moore:

You suggest that your results indicate that subjects do not use a within-channel strategy, but rather extract the spectral profile and detect changes in that profile. However, it would be possible for the subjects to perform the task using a within-channel strategy. Consider the behaviour of the second harmonic, at 1350 Hz. For one stimulus, increases in frequency are coupled with increases in amplitude, while for the other increases in frequency are coupled with decreases in amplitude. If the subject were to listen to the output of an auditory filter centred somewhat below 1350 Hz, say at 1100 Hz, then the depth of modulation at the output of that filter would differ for the two stimuli; it would be greater for the second than for the first. Thus the depth of modulation within a channel would provide a cue.

Reply by McAdams and Rodet:

This is a reasonable criticism which reflects more on the nature of the experimental task (2 IFC with feedback - which allows the development of such listening strategies) than on real-world behavior. If we assume a slope of 27 dB/Bark on the lower side of the activity pattern resulting from stimulation at 1350 Hz (Zwicker and Feldkeller, 1967), the amplitude modification depth of the activity in a frequency channel at 1100 Hz may be estimated for SE 1 as approximately four times that for SE 2 at any of the vibrates width used in this experiment (see Fig.C1). Since the slope is independent of the sound pressure level of the component, the difference in modulation depth between SE 1 and SE 2 is independent of the global amplitude and would thus be unaffected by amplitude roving. For this cue to be usable, the absolute level of activity in this channel needs to be detectable. Based on the above slope estimate and a 58 dB level of the component, the level of stimulation at 1100 Hz varies around a value of 21.5 dB. It is also necessary that the modulation depth be sufficient to be detectable. The estimated depths for stimuli with vibrato widths around threshold discrimination are listed below:

	SE 1	SE 2
4%	10.9 dB	2.8 dB
2%	5.4 dB	1.4 dB
1%	2.7 dB	0.7 dB

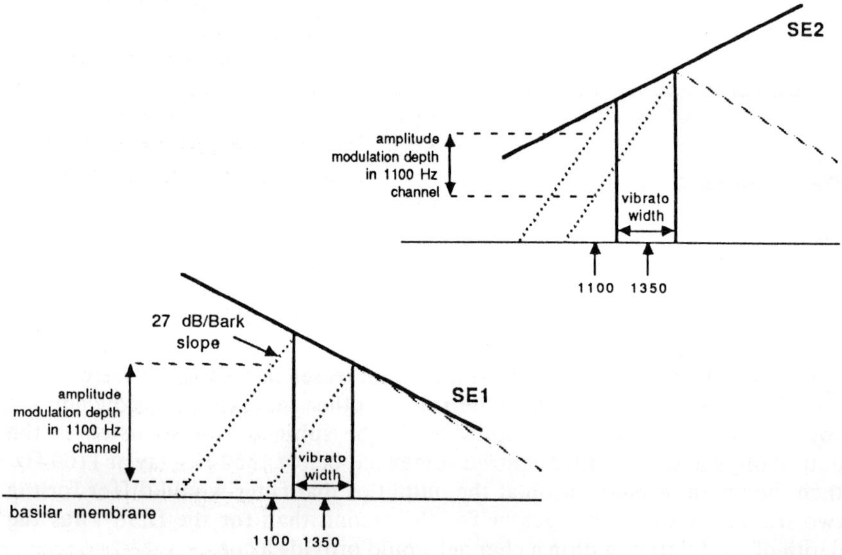

Figure C1. Frequency modulation of the basilar membrane activity pattern due to the component at 1350 Hz yields amplitude modulation depth in a channel at 1100 Hz that are larger for SE1 than for SE2.

If a listener attends to this channel, the amplitude modulation should always be detectable, at least for SE 1. However, no subject reached threshold discrimination at 1%. Also, if this cue was responsible for the discrimination observed, there should be no difference in performance between sine and complex tone conditions. Such a difference does exist for 2 Ss, though it is small. One of the subjects for whom there is no difference has very high thresholds, perhaps indicating that this information is not used. In any case, for these spectral envelopes, even roving the $F_0 \pm 5\%$ across tones in a trial would not succeed in completely thwarting the possibility of using this kind of listening strategy. Different envelopes would need to be chosen to allow a greater frequency roving range.

Houtsma:

As shown in your figure you have chosen your stimuli such that for zero % vibrato width the stimuli were identical and, consequently, indiscriminable. Could you tell what would happen if for zero% modulation the second harmonics of the alternative signals are made unequal? This would allow us to assess the relative importance of frequency modulation compared with fixed differences between partials in the complex-tone discrimination task.

Reply by McAdams:

That would, of course, be more like the steady-state profile analysis experiments with wide component spacing and a small number of components, but with harmonic frequencies and a multi-formant profile. We have planned some studies to compare modulated and steady-state thresholds in spectral envelope discrimination and to compare performance on harmonic, multi-formant stimuli with the inharmonic flat spectrum used by Green and colleagues.

Pitch and pitch strength of peaked ripple noise

H. Fastl

Institute of Electroacoustics
Technical University München, F.R. Germany

Introduction

When adding delayed versions of a noise to the undelayed noise, a power spectrum can be produced, which shows a cosine shape when plotted on linear coordinates. Therefore, this noise frequently is called "cosine noise" (e.g. Bilsen, 1966; Bilsen and Wieman, 1980; Buunen, 1980; Yost and Hill, 1978; Yost, 1980, 1982). On the other hand, the delayed noise can be fed back to the input, leading to a noise with sharp peaks in its spectrum. Bilsen and Wieman (1980) as well as Bilsen and Raatgever (1983) call this noise "comb filtered noise". However, as pointed out by Wilson (1980), some colleagues use the term "comb filtered noise" for "cosine noise". In order to avoid further confusion, in this paper we call the noise produced by feedback of delayed noise "peaked ripple noise".

Experiments on the pitch and the pitch strength of rippled noise spectra have a long tradition (e.g. Bilsen, 1966; Wilson, 1967; Bilsen and Ritsma, 1970; Ritsma and Bilsen, 1970; Yost and Hill, 1978; Yost *et al.*, 1978; Bilsen and Wieman, 1980; Buunen, 1980; Yost, 1980, 1982; Bilsen and Raatgever, 1983). While the pitch strength of "cosine noise" amounts only to some 15% in comparison to the pitch strength of a pure tone (Fastl and Stoll, 1979), ripple noise with distinct spectral peaks can produce much larger pitch strength. This notion can be inferred from results of Bilsen and Raatgever (1983), who showed that the JND in frequency for peaked ripple noise is equal to the JND for a periodic pulse.

In this paper, we describe the dependence of the pitch strength of peaked ripple noise on the spectral modulation depth, on the frequency spacing of the peaks, and on level. We use a direct method, in which numbers are assigned to the perceived pitch strength which has proven successful for the description of the pitch strength of various sounds (Fastl and Stoll, 1979; Fastl 1980, 1981), and was adopted by our colleagues in the States (Lundeen and Small, 1984). Moreover, the pitch strength of peaked ripple noise is directly compared to the pitch strength of a pure tone producing the same pitch as the peaked ripple noise. In addition, results of pitch matches between pure tones and peaked ripple noise are given, and compared to predictions by a model of virtual pitch (Terhardt *et al.*, 1982).

Experiments

All experiments were performed by eight normal hearing subjects. Their age was between 25 and 38 years (median 27 years). Sounds were presented diotically in a sound proof booth through electrodynamic earphones (Beyer DT 48) with freefield equalizer (Zwicker and Feldtkeller, 1967, p. 40).

The peaked ripple noises were produced by feeding back inverted, delayed broadband noise to the input. Bilsen and Raatgever (1983) give a detailed description of this type of noise. However, while they directly fed back the delayed noise to the input, we inverted the delayed noise before feedback. In this way, spectra are produced which show sharp peaks at $(n - 0.5)/\Delta t$ for $n = 1, 2, 3...$ and minima at $n/\Delta t$ for $n = 0, 1, 2...$, with Δt representing the delay time. Fig. 1a shows a schematic diagram of the network used to produce peaked ripple noise. Fig. 1 b illustrates the spectral distribution for 1 ms delay time and 0.4 dB attenuation, leading to a spectral modulation depth $\Delta L = 33$ dB, and Fig. 1c shows the spectrum for 6 dB attenuation, corresponding to $\Delta L = 9$ dB. The delay was realized in a microcomputer by AD-converting, delaying and DA-converting the noise. To avoid aliasing, before AD-conversion, the broadband noise was low-pass filtered at 9 kHz. Because of phase shifts due to this antialiasing filter, with increasing frequency, the peaks in the peaked ripple noises got broader and lower (see Fig. 1b). In order to assess possible influences of low-pass filtering on the pitch strength of peaked ripple noise at high frequencies, in separate sessions, the pitch strength of peaked ripple noise was measured with noises showing peaks of same height up to 19 kHz.

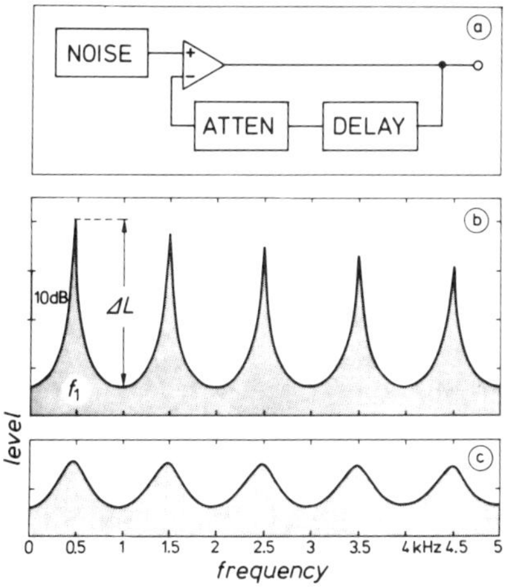

Figure 1: Schematic diagram of a circuit to generate peaked ripple noise (a) and spectral distributions for 1 ms delay time and spectral modulation depths of $\Delta L = 33$ dB (b) and $\Delta L = 9$ dB (c).

For the evaluation of pitch strength, a method of magnitude estimation with anchor sound was used. Sounds of 800 ms duration were presented in pairs with 600 ms silent interval. The first sound of a pair (anchor sound) was kept constant and assigned a number, representing its pitch strength. Relative to this anchor sound, the pitch strength of the second sound of each pair had to be scaled. For further details about the method see e.g. Fastl and Stoll (1979). Each subject evaluated each stimulus condition four times, leading to a total of 32 data points, from which medians and interquartiles were calculated, which are displayed in the figures.

The pitch of peaked ripple noise was assessed by a method of adjustment. Pairs of peaked ripple noise and pure tone with 800 ms stimulus duration and 600 ms silent interval were presented. The subject varied the frequency of a tone generator, until the pitch of the pure tone matched the pitch of the peaked ripple noise. At each delay time, each subject performed four pitch matches. From the resulting 32 data points, distributions of the comparison frequency were derived, by shifting a window with 0.2 Bark bandwidth along the frequency scale.

Results

Figure 2 shows the dependence of the pitch strength of peaked ripple noise on spectral modulation depth. In each panel, the pitch strength was normalized relative to the maximum value. The delay time was 2, 1, and 0.5 ms, respectively, leading to the first peak in the spectrum at 250, 500, and 1000 Hz as indicated in the different panels of Fig. 2. At each delay time, two sets of experiments were performed: one with an anchor sound with $\Delta L = 18$ dB spectral modulation depth (□) and another with $\Delta L = 33$ dB spectral modulation depth (○). The respective anchor sounds are indicated in Fig. 2 by filled symbols. All peaked ripple noises had the same sound pressure

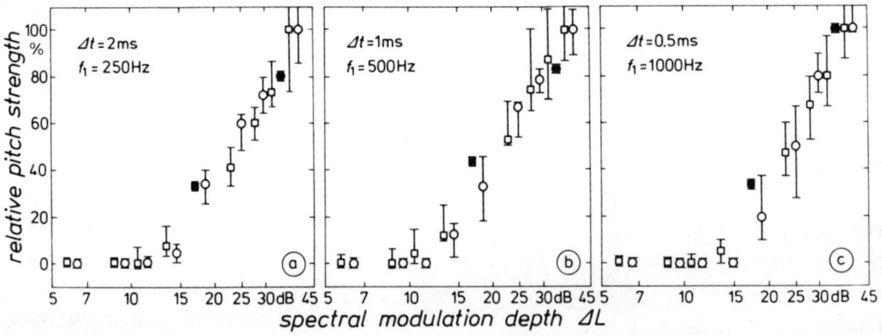

Figure 2: Relative pitch strength of peaked ripple noise as a function of spectral modulation depth. Sound pressure level 60 dB, delay times Δt, and correlated frequencies of the first peak in the spectrum f_1 as indicated in the panels. Spectral modulation depth of anchor sound 18 dB (□) or 33 dB (○).

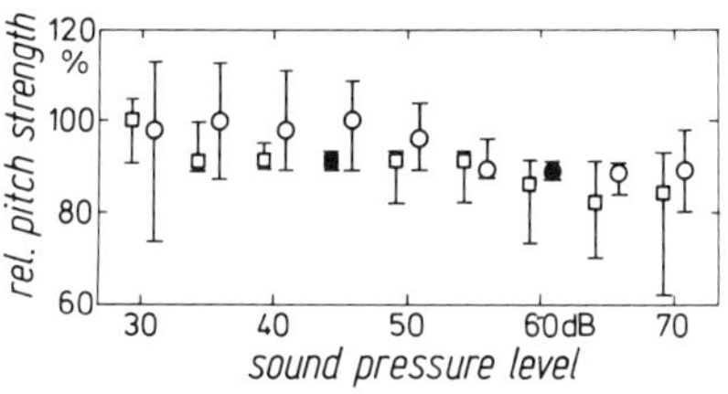

Figure 3: Relative pitch strength of peaked ripple noise as a function of sound pressure level. Delay time Δt = 1 ms (f_1 = 500 Hz), spectral modulation depth ΔL = 33 dB. Sound pressure level of anchor sound 45 dB (□) or 60 dB (○).

level of 60 dB.

The results displayed in Fig. 2 suggest that at all frequencies considered, up to a spectral modulation depth of about 10 dB, peaked ripple noise produces no pitch strength. At higher spectral modulation depth ΔL, pitch strength increases with ΔL. Half of the maximum pitch strength is reached for ΔL around 20 to 25 dB. A comparison of the data illustrated in Fig. 2 by squares vs circles reveals that the results are not much influenced by the choice of the anchor sound. Larger interquartile ranges, in particular in Fig. 2c are due to interindividual differences.

Figure 3 shows the dependence of the pitch strength of peaked ripple noise on sound pressure level. All peaked ripple noises had a delay time of Δt = 1ms (f_1 = 500 Hz), and a spectral modulation depth of ΔL = 33 dB. Two anchor sounds were used: one with a sound pressure level of 45 dB (□) and another with 60 dB SPL (○).

The results displayed in Fig. 3 indicate that the pitch strength of peaked ripple noise decreases somewhat with increasing sound pressure level. Both anchor sounds (squares vs circles) lead to similar results. Again, the magnitude of the interquartile ranges is primarily due to interindividual differences.

Figure 4 shows the dependence of the pitch strength of peaked ripple noise on the frequency f_1 of the first peak in the spectrum as well as the correlated delay time Δt. All peaked ripple noises had a sound pressure level of 60 dB and a spectral modulation depth of ΔL = 33 dB. As anchor sound, peaked ripple noise with f_1 = 0.5 kHz (○) or f_1 = 1 kHz (□) was used. Each symbol in Fig. 4 represents a median, derived from 24 data points of six subjects.

The results displayed in Fig. 4 suggest that with increasing frequency f_1 of the first peak in the spectrum, the pitch strength of peaked ripple noise decreases. However, it has to be mentioned that two of the eight subjects produced a more bandpass-like dependence of pitch strength on f_1, with a maximum around f_1 = 1 kHz. At f_1 = 3 kHz they report a pitch strength which is about a factor of three smaller than the pitch strength at f_1 = 1 kHz, a result which is in line with the data of the remaining six subjects as displayed in Fig. 4. However, in comparison to the pitch strength for f_1 = 1 kHz, the group of six subjects scales the pitch strength of peaked ripple noise at f_1 = 0.125 kHz almost by a factor of two **larger** , but the group of two subjects by more than a factor of two **smaller**.

In order to get more information about the two groups of subjects, peaked ripple noise was compared with respect to pitch strength to pure tones with

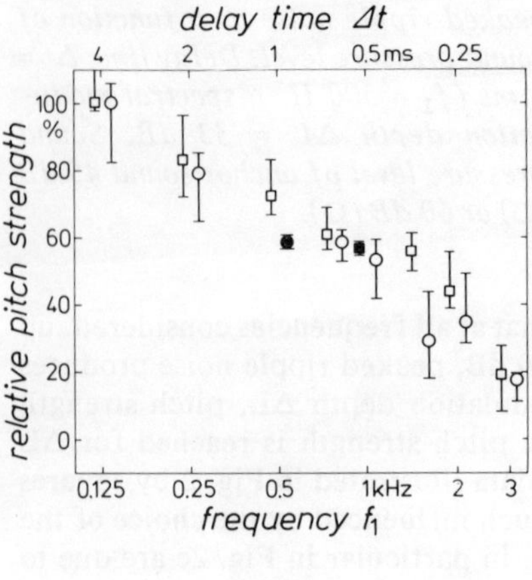

Figure 4: Relative pitch strength of peaked ripple noise as a function of both the frequency f_1 of the first peak in the spectrum and the correlated delay time Δt. Sound pressure level 60 dB, spectral modulation depth ΔL = 33 dB. Frequency f_1 of anchor 0.5 kHz (○) or 1 kHz (□).

60 dB and a frequency $f_T = f_1$ (approximately same pitch). For the six subjects, at f_1 = 0.125, 1, and 3 kHz the peaked ripple noise produced a pitch strength, which is 0.83, 0.5, and 0.2 times the pitch strength of a pure tone of equal pitch. These data are in line with the relative pitch strength data displayed in Fig. 4. For the remaining two subjects, peaked ripple noise at f_1 = 0.125, 1, and 3 kHz produced a pitch strength 0.1, 0.4 and 0.2 times the pitch strength of a pure tone. The correlated factors of pitch strength are in line with the relative pitch strength data at low f_1, but are too high at high f_1. Further studies will be necessary to arrive at firm conclusions with respect to the pitch strength perceived by the group of two subjects.

Since the spectra of the peaked ripple noises were low-pass filtered at 9 kHz (antialiasing), at f_1 = 1.5 kHz only three peaks are within the passband, and at f_1 = 3 kHz only one peak. Therefore, it was checked, whether the pitch strength at high values of f_1 increases, if the bandwidth is increased from 9 to 19 kHz. For the six subjects, whose results are displayed in Fig. 4, the pitch strength increased by 8% at f_1 = 1.5 kHz and by 12% at f_1 = 3 kHz. For the remaining two subjects the increase in bandwidth led to a **decrease** in pitch strength by about 20% at both values of f_1. Obviously, for these subjects additional spectral peaks do not enhance the pitch strength.

Fig. 5 shows the distributions of the frequencies of comparison tones matched in pitch to peaked ripple noises with different frequencies f_1 of the first spectral peak. For the frequencies f_1, "odd" numbers were chosen to avoid musically meaningful intervals like octaves or fifths. The peaked ripple noises had a spectral modulation depth of ΔL = 38 dB and a sound pressure level of 60 dB. The level of the comparison tone was also 60 dB. For each peaked ripple noise, the most prominent pitch was calculated according to the virtual pitch theory (Terhardt *et al.*, 1982). Calculated pitch values are displayed at the upper abscissa in each panel. Arrows pointing downward indicate virtual pitches, arrows pointing upward spectral pitches.

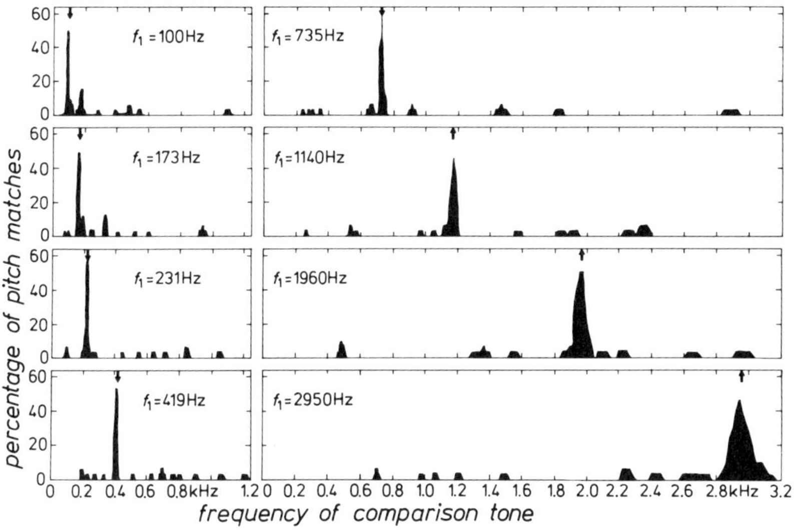

Figure 5: Distributions of the frequencies of comparison tones matched in pitch to peaked ripple noise with frequencies f_1 of the first spectral peak. Percentage of pitch matches within a frequency window of 0.2 Bark bandwidth. Downward pointing arrows represent virtual pitch values, upward pointing arrows spectral pitch values as calculated according to Terhardt et al. (1982).

The results displayed in Fig. 5 show that the maxima in the histograms of the comparison frequency coincide with the frequency f_1 of the peaked ripple noise. At f_1 = 100 Hz and 173 Hz, side maxima show up, which lie an octave above the main maximum. More detailed inspection reveals that at low f_1, the maximum of the histogram lies somewhat below the frequency f_1, indicating a negative pitch shift as usual for virtual pitches of complex tones. A comparison of the maxima of the distributions and the arrows in each panel of Fig. 5 shows that the virtual pitch theory nicely predicts the pitch of peaked ripple noise. Up to a frequency of f_1 = 735 Hz the pitch is classified as virtual pitch (downward pointing arrows), at higher values of f_1, the theory predicts spectral pitches (upward pointing arrows).

Conclusion

When feeding back delayed versions of a noise to the input, rippled noise with sharp spectral peaks can be produced. Peaked ripple noise with a spectral modulation depth ΔL = 33 dB can elicit a pitch strength, which amounts to about 0.85 times the pitch strength of a pure tone of same pitch. For spectral modulation depths below about 10 dB, peaked ripple noise produces no pitch strength, however, a distinct colouration (e.g. Bilsen and Raatgever, 1983). For spectral modulation depths above about 10 dB, pitch strength increases with ΔL. With increasing sound pressure level, the pitch strength of peaked ripple noise decreases somewhat. With increasing frequency of the first peak in the spectrum, and hence with increasing peak spacing, the pitch strength of peaked ripple noise decreases almost linearly with the logarithm of frequency. For some subjects, a more bandpass-like dependence may occur. The pitch of peaked ripple noise corresponds to the frequency of the first peak in the spectrum. This pitch can be predicted by means of the virtual pitch model (Terhardt *et al.* 1982), despite the fact that this theory was originally designed for line spectra and not for continuous spectra.

Although the pitch of peaked ripple noise corresponds numerically to a distinct **spectral** feature of this sound, i.e. the first peak in the spectrum at the frequency f_1, the virtual pitch theory predicts a virtual pitch for peaked ripple noises with frequencies f_1 up to 735 Hz. There are several indicators which suggest an interpretation of the pitch of peaked ripple noise as a **virtual** pitch, like the octave ambiguities and pitch shifts at low frequencies, and the slight decrease of pitch strength with level. In addition, Bilsen and Raatgever (1983) showed JND's in frequency for peaked ripple noise as low as 0.2% at 100 Hz peak spacing which are typical for virtual pitch, but too small for spectral pitch. Therefore, an interpretation of the pitch of peaked ripple noise as a virtual pitch seems to be appropriate, at least for peak spacings up to about 750 Hz.

References

Bilsen, F.A. (**1966**). " Repetition pitch: monaural interaction of a sound with the repetition of the same, but phase shifted sound." Acustica **17**, 295-300.

Bilsen, F.A. and Raatgever, J. (**1983**). "Monotic and dichotic pitch JND's compared." In: *Hearing-Physiological Bases and Psychophysics*, edited by R.Klinke and R.Hartman (Springer, Berlin).

Bilsen, F.A. and Ritsma, R.R. (**1970**). " Some parameters influencing the perceptibility of pitch." J.Acoust.Soc.Am. **47**, 469-476.

Bilsen, F.A. and Wieman, J.L. (**1980**). "A tonal periodicity sensation of comb filtered noise signals." In: *Psychophysical, Physiological and Behavioural Studies in Hearing*, edited by G. van den Brink and F.A. Bilsen (Delft University Press), pp. 379-382.

Buunen, T.J.F. (**1980**). "The effect of stimulus duration on the prominence of pitch." In: *Psychophysical, Physiological and Behavioural Studies in Hearing*, edited by G. van den Brink and F.A. Bilsen (Delft University Press), pp. 374-377.

Fastl, H. (**1980**). "Pitch strength and masking patterns of low-pass noise." In: *Psychophysical, Physiological and Behavioural Studies in Hearing*, edited by G. van den Brink and F.A. Bilsen (Delft University Press), pp. 334-339.

Fastl, H. (**1981**). "Ausgeprägtheit der Tonhöhe pulsmodulierter Breitband-

rauschen." In: Fortschritte der Akustik, DAGA'81, VDE-Verlag Berlin, 725-728.
Fastl, H. and Stoll, G. (**1979**). "Scaling of pitch strength." Hearing Res. **1**, 293-301.
Lundeen, C. and Small, A.M.Jr. (**1984**). "The influence of temporal cues on the strength of periodicity pitches." J.Acoust.Soc.Am. **75**, 1578-1587.
Ritsma, R.R. and Bilsen, F.A. (**1970**). "Spectral regions dominant in the perception of repetition pitch." Acustica **23**, 334-339.
Terhardt, E., Stoll, G. and Seewann, M. (**1982**). "Algorithm for extraction of pitch and pitch salience from complex tonal signals." J.Acoust.Soc.Am. **71**, 679-688.
Wilson, J.P. (**1967**). "Psychoacoustics of obstacle detection using ambient or self-generated noise." In: *Animal Sonar Systems*, edited by R.G. Russel. (Jony-en-Josas) pp. 89-114.
Wilson, J.P. (**1980**). "Comment to the paper by F.A. Bilsen and J.L. Wieman." In: *Psychophysical, Physiological and Behavioural Studies in Hearing*, edited by G. van den Brink and F.A. Bilsen (Delft U.P., The Netherlands).
Yost, W.A. (**1980**). "Temporal properties of the pitch and pitch strength of ripple noise". In: *Psychophysical, Physiological and Behavioural Studies in Hearing*, edited by G. van den Brink and F.A. Bilsen (Delft U.P., The Netherlands).
Yost, W.A. (**1982**). "The dominance region and ripple noise pitch: A test of the peripheral weighting model." J.Acoust.Soc.Am. **72**, 416-425.
Yost, W.A. and Hill, R. (**1978**). "Strength of the pitches associated with ripple noise." J.Acoust.Soc.Am. **64**, 485-492.
Yost, W.A., Hill, R. and Perez-Falcon, T. (**1978**). "Pitch and pitch discrimination of broadband signals with rippled power spectra." J.Acoust.Soc.Am. **64**, 1166-1173.
Zwicker, E. and Feldtkeller, R. (**1967**). *Das Ohr als Nachrichtenempfänger*. 2. erw. Auflage (Hirzel-Verlag, Stuttgart).

Comments

Bilsen:

According to dr. Fastl's Fig. 2 peaked ripple noise, up to a spectral modulation depth of about 10 dB, does not produce pitch strength. This seems in contradiction with the threshold of perceptibility of repetition pitch (i.e. the "virtual pitch" of cosine ripple noise), viz. a spectral modulation depth of about 1 dB, as found by Bilsen and Ritsma (1970). The discrepancy might be due to the fact that dr. Fastl uses a stationary stimulus rather than a dynamic ("musical") stimulus.

Investigating spectral dominance, Raatgever *et al.* (1986) performed pitch matchings for the same stimulus as used by dr. Fastl, viz. anharmonic peaked comb noise, though with a periodic pulse in a background noise as a matching signal instead of a pure tone. Their (averaged) results of three trained subjects can roughly be summarized as follows (see figure). For $\Delta t > 4$ ms, pitch values were found equal to $1.10/\Delta t$ and/or $0.90/\Delta t$ (95%-confidence interval $\pm$ 0.02). For $\Delta t < 5$ ms, pitch matchings centered around $0.500/\Delta t$ (95%-confidence interval $\pm$ 0.005), thus around a frequency equal to the lowest peak (f_1) present in the spectrum. Basically, the same results were found for cosine comb noise. Inspecting dr. Fastl's Fig. 5, pitch matchings are found mainly around f_1 for *all* values of Δt, and around $2f_1(=1/\Delta t)$ for $\Delta t > 5$ ms (roughly taken). It cannot be read from this figure whether the latter results are in agreement with those from Raatgever *et al.* or not.

However, the interpretation of the results by dr. Fastl on the basis of the virtual pitch theory puzzles me, viz. the fact that "up to a frequency of f_1 = 735 Hz the (f_1)pitch is classified as virtual pitch", and only as spectral pitch for higher f_1-values. I would expect that a theory based on a best harmonic spectral fit (e.g. Central Spectrum Theory, or Optimum Processor Theory) would predict the virtual pitch to be equal to something like $1.1/\Delta t$ and/or $0.9/\Delta t$, so roughly speaking one octave higher. Do the theories predict differently, or is the "dominance region" incorporated differently?

Raatgever, J. and Bakkum, M.J. (1986). "Spectral dominance for noise signals with monaural and dichotic comb spectra". Proc. 12th Int. Congr. Acoust., Toronto, B2-4.

PITCH OF PEAKED COMB NOISE

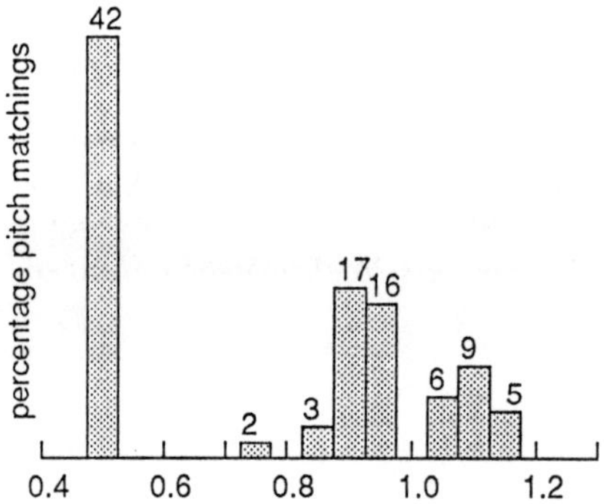

Reply by Fastl:

Peaked ripple noise with spectral modulation depths smaller than ΔL=10dB shows a distinct colouration which may account for the threshold of perceptibility at small values of ΔL.

Figure 5 in my paper shows that, in agreement with the data of Raatgever and Bakkum (1986), most pitches are matched to the first peak in the spectrum of peaked ripple noise. From our 32 pitch matches we can not decide, whether in the panel for f_1=100 Hz, the second maximum around 200 Hz can be split up further.

The virtual pitch theory predicts several pitches of different weight. All arrows in Fig.5 indicate the pitch with the **largest** weight for the respective peaked ripple noise. Pitches, which are roughly one octave higher are also predicted by the virtual pitch model, however with smaller weight.

Schroeder:

The following standard designations suggest themselves for the two kinds of rippled noises mentioned by Fastl. The "peaked ripple" noise obtained by a feedback filter with an **infinite** impulse response, commonly designated by the letters IIR. The "cosine" noise is obtained by a **finite** impulse response, or FIR, filter. Thus, the two noises might be called IIR- and FIR-noises, respectively, in agreement with standard electrical engineering nomenclature.

Houtsma:

The measure one obtains for pitch strength of a sound may be very much dependent on the operational definition of pitch strength and, consequently on the way one measures it. Besides the method of scaling you employed, one could also assess pitch strength by the size of the pitch JND, by the magnitude of the delayed noise image necessary for detection (Yost and Hill, 1978) or by the degree to which subjects can correctly identify the notes of a random melody played with such sounds (Houtsma,1983). As long as different methods lead to different results, I feel we do not really understand the concept of pitch strength.

Houtsma, A.J.M., "Pitch salience for various complex sounds", Music Perception (1983)

Reply by Fastl:

I agree with Dr. Houtsma that there exist several methods to assess the pitch strength of sounds. We chose the method of magnitude estimation, since it is the only one of the methods mentioned, which yields a *direct* estimate of pitch strength. With the other methods, the pitch strength has to be derived from the data using additional assumptions.

The influence of duration on the perception of single and simultaneous two-tone complexes

John G. Beerends and Adrianus J.M. Houtsma

Institute for Perception Research / IPO
P.O. Box 513, NL 5600 MB Eindhoven, The Netherlands

Introduction

When the duration of a bandlimited signal is shortened, its spectrum is broadened. This can be represented, under certain conditions by the equality $\Delta f \Delta t = constant$. One perceptual consequence of this relation is that the pitch of short tones is less salient than the pitch of longer ones. The effect of stimulus duration on the pitch of pure tones has been investigated by several authors (Moore, 1973; Majernik and Kaluzny, 1979). The effect of duration on the pitch of complex tones has been investigated to a lesser extent. The evidence nevertheless suggests that complex tones are affected by duration in a similar manner as pure tones (Ritsma *et al.*, 1966).

All these studies, however, focussed on the frequency uncertainty Δf, measured as a just noticable difference in a discriminative task, or a standard deviation in a pitch matching task. It is now common believed that the pitch percept of a complex tone results from a pattern recognizer. In the Optimum Processor theory of Goldstein (1973) the accuracy with which this pattern recognizer operates is specified by a noise function (the "sigma function"), which is the model's only free parameter. One of the objectives of this study is to investigate the dependence of that sigma function on stimulus duration. Two experiments are discussed. The first one studies the effect of tone duration on the pitch percept of isolated complex tones. The second one explores the influence of tone duration on the pitches of two simultaneously presented complex tones.

Experiment 1

Subjects were asked to identify single notes represented by two harmonics $f_1 = mf_{01}$ and $f_2 = (m+1)f_{01}$, where the fundamental f_{01} was 200, 225, 250, 267, or 300 Hz with equal probability. This choice of fundamental frequencies musically produces the notes "do, re, mi, fa, so" in just temperament. The harmonic numbers m were randomly chosen between 2 and 10 on each trial, so that the total stimulus set contained 45 elements, each of

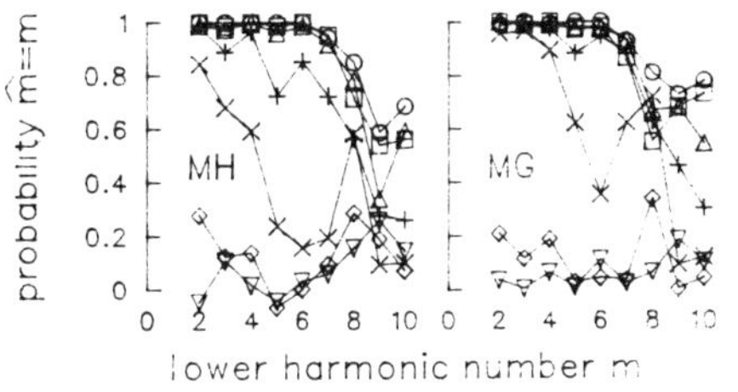

Figure 1. Probability of a correct harmonic number estimate, $Pr[\hat{m} = m]$ for two subjects and 7 durations. ○ = 600 ms, □ = 100 ms, △ = 50 ms, + = 20 ms, × = 10 ms, ◇ = 5 ms, ▽ = 2 ms, excluding the ramps of 2 ms.

which was presented about 20 times. Duration of the complex tones was varied from 600 ms to 2 ms, using a linear on/offset ramp of 2 ms, but was held constant within runs. The stimuli were gated on and off at random phase to prevent identification on artifacts caused by transients. All stimuli were presented diotically, 20 dB above masked threshold, with 30 dB SL broadband white noise (50-5000 Hz) as masking background. This procedure roughly yields equally loud tones within each given run, while the noise masks aural distortion products that might arise as unwanted partials.

Subjects seated in a sound-proof chamber were instructed to play each note back on a five-note keyboard. They were given unlimited response time, no feedback, and their response triggered presentation of the next stimulus with some fixed delay. All four subjects were first tested for their ability to identify the five notes when they were represented by pure tones of 600 ms and frequency f_{01}. They scored better than 99 percent correct, which indicated that they possessed the musical skill to perform the task.

Results

Responses to the various fundamental frequencies (or notes) were pooled for each lower harmonic number m to reduce the data to a count of correct identification as a function of m. With these scores the optimum processor's probabilities of correctly estimating the harmonic number m, $Pr[\hat{m} = m]$, were computed (Beerends and Houtsma 1986), from which one can easily calculate the sigma function of the central processor (Goldstein 1973). The results

Table I. Uncertainty products $\sigma\Delta t$ for different frequencies and durations averaged over two subjects.

Duration Δt (ms)	Frequency (Hz) 750	1000	1250	1500	1750	2000	2250	2500	2750
100	1.2	0.6	0.7	0.7	0.8	0.8	0.9	1.0	1.2
50	0.8	0.3	0.3	0.4	0.4	0.4	0.5	0.6	0.7
20	0.4	0.2	0.2	0.2	0.2	0.3	0.3	0.4	0.6
10	0.3	0.3	0.3	0.3	0.3	0.3	0.4	0.4	0.5
5	1.1	0.9	0.8	0.8	0.8	0.7	0.5	0.4	0.3

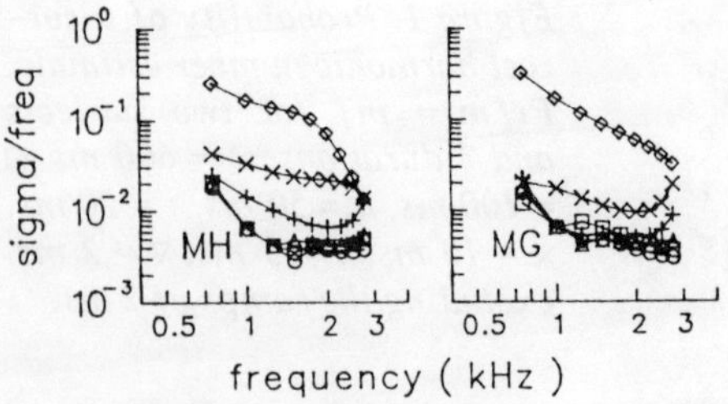

Figure 2. Sigma functions, σ/f, representing frequency coding noise, for two subjects and the 6 longest durations (see Fig. 1).

shown in Fig. 1 indicate that, when two-tone complexes are shortened, the dependence of $\Pr[\hat{m} = m]$ becomes non monotonic. This is seen most prominently for stimulus durations of 10 ms where $\Pr[\hat{m} = m = 6]$ is about 0.3 whereas the scores for $m = 8$ are about 0.6. The most logical explanation for this effect is that, for short complex tones, subjects tend to switch to the analytic mode of perception. For stimuli where none of the partials has an octave relationship to the missing fundamental (for instance when m equals 5 or 6), analytic listening always leads to a wrong pitch estimate. On the other hand, when one of the partials has an octave relationship to the missing fundamental (m equals 7 or 8) analytic listening tends to lead to correct responses.

The effect of analytic listening confounds a simple interpretation of the data in terms of the Optimum Processor model, because this model only describes the synthetic mode of pitch perception. The effect of duration on the "synthetic" pitch can be estimated by fitting a parabolic function through the data points of Fig. 1 and calculating the corresponding sigma values from these fitted functions. Sigma functions thus calculated are given in Fig. 2. From these sigma values we calculated the uncertainty products $\sigma\Delta t$ as given in Table I.

Experiment 2

In this experiment the same subjects were asked to identify the pitches of two simultaneously sounding diotic notes, each represented by two harmonics, $f_1 = mf_{01}$, $f_2 = (m+1)f_{01}$, $f_3 = nf_{02}$ and $f_4 = (n+1)f_{02}$. The fundamentals f_{01} and f_{02} were both elements of the same stimulus set "do, re, mi, fa, so" (200, 225, 250, 267, 300 Hz) that was used in the first experiment and could not be the same. Both (lower) harmonic numbers m and n varied randomly between values of 2 and 10, although within an experimental run they were limited to ranges of 3, independent for m and n. Each of the 810 physically different stimuli was, on the average, presented about three times.

Stimuli were presented under the same conditions as in experiment 1. The subjects were first tested for their ability to perform the two-note identification task with both fundamentals f_{01} and f_{02} represented by single sinusoids of 600 ms. All subjects produced an essentially perfect score (better than 99 percent correct).

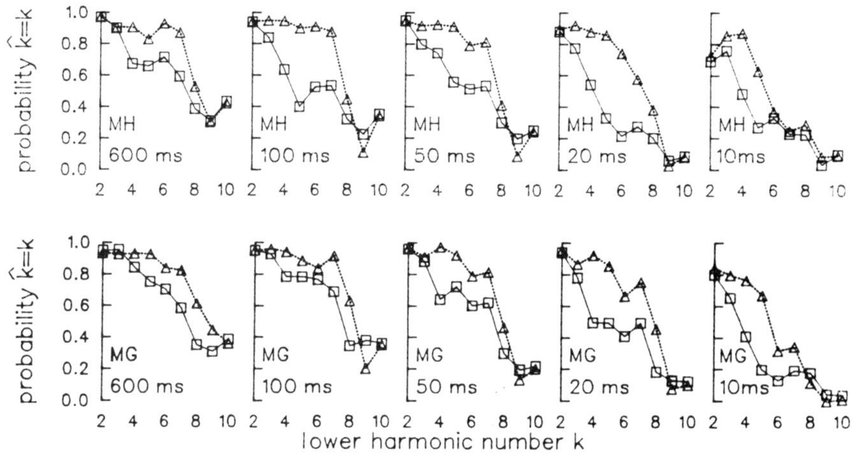

Figure 3. Two sets of underlying probabilities of correctly estimating the harmonic number of one complex tone for two subjects and 5 durations in a two-note identification task. The first set, △, gives the probabilities of correctly estimating the harmonic number k when the complex tone has the most salient pitch, i.e. the one with the lowest harmonic numbers. The second set, □, gives the same probabilities but for the less salient one. The harmonic numbers k can represent m or n depending on the context.

Results

The raw data of this experiment consisted of a record for each trial of the presented fundamentals f_{01} and f_{02}, their lower harmonic numbers m and n, and the subject's two responses R_a and R_b. The responses to the notes were pooled and analysed in terms of identification of individual notes.

From this analysis we can calculate two sets of underlying probabilities of correct identification, one describing the identification of the most salient pitch, i.e., the pitch of the complex which is represented by the lowest harmonic numbers, and another describing the identification of the less salient pitch, the one represented by the higher harmonic numbers. Figure 3 shows these probability functions for the subjects for five different durations. As can be seen, the effect of nonmonotonic behaviour is much less pronounced than in the single identification experiment indicating that subjects used mainly synthetic pitch cues for the identification of the two notes. These two sets of underlying processor probabilities show that the identification performance for the less salient pitch is more affected by the shortening of the notes. This effect is for subject MH already noticable with durations of about 100 ms where the $\Pr[\hat{k} = k]$ for the less salient pitch in the region of $k = 5,6$ drops from about 0.7 to 0.45 while the performance for the most salient one remains about the same. In the single identification experiment the shortening of the notes from 600 to 100 ms did not affect the identification performance. This effect although less prominent can also be seen with the other subject MG.

From the correct identification scores for the most salient pitch we calculated again a set of sigma functions for the different durations in the simultaneous identification experiment. The sigma values for durations longer than 10 ms were about twice as large as those obtained in the single note identification experiment, while for the duration of 10ms they were about the same.

Two main conclusions can be drawn from the quantitative results shown in Table I and in Fig. 1-3. (i) When isolated complex tones are shortened subjects often switch to the analytic mode of perception. (ii) When simultaneous complex tones are shortened the less salient pitch is affected first.

Acknowledgement

This work was supported by the Netherlands Organisation for Scientific Research (N.W.O.), through the foundation Psychon, grant# 560-260-009.

References

Beerends, J.G., and Houtsma, A.J.M. (**1986**). "Pitch identification of simultaneous dichotic two-tone complexes," J.Acoust.Soc.Am. **80**, 1048-1055.

Goldstein, J.L. (**1973**). "An optimum processor theory for the central formation of the pitch of complex tones," J.Acoust.Soc.Am. **54**, 1496-1516.

Majernik, V., and Kaluzny, J. (**1979**). "On the auditory uncertainty relations," Acustica **43**, 132-146.

Moore, B.C.J. (**1973**). "Frequency difference limens for short-duration tones," J.Acoust.Soc.Am. **54**, 610-619.

Ritsma, R.J., Cardozo, B.L., Domburg, G., and Neelen, J.J.M. (**1966**). "The build-up of the pitch percept," IPO Annual Progress Report **1**, 12-15.

Comments

Moore:

You suggest that the non-monotonic functions relating performance to harmonic number for short-duration tones can be explained by assuming that subjects switch to an analytic mode of perception (hearing individual partials) for short tones. However, several sets of results suggest exactly the opposite; analytic perception becomes less likely for short tones. For example, Moore *et al.* (1986) measured the degree of mistuning from a harmonic frequency required for a partial to be heard as a separate component in a complex tone. They found that the degree of mistuning increased as the duration decreased.

In other words, the tones were more likely to fuse into a single percept at short durations. I think that you must seek some other explanation for your non-monotonic functions.

Moore, B.C.J., Glasberg, B.R. and Peters, R.W. (1986). "Thresholds for hearing mistuned partials as separate tones in harmonic complexes," J.Acoust.Soc.Am. 80, 479-483.

Reply by Beerends and Houtsma:

I am afraid we are employing a somewhat different operational definition of analytic and synthetic hearing compared with Moore *et al.* (1986). The empirical fact that the frequency coding noise "sigma" increases with decreasing stimulus duration, is quite consistent with Moore *et al.*'s finding that perceptual tolerance for a frequency-shifted partial of a harmonic tone complex increases as well. Our notion of synthetic listening in pitch perception focusses on "hearing the missing fundamental" rather than on "do all partials integrate to one percept". Because the evidence in our experiment is rather indirect we did the following preliminary experiment. Subjects were presented the same stimuli as in experiment 2 except that they were presented sequentially. In each presentation a random duration of 1-500 ms was presented. The task of the subject was to determine whether the pitch went up or down. In stimuli where frequencies and missing fundamental both went up the correct identification was about 99% (Fig.C1, circles). For stimuli where the frequencies moved opposite to the missing fundamental we plotted the percentage of trials in which the frequency direction of the partials was identified correctly (Fig.C1, crosses). The results show that for long durations synthetic hearing dominates the pitch percept, whereas for short durations spectral features seem to dominate.

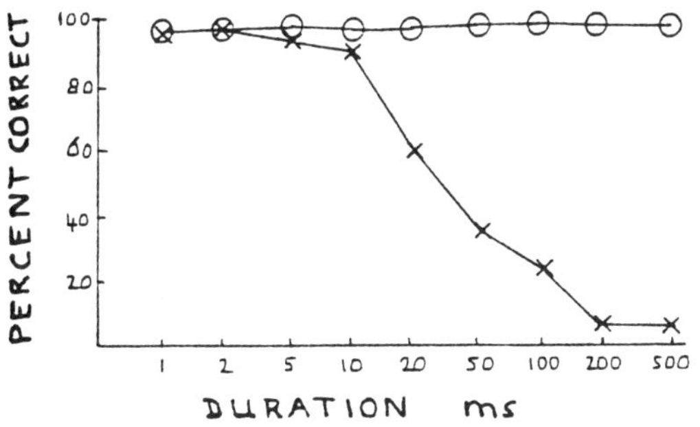

Figure C1.

Multiple images - psychoacoustical data and model predictions

W. Gaik and S. Wolf

Lehrstuhl für allgemeine Elektrotechnik und Akustik
Ruhr-Universität Bochum, Fed. Rep. of Germany

Introduction

To determine the angle of incidence of sounds, the binaural system mainly evaluates two parameters: the interaural arrival time difference (ITD) and the interaural intensity difference (IID). The interaural parameters are integrated over frequency ranges which correspond to the well known critical bands (Scharf et al., 1976).

Examining the lateralization of narrow band noise it can be observed that certain combinations of ITD and IID result in the perception of two auditory events. This was already reported in the literature (e.g. Whitworth and Jeffress, 1961; Ruotolo, Stern and Colburn, 1979; Lindemann, 1986), but quantitative results are still rare and sometimes even contradictory. Therefore lateralization experiments have been carried out with special attention to the rise of additional images. The results of the experiments have been compared with predictions of two different models.

The experiment

Experimental setup

Signals were generated (Fig.1) by a noise generator (pink noise) and passed

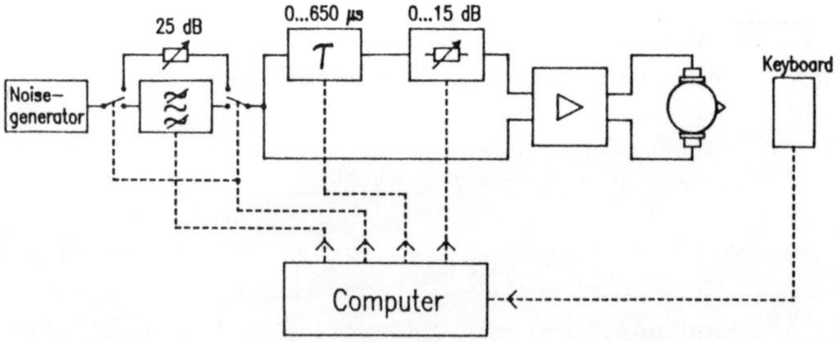

Figure 1. Experimental setup for the lateralization experiment.

Table 1. Parameters used in the experiment. Each interaural difference (delay-time or attenuation) was used in combination with each filter setting.

	Filter settings	Delays	Attenuations
1	200 Hz....300 Hz	0.00 ms	3 dB
2	400 Hz....510 Hz	0.20 ms	6 dB
3	630 Hz....770 Hz	0.35 ms	9 dB
4	997 Hz, 20% bandwidth	0.50 ms	12 dB
5	1.37 kHz, 20% bandwidth	0.65 ms	15 dB
6	1.85 kHz, 20% bandwidth		
7	2.50 kHz, 20% bandwidth		
8	3.41 kHz, 20% bandwidth		

through a bandpass filter (90 dB/oct). The filter output was used as the right channel of the test signal, its delayed or attenuated version as the left one. Both channels were amplified and presented to the subjects via earphones (Sennheiser HD 424) at a level of approx. 70 dB (SPL). Prior to every experimental run, pink noise was presented diotically to let the subject center the image by adjusting the balance of the amplifier. For this purpose the filter was bypassed using a programmable switch. Filter, delay, attenuator, and switch were controlled by a computer (Siemens PC 16-11) via an IEEE-488 interface.

Method

Five different delay-times and five attenuations were used, giving a total of ten interaural conditions in eight critical bands (Tab.1). Each of the eighty stimuli was presented with two preceding reference signals, namely the diotic and monotic noise signals in the corresponding critical band. The reference signals lasted one second each, whereas the subjects could listen to the test signal as long as they wanted. Each triple of stimuli could be repeated several times, if desired. The subjects were asked to report the laterality of the perceived auditory event or, in case of two auditory events, the laterality and the relative loudness of both. The lateral position of the images was described on a scale from -10 (left) to +10 (right); relative loudness of each image was reported in percentage of total loudness. The subjects' responses were directly entered into the computer. Four subjects took part in the experiment; three of them were experienced in lateralization and other psychoacoustic experiments (HS, SW and WG). All subjects ran the test twice.

Results and discussion

The reported images may be classified into different categories: the central auditory event and a second image, which appeared only at the very right position. One of the subjects (SW) also reported an additional image on the left in the case of ITDs greater than 0.35 ms in the third, fourth and fifth

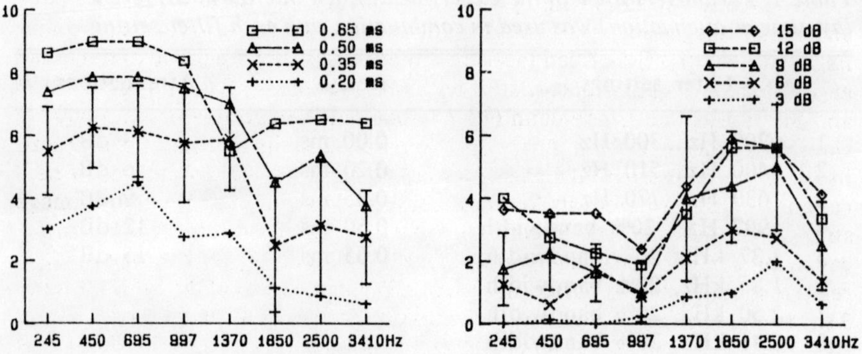

Figure 2. Averaged lateralization of the central image as a function of frequency. Parameters are ITD (left) or IID (right). To avoid confusion the standard deviation is plotted only for one curve.

frequency band (Tab.1). Due to the quasi periodic shape of the bandpass filtered signals, these images appear to be closely related to the ambiguities also observed by other authors (e.g. Yost, 1981; Sayers, 1964; for a detailed discussion see Blauert, 1983). Cross-correlation models of binaural hearing show similar behaviour with respect to the formation of side-lobes.

The lateral position of the central image (also referred to as "binaural image" in this text) is determined by the value of ITD or IID. Like other authors (e.g. Trahiotis and Bernstein, 1986), we found that with respect to fixed ITD lateral displacement decreases with increasing frequency (Fig.2, left). In case of IID the reported displacement of the binaural image slightly increases with frequency (Fig.2, right).

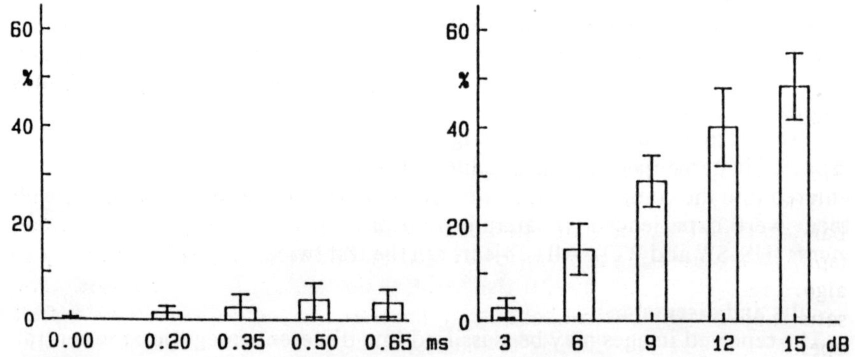

Figure 3. Averaged rel. loudness of monaural image as a function of ITD (left) and IID (right). Dotted line: 1st run of subject DM ignored.

As already observed in preliminary experiments, the detection of additional images was extremely facilitated by preceding reference signals. Especially the IID signals led to second images, which were mainly lateralized at position 10. This is in accordance with observations by Ruotolo et al. (1979) and the results that Lindemann (1986) obtained in experiments with 500 Hz sinusoids. Due to the similarity to the perception in monotic hearing this image is called "monaural image". Its lateral position was found not to be a function of IID, whereas its loudness compared to that of the binaural image strongly depends on IID. Except for the first run of subject DM, a significantly higher number of monaural images and also a higher average of their relative loudness was reported in case of IID compared to ITD (Tab.2). Figure 3 shows the relative loudness of the monaural images as a function of ITD and IID, averaged over all subjects and frequency bands (relative loudness was assumed to be zero if no monaural image was reported). It is obvious that with IIDs monaural images were much more prominent than with ITDs.

Table 2. Number of reported monaural images (n) and their averaged relative loudness (LR) for stimuli with pure time/intensity difference. Total number of signals was 32/40 (zero delay was not taken into account).

	1st run		2nd run	
Subject	n	LR (%)	n	LR(%)
DM	10/17	61/46	1/15	10/53
HS	5/27	16/41	4/32	29/45
SW	10/31	21/40	8/30	20/33
WG	2/31	15/36	4/31	19/31

Model predictions

Two models of binaural hearing were involved in the simulation of the above mentioned psychoacoustical data. Both are based on the interaural cross-correlation function extended by contralaterally acting inhibitory processes.

Simulations with the probabilistic model

The probabilistic lateralization model uses the ear input signals (after bandpass filtering and half-wave rectification) to generate series of impulses (spikes), representing neural activity in the auditory nerve. This is done by an algorithm (Duifhuis, 1972) that takes into account refractoriness and saturation. In each critical band several hundred of these spike generators are operating in parallel. Similar to the model suggested by Jeffress (1948), the spikes from left and right are running along delay lines and lead to coincidences. A running integration is performed over the coincidences at each tap of the delay line, which results in a timevarying coincidence pattern.

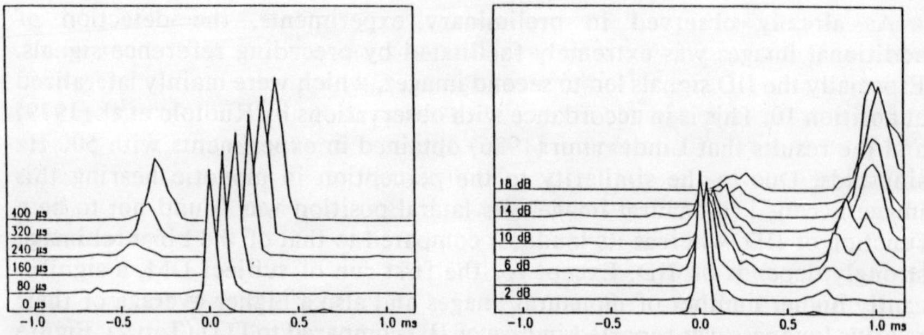

Figure 4. Model predictions (probabilistic model) for sinusoidal signals with interaural time (left) and intensity differences (right).

The location of each peak in the pattern is identified with the lateral position of an auditory event. In order to get correct model predictions for signals with interaural time as well as intensity differences, an additional mechanism was introduced which cancels each pair of spikes that has led to a coincidence. The resulting effect is comparable to the inhibition mechanism of the deterministic model described below: suppression of side-lobes in the coincidence pattern, increased sharpness of the peaks (contrast enhancement), and enabling of the identification of each peak with an auditory event.

The model is implemented on a computer and, caused by the poisson process that is part of the spike generating algorithm, produces one realization of a stochastic process each time it is run (Wolf, 1987).

Figure 4 shows model predictions for sinusoidal signals (1 kHz) with ITDs of 0 to 0.4 ms and IIDs of 0 to 18 dB. For increasing ITD, the central image is shifted accordingly, with a second image arising on the contralateral side. For increasing IID, the central image moves to the side and decreases in amplitude, with a second image appearing on the ipsilateral side and growing in amplitude. Both model predictions are consistent with the results of the lateralization experiment.

Simulations with the deterministic model

Our deterministic model is a further development of the model proposed by Lindemann (1986). It consists of parallel structures allowing the calculation of activity patterns over the whole audio frequency range. The input section splits the incoming signals into bandpass signals according to the critical bands given by Zwicker and Feldtkeller (1967). In contrast to the probabilistic model described above, time functions are calculated which approximately represent the firing probabilities of nerve fibers in each critical band. This preprocessing stage mainly consists of half-wave rectification and bandpass filtering to obtain the envelopes instead of the signal's fine structure in higher frequency ranges. A non linear component with regard to saturation effects in firing probability was simply introduced by extracting the square root of the obtained functions. Hence it is obvious that the signal preprocessing technique used in this model was not designed as an accurate reproduction of the peripheral system but as a compromise between simulation of the peripheral auditory system and reasonable computational effort.

The preprocessed signals are then fed into parallel "binaural processors". Within each critical band the corresponding signals from both ears are passed through delay lines. Interaction of the two signals is achieved by contralateral inhibition. After each sampling interval the "inhibited cross-correlation function" is calculated by multiplying and integrating the contents of the delay lines.

Contralateral inhibition does not only increase the contrast in the resulting patterns, but also leads to a dependence upon IID in addition to the cross-correlation function's dependence on ITD. The inhibition mechanism developed by Lindemann had to be changed to avoid the undesireable influence of signal amplitude on model performance. An adaptive algorithm was introduced to adjust the strength of the contralateral inhibition to the long-term spectrum of the input signal.

Since cross-correlation models fail in simulating monotic listening situations, detectors for monaural auditory events have to be implemented (models of binaural unmasking also use monaural processors, see the survey by Colburn and Durlach, 1978). In this model signal components arriving at the end of the delay lines contribute to the formation of monaural auditory events. This provides a simple explanation of the psychoacoustical data reported above. With respect to the model, binaural fusion is equivalent to complete mutual inhibition of the signals. Differences in intensity produce an asymmetrical inhibition, which is equivalent to incomplete fusion. Hence some energy is left in the more intense signal, which then proceeds to the end of the delay line, causing a second relative maximum in the pattern. Model runs with the signals used in the psychoacoustical experiment have been carried out. The results show high correspondence with the psychoacoustical data (Gaik, 1987).

The explanation given above of the rise of monaural images fails if natural signals are taken into account, which almost always contain IIDs without yielding any monaural images. Hence the asymmetrical effect of the inhibition must be eliminated if the coincidence of the signals takes place at a position on the correlation axis, which corresponds (in terms of interaural delay) in a natural manner to the amount of IID. Meanwhile our deterministic model was extended by a mechanism which makes use of the knowledge of natural combinations of interaural parameters. Figure 5 shows model results obtained with a dummy head recorded noise signal in the frequency range from 400 to 510 Hz with an IID of 4.2 dB and an ITD of 0.5 ms, which represent one natural combination of interaural parameters for the dummy head we used. The solid line shows the inhibited cross-correlation function. Increasing the level in the contralateral ear gives rise to a second relative maximum representing the monaural image. Also the binaural image is shifted closer to the center and becomes broader because of the reduced strength of inhibition. These phenomena correspond very much to the

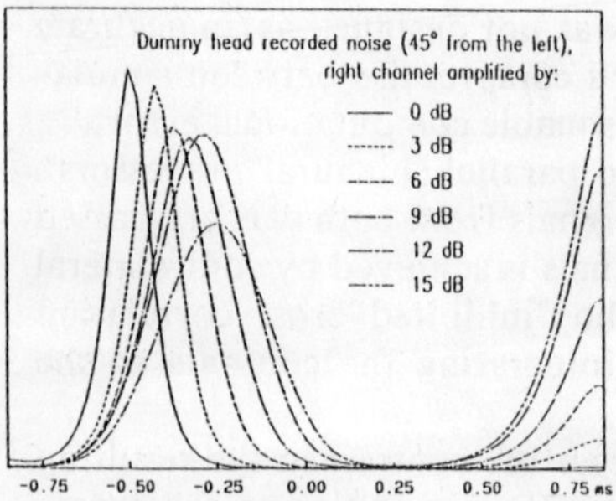

Figure 5. Model results, illustrating the formation of a monaural image. The scale (in ms) corresponds to the correlation axis.

perception which can be observed when trying to recenter an image by means of changing the IID.

Summary

Our results can be summarized as follows:

(1) The configuration of two reference signals (diotic and monotic) preceding the test signal facilitates the detection of multiple images by focusing the subjects' attention on monaural images.

(2) ITDs in narrow band noise signals yield a shift of the perceived image depending on frequency and amount of ITD. Because of the quasi periodic shape of the stimuli, second central (contralateral) images occur in certain frequency ranges.

(3) The perceived auditory events, when using IID stimuli, may be described as follows. With low IIDs only one image can be detected. With increasing IID this image moves towards the ear stimulated by the more intense signal and decreases in loudness monotonously. Simultaneously a second (the monaural) image originates at the ear receiving the higher intensity, not changing its location but growing in loudness with increasing IID.

(4) Models of binaural hearing, which make use of mechanisms of contralateral inhibition offer plausible explanations of the observed psychoacoustical phenomena.

References

Blauert, J. (1983). *Spatial hearing - the psychophysics of human sound localization.* (MIT Press, Cambridge, MA).

Colburn, H.S., and Durlach, N.I. (1978). "Models of binaural interaction." *Handbook of perception*, edited by Carterette and Friedman (Academic Press, NY), Vol. IV, pp 467-518.

Duifhuis, H. (1972). *Perceptual analysis of sound*. PhD-thesis, Techn. Hogeschool, Eindhoven, The Netherlands.

Gaik, W. (**1987**). "Simulation binauraler Signalverarbeitung auf der Basis eines Kreuz-Korrelationsmodells: die Lateralisation frequenzgruppen-breiten Rauschens." *Fortschritte der Akustik*, DAGA '87, VDI-Verlag, Düsseldorf, pp 529-532.

Jeffress, L.A. (**1948**). "A place theory of sound." J.Comp.Physiol.Psychol. **61**, 468-486.

Lindemann, W. (**1986**). "Extension of a binaural cross-correlation model by contralateral inhibition. I. Simulation of lateralization for stationary signals." J.Acoust.Soc.Am. **80**, 1608-1622.

Ruotolo, B.R., Stern, R.M., and Colburn, H.S. (**1979**). "Discrimination of symmetric time-intensity traded binaural stimuli. J.Acoust.Soc.Am. **66**, 1733-1737.

Sayers, B. McA. (**1964**). "Acoustic-image lateralization judgements with binaural tones." J.Acoust.Soc.Am. **36**, 923-926.

Scharf, B., Florentine, M., and Meiselman, C.H. (**1976**): "Critical Band in auditory lateralization. Sensory Processes **1**, 109-126.

Trahiotis, C., and Bernstein, L.R. (**1986**). "Lateralization of bands of noise and sinusoidally amplitude-modulated tones: Effects of spectral locus and bandwidth. J.Acoust.Soc.Am. **79**, 1950-1957.

Whitworth, R.H., and Jeffress, L.A. (**1961**). "Time versus intensity in the localization of tones. J.Acoust.Soc.Am. **33**, 925-929.

Wolf, S. (**1987**). "Ein probabilistisches Modell zur Simulation binauraler Phänomene. *Fortschritte der Akustik*, DAGA '87, VDI-Verlag, Düsseldorf, pp 533-536.

Yost, W.A. (**1981**). "Lateral position of sinusoids presented with interaural intensive and temporal differences." J.Acoust.Soc.Am. **70**, 397-409.

Zwicker, E., and Feldtkeller, R. (**1967**). *Das Ohr als Nachrichtenempfänger.* S. Hirzel Verlag, Stuttgart.

Discrimination of direction for complex sounds presented in the free-field

Ervin R. Hafter, Thomas N. Buell, David A. Basiji and Elizabeth E. Shriberg

Department of Psychology, University of California
Berkeley, California, USA

Introduction

The study of sound localization seeks to explain our ability to orient with respect to stimuli encountered in the acoustic environment. With limited exceptions (e.g. Mills, 1958), the majority of what we know about the primary cues for localization, the Interaural Differences of Time and Level (IDTs and IDLs) due to the presence of the head has come from manipulation of signal parameters through earphones.

Whereas listening in the open field is more natural, there are a variety of reasons for using earphones. For one, it is more difficult to model results gathered in the free field where one lacks the independent control over interaural cues easily accomplished with earphones. Therefore, it is hardly surprising that the most widely cited study of localization (Mills, 1958) was restricted to the use of pure tones. Another reason for avoiding loudspeakers is that their frequency-responses are usually more irregular than those of earphones, making it harder to specify the actual nature of the stimulus. And finally, there is the problem that no two loudspeakers have completely identical spectral responses. One can control for the unwanted cues introduced by dissimilarity between the transducers by using a single speaker that is moved between observations (Mills, 1958); another way is to select individual loudspeakers that are indistinguishable in their spectral responses (Banks & Green, 1973), though the adequacy of such selection is open to question and depends on the bandwidths to be tested.

The most effective way to correct for the spectral idiosyncracies of loudspeakers is to preprocess the electrical signals with inverse filters built to counter the resonances in each speaker. To this end, Leiman and Hafter (1973) used computer-controlled attenuators to set the levels of pure tones presented in the free-field. In a reversal on this theme, Wightman and Kistler (1980) and Poesselt, Schroeter, Optiz, Divenyi and Blauert (1986) placed probe microphones in the external auditory meatus to record the spectral effects of the listener's head and ears, and then modified the signals so that when heard through earphones they would mimic those heard in the free-field.

The goal of the current study has been to develop a relatively simple paradigm in which the psychophysics of direct comparison (forced choice) can be used to study sensitivity to direction with *complex signals*. The hope has been to avoid the arduous task of generating a model of the external ear for every possible direction by using inverse filters to flatten the amplitude and phase responses of the individual loudspeakers. In this way, we reap two benefits. First, we can present stimuli as specified, regardless of the characteristics of the speakers. And second, we can feel confident that discriminations are based on differences in azimuth and not on idiosyncratic differences between spectra.

The paper reports preliminary data derived by this method. Among the first measures were Minimum Audible Angles (MAA) taken at three different azimuths. Since studies using earphones have shown that interaural information at the beginning of a stimulus is especially effective, we also examined the ability to integrate interaural information across the duration of the signal (Hafter and Dye, 1983; Hafter, Dye and Wenzel, 1983; Hafter, Buell and Richards, 1988).

Method

Listening Environment

These experiments were conducted in a commercial anechoic chamber (Eckels Corp., 8.3 x 5.4 x 4.0 m) in Tolman Hall at the Univ. of California. As depicted in Figure 1, the listener sat on a height-adjustable chair with his ears at the level of the loudspeakers. His head was at the center of the circle (radius = 1.68 m) on which the speakers were located. The small size of this circle was determined by limitations of the room; however, the acoustics of the far-field were maintained by restricting stimuli to a region above 1 kHz. As seen in the drawing, individual loudspeakers were mounted on tubular rods, each filled with sand to provide damping. The rods were bolted to an iron ring, also filled with sand and oil and placed 1.24 m below the listening plane. The loudspeakers (Audax MHD12P25 FSM-SQ) had radii of 9 cm, which at the distance presented limited the smallest possible angle that could be tested to 3.5°.

Fixation of the head

The most common way to fix an observer's head in sensory experiments is to use dental impressions mounted on a "bite bar." While this is fine for studies of vision, it can reduce control in studies of hearing if biting down on the bar varies tensions in the middle ear muscles (Carmel and Starr, 1963). For this reason we have constructed the optical centering device (OCD) shown in Figure 1. It consists of a plastic head-frame taken from a protective mask used in arc welding. Attached to the top of the frame is a small telescope focussed on a 3-Watt light bulb placed 1.42 m behind the subject's head. Differential diodes within the telescope are used to compute the optical angle

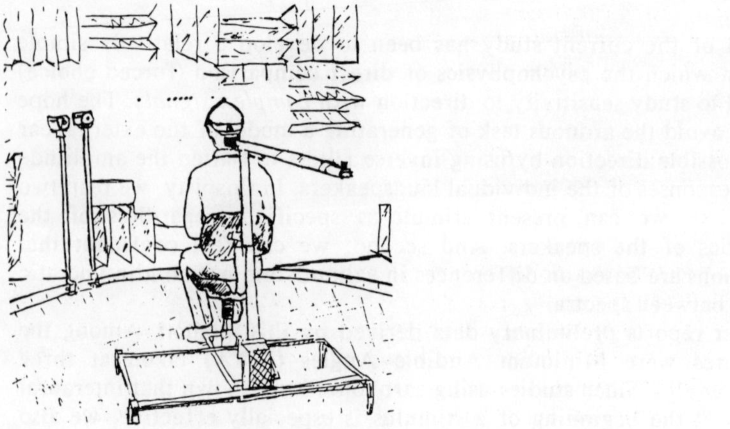

Figure 1. Tracings from a photograph of a listener in the apparatus.

of the telescope. The subject sits comfortably with his neck placed against a rubber cushion and "points" the OCD toward the light using a visual display on the facing wall. The display contains five light emitting diodes (LEDs), the center one green and two on either side red. A true point (within 1° of arc) is signaled when only the green LED is lit, with turns to either side marked by the red LEDs. Subjects report that the OCD offers an easy and relaxed way to maintain alignment.

Stimuli

In these first experiments, the stimuli were restricted to complex sounds about which a great deal was already known from previous studies with earphones; they were high-frequency filtered clicks presented either singly or in trains. The waveform for each click was subjected to an *inverse digital filter* derived for the particular loudspeaker to be used. Inverse filters were obtained by applying a 60-μs pulse to each loudspeaker and using a Hewlett-Packard 3582A FFT spectrum analyzer to compute the cross-spectrum between the pulse and the output of the loudspeaker. Signals generated in the PDP-11/73 computer were converted with 16-bit Digital-to-Analogue circuits at a sampling rate of 50 kHz and reconstructed with 48 dB/octave lowpass filters set to 16 kHz.

Prior to correction for characteristics of the loudspeakers, single clicks were defined by the idealized impulse responses of Gaussian filters. The bandwidths of these filters at the $\pm 1\sigma$ points were ±700 Hz. Of experimental interest were: a) the center frequencies (f_cs) of the clicks; b) the number in a train (n); c) for numbers greater than 1, the Interclick Intervals (ICIs); and d) the azimuth of the pairs of speakers relative to center. Table I lists values of the various parameters.

High sensation levels (SLs) could not be used because, with the pair of speakers set to the minimum separation (3.5°), discrimination was often

Table I. List of tested conditions

f_c (Hz):	2050; 4050; 6050
n:	1; 9; 18
ICI (ms):	4; 12
Azimuth (degrees):	0; 30; 60

perfect. Thus testing was done with clicks which when heard singly were at 10 dB SL. The levels for each f_c and azimuth were established using a "method of limits". Even with these very weak signals, directional discrimination was sometimes well above the classical definition of threshold, which meant that the MAA could be estimated only by extrapolating psychometric functions having no measurable low ends. The low SPLs of the stimuli in combination with the extreme directionality of the speakers ensured that reflections from the walls of the chamber were insignificant.

Task

The subject was a highly trained listener with considerable experience in lateralizing trains of clicks using earphones. Both at the beginning and halfway through the study, the loudspeakers were mounted one above the other to make certain that the signals were not being discriminated on the basis of spectral differences. For each test of localization, a pair of the spectrally equated loudspeakers was placed on either side of the azimuth being studied. The listener maintained head position using the OCD. If at any time the alignment was lost, the computer aborted the trial and waited for him to realign. A two-alternative forced choice paradigm was used to measure performance for each angular setting; the percents correct were converted to d' and a linear fit between d' and angle was used to define thresholds (at a d' of 1.0). Occasional two-point psychometric functions were gathered in order to test the assumption of linearity.

Results and discussion

It is difficult to capture the results of a multi-parameter experiment in any single plot. In order to allow individual drawings to stress specific comparisons, there is some repetition of data in the figures.

Minimum Audible Angles

Figure 2 plots MAAs for f_cs of 2050, 4050 and 6050 Hz at azimuths 0°, 30° and 60°. Only the conditions with ICIs of 12 ms are included. The lines, taken from Mills (1958), are included for comparison. The most prominent feature here is the strong improvement in performance from single clicks to trains. Of course, lower thresholds are to be expected if information is accumulated across the duration of a train and this factor is discussed in more detail below.

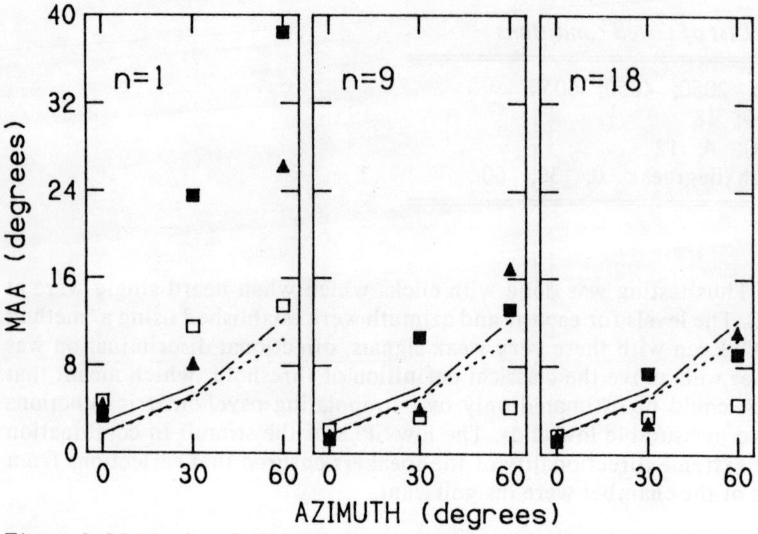

Figure 2. MAAs for clicks with f_cs of 2050 (open square), 4050 (triangle) and 6050 Hz (filled square). For trains, the Interclick Interval was 12 ms. The lines are Mills' (1958) data for tones: solid for 2 kHz, dotted for 4 kHz and dashed for 6 kHz.

It is difficult to know just how to compare Mills' (1958) data with tones to those found here. Whereas his signals lasted 1s, our trains of clicks ranged in duration from 3 to 207 ms; and whereas his signals were presented at 50 dB SPL, ours were just above threshold. Although the similarity between Mills' data and ours for *n*=18 may seem striking, it is probably misleading. For one, his listeners were unable to localize the 2-kHz tones at 60°, whereas our subject found this to be fairly easy, even for *n*=1. What is more, Dye and Hafter (1986), using earphones, showed that lateralization improved by a factor of as much as four over a 40-dB range. Undoubtedly, the MAAs found in the current paper would have been even smaller with higher SPLs and longer durations. This is a conjecture that will have to wait until smaller loudspeakers can be integrated into the experiment.

"Binaural Adaptation" and the accumulation of information over duration

In numerous studies using earphones, it has been shown that the efficiency with which interaural information can be derived from the envelopes of high-frequency stimuli depends upon the rate of stimulation. When periods between peaks in the envelope are comparatively long, as with the 12-ms ICIs used here, the auditory system performs efficiently, extracting interaural differences equally from each click. As the rate of presentation is increased, successive clicks become less effective, thus increasing dependence on the signal's onset for lateralization. In the model that we have offered for these results, the information used for detection is related to the number of clicks in

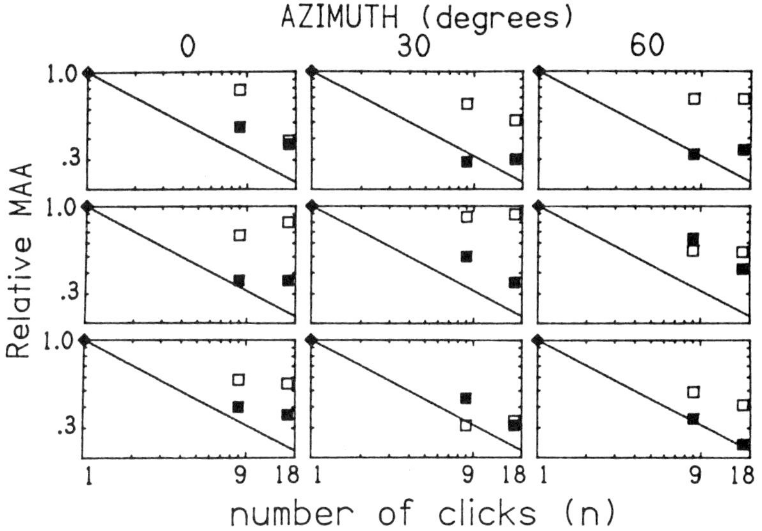

Figure 3. Logarithmic plots of the MAA relative to those found with single clicks vs. the number in a train. The lines have a slope of -0.5. The closed symbols represent ICIs of 12 ms, the open symbols ICIs of 4 ms. The first, second and third rows represent f_cs of 2050, 4050 and 6050 Hz, respectively.

a train by a compressive power function whose exponent is less than 1.0 and is inversely related to the click-rate. Hafter, Dye and Nuetzel (1980) have shown that the decreased usefulness of post-onset information hold for both IDT and IDL presented with earphones; one would presume that the same should hold true for the combined interaural cues encountered in the free-field. However, Blauert, Canevet and Voinier (1987) have recently suggested that some features of "binaural adaptation" (as we have begun to call the effect of high envelope-rates; Hafter *et al.*, 1988) may be different for earphone and free-field listening.

Figure 3 contains results from both short and long ICIs plotted as log thresholds vs. log n. The ordinates show relative MAAs, computed by dividing each threshold by the MAA found using a single click. The lines with slopes of -0.5 show ideal performance, that is, what should occur if the transmission of information is uniform throughout the duration of a train. The -0.5 reflects the square-root decrease in the standard error of the internal noise with repeated sampling. The fact that the slopes are more shallow than -0.5 exemplifies the compressive power functions discussed above. While slopes were surprisingly shallow for an ICI as long as 12 ms, it was nevertheless encouraging to replicate the form of the data found with earphones.

Summary

A program of research on the directional discriminability of complex sounds has begun with the creation of an anechoic environment in which computer-controlled digital filters flatten the spectral responses of loudspeakers. Preliminary results with trains of high-frequency clicks show that directional sensitivity is extremely good, even when the stimuli are just above the threshold of audibility. As expected, MAAs decline away from the median azimuth. Discrimination improves with increased numbers of clicks in the train, though the amount of the improvement depends upon the click-rate, as has been shown in studies using earphones. Work in the free-field has also begun on a study of the active recovery from adaptation previously shown using headphones (Hafter, Buell and Richards, 1988). In the present case we have found that the MAA for a long train of clicks presented with an ICI of 4 ms is reduced by presenting a 5-ms burst of noise during the middle of the train. Presumably this "triggering" stimulus ends the adaptation, allowing the binaural system to resample the spatial information. Long-range plans call for the introduction of artificial echoes generated from additional loudspeakers in order to allow for direct observation of the effects of multiple acoustic pathways on localization.

Acknowledgements

We wish to express great thanks to engineers Ted Krum, Robert Drucker and Steve Lones and to computer programmer Ephram Cohen for their advice and assistance throughout the project.

References

Blauert, J., Canevet, G. and Voinier, T. (**1987**). "The precedence effect: no evidence for an 'active' release process found" (pers. comm.)

Banks, S. M., and Green, D. M. (1973). "Localization of high- and low-frequency transients," J.Acoust.Soc.Am. **53**, 1432-1433.

Carmel, P. W., and Starr, A. (1963). "Acoustic and nonacoustic factors modifying middle-ear muscle activity in waking cats," J.Neurophysiol. **26**, 599-616.

Dye, R. H. Jr. and Hafter, E. R. (**1984**). "The effects of intensity on the detection of interaural differences of time in high-frequency trains of clicks," J.Acoust.Soc.Am. **75**, 1593-1598.

Hafter, E. R., Buell, T. N., and Richards, V. M. (**1988**). "Onset-coding in lateralization: Its form, site, and function," in *Functions of the Auditory System*, edited by G.M.Edelman, W.E.Gall, and W.M.Cowan (Wiley, New York).

Hafter, E. R., and Dye, R. H. Jr. (**1983**). "Detection of interaural differences of time in trains of high-frequency clicks as a function of interclick interval and number," J.Acoust.Soc.Am. **73**, 644-51.

Hafter, E. R., Dye, R. H. Jr., and Wenzel, E. W. (**1983**). "Detection of interaural differences of intensity in trains of high-frequency clicks as a function of interclick interval and number," J.Acoust.Soc.Am. **75**, 1708-1713.

Hafter, E. R., Dye, R. H. Jr. and Nuetzel, J. M. (**1980**). "Lateralization of high-frequency stimuli on the basis of time and intensity" in *Psychophysical, Physiological and Behavioural Studies in Hearing*, edited by G. van den Brink and F. A. Bilsen, (Delft University Press, Delft, The Netherlands).

Leiman, A. L., and Hafter, E. R. (**1972**). "Responses of inferior colliculus neurons to free field auditory stimuli," Experimental Neurology **35**, 431-449.

Mills, A. W. (**1958**). "On the minimum audible angle," J.Acoust.Soc.Am. **30**, 237-246.

Poesselt, C., Schroeter, J., Optiz, M., Divenyi, P., and Blauert, J. (**1986**). "Generation of binaural signals for research and home entertainment," Proceedings of Int.Cong.Acoust. - XII **1**, B1-6.

Wightman, F. L. and Kistler, D. J. (**1980**). "A new look at auditory space perception," in *Psychophysical, Physiological and Behavioural Studies in Hearing*, edited by G. van den Brink and F.A.Bilsen, (Delft University Press, Delft, The Netherlands).

Section 6

Hearing impairment research

Understanding of sensory-neural hearing impairment is an essential prerequisite for optimal rehabilitation. This section contributes to the necessary information. The first five papers investigate several psychophysical aspects, the final two present results from neurophysiological studies in the area.

Nonlinearities of cochlear filtering in normal hearing

Wouter A. Dreschler, Joost M. Festen[1], A. Rens Leeuw

Clinical Audiology, Academic Medical Center, University of Amsterdam, Amsterdam, The Netherlands
[1] *Experimental Audiology, ENT department, Free University Hospital, Amsterdam, The Netherlands.*

Introduction

An important question in auditory nonlinearity is whether the auditory filter should be described with constant-input pattern data or with constant-output pattern data (Verschuure, 1981). Knowledge about the order of events in the filtering process is a prerequisite for a correct way of measuring it. Although the measuring technique with notched noise, developed by Patterson and Nimmo-Smith (1980), has been widely accepted as the best method to take the off-frequency listening phenomenon (Patterson, 1976) into account, comparative data of constant-input pattern results and constant-output pattern results with this technique are only available for simultaneous masking (Lufti and Patterson, 1984). This has been the reason to measure auditory filter shapes with both techniques in forward and simultaneous masking for a group of 14 normal-hearing listeners.

Also, the role of lateral suppression in auditory frequency selectivity is still unclear. This highly nonlinear phenomenon, first shown psychophysically by Houtgast (1974), may be responsible for the sharpening of the auditory filters in nonsimultaneous masking. Unfortunately, also the psychophysical method to measure lateral suppression is subjected to procedural limitations. In studies applying forward masking procedures off-frequency listening may have played a role again. Moreover, qualitative differences between the reference condition with a single-tone masker and the actual suppression measurements with a two-tone masker may have introduced extra cues, overestimating the amount of suppression. By means of an improved measuring technique the effects of lateral suppression have been re-examined for the same group of listeners.

Experiment 1

Frequency resolution at 1000 Hz was measured with a notched-noise masker, consisting of two 400-Hz wide bandpass noises with a spectral notch in between. The noise had a flat spectrum in the passband and equal levels in both bands. In 5 conditions the noise bands were located symmetrically (on a linear frequency scale) around the center frequency of 1000 Hz with a notch width of 0, 100, 200, 400, and 800 Hz, respectively. In 8 asymmetrical conditions either the lower-frequency band or the higher-frequency band was shifted an extra 200 Hz away from the center frequency, resulting in notch widths of 300, 400, 600, and 1000 Hz, respectively. The masking noise was presented in 300-ms intervals with 5-ms rise and fall times and the probe was a 1000-Hz tone burst with 6-ms steady-state and 5-ms rise and fall times. In simultaneous masking the tone burst was switched off 11 ms before the noise. In forward masking the rising flank of the tone burst started 9 ms after the masker was switched off completely. For the constant-output measurements the probe-tone level was fixed at 10 dB SL both in simultaneous and in forward masking and the masker level was varied. For the constant-input measurements the masker level was fixed at the level, just masking the probe in the constant-output measurements for the widest symmetrical notch in forward masking and the probe level was varied. In order to compensate for the listener-dependent decay of masking, the forward masking thresholds

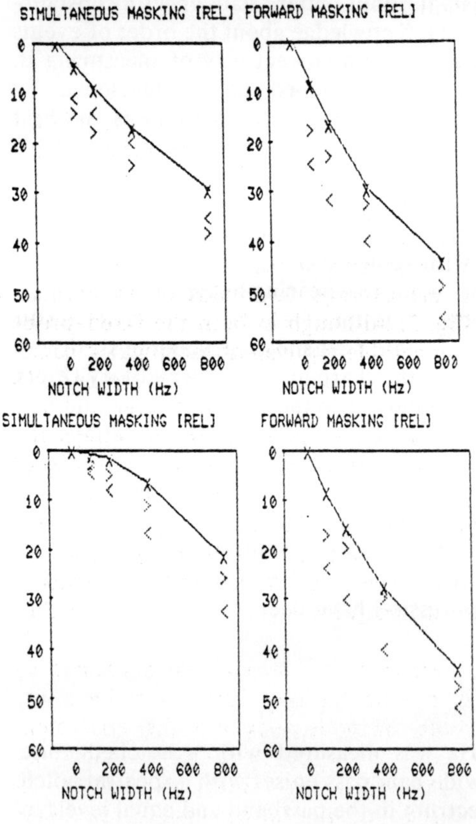

Figure 1. Average thresholds for the measurements with a fixed probe level (constant output, CO, upper panels) and with a fixed masker level (constant input. CI, lower panels) for simultaneous masking (left-hand panels) and forward masking (right-hand panels). All data are plotted as functions of the deviations of the near noise edge from the signal: in symmetrical conditions by crosses, connected by drawn lines, in asymmetrical ones by < and > in case of a shift of the lower or higher frequency band, respectively.

have been transformed to the level of a white noise with the same masking effect by means of an individual transformation curve. Thresholds were found by means of an adaptive 3AFC-method. The average results for 14 normal-hearing subjects are presented in Fig. 1. From this plot it can be seen that in comparable types of measurements the masking effectiveness decreases more rapidly with notch width in forward masking, indicating that the auditory filter in forward masking is sharper. Secondly, the amount of unmasking in case of shifting one of the noise bands away from the probe frequency depends upon the choice of the band. This means that the auditory filter is asymmetrical, but the patterns found are not identical for all types of measurements.

These thresholds were analyzed with the assumption that they represent conditions of equal S/N-ratio at the output of some auditory filter, whose form is independent of either masker level (constant-output filter) or probe level (constant-input filter). The filter acts upon the input signal as an intensity weighting function and its general form is assumed to be composed of two rounded exponential functions, as described by Patterson *et al.* (1982). The branches of the filter are represented by:

$$W(g) = (1-r).(1+p.g).\exp(-p.g) + r$$

where g is the relative deviation from the filter center frequency, p is the parameter which defines the steepness of one of the filter slopes, and r places a limit on the dynamic range of the filter. The parameters of the filter were obtained from a least-squares fit of predicted thresholds to the measured thresholds. In each condition the central frequency of the auditory filter in the model is shifted in order to maximize signal-to-noise ratio.

The auditory filters based upon the average thresholds of 14 normal-hearing listeners are presented in Fig. 2. Although in both the fixed-probe and the fixed-masker techniques comparable equivalent rectangular bandwidth values were found (181 and 207 Hz in simultaneous masking and 118 and 108 Hz in forward masking, respectively), it can be seen that the auditory filter shapes vary for different measuring techniques. Plotted on a logarithmic frequency scale, in simultaneous masking a relatively symmetrical constant-output filter is obtained, while the constant-input filter is more asymmetrical: a shallower low-frequency skirt and a steeper high-frequency skirt. In forward masking the filter shapes are considerably more similar for both measuring techniques and asymmetrical filters are found. The equivalent rectangular bandwidths in forward masking are 35% and 48% smaller than in simultaneous masking.

However, in the individual data there is less agreement than suggested by the average results: the steepness of the various filter skirts are not significantly correlated between both methods, nor are the equivalent rectangular bandwidths. Moreover, for the constant-input filters no significant correlations between corresponding filter parameters in simultaneous and forward masking were found. For the constant-output filter

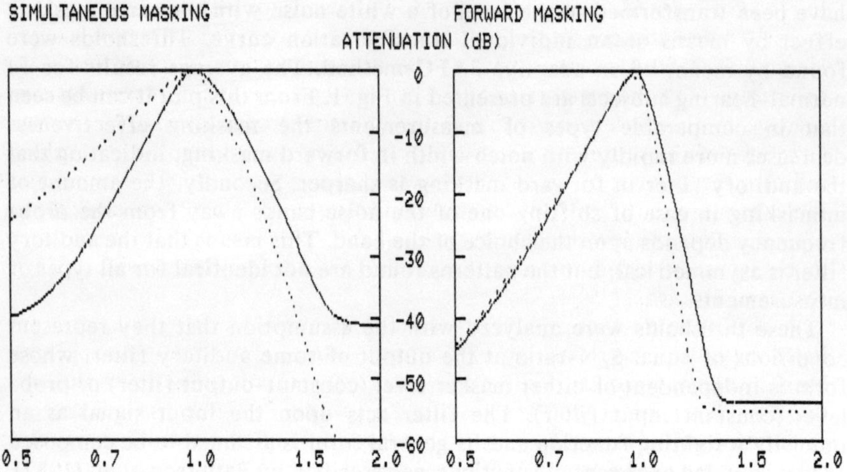

Figure 2. Auditory filter shapes for fixed probe (CO, drawn lines) and fixed masker level (CI, dotted lines) measurements in simultaneous (left-hand panel) and forward masking (right-hand panel).

data the steepness parameters in simultaneous and forward masking show a significant correlation, resulting in a significant relation between the equivalent rectangular bandwidths (r=0.63).

Experiment 2

In experiment 2 lateral suppression was measured psychophysically in the same subjects. By switching a noise together with the single-tone and two-tone maskers, qualitative differences between masker and probe have been introduced in all conditions. So, effects of cueing may be assumed to be minimal. In addition, off-frequency listening was restricted by the application of a notched-noise masker with a 150-Hz wide interval between the two bandpass noises.

The amount of unmasking due to a suppressing tone added to a single-tone masker presented together with the notched noise was measured in forward masking for a 1000-Hz tone burst. The probe tone had 5 ms rise and fall times with a 6 ms steady-state and was presented at a level of 20 dB SL. The first masker component was a 1000-Hz tone, the second component (the suppressor) was a tone of either a higher frequency (at 1100, 1200, 1300, 1400, and 2500 Hz) or a lower frequency (at 900, 800, 700, and 600 Hz). The level of the second component was 20 dB higher than the level of the first component and the levels of both tones were varied together, leaving the 20-dB difference unaffected. The level of the notched noise was the level at which a probe burst of 10 dB SL was just masked. For each subject the average value measured for the conditions without a suppressor and with the supressor located at 2500 Hz was taken as the no-suppression baseline level. The thresholds with the suppressor at the remaining frequencies were considered relative to this baseline. In Fig. 3 the average group results are shown as functions of the suppressor frequency. Values below zero on the vertical scale indicate the amount of unmasking due to the introduction of a suppressor. It is clear that in the area of investigation the high-frequency suppressor is more effective than the low-frequency one. On the other hand, the lower one seems to be more extended towards the lower frequencies, comparable with the results of Houtgast (1974).

A confounding factor in this way of presentation is that the suppressor itself may also cause masking of the probe tone, raising the no-suppression baseline above zero. Especially in listeners with relatively shallow filter skirts this may have influenced the results. Therefore, for each listener a second calculation of the amount of suppression was made relative to a new baseline, calculated by applying the individual auditory filters from experiment 1 to the two-tone masker plus notched noise as used in this experiment. In view of the fixed probe level in the suppression experiment, we used the constant-output filter in forward masking for this purpose. Based upon this filter the degree of off-frequency listening was calculated by optimizing the signal-to-noise ratio for each masker configuration. The amount of masking was obtained from the correspondingly shifted filters.

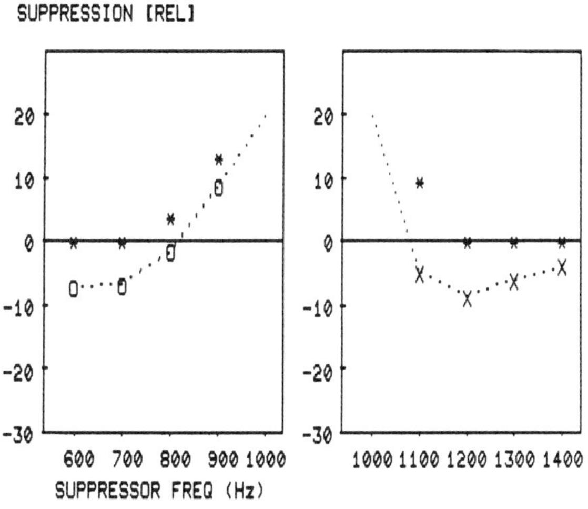

Figure 3. Average thresholds for the measurement of lateral suppression for the suppressor at a lower frequency (left-hand panel) and for the suppressor at a higher frequency (right-hand panel) as a function of suppressor frequency. Suppression is calculated relative to the uncompensated baselines (drawn lines) or relative to the compensated ones, indicated by asterisks (see text).

One assumption in this approach is that the auditory filter, derived with noise bands, is also valid for pure-tone maskers. Another assumption is that the effect of the small differences between the probe levels in the filter measurements (10 dB SL) and in the suppression measurements (20 dB SL) may be assumed to be negligible (Glasberg and Moore, 1982). For several listeners, this method to compensate the baseline for masking due to the relatively loud suppressor resulted in considerably more suppression. The average new baselines are indicated by asterisks in Fig. 3.

Relation between frequency resolution and suppression revisited

It is possible to reexamine the relation between frequency resolution and lateral suppression by means of the data presented here. In this study both constant-input and constant-output data are available and our results on lateral suppression were obtained by an improved protocol, minimizing the effects of off-frequency listening and cueing. Finally, in further analysis masking effects from the suppressor can partly be compensated for.

By using individual results on the experiments outlined before, we can investigate underlying relations by correlation analyses. The correlation coefficients between constant-output filter parameters and the sum of the amount of suppression for the 4 suppressor frequencies, either on the low-frequency side or on the high-frequency side of the probe tone, are given in Table I. As far as possible, the compensated suppression measures have been used, but in the correlations with forward-masking parameters the same data have been used for the compensation procedure itself. So, for some cells the uncompensated suppression values are given, as is indicated by quotes. In simultaneous masking, the steepness of the low-frequency skirt is significantly correlated to lf-suppression ($p<0.10$) and the steepness of the high-frequency skirt to hf-suppression ($p<0.01$). In forward masking only the uncompensated suppression values could be used and an unexplained significant correlation was found between lf-suppression and the steepness of the high-frequency skirts of the filters. In the correlations between suppression and constant-input parameters no significant correlations were present at all (see Table II).

Discussion and conclusions

Considerable differences between constant-output and constant-input filters have been found in simultaneous masking: constant-input data yield shallower lf-skirts and steeper hf-skirts. This is in agreement with the higher presentation levels used in the constant-input protocol especially for the narrow-notched maskers. In forward masking the average filter functions are nearly independent of the measuring technique. This in agreement with the findings of Glasberg and Moore (1982). They also showed that the level effect in forward masking is rather small. So, at least part of the nonlinearities

Table I: Relation constant-output filter and suppression: rank-order correlation coefficients between the steepness-values (pl and ph) in simultaneous and forward masking and suppression. Dpl and dph are the differences in steepness between simultaneous and forward masking for pl and ph, related to the sharpening of the filter skirts in non-simultaneous masking. Correlation coefficients based upon uncompensated suppression values are denoted by quotes (').

	pl(sim)	pl(fm)	dpl	ph(sim)	ph(fm)	dph
lf-suppression	*0.49*	0.19'	-0.44'	-0.06	0.56'	0.58'
hf-suppression	0.03	-0.23'	0.11'	*0.76*	0.39'	0.40'

Table II. As Table I, but for constant-input filter parameters.

	pl(sim)	pl(fm)	dpl	ph(sim)	ph(fm)	dph
lf-suppression	-0.35	-0.04	0.09	0.26	0.15	0.09
hf-suppression	-0.03	-0.05	-0.13	0.05	-0.06	0.00

involved in auditory filtering can be avoided by measuring the frequency resolution in forward masking.

By means of the improved measuring technique with notched noise fair amounts of lateral suppression could be shown psychophysically. A further analysis of the results in relation to the constant-output filter shapes suggests that, apart from stimulus configurations with masking and stimulus configurations with suppression, also stimulus conditions could be found in which both masking and suppression are present. However, this finding contrasts with the conclusions of Shannon (1976) based upon his measurements with one-tone maskers. Our results imply that the amount of suppression can be underestimated due to masking from the suppressor, especially in listeners with shallow filter skirts.

With respect to the suggested relation between suppression and the sharpening of the auditory filter in nonsimultaneous masking we did not find significant correlations to support this hypothesis. This is in agreement with earlier findings (Dreschler and Festen, 1986), although in the latter results the suppression parameters possibly have been influenced by masking effects from the suppressor.

Unexpectedly, significant correlations with filter parameters are found only in simultaneous masking. All theories advocated thus far assume that the suppression phenomenon in simultaneous masking affects the probe and the masker equally (Houtgast, 1974; Shannon, 1976). This assumption may not be valid for all combinations of maskers and probe tones. The effects of suppression in noise bands with a complex pattern of interactions between masker components are unknown. For noise bands positioned in different frequency areas as the probe tone as used in the filter measurements these effects may play a role and they may depend upon presentation level.

This tentative hypothesis should be tested with direct measurements on suppression in simultaneous masking for complex maskers as a function of presentation level. However, if the amount of suppression in simultaneous masking is not necessarily equal for all masker and probe combinations, the correlations found may be related to effects of the masker level, which varies in the constant-output measurements but not in the constant-input measurements. In that case, the discrepancies between constant-input and constant-output filters in simultaneous masking rather than the discrepancies between corresponding filters in simultaneous and forward masking can be ascribed to lateral suppression.

Acknowledgements

This research was financially supported by the Heinsius Houbolt Fund.

References

Dreschler, W.A., and Festen, J.M. (**1986**). "The effect of hearing impairment on auditory filter shapes in simultaneous and forward masking." In: *Auditory Frequency Selectivity*, edited by B.C.J. Moore and R.D. Patterson, (Plenum Press) pp. 331-340.

Glasberg, B.R., and Moore, B.C.J. (**1982**). "Auditory filter shapes in forward masking as a function of level," J.Acoust.Soc.Am. **71**, 946-949.

Houtgast, T. (**1974**). *Lateral suppression in hearing*. Doct. thesis, Utrecht.

Lufti, R.A., and Patterson, R.D. (**1984**). "On the growth of masking asymmetry with stimulus intensity," J.Acoust.Soc.Am. **76**, 739-745.

Patterson, R.D. (**1976**). "Auditory filter shapes derived with noise stimuli," J.Acoust.Soc.Am., **59**, 640-654.

Patterson, R.D., and Nimmo-Smith, I. (**1980**). "Off-frequency listening and auditory-filter asymmetry," J.Acoust.Soc.Am., **67**, 229-245.

Patterson, R.D., Nimmo-Smith, I., Weber, D.L., and Milroy, R. (**1982**). "The deterioration of hearing with age: frequency selectivity, the critical ratio, the audiogram, and speech threshold," J.Acoust.Soc.Am. **72**, 1788-1803.

Shannon, R.V. (**1976**). "Two-tone unmasking and suppression in a forward-masking situation," J.Acoust.Soc.Am. **59**, 1460-1470.

Verschuure, J. (**1981**). "Pulsation patterns and nonlinearity of auditory tuning II. Analysis of psychophysical results," Acustica, **49**, 296-306.

Comments

Scharf:

A clarification is needed of why in the first panel of Fig.1 an asymmetrical shift of the masking band results in a greater drop in masking when the shift is more toward the high-frequency than toward the low frequency side.

Reply by Dreschler et al.:

The reason may be the rather low presentation level used in the fixed-probe measurements (probe level is 10 dB SPL). Several authors report a reversed asymmetry at low presentation levels and this results in the phenomenon you noticed in the first panel of Fig.1. It is important to note that this asymmetry is also present in the left panel of Fig.2, although not clearly because of the log frequency scale.

Delgutte:

Your observation that significant correlation between suppression and slopes of auditory filters is found in simultaneous masking but not in forward masking fits well with the physiological results reported in my paper. It is shown that suppression of responses to a tone signal by a tone masker has a major effect on the slope of physiological masking patterns measured in simultaneous masking, particularly for signal frequencies well above the masker. If these results for single-tone maskers can be extended to notched-noise maskers, masker-to-signal suppression should also affect the skirts of auditory filters in simultaneous masking. On the other hand suppression of a signal by a masker does not occur if the two stimuli are not simultaneous, so that auditory filters obtained in forward masking should not be influenced by suppression.

Temporal and spectral processing in cochlear and partially simulated impairments

M. Florentine[1] and S. Buus[2]

[1]*Communication Research Laboratory (133 FR)*
[2]*Communication and Digital Signal Processing Center (409 DA)*
Northeastern University Boston, MA 02115, U.S.A.

Introduction

The purpose of this paper is to examine a method for comparing psychoacoustical measurements in normal listeners and listeners with cochlear impairments. When evaluating results for listeners with cochlear impairments, the experimenter must choose whether to compare their performance with that of normal listeners tested at the same SL, the same loudness, or the same SPL. Obtaining psychoacoustical measurements in the presence of a masking noise offers a possibility of equating SL, loudness, and SPL in normal and impaired listeners. We call the masked normal ear a partially simulated impairment when the level and spectral shape of the masking noise is chosen to produce thresholds similar to those of an impaired listener.

Masking a normal ear produces altered intensity perception similar to that of cochlear impairments. For example, masked normal listeners have elevated thresholds, rapid growth of loudness, and reduced dynamic range (Steinberg and Gardner, 1937). On the other hand, temporal integration (Zwicker and Wright, 1963), temporal resolution (Florentine and Buus, 1984), and frequency selectivity (Green, Shelton, Picardi, and Hafter, 1981) all appear relatively unaffected by masking. Therefore, we believe that comparisons of real and partially simulated impairments may help separate the effects of the impaired listeners' altered intensity perception from the effects of possible alterations in their temporal and/or spectral processing.

In this paper, we wish to demonstrate the utility of this approach by reviewing some data on temporal and spectral processing. Temporal processing will be discussed in terms of temporal integration, as measured by detection of tones as a function of duration, and in terms of temporal resolution, as measured by gap detection. Spectral processing will be discussed in terms of frequency selectivity, as measured by psychoacoustical tuning curves.

Temporal integration: detection threshold as a function of duration

Method

Detection thresholds at 0.25, 1, and 4 kHz were measured monaurally for stimulus durations from 2 to 500 ms. The shortest durations were not used at the low frequencies to reduce the effects of spectral splatter. The raised cosine onsets and offsets had durations of 1 ms. An adaptive procedure and a two-interval, two alternative forced-choice (2I, 2AFC) paradigm with feedback was used.

The two impaired listeners (PM and RT) had mildly sloping, moderate high-frequency hearing losses of primarily cochlear origin. Their thresholds are quite similar and differ no more than 15 dB at any test frequency between 0.25 and 18 kHz. Below 1 kHz, their audiograms show nearly normal thresholds. Above 1 kHz, their thresholds increase to about 50 dB HL at 4 kHz. The two normal listeners, who simulated RT's hearing impairment, had thresholds within 10 dB HL at all audiometric test frequencies (ANSI, 1969). All four listeners were young university students and had no medical history of conductive or retrocochlear lesions. [Further details of the procedure and audiometric data for the impaired listeners can be found in Florentine, Fastl, and Buus, 1988.]

Results and Discussion

Figure 1 shows results at three frequencies from the two impaired listeners

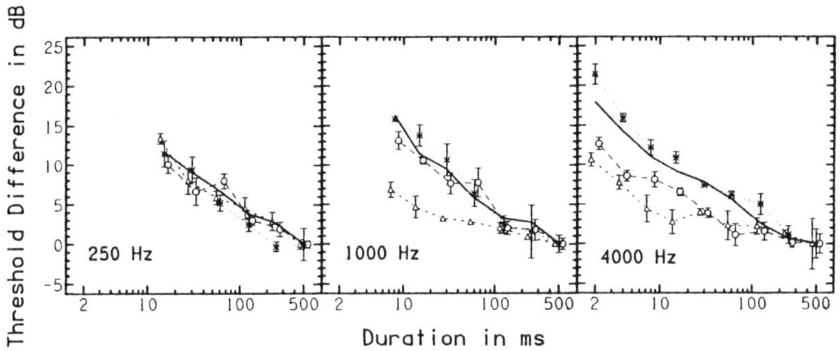

Figure 1. The threshold difference in dB (normalized re 500 ms) plotted as a function of stimulus duration at 0.25, 1, and 4 kHz. Individual data are shown from two impaired listeners (PM by the circles and RT by the triangles) and average data are shown from two listeners with simulations of RT's audiogram (asterisks). The average data are shown from the two simulations because the individual data are similar. In cases where the points overlap, they have been shifted along the abscissa. The vertical bars show plus and minus 1 SE. For comparison, average data from five normal listeners tested in the quiet are also shown (solid line). [Data are replotted from Florentine et al., 1988.]

(PM and RT), two normal listeners with partially simulated impairments, and five normal listeners tested in the quiet. At 250 Hz, temporal integration appears similar in the normal and impaired listeners. At 1 kHz, temporal integration is reduced in one impaired listener, but normal in the other. At 4 kHz, temporal integration is reduced for both impaired listeners.

The reduced temporal integration in the impaired listeners is probably not caused by increased test levels and/or increased audibility of spectral splatter. Both the test level and the audibility of spectral splatter should be the same in real and simulated impairments, but the listeners with partially simulated impairments show the same amount of temporal integration as the normal listeners tested in the quiet. Therefore, it appears that temporal integration is truly reduced in listener RT at 1 and 4 kHz and in listener PM at 4 kHz. It is noteworthy that listener PM has normal temporal integration at 1 kHz where his threshold is 35 dB HL. In contrast, listener RT has reduced temporal integration and a threshold of only 20 dB HL. This finding suggests that temporal integration for individual impaired listeners cannot be predicted from the threshold alone. Similar results have been obtained in other impaired listeners (see Florentine *et al*., 1988).

Temporal resolution: gap detection

Method

The minimum detectable gap duration, MDG, in a low-pass (cut-off 7 kHz) noise was measured monaurally as a function of SPL in the same listeners used in the previous experiment. An adaptive procedure and a 2I, 2AFC paradigm with feedback was used. The gap was produced by turning off and on the noise with fall and rise times of 1 ms. [For details of this procedure, see Florentine and Buus (1984).]

Results and Discussion

Figure 2 shows the results from the two impaired listeners (PM and RT), two listeners with simulations of PM's impairment, and six normal listeners tested in the quiet. Listener PM's MDGs are elevated near threshold, but decrease rapidly with increasing level and above 80 dB SPL they are identical to the MDGs for normal listeners. His results are very similar to those obtained with the partially simulated impairments. Therefore, it seems that PM has normal temporal resolution and the elevation of his MDGs near threshold result from the decreased sensation level of the noise at high frequencies where temporal resolution is best (Fitzgibbons, 1983; Florentine and Buus, 1983; Shailer and Moore, 1983; Buus and Florentine, 1985; Bacon and Viemeister, 1985). Listener RT's MDGs also are enlarged near threshold and decrease rapidly with increasing level. In contrast to the MDGs for PM, however, RT's MDGs are elevated at high levels. At 80 and 90 dB SPL, her MDGs are 1.5-to-2 times greater than those for PM's real and partially simulated impairments, despite the similarity in age and audiograms. Therefore, it appears that RT has reduced temporal resolution although most of the enlargement of her MDGs at low and moderate levels probably results from the reduced sensation level of the noise. The comparison of normal and impaired listeners in the quiet could be interpreted as both impaired listeners having reduced temporal resolution. However, the comparison of partially simulated and real impairments clearly shows that only one of the listeners truly has reduced temporal resolution. Further measurements with octave-band noises confirm this conclusion [see Buus and Florentine (1985)]. Also, similar results have been obtained for other impaired listeners [see Florentine and Buus (1984)].

Frequency selectivity: psychoacoustical tuning curves

Method

Tuning curves were measured monaurally using an adaptive procedure and a 2I, 2AFC paradigm. The probe was set to 10 dB SL and the level of a narrow-band noise masker necessary to mask the probe was measured for each of six masker frequencies. The masker frequencies were 0.43, 0.78, 0.92, 1.08, 1.23, and 1.48 times the probe frequency. The masker was pulsed to mark the observation intervals; it had a duration of 750 ms and an interstimulus interval of 250 ms. The probe was a double pulse consisting of two 150-ms tone bursts separated by a 150-ms interstimulus interval. The onset of the first tone pulse was 200 ms after the beginning of the masker. The rise and fall times were 20 ms for both masker and probe. [For further details of the procedure, see Buus, Florentine, and Mason (1986).]

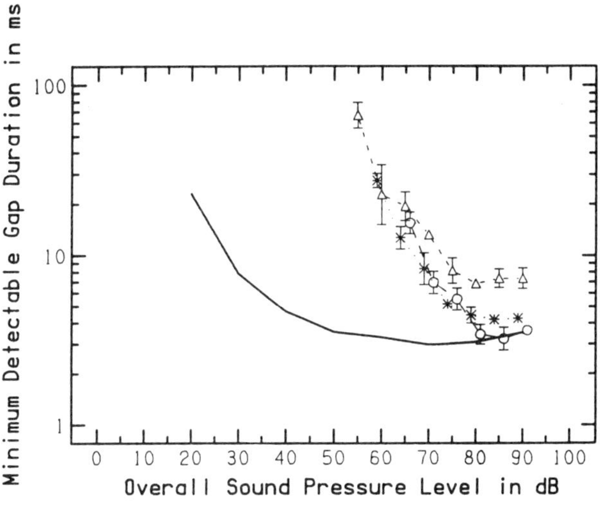

Figure 2. The minimum detectable gap is plotted as a function of level. The data are plotted in the same manner as Fig. 1, except that the vertical bars are plus and minus 1 SD. [Data are replotted from Florentine and Buus, 1984.]

Two impaired listeners were used in this experiment. Listener RT, who served in the previous experiment, and listener AJ, who had a unilateral impairment of cochlear origin. Thresholds in her impaired ear were relatively constant at 75 dB SPL across frequency. Thresholds in her good ear were within normal limits (ANSI, 1969) in the test frequency range.

Results and Discussion

Figure 3 shows results from impaired listener RT and two normal listeners tested in simulation noise and in the quiet. In comparison to the normal listeners tested in the quiet, the low side of RT's tuning curves appears flatter than normal, which might be taken to indicate that her frequency selectivity

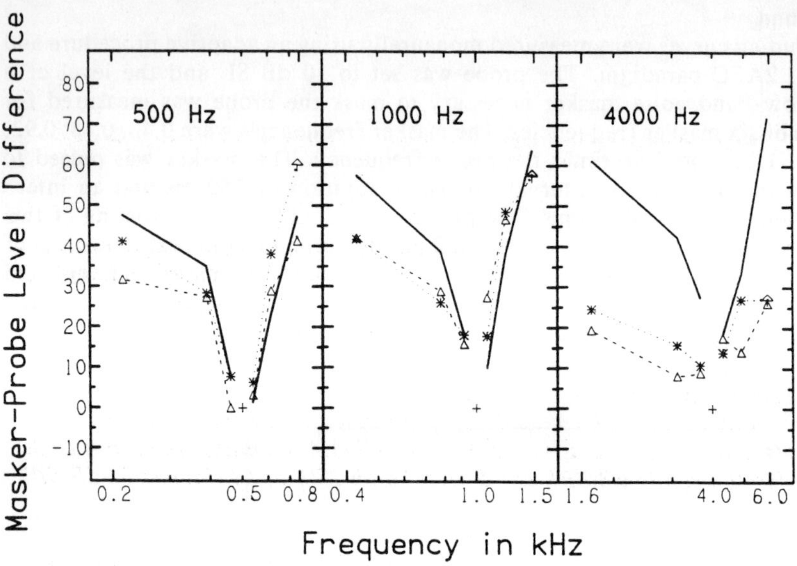

Figure 3. Psychoacoustical tuning curves at 0.5, 1, and 4 kHz for impaired listener RT (triangles) and for two listeners with simulations (asterisks) of RT's hearing loss. For each tuning curve, the average level difference between the masker and probe (plusses) obtained in two measurements is plotted as a function of the masker's frequency. In most cases the two measurements differ less than 4 dB. The up-arrows indicate masker levels greater than 102 dB, which was the upper limit for our measurements. For readability, the up-arrows have been connected to the adjacent points on the tuning curve although such lines give an incorrect visual representation of the shape of the tuning curve. For comparison, the solid line shows the average tuning curves for the normal listeners tested in the quiet. For the normal listeners tested in the quiet, the probe levels were 14 dB SPL at 0.5 kHz, 9 dB SPL at 1 kHz, and 17 dB SPL at 4 kHz. For the real and simulated impairments, the probe levels were 42 dB SPL at 0.5 kHz, 45 dB SPL at 1 kHz, and 75 dB SPL at 4 kHz.

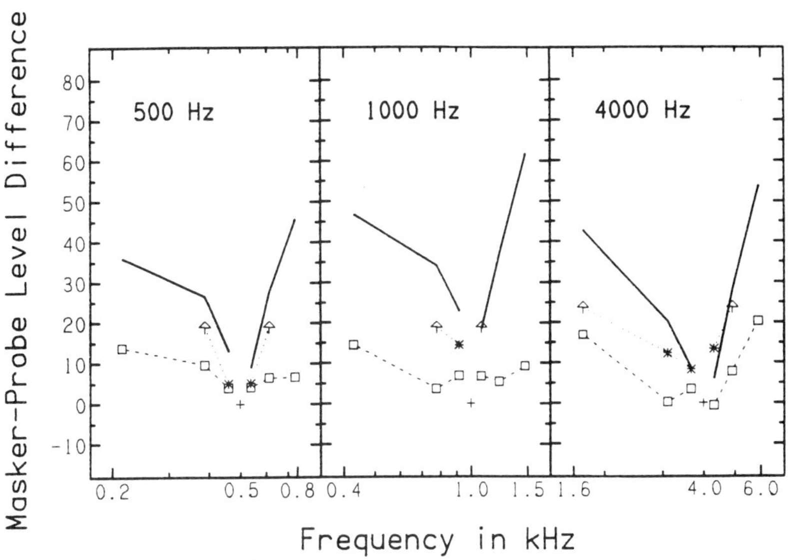

Figure 4. Psychoacoustical tuning curves at 0.5, 1, and 4 kHz for the impaired ear (squares) and the normal ear with simulation noise (asterisks) of unilaterally impaired listener AJ. Her tuning curves are plotted in the same manner as the previous figure. Each point is the average of two measurements which, in most cases, differ less than 4 dB. For comparison, the solid line shows the tuning curves for her normal ear obtained in the quiet. For her normal ear tested in the quiet, the probe levels were 30 dB SPL at 0.5 kHz, 22 dB SPL at 1 kHz, and 28 dB SPL at 4 kHz. For the real and simulated impairments, the probe levels were 86 dB SPL at 0.5 kHz, 86 dB SPL at 1 kHz, and 81 dB SPL at 4 kHz.

is somewhat reduced. However, the comparison with partially simulated impairments clearly indicates that most of the flattening results from elevated test levels and altered intensity perception. At 0.5 and 1 kHz, listener RT's tuning curves are reasonably similar to those from the listeners simulating her impairment. At 4 kHz, her tuning curve is somewhat flatter than that for the partially simulated impairments, but the difference is greater on the high side than on the low. Therefore, it appears that RT has relatively normal frequency selectivity, except at 4 kHz where the high side of her tuning curve is flatter than that for the simulated impairments.

Figure 4 shows tuning curves from listener AJ. Her unilateral impairment enables us to use her as her own control by partially simulating her unilateral hearing impairment in her good ear. Whereas the top of the tuning curves in her partially simulated impairment are relatively sharp, they are rather flat in her impaired ear. This demonstrates that her impaired ear has reduced frequency selectivity, although some flattening is evident in the tuning curves for her simulated impairment.

The results from the impaired listeners shown in Figs. 3 and 4 range from normal to clearly impaired frequency selectivity. They also show how comparisons between real and partially simulated impairments can lead to conclusions different from those obtained by direct comparison between normal and impaired hearing in the quiet.

General discussion

The comparison of cochlear and partially simulated impairments appears to be a useful tool in the study of auditory processing of impaired listeners. It solves the problem of whether to compare impaired and normal hearing at equal SL, equal loudness, or equal SPL and permits us to separate the effects of possible reductions in temporal and/or spectral processing from the effects of altered intensity perception. Whereas comparisons between impaired and normal listeners tested in the quiet could be interpreted as almost all impaired listeners having reduced temporal and spectral resolution, the comparison with partially simulated impairments indicates that temporal and spectral processing, per se, are normal in some impaired listeners and reduced in others.

Although the simulation data provide a compelling comparison, we should be cautious not to assume that the simulation noise alters the auditory system in the same manner as a cochlear hearing impairment. The similar effects that may be obtained in partially simulated and real hearing impairments may result from very different neural responses. In addition, we should also be cautious to realize the effects of practice. For example, an impaired listener, who has listened through a hearing loss for several decades, may be more practiced than a normal listener, who has listened through a simulated loss for only a short period of time. We believe that for simple tasks, such as those discussed in this paper, the effect of practice is small. But, for more complicated tasks, such as speech perception, the effects of practice could be very important and give impaired listeners an advantage over their simulated loss counterparts.

Although noise masking may alter the auditory system differently than hearing impairment, noise simulation appears to be a useful concept in modeling cochlear impairment. For example, Zwicker's (1958) model of loudness summation can be applied successfully to listeners with noise-induced hearing loss when reduced frequency selectivity is taken into account and the elevated threshold is modeled as a masking noise. [For details, see Florentine and Zwicker (1979).]

In conclusion, despite the caveats, we believe that if we exercise caution interpreting the data, the comparison of the partly simulated and real impairments is a very useful tool in the study of auditory processing of cochlearly impaired listeners. The present results show that modeling impaired listeners' threshold elevations and altered intensity perception by means of a simulation noise can explain changes in the shape of their gap-detection functions and tuning curves in some cases. However, in other cases the changes exceed what can be explained by noise simulation and it appears necessary to assume that changes in temporal and/or spectral processing result from the hearing impairment.

Acknowledgments

This work is supported, in part, by NIH-NINCDS grant RO1NS18280. Dr. R.P. Carlyon gave helpful comments on an earlier version of this paper.

References

ANSI (**1969**). American National Standard specifications for audiometers (ANSI S3.6-1969), New York: American National Standards Institute.

Bacon, S. P., and Viemeister, N. F. (**1985**). "Temporal modulation transfer functions in normal-hearing and hearing-impaired listeners," Audiology **24**, 117-134.

Buus, S., and Florentine, M. (**1985**). "Gap detection in normal and impaired listeners: the effect of level and frequency," in *Time Resolution in uditory Systems*, edited by A. Michelsen (Springer, New York) pp.159-177.

Buus, S., Florentine, M., and Mason, C. (**1986**). "Psychoacoustical tuning curves and absolute thresholds at high frequencies," in *Auditory Frequency Analysis*, edited by B.C.J.Moore and R.D.Patterson (Plenum, New York), pp.341-350.

Fitzgibbons, P. (**1983**). "Temporal gap detection in noise as a function of frequency, bandwidth, and level," J.Acoust.Soc.Am. **74**, 67-72.

Florentine, M., and Buus. S. (**1983**). "Temporal resolution as a function of level and frequency," Proc. 11th Int.Cong.Acoust. **3**, 103-106.

Florentine, M., and Buus, S. (**1984**). "Temporal gap detection in sensorineural and simulated hearing impairments," J. Speech and Hearing Res. **27**, 449-455.

Florentine, M., Fastl, H., and Buus, S. (**1988**). "Temporal integration in normal hearing, cochlear impairment, and impairment simulated by masking," J.Acoust.Soc.Am., in press.

Florentine, M., and Zwicker, E. (**1979**). "A model of loudness summation applied to noise-induced hearing loss," Hearing Res. **1**, 121-132.

Green, D. M., Shelton, B. R., Picardi, M. C., and Hafter, E. R. (**1981**). "Psychophysical tuning curves independent of signal level," J.Acoust.Soc. Am. **69**, 1758-1762.

Shailer, M. J., and Moore, B. C. J. (**1983**). "Gap detection as a function of frequency, bandwidth, and level," J.Acoust.Soc.Am. **74**, 467-473.

Steinberg, J. C., and Gardner, M. B. (**1937**). "The dependence of hearing impairment on sound intensity," J.Acoust.Soc.Am. **9**, 11-23.

Zwicker, E., and Wright, H. N. (**1963**). "Temporal summation for tones in narrow-band noise," J.Acoust.Soc.Am. **35**, 691-699.

Comments

Tyler:

I've always been concerned about using masking noise to simulate hearing impairment. Masking noise presented to a normal ear results in widespread neural activity across many auditory-nerve fibers. In contrast, the nerve fibers in a hearing-impaired ear usually show decreased spontaneous activity. It seems like these are two very different situations. While some psychophysical tasks produce results that appear similar between hearing-impaired subjects and normals presented with masking noise, I never know how far to interpret the analogy.

Reply by Florentine:

We would expect that the physiological response in impaired listeners and in normal listeners with partially simulated impairments would be different for several reasons. One of the most compelling reasons is that impaired listeners have additional alterations in their abilities to process frequency and time-varying amplitude than normal listeners. When we understand more about neural coding in normal and impaired listeners, we expect to better be able to interpret these data. Until then, the partial simulation are the best method of which we are aware to **psychoacoustically** separate the effects of impaired listeners altered intensity perception from other alterations in their auditory processing.

Effects of the relative phase of the components on the pitch discrimination of complex tones by subjects with unilateral cochlear impairments

Brian C.J. Moore and Brian R. Glasberg

Department of Experimental Psychology, University of Cambridge, Downing Street, Cambridge CB2 3EB, England

Introduction

A number of theories of the perception of the pitch of complex tones hold that the resolution of spectral components is an essential first stage; the pitch of a complex tone is assumed to be derived from the frequencies or pitches of its resolved components (Goldstein, 1973; Terhardt, 1974). We will refer to these theories as spectral theories (even though the frequencies of the components may be coded by temporal means). For a complex tone with equal-amplitude harmonics, only the first five or six harmonics are resolved (Plomp, 1964; Moore, Glasberg and Shailer, 1984). Hence these theories predict that the pitches of such complex tones should be determined primarily by the first five or six harmonics, and pitch perception should be poor if those harmonics are absent. In addition, the pitches of complex tones should be unaffected by the relative phases of the components. Finally, for subjects with cochlear impairments, who usually have reduced frequency selectivity, fewer components should be resolvable, and so pitch perception should be impaired.

Alternative theories (called here spectro-temporal theories) propose that the pitch of complex tones is derived from both spectral and temporal information (Moore, 1982; Srulovicz and Goldstein, 1983; Moore and Glasberg, 1986; Patterson, 1987); the spectral analysis performed in the auditory filters is followed by an analysis of the time pattern of the output of each filter, as represented in the patterns of phase locking in the auditory nerve. According to these theories, the pitches of complex tones can be extracted from unresolved as well as resolved components. Hence pitch perception and discrimination will not necessarily be impaired by removing the lower harmonics. Also, for high harmonics, which are not resolved by the auditory filters, the relative phases of the components may affect pitch perception (Moore, 1977). For subjects with cochlear impairments, pitch perception may be impaired both because the temporal information conveying the pitch is more ambiguous (Rosen and Fourcin, 1986) and because temporal analysis is impaired. The spectro-temporal theories also predict that impaired subjects should be more affected by relative phase than normally hearing subjects, since the reduced frequency selectivity of the former means that even the low harmonics may interact at the output of the auditory filters (Rosen and Fourcin, 1986).

In a previous paper (Moore and Glasberg, 1987) we presented preliminary data intended to evaluate the two classes of theory. Difference limens (DLs) for the fundamental frequency, F_0, of harmonic complex tones with equal-amplitude components were measured for each ear of ten subjects with unilateral cochlear impairments and twelve subjects with bilateral cochlear impairments. One complex tone contained the lower resolvable harmonics while the other did not. The components were added in two different phase relationships, designed to give waveforms with markedly different degrees of "peakedness". The fundamental frequency was always 200 Hz. The DLs were generally larger for the impaired ears than for the normal ears. However, contrary to the predictions of the spectral theories, the DLs were not usually larger when the first five harmonics were removed, and the DLs were affected by the relative phases of the components.

In this paper we present the results of more detailed measurements using four subjects with unilateral cochlear impairments. DLs were measured for four F_0's, three phase relationships of the components, and three types of harmonic complex. The results suggest that the pitch discrimination of complex tones depends at least partly on temporal coding.

Method

Stimuli

All stimuli were computer synthesized using a 12-bit digital-to-analogue converter (DAC) and either a 10-kHz or 20-kHz sampling rate; the latter was used for F_0 = 400 Hz. The output of the DAC was low-pass filtered at 0.4 times the sampling rate. The complex tones had a mean F_0 of 50, 100, 200 or 400 Hz. They contained either harmonics 1-5 or 1-12 or 6-12, and the level of each harmonic was 70 dB SPL (subjects AW and DJ were also tested at a level of 80 dB SPL per component (dB/c); results were similar to those obtained at 70 dB/c). The components were added in three different phase relationships. For the cosine-phase condition, all components started in cosine phase, giving a very "peaky" waveform. For the alternating-phase condition, the odd numbered harmonics started in cosine phase and the even numbered harmonics in sine phase, giving a less "peaky" waveform, but with two major peaks per period (see Moore and Glasberg, 1987, fig. 1). For the Schroeder-phase condition the phases were chosen according to a formula given by Schroeder (1970) so as to give a waveform with a very flat envelope. For this condition, the instantaneous frequency swept upwards within each period, giving a so-called "up chirp". Each tone had a steady-state portion of 200 ms and 10-ms rise/fall times, shaped with a half-cycle of a raised-cosine function. The silent interval between the two tone bursts in a trial was 500 ms. Signals were presented to one ear at a time using Sennheiser HD414 earphones.

According to the spectro-temporal theories, the temporal structure of the waveforms at the outputs of the auditory filters is important for pitch perception. Simulations of auditory filtering, assuming filters with linear phase responses, showed that, for a filter centered at the fifth harmonic, the cosine-phase wave usually has well defined envelope peaks which would be expected to give clear information about F_0. The alternating-phase wave gives a much flatter envelope, so that F_0 is less well represented. After filtering, the Schroeder-phase wave often appears similar to the cosine-phase wave (see Moore and Glasberg, 1987, fig. 1). These difference between the waves are also found when the simulated filter is centered on higher harmonics. In the case of an impaired ear, with reduced frequency selectivity the temporal structure at the output of the filter is very different for the alternating-phase wave and the other two waves, the alternating-phase wave having peaks separated by times not corresponding to the period of F_0. The spectro-temporal theories predict that such a wave should have an ambiguous pitch and should be poorly discriminated. It should be noted that if the phase responses of the auditory filters are markedly nonlinear, the waveforms after filtering would be quite different from those described above. In addition, the amplitude and phase response of the earphone and outer/middle ear will affect the waveforms. However, we would still expect the different phase conditions to give rise to different waveforms at the outputs of the auditory filters.

Procedure

Frequency DLs were measured using an adaptive two-alternative forced-choice procedure. On each trial the subject heard two successive complex tones differing in F_0, and was required to indicate which had the higher pitch. Feedback was provided by lights. A run started with a large difference in F_0 between the tones. After two consecutive correct responses the difference in F_0 was decreased by a factor of 1.4. After one incorrect response the difference was increased by a factor of 1.4. Testing continued until twelve

Table 1. Audiometric data for each subject.

				Threshold, dB HL						
Subj.	Age	Sex	Ear	0.25	0.5	1.0	2.0	4.0	8.0	Diagnosis
DJ	48	M	Normal	5	10	0	5	15	10	Ménière's
			Impaired	65	70	60	55	70	80	
PM	69	F	Normal	20	15	10	15	30	60	Ménière's
			Impaired	65	60	55	50	55	70	
AW	72	M	Normal	20	15	10	15	30	50	?
			Impaired	50	55	55	40	30	50	
GB	59	F	Normal	10	15	25	35	45	55	?
			Impaired	50	55	55	55	60	70	

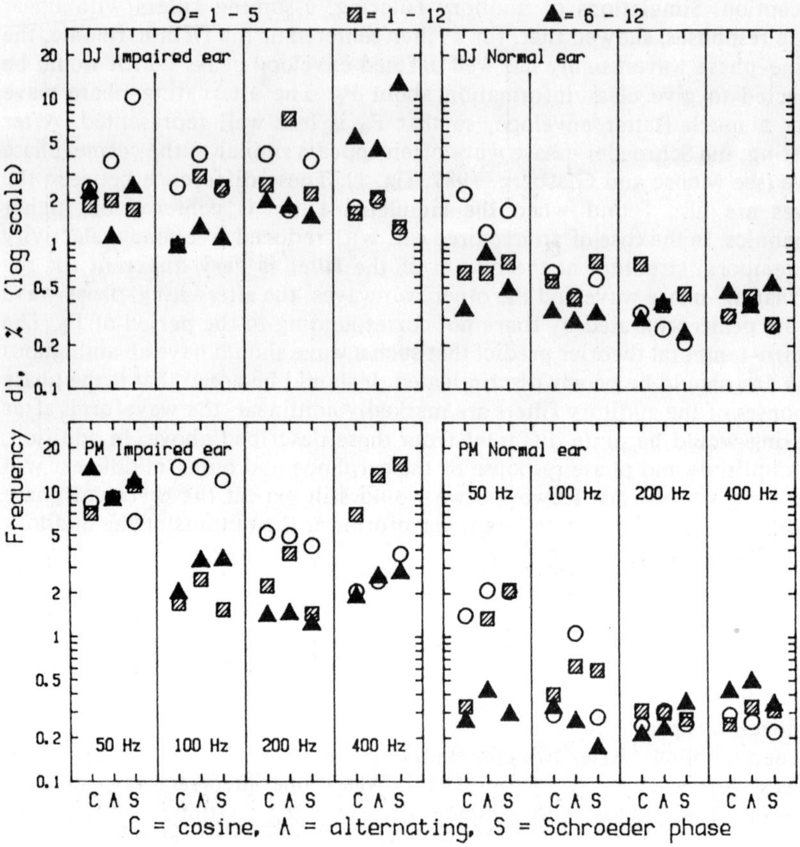

Figure 1. Frequency DLs for subjects DJ and PM.

"turnarounds" had occurred. Threshold was taken as the geometric mean of the values at the last eight turnarounds. Each threshold reported is the mean of at least three estimates.

Subjects

Four subjects with unilateral cochlear hearing losses were tested. They were carefully screened to exclude conductive or retrocochlear losses. The impaired ears were selected to have relatively flat losses as a function of frequency. The normal ears had absolute thresholds within normal limits given the ages of the subjects. Table 1 gives audiometric data for each subject. All subjects had extensive practice in psychoacoustic tasks.

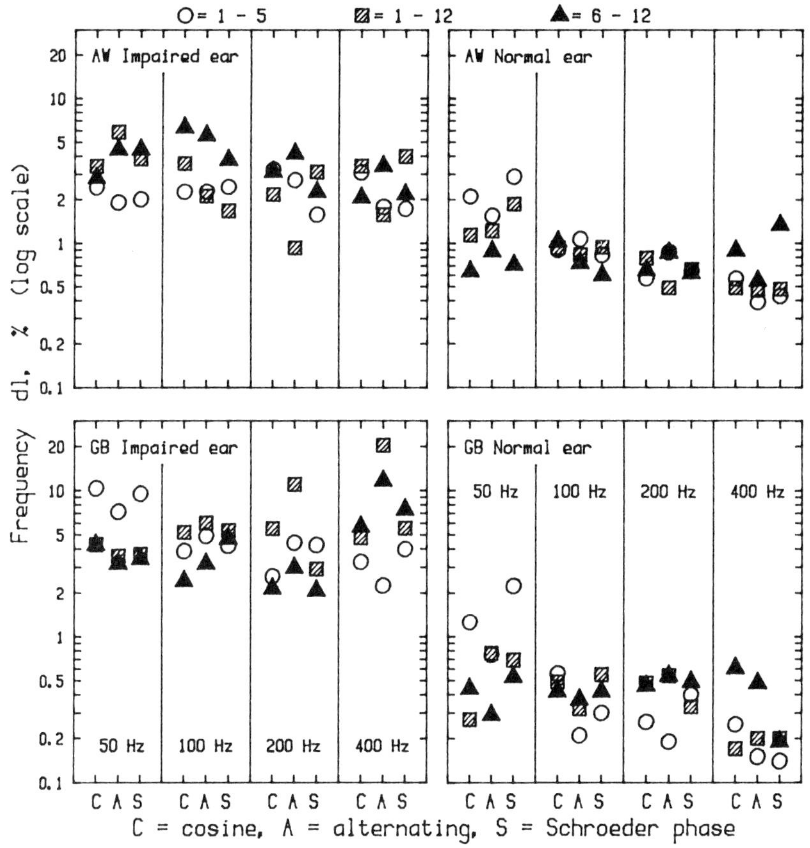

Figure 2. Frequency DLs for subjects AW and GB. See text for details.

Results

The results are shown separately for each subject in figures 1 and 2 (70-dB data only). The key to the symbols is at the top of the figure. Consistent with earlier work, the frequency DLs are larger than normal for the ears with cochlear impairments (Hoekstra and Ritsma, 1977; Moore and Glasberg, 1987; Horst, 1987). For F_0's from 100 to 400 Hz, the DLs for the normal ears are typically between 0.15 and 1%; the DLs increase somewhat for $F_0 = 50$ Hz. For the impaired ears, the DLs are typically between 1.5 and 15%, an order of magnitude larger. This is consistent both with the spectral theories and with the spectro-temporal theories.

Consider now the effect of the presence or absence of the first five harmonics. For F_0's of 200 and 400 Hz, the DLs for the normal ears show no consistent effect of harmonic content; the complex tones containing only higher harmonics (6-12) are discriminated about as well as the tones containing harmonics 1-12. For F_0 = 50 Hz (and 100 Hz for subject DJ) the complexes with harmonics 6-12 generally give smaller DLs than the complexes with harmonics 1-12. The complex tones containing harmonics 1-5 tend to be rather poorly discriminated. Thus, at least for low fundamentals, the higher harmonics seem to make an important contribution to pitch discrimination, consistent with the spectro-temporal models.

For the impaired ears, the effects of harmonic content vary considerably across subjects and fundamental frequency, but some consistent within-subject trends can be observed. For subject PM at F_0 = 400 Hz, the complex with harmonics 1-12 gives larger DLs than either of the other complexes, for all phase conditions. For subject DJ at F_0 = 200 Hz, the complex with harmonics 1-12 gives larger DLs than the complex with harmonics 6-12, for all phase conditions. This is also true for the data obtained at a level of 80 dB SPL per component. For subject GB in the alternating-phase condition, the complex with harmonics 1-12 gives larger DLs than the complex with harmonics 6-12 for all values of F_0. Thus, cases can be found where the first five harmonics actually impair performance. A few cases can also be found where the lower harmonics lead to better performance, e.g. subject DJ at F_0 = 400 Hz.

For the normal ears, there are no consistent effects of relative phase. For the impaired ears, there are large individual differences, but some consistent within-subject trends can be observed. For subjects PM and DJ, the complex with harmonics 1-12 gives DLs which are larger for the alternating-phase condition than for the cosine-phase condition at all values of F_0. This is also true for subject GB at F_0's of 100, 200 and 400 Hz, but AW shows an effect in the opposite direction. Phase effects also occur in other cases, but not in a consistent pattern.

The following analysis shows that the phase effects are not just the result of random errors of measurement. We will consider the logarithms of the DLs, rather than the DLs themselves, since each DL was calculated as the geometric mean of three estimates, and the variability is roughly constant when expressed in terms of log values. The standard error (SE) of the three estimates for a given condition has an average value of 0.07 for the normal ears and 0.08 for the impaired ears. If relative phase has no effect on the DLs, then the standard deviation (SD) of the DLs across phase conditions for a given complex, subject and fundamental frequency should not be significantly greater than the above SEs, as determined by an F-test. In fact, the SD has an average value of 0.11 for the normal ears, slightly but significantly ($p < 0.01$) greater than would be expected from errors of measurement. The corresponding SD for the impaired ears is 0.18, considerably and significantly ($p < 0.001$) greater than would be expected from errors of measurement. Thus, changes in the relative phases of the components produce significant changes in the DLs.

Discussion and conclusions

Our results confirm that cochlear hearing loss impairs the discrimination of the pitch of complex tones. Removing the lower harmonics does not consistently result in larger DLs, either for normal or impaired ears, suggesting that pitch can be extracted from the temporal pattern of the higher unresolved harmonics. For some impaired subjects, adding the lower harmonics gives larger DLs. This may arise in the following way. The impaired ears have auditory filters which are much broader than normal. This was confirmed by measurement of the auditory filter shape using a notched-noise masker (Glasberg and Moore, 1986). At a center frequency of 500 Hz, AW, PM and GB had auditory filters too broad to be measured and DJ had a filter bandwidth of 250 Hz, much broader than normal. At 1000 Hz, filter bandwidths for AW, PM and GB were 2 -4 times wider for the impaired ears than for the normal ears, and DJ had no measurable filter. Under these conditions it seems likely that none of the harmonics in the complexes would have been well resolved. The output of each auditory filter would be a complex waveshape, which might make the subsequent temporal analysis more difficult. Adding the lower harmonics may have the effect of making the waveshape even more complex, with multiple peaks per period, thereby adding even more to the difficulty of temporal analysis.

The relative phases of the components can influence DLs for F_0, and the effect of phase is larger for impaired ears than for normal ears. A similar result has been found previously for subjects with more severe hearing losses (Rosen, 1987). This can be explained in terms of the broadened auditory filters for the impaired ears, which would result in strong interactions of the harmonics. Again, this suggests that temporal processing is involved in the extraction of pitch. The variation of the phase effects across subjects and F_0's may result from variations in the amplitude and phase responses of the auditory filters. The results are not readily explained by spectral models of pitch perception.

Acknowledgement

This work was supported by the MRC (U.K.). We thank Stuart Rosen, Roy Patterson and Andrew Faulkner for useful comments on an earlier version of this paper.

References

Glasberg, B.R. and Moore, B.C.J. (**1986**). "Auditory filter shapes in subjects with unilateral and bilateral cochlear impairments," J.Acoust.Soc.Am. **79**, 1020-1033.

Goldstein, J.L. (**1973**). "An optimum processor theory for the central formation of the pitch of complex tones," J.Acoust.Soc.Am. **54**, 1496-1516.

Hoekstra, A. and Ritsma, R.J. (**1977**). "Perceptive hearing loss and frequency selectivity," in *Psychophysics and Physiology of Hearing*, edited by

E.F.Evans and J.P.Wilson (Academic Press, London).
Horst, J.W. (1987). "Frequency discrimination of complex signals, frequency selectivity, and speech perception in hearing-impaired subjects," J.Acoust. Soc.Am. **82**, 874-885.
Moore, B.C.J. (**1977**). "Effects of relative phase of the components on the pitch of three-component complex tones," in *Psychophysics and Physiology of Hearing*, edited by E.F.Evans and J.P.Wilson (Academic Press, London).
Moore, B.C.J. (**1982**). *An Introduction to the Psychology of Hearing*, (Academic Press, London).
Moore, B.C.J. and Glasberg, B.R. (**1986**). "The role of frequency selectivity in the perception of loudness, pitch and time," in *Frequency Selectivity in Hearing*, edited by B.C.J.Moore (Academic Press, London).
Moore, B.C.J. and Glasberg, B.R. (**1987**). "Pitch perception and phase sensitivity for subjects with unilateral and bilateral cochlear hearing impairments," in *Clinical Audiology '87*, edited by A.Quaranta (Laterza, Bari, Italy, in press).
Moore, B.C.J., Glasberg, B.R. and Shailer, M.J. (**1984**). "Frequency and intensity difference limens for harmonics within complex tones," J.Acoust. Soc.Am. **75**, 550-561.
Patterson, R.D. (**1987**). "A pulse ribbon model of peripheral auditory processing," in *Auditory Processing of Complex Sounds*, edited by W.A.Yost and C.S.Watson (Erlbaum, New Jersey).
Plomp, R. (**1964**). "The ear as a frequency analyzer," J.Acoust.Soc.Am. **36**, 1628-1636.
Rosen, S. (**1987**). "Phase and the hearing impaired," in *The Psychophysics of Speech Perception*, edited by M.E.H.Schouten (Nijhoff, Netherlands).
Rosen, S. and Fourcin, A.J. (**1986**). "Frequency selectivity and the perception of speech," in *Frequency Selectivity in Hearing*, edited by B.C.J. Moore (Academic Press, London).
Schroeder, M.R. (**1970**). "Synthesis of low peak-factor signals and binary sequences with low autocorrelation," IEEE Trans.Inf.Th., **IT-16**, 85-89.
Srulovicz, P. and Goldstein, J.L. (**1983**). "A central spectrum model: a synthesis of auditory-nerve timing and place cues in monaural communication of frequency spectrum," J.Acoust.Soc.Am. **73**, 1266-1276.
Terhardt, E. (**1974**). "Pitch, consonance and harmony," J.Acoust.Soc.Am. **55**, 1061-1069.

Comments

Houtsma:

I think one has to be very careful drawing any general conclusions from this experiment. Although it was presented as a discrimination experiment for f_0, no effort was made to prevent subjects from using frequency changes in the partials as discrimination clues. The fact that the data show almost no systematic dependance on phase configuration and spectral composition suggests to me that indeed frequency changes, and not the percept of the (missing) fundamental f_0, were the dominant clue.

Reply by Moore

For the complex tones containing harmonics 6-12, it is unlikely that the harmonics 7-11 moved have been resolvable. However, it is possible that subjects could have listened to "edge pitches" associated with the 6th or 12th harmonics and used these to perform the task. We performed two experiments to check on this. In the first, the complex tones were presented in a complementary band-stop noise. For the normal ears, this produced only a small impairment in discrimination of f_0. For the impaired ears, the DLs for f_0 were affected somewhat more (which is to be expected from their reduced frequency selectivity), but the pattern of phase effects was not altered. In the second experiment, the spectral envelope of the complex tones was made to tail off gradually instead of having abrupt edges. Again, this had only marginal effects on performance. These experiments lead to the conclusion that the results reported in our paper were not strongly influenced by cues related to the sharp spectral edges of the stimuli. We believe that our subjects were discriminating the stimuli on the basis of residue pitch, and that our results are difficult to explain in terms of spectral models of pitch perception.

Green:

Dr. Houtsma has raised the objection that your listeners may be comparing individual components in your complex waves rather than comparing their residue on virtual pitch. Would the following procedure remove that objection? Suppose, in one interval of a forced-choice trial, we present a single component at the fundamental frequency. In the other interval, we present a harmonic complex consisting of several higher harmonics **without** the fundamental. For example, in one interval, the listener might hear 200 Hz. In the second interval, the listener might hear a complex consisting of 404, 606, 808, 1010, 1212 and 1414 Hz. The correct answer, based on the pitch of the waveform would be that the second interval has a higher pitch (202 > 200 Hz). If the listener can reliably perform such discriminations then their judgment cannot be based on a comparison of individual components since none occupy the same frequency region.

Reply by Moore:

We have not done exactly the experiment you describe, but we have done something similar. We have required subjects to discriminate differences in f_0 of two complex tones which have no harmonics in common. For example, one complex tone might contain harmonics 1, 4, 5, 8, 9 and 12, while the other would contain harmonics 2, 3, 6, 7, 10 and 11. Unfortunately, the large difference in timbre between the two tones makes the task very difficult; the small differences in pitch are much less salient than the differences in timbre. As a consequence, large practice effects are observed. Well-practiced, highly-motivated subjects (e.g. myself) can achieve DL's for f_0 of less than 0.4% for values of f_0 of 100, 200 and 400 Hz. These DL's are similar to those obtained for complex tones with harmonics in common. However, other subjects seem to have great difficulty in ignoring the differences in timbre. I don't think it would be practical to use this method with hearing-impaired subjects.

Horst

You describe the effect of cochlear filtering on your stimuli by referring to your simulations rather than to single-fiber responses (Horst *et al.*, 1986) to these types of stimuli. Does this mean that you prefer simulations to single-fiber responses as a model of the human cochlea?

Horst, J.W., Javel, E. and Farley, G.R (1986). "Effects of phase and amplitude spectrum in the nonlinear processing of complex stimuli in single fibers of the auditory nerve". In: Auditory frequency selectivity, B.C.J. Moore and R.D. Patterson, eds. (Plenum).

Reply by Moore:

We feel that there are difficulties in comparing psychophysical data obtained in man with neural responses obtained in animals, since there may be qualitative differences in degree of frequency selectivity and of nonlinearity. For this reason, we tend to prefer simulations based on psychophysical measures of frequency selectivity obtained in man. However, we would not deny the usefulness of comparison with neural data such as yours. Where such comparisons are made, we feel that they should take account of differences in the audible frequency range between man and the animal being studied. Comparison at corresponding points on the basilar membrane may be appropriate, with frequencies of stimuli scaled appropriately.

Horst:

Your paper suggests that the controversy between spectral and temporal theories is fairly young. It will be of interest to the reader who is not familiar with the subject, to note that in the nineteenth century this issue was already debated by Seebeck ("spectro-temporal") and Ohm ("spectral"). In the present century e.g. Schouten made important contributions to the spectral-temporal theory (e.g. Schouten, 1940).

Ohm, G.S. (1843): "Ueber die Definition des Tones nebst daran geknüpfter Theorie der Sirene und ähnlicher tonbildender Vorrichtungen." Ann.Phys.Chem. 59, 513-565.

Schouten, J.F. (1940). "The residue, a new component in subjective sound analysis." Proc.Kon. Ned.Akad.Wetensch. 43, 356-365.

Seebeck, A. (1843). "Beobachtungen über einige Bedingungen der Entstehung von Töne." Ann. Phys. Chem. 53, 417-436.

Temporally-based auditory sensations in the profoundly hearing-impaired listener

Stuart Rosen & David A. J. Smith

Department of Phonetics and Linguistics, University College London
4 Stephenson Way, London NW1 2HE

Introduction

In considering the residual auditory capacities of listeners with an acquired loss of profound degree, attention has been primarily focussed on the extent of degradation suffered in hearing ability. We have recently begun a project to determine what abilities remain, in order, among other aims, to guide the development of appropriate hearing aids. As evidence from measurements of psychoacoustical tuning curves suggests severe or total degradation in "place"-based processing for frequency selectivity (Faulkner *et al.*, in press), the role of time-based processes comes to the fore.

One experimentally convenient way to alter the temporal properties of a signal is through a manipulation of its phase spectrum, as this leaves the amplitude spectrum unchanged. When stimulus components are relatively close, phase changes are reflected in relatively slow fluctuations in various stimulus properties - that is, in gross temporal structure. Such stimuli may prove useful in determining temporal acuity in a frequency-specific manner. Gap detection tasks which attempt to do this introduce gaps in relatively narrow bands of noise, using band-stop noises straddling the signal in frequency to mask off-frequency splatter (e.g. Fitzgibbons & Wightman, 1982). However, the performance of impaired listeners may be degraded by widened auditory filters which allow the masking noise to "leak" into channels in the stimulus frequency region. The use of stimuli which need no masking of extraneous cues may avoid such difficulties of interpretation.

For harmonic components that are relatively far apart, phase changes evidence themselves as changes in waveshape - that is, in fine temporal structure. Such stimuli may prove useful in determining the role of temporal cues in pitch and timbre perception, and thus introduce a new stimulus parameter to be controlled in practical hearing aids (Rosen, 1987).

Listeners

The impaired listeners form a fairly homogeneous group in having a long

Table 1: Hearing Levels (ISO) for the impaired listeners.

	frequency (Hz)						
listener	125	250	500	1000	2000	4000	8000
C	70	100	105	115	115	>120	>100
K	45	65	85	100	>120	>120	>100
L	70	85	100	115	>120	>120	>100
R	35	60	95	110	120	>120	>100
S	75	85	100	120	>120	>120	>100
T	75	95	120	>120	115	120	>100

history of normal or near-normal hearing, and a loss of profound degree acquired in adulthood. All have "left-hand corner" audiograms, with best hearing levels at 125 Hz, which worsen with increasing frequency (Table 1). Dynamic range is best at the low frequencies, and shrinks to only a few dB (or is nonexistent) within the frequency range 0.5 - 2 kHz (Rosen *et al.*, 1987).

General methods

To ensure accurate reproduction of low frequency sounds, Rosen and Nevard (1987) have developed a technique that measures the sound pressure waveform delivered by headphones while the listener wears them. Measurements on an acoustic manikin (KEMAR) indicate that a small electret microphone mounted on the earphone grid gives an accurate measure of the sound field at the tympanic membrane up to frequencies of 2 kHz (within about 5 dB and 10°).

Connevans CE8 headphones, chosen for their relatively low nonlinear distortion at high levels and low frequencies, were used in all tests. Stimuli were synthesized digitally at a sampling frequency of 10 kHz. Except where noted, the phase and amplitude of each stimulus component was corrected for the linear phase and amplitude distortions of the headphones, determined for each listener using a spectrum analyzer. The resulting transfer function was sent via an interface to a digital computer for subsequent use in determining appropriate corrections for synthesis of the stimuli.

Detecting phase changes among closely spaced components

Our test of abilities to resolve relatively slow changes in temporal structure, was based on sinusoidally-*a*mplitude *m*odulated (AM) and so-called *q*uasi-*f*requency *m*odulated (QFM) sounds of low modulation rate. These signals contain three sinusoidal components, a carrier and two sidebands, and have the general form:

$$s(t) = \cos(ct + d) + 0.5\cos[(c-m)t] + 0.5\cos[(c+m)t] \qquad (1)$$

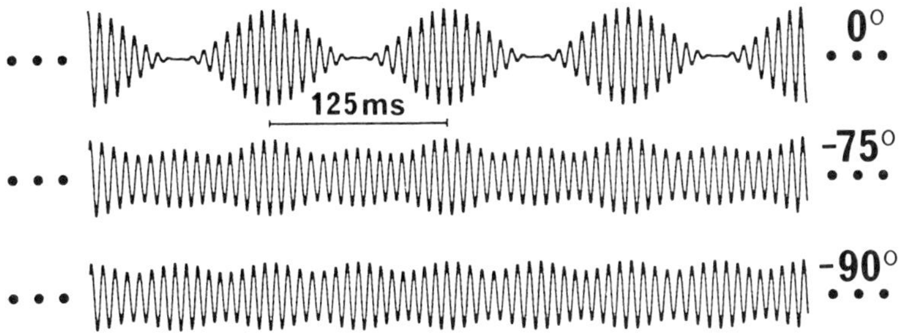

Figure 1. Examples of the PSC-AM waveforms for a carrier frequency of 125 Hz, a modulating frequency of 8 Hz, and three values of d. Most listeners are able to distinguish the lower two sounds.

Here c and m are the angular frequencies of the carrier and modulator, respectively (in radians/s) and d is the difference in phase between the carrier and each of the two sidebands. When d = 0, all three components are in cosine phase (simple AM). When d = -90°, the resulting spectrum approximates that obtained by frequency modulation (hence QFM). Both because the approximation of QFM to true FM is not all that good for these stimuli, and because non-zero values of d other than -90° will be frequently used, we prefer a more accurate term - phase-shifted carrier AM of d degrees (PSC-AM:d). Hence QFM sounds will now be labelled PSC-AM:-90.

In any particular experimental test, both the carrier and modulation frequencies were fixed. Stimuli were presented in a 3-interval 2-alternative forced-choice (3I-2AFC) task in which the first stimulus and either the second or the third were the PSC-AM:-90. The listener indicated whether the "different" stimulus occurred in intervals two or three, and this was varied randomly from trial to trial. Feedback (as to the correctness of response) was given after each trial. All sounds had a total duration of 1 s, with 50 ms raised-cosine rises and falls. At the start of each session the "different" stimulus was AM (PSC-AM:0) and the carrier phase was varied adaptively to find the minimum phase difference which the listener could discriminate about 79% of the time.

Figure 1 shows the effect of varying the relative phase of the carrier (d) on the stimulus waveform. A crucial stimulus feature which varies with d is the amplitude envelope, an expression for which can be obtained from (1) using the so-called analytic signal, constructed via a Hilbert transform:

$$\text{Envelope}(t) = \sqrt{0.5\cos(2mt) + 2\cos(d)\cos(mt) + 1.5} \qquad (2)$$

Note that this does not depend on carrier frequency. When d = 0° (AM) the amplitude envelope is sinusoidal with frequency m. When d = -90°, the envelope is periodic with frequency 2m rads/s, and a 3-dB variation between maxima and minima. For phase values between these extremes, the envelope is periodic with frequency m rads/s, with a major and minor peak per period

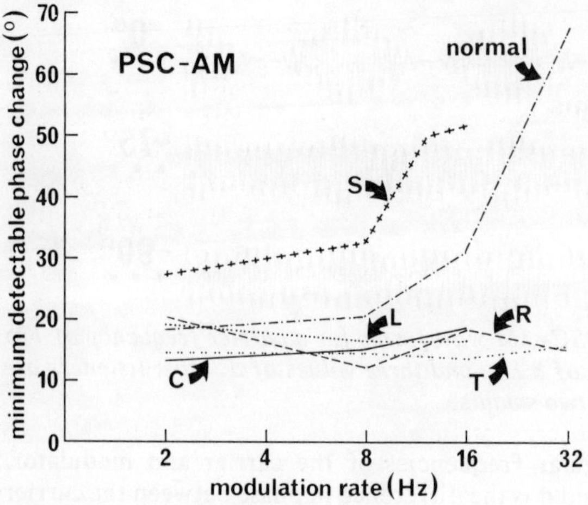

Figure 2. Minimum detectable phase change from a PSC-AM:-90 sound. Each point is the average of 1 to 6 (mean of 3.3) adaptive runs.

(as seen for d = -75° in Figure 1). As d decreases from 0 to -90°, the size of the major peak decreases while that of the minor increases, until they are equal at d = -90°.

A number of normal and profoundly impaired listeners have participated in this task at a carrier frequency of 125 Hz (Figure 2). For normal listeners (carrier at 60 dB SPL), there is a range of low modulation frequencies over which performance is fairly constant. In this region, spectral components are not resolved by peripheral filtering, and it is presumably purely the temporal aspects of the stimuli that are determining performance.

At higher modulation frequencies, performance worsens precipitously. Here spectral components are presumably segregated into separate auditory filters, thus the envelope modulation (which requires the interaction of components) does not arise. Support for this view is also found in initial tests at a carrier frequency of 1 kHz which show that the modulating frequency at which good discrimination is still possible is much higher than it is at a carrier of 125 Hz, corresponding to the way in which it is known that the bandwidth of auditory filters varies with frequency. Sensitivity to phase changes has, of course, been understood in this way for many years (e.g. Mathes & Miller, 1947).

Most of the profoundly impaired listeners perform about as well as normal listeners at low modulation rates, albeit with sounds considerably more intense (always at a listener-determined "comfortable" level). At relatively high modulation rates they generally do better. That impaired listeners can be more sensitive to phase changes than normals has already been reported by Rosen (1986, 1987) for moderately impaired listeners, and almost certainly results from impaired auditory filtering allowing increased interaction among stimulus components. These results bode well for even profoundly impaired listeners' abilities to follow the time course of amplitude fluctuations in speech, which Plomp (1983) reports to fall in the region 0.3 - 15 Hz. One listener ("S"), however, shows a pattern that may indicate temporal abilities considerably more degraded than those of the other impaired listeners, as his performance steadily worsens with increasing modulation frequency.

Rather less easy to explain are some preliminary results obtained at higher carrier frequencies. We have tested "C", "L" and "T" at carrier frequencies of 500 Hz and find essentially similar results to those they obtained at 125 Hz. At 1 kHz, however, "C" shows better performance at a modulation frequency of 32 Hz (with a minimum detectable change of 13°) than at 2 or 16 Hz (where changes of about 36° are necessary). It may be that there is abnormal tone decay at this frequency, a possibility which we are currently investigating.

There is also a troubling aspect to this finding. If listeners like "C" have no frequency selective mechanisms remaining, as seems to be the case, we might expect that the perception of all sinsuoids, no matter their frequency, would be mediated through the same auditory nerve fibres. If that is so, why is temporal resolution, as measured here, so different at 125 and 1000 Hz and low modulation rates, given that the amplitude envelopes of the two stimuli are identical?

One other point remains. Although subjectively, amplitude envelope cues seem to be primary in this task, there are variations in instantaneous frequency as well (also determined via the analytic signal), given by:

$$\mathrm{IF}(t) = c + [m \sin(d) \sin(mt)]/\mathrm{Envelope}^2(t) \qquad (3)$$

When d = -90°, the instantaneous frequency varies periodically with frequency m rads/s and maximum deviations of m from the carrier frequency. Thus, the faster the modulation rate, the greater the deviations from the carrier (this holds for all non-zero d). That instantaneous frequency is likely to be an important feature for at least some sounds is supported by the fact that a physiologically plausible operation like peak-picking will, on average, lead to interspike times whose reciprocal is an approximation to instantaneous frequency. This requires both sufficiently high waveform amplitude and a significant degree of interaction among spectral components within a single auditory filter.

Currently, these tests are being extended to more listeners, and over a wider range of carrier frequencies. In order to determine exactly what stimulus attributes are being utilized by listeners (and in particular, the role of instantaneous frequency), we plan to investigate the perception of pure FM and AM signals of similar modulation rates.

Phase changes in harmonic complexes

Although it is clear that alterations in phase spectrum are of relatively minor perceptual importance in comparison to changes in the amplitude spectrum for normal listeners (e.g. Plomp & Steeneken, 1969), we have argued

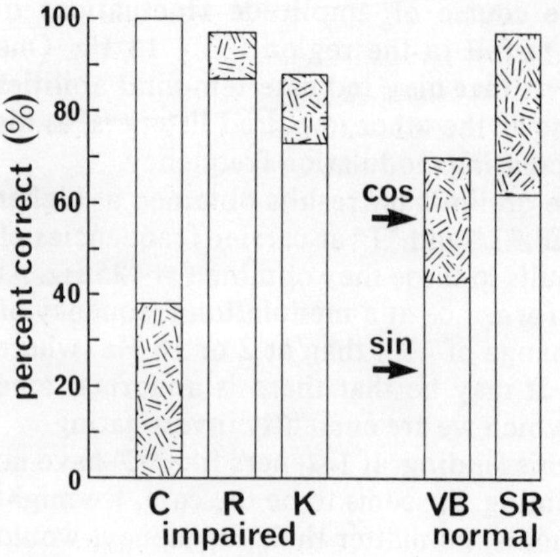

Figure 3. Percent correct in a fixed-level AM/QFM discrimination task in which the nominal phases of the AM stimulus were sine or cosine. In fact, inspection of the output of the headphones showed the nominally cosine stimulus to be in sine phase, and the nominally sine stimulus to be in -cosine phase.

previously that phase is likely to play a more important role in determining the percepts of impaired listeners (Rosen, 1987; Rosen & Fourcin, 1986). Our initial investigations, for historical reasons, used AM/QFM stimulus pairs. To make the stimuli more relevant to speech perception, the stimulus components were the first three harmonics of a fundamental of 250 Hz. Testing used a 3I-3AFC paradigm in which, during a particular session, the two sounds whose discriminability was being tested remained constant. To counteract the effect of the headphones, a set of mean amplitude corrections was used (determined from 8 ears), but phase was not corrected. Figure 3 shows the performance obtained by three profoundly impaired, and two normal listeners, for a 90° phase shift of the carrier as a function of the reference phase of the complex. Reference phase clearly has an effect on the relative detectability of the phase change (Rosen, 1986). Furthermore, the impaired listeners do about as well as the normal listeners (SR being highly practiced), and better for sine phase stimuli. The intensity levels for normal listeners are considerably lower than those for the impaired listener, but it is not possible to use such high levels with the normals. If equal SL levels were used, the performance of normal listeners would considerably worsen (Goldstein, 1967).

In more recent work, we have made all three stimulus components of equal amplitude, to increase the degree of interaction among harmonics in an auditory filter centred on the "carrier". We have also used adaptive techniques to find the minimum detectable phase change in the central component in a 3I-2AFC task, as for PSC-AM. The standard complex has all components either in sine or cosine phase, while the test complex starts with its central component 90° out of phase. Table 2 shows initial results for two normal and one impaired listener.

Reference phase again affects performance significantly, in a way which varies across individuals. Presumably, phase characteristics of auditory filters will vary from person to person, putting the stimulus components into a phase

Table 2: Results from a phase discrimination task for three equal amplitude harmonics of 125, 250 and 375 Hz. Levels were 80 dB SPL/ component for the normal listeners and 118 dB SPL for the impaired listener "C". Each value is based on 2-3 adaptive runs. For sine phase sounds, "C" was unable to identify the maximum 90° phase shift at better than chance level.

	minimum detectable phase change (°)	
listener	sine phase	cosine phase
SR	49.1	29.4
DAJS	39.5	54.7
C	>90	15.4

relationship which may help or hinder discrimination performance. Also, for the cosine complex, the performance of the profoundly impaired listener is far superior.

At least as interesting as the ability to discriminate phase changes is the way in which listeners describe the perceptual attributes they are using to perform this task. Often a change in "pitch" is ascribed, but just as frequently, there is said to be change in the quality or "tone" of the sound. One profoundly impaired listener ("R"), in the tests of Figure 3 claimed the AM and QFM sounds in cosine reference phase were heard as different vowels. This has implications both theoretically, for models of timbre perception that stress the importance of temporal factors, and practically, in providing a new way of signalling vowel colour (for fuller discussions, see Rosen & Fourcin, 1986; Rosen, 1987).

For this to be possible, however, a more accurate way for listeners to "describe" their experiences is necessary. We have recently begun working with a paradigm in which listeners are asked to adjust (using a joystick and rotatable wheel), the spectral slope, fundamental frequency and intensity of a stimulus with three harmonic components in (say) sine phase, to a stimulus consisting of three equal-amplitude harmonics in which the phase relationship of the central component is varied from trial to trial, while the flanking components remain in sine phase. One striking feature of our pilot investigations is the ease of making the match when the reference and adjustable complex were identical in phase spectrum, and the difficulty experienced when the phase of the central components differed. Also, a phase shift of -90° led to changes in all three stimulus attributes being adjusted. The extent to which the "matched" sound is perceptually close to a sound with altered phase will be tested in discrimination experiments looking for trading relationships between phase and the other stimulus attributes.

Final remarks

Current evidence suggests that phase will play a much greater role in determining the percepts of hearing impaired, than of normal, listeners. In some sounds, manipulations of phase may prove useful in examining aspects of relatively gross temporal acuity. For harmonic complexes, we hope to determine the relationship between manipulations of relative phase and subjective changes in timbre, pitch and/or loudness. For profoundly impaired listeners, this may lead to hearing aids that use phase intentionally to signal aspects of vowel colour. For normal listeners, mapping out such relationships will doubtless provide important ways of testing models for the coding of pitch and timbre.

Acknowledgements

First thanks to the hearing-impaired listeners for their participation in what one has called "soporific" tests. David Seggie and Ian Howard assisted in sorting out the mathematical and computational aspects of analytic signals. Andrew Faulkner and Brian Moore made useful comments on the manuscript. This work is supported by the Medical Research Council of Great Britain, and by a special travel grant from the Heinz and Anna Koch Foundation.

References

Faulkner, A., Ball, V., Rosen, S., Moore, B.C.J. & Fourcin, A.J. (**in press**). "Auditory acuity with residual low-frequency hearing," Brit.J.Audiol. (abstract).

Fitzgibbons, P.J. & Wightman, F.L. (**1982**). "Gap detection in normal and hearing-impaired listeners," J. Acoust. Soc. Am. **72**, 761-765.

Goldstein, J.L. (**1967**). "Auditory spectral filtering and monaural phase perception," J. Acoust. Soc. Am. **41**, 458-479.

Mathes, R.C. and Miller, R.L. (**1947**). "Phase effects in monaural perception," J. Acoust. Soc. Am. **19**, 780-797.

Plomp, R. (**1983**). "The role of modulation in hearing," in Hearing - Physiological Bases and Psychophysics, edited by R. Klinke & R. Hartmann (Springer-Verlag, Berlin).

Plomp, R. and Steeneken, H.J.M. (**1969**). "Effect of phase on the timbre of complex tones," J. Acoust. Soc. Am. **46**, 409-421.

Rosen, S. (**1986**). "Monaural phase sensitivity: Frequency selectivity and temporal processes," in Auditory Frequency Selectivity, edited by B.C.J. Moore & R.D. Patterson (Plenum, New York).

Rosen, S. (**1987**). "Phase and the hearing-impaired," in The Psychophysics of Speech Perception, edited by M.E.H. Schouten (Martinus Nijhoff, Dordrecht).

Rosen, S. & Fourcin, A.J. (**1986**). "Frequency selectivity and the perception of speech," in Frequency Selectivity in Hearing, edited by B. C. J. Moore (Academic, London).

Rosen, S. and Nevard, S. (**1987**). "A headphone monitoring system for low-

frequency psychoacoustics," Brit. J. Audiol. **21**, 108-109 (abstract).
Rosen, S., Walliker, J.R., Fourcin, A. & Ball, V. (**1987**). "A microprocessor-based acoustic hearing aid for the profoundly impaired listener," J. Rehab. Res. Dev. **24**, 239-260.

Comments

Narins:

Did you adjust the total power of your QFM stimulus to compensate for changes in modulation depth? This would be important to avoid introducing signal level changes which could provide unintentional cues to aid in discrimination.

Reply by Rosen:

For given carrier and modulation frequencies, all the PSC-AM sounds have identical power spectra - the changes in amplitude envelope result purely from a change in the phase spectrum of the sounds. These changes in envelope are thus different to those in which a sinusoid is amplitude modulated, a process which does introduce changes in the power spectrum in the form of sidebands.

Simultaneous and forward-masking patterns of a formant transition

Richard S. Tyler[1,2], Karen Iler Kirk[2], Nancy Tye-Murray[1]

[1]*Department of Otolaryngology--Head & Neck Surgery*
[2]*Department of Speech Pathology & Audiology*
The University of Iowa, Iowa City, IA 52242

Introduction

Determining the peripheral auditory representation of speech sounds might help us to understand the perception of natural and distorted speech, and the consequences of hearing loss.

One technique used to study the peripheral representation of speech in humans is to obtain vowel-masking patterns. A steady-state vowel is used as a masker, and pure-tone signal thresholds are obtained for a variety of signal frequencies. The resulting masking pattern likely reflects the amount of neural activity in different frequency regions produced by the vowel. The greater the signal threshold, the greater the assumed neural activity in a particular frequency region (Tyler, 1988).

Several investigators have observed the preservation of formant-frequency locations in vowel-masking patterns in normal listeners (Bacon and Brandt, 1982; Houtgast, 1974; Moore and Glasberg, 1983; Sidwell and Summerfield, 1985; Tyler and Lindblom, 1982). The formant locations are more clearly defined in non-simultaneous masking procedures than in simultaneous masking, probably due to the effects of suppression which are revealed in the former (Moore and O'Loughlin, 1986).

The vowel-masking patterns in the hearing impaired do not always show a preservation of the formant locations (Bacon and Brandt, 1982; Sidwell and Summerfield, 1985; Tyler, 1986). This is consistent with poor frequency resolution, commonly observed in the hearing impaired (e.g., Dreschler and Festen, 1986; Florentine *et al.*, 1980; Pick, Evans, and Wilson, 1977; Stelmachowicz *et al.*, 1985; Tyler, 1986).

Measuring the masking patterns of consonants presents methodological problems, because consonants change their acoustic characteristics over time.

Lacerda and Moreira (1982) obtained simultaneous masking thresholds at three frequencies at different time delays throughout a sinusoidal frequency transition. They noted that the masking produced by the transition in an upward direction was different from that obtained when the transition was in a downward direction. They attributed these differences to asymmetrical differences in suppression.

Sidwell and Summerfield (1986) measured simultaneous masking patterns using consonant-vowel-consonant syllables as maskers. Although not the primary thrust of their paper, they observed that the masking patterns obtained at the beginning of a transition were different from those obtained at the end of a transition.

Spiegel (1987) measured simultaneous masking patterns in vowel-consonant-vowel and in consonant-alone stimuli. He noted that thresholds obtained during the consonant were sometimes higher when the neighboring vowels were present, suggesting the adjacent vowels had some forward and backward masking effects.

It is known that with simultaneous masking there are interactions between the signal and the masker that confound the interpretation of the masking pattern. These confounding factors include beats, combination tones, and lack of suppression effects. To avoid these effects, nonsimultaneous paradigms, such as forward masking, have been used. Because the signal follows the masker, beats and combination tones are avoided, and suppression effects among components of the masker can be observed (see Moore and O'Loughlin, 1986).

A forward-masking pattern obtained after the termination of a consonant

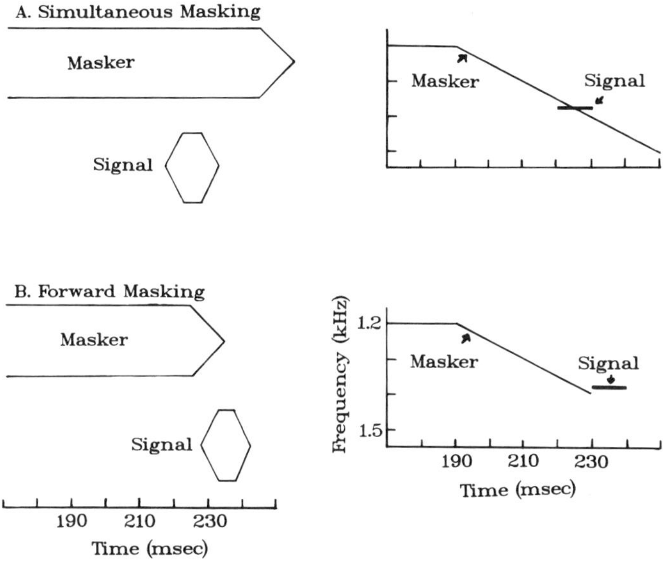

Figure 1. Schematic representation of the temporal and spectral relationship between the formant-transition masker and the signal (for one time delay, as an example) in the simultaneous (top) and forward-masking paradigm (bottom). Only the last 60 ms of the stimuli are shown.

would reflect some weighted representation of the latter portion of the transition. It would be of greater interest to obtain masking patterns at different time intervals throughout the consonant. In this way the auditory spectral representation could be tracked in time.

Our approach (shown in Figure 1) was to measure forward masking with different segments of the consonant. Only the last 60 ms of the stimuli are shown. On the left, we see the temporal relationship between the signal and masker. On the right, we show a schematic spectrogram. As an example we have chosen a condition where the signal onset occurs 210 ms after the onset of the transition in the simultaneous paradigm (top). The simultaneous masking pattern should represent the auditory spectrum from about 220 to 230 ms. In forward masking (bottom), the masker is terminated after 230 ms, when the signal is turned on. The forward masking pattern should represent the auditory spectrum of the masker just before it was terminated, also from about 220 to 230 ms.

In the preliminary experiment reported here, we measured the masking pattern of a formant transition with both a simultaneous and nonsimultaneous masking procedure at four different time delays during the transition.

Methods

A synthetic formant transition (bandwidth = 100 Hz) was used as the masker. The center frequency increased from 1200 to 1500 Hz from 0 to 60 ms; remained at 1500 Hz from 60 to 190 ms; and then decreased from 1500 to 1200 Hz from 190 to 250 ms. A noise source was used for excitation to avoid beats between the signal and masker in the simultaneous paradigm. The masker level was 85 dB SPL.

Two normal-hearing listeners served as subjects. They received about one hour of practice before testing.

An adaptive three-interval two-alternative procedure was used. Three correct responses resulted in a decrease in signal level, and one incorrect response resulted in an increase in signal level. The step size was 6 dB, which was reduced to 2 dB after 4 reversals. A threshold run was terminated after nine reversals. The average of the last 5 reversals was defined as threshold. At least three independent estimates were obtained for each threshold. If these differed by more than 6 dB, then additional threshold estimates were obtained until three threshold estimates were within a 6 dB range. The average values of the three lowest threshold estimates are shown in the figures.

The formant masker was 250 ms in duration (between 50% points on the envelope) for simultaneous masking, and was shaped with an external gate with a 10-ms rise/fall time (between 10 and 90% points on the envelope). The signal was a 10-ms duration tone with a 5 ms rise/fall time. In the forward-masking paradigm, there was a 0 ms delay between the 50% points of the envelope of the masker offset and signal onset.

For the simultaneous masking condition, the signal was turned on 180, 200, 220, and 240 ms after the onset of the masker. For the forward masking

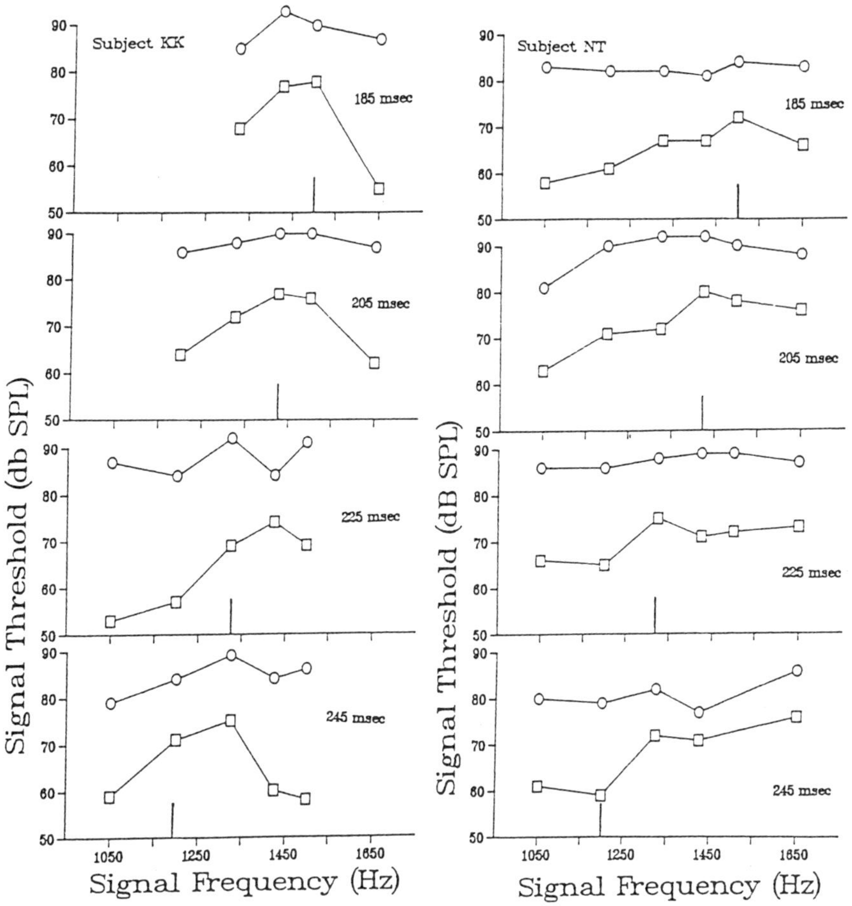

Figure 2. Simultaneous (○) and forward-masking (□) patterns for normal-hearing subject NT (left) and subject KK (right) at four different times during the transition. Times on the right indicate the temporal center of the signal in the simultaneous masking condition relative to the onset of the masker. The vertical lines indicate the formant locations.

conditions, the signal was turned on 190, 210, 230, and 250 ms after the onset of the masker.

Results

The results are shown for two normal-hearing subjects in Figure 2. From top to bottom, each panel represents a successive 20-ms segment of the auditory representation of the transition.

For subject KK, the simultaneous-masking patterns show broad, shallow peaks in the region of the formant transition. The forward-masking patterns show more well-defined peaks, with larger threshold differences between signal frequencies at peaks compared to those at neighboring frequencies. Furthermore, the peak follows the transition. For example, at 185 ms, the peak is at around 1425-1500 Hz. At 245 ms, the peak has shifted to 1325 Hz. The threshold at 1500 Hz decreases from 78 dB SPL at 185 ms to 58 dB SPL at 245 ms. Also note that masked thresholds at frequencies higher than the formant-transmission remain elevated after the formant has passed through that frequency region.

For subject NT, the simultaneous masking pattern also shows poorly defined, broad peaks, if they exist at all. Peaks in the forward-masking patterns are more easily identifiable, and shift according to the frequency of the transition. Again, the thresholds obtained at frequencies where the formant transition has already passed remain elevated for a time.

Conclusions

We have attempted to determine the auditory representation of a formant transition by measuring simultaneous and forward masking patterns at different times during the transition. The simultaneous masking patterns do not reflect the acoustic spectra as well as the forward-masking patterns. We interpret the series of forward-masking patterns as a better representation of the auditory spectrum changing in time. It is likely that the better representation of the spectra in the forward-masking patterns are a reflection of suppression.

There are spectral and temporal limitations to this approach. Spectrally, the signal is smeared in the frequency domain by its brief duration and rise/fall time. In the forward-masking condition, the spectrum of the transition is also smeared because it is gated off. This gating also attenuates the latter portion of the transition.

Temporally, the signal does not represent a single point in time because of its 10-ms duration. Therefore in simultaneous masking, thresholds represent activity over a 10-ms period while the masker spectrum is changing. In forward masking, the signal threshold will be influenced by maskers that occur within 40-50 ms of the sinal (Elliott, 1962), but should be primarily dependent upon maskers that occur within 10-15 ms.

Simultaneous masking may have one advantage over forward masking in this application. The masking pattern obtained with simultaneous masking will include the effects of the excitation produced after the signal (backward masking) (Spiegel, 1987), which is not accounted for in a forward-masking paradigm.

The representation of a transition in the auditory system will be influenced by the excitation and adaptation produced by the formants and the suppression effects on adjacent frequency regions. Suppression could function to emphasize spectral contrasts, by 1) suppressing simultaneously intraformant valleys, and 2) decreasing the excitation in 'valleys' into which the formants will move at a later time during the transition.

These psychophysical results are also qualitatively consistent with the response of auditory neurons, which have been shown to follow the formant peaks during consonant transitions (Delgutte and Kiang, 1984; Miller and Sachs, 1983).

References

Bacon, S.P., and Brandt, J.F. (**1982**). "Auditory processing of vowels by normal-hearing and hearing-impaired listeners," J.Acoust.Soc.Am. **25**, 339-347.

Delgutte, B., and Kiang, N.Y.S. (**1984**). "Speech coding in the auditory nerve: IV. Sounds with consonant-like dynamic characteristics," J.Acoust.Soc. Am. **75**, 897-907.

Dreschler, W.A., and Festen, J.M. (**1986**). "The effect of hearing impairment on auditory filter shapes in simultaneous and forward masking," in *Auditory Frequency Selectivity*, edited by B.C.J.Moore and R.D.Patterson (Plenum Press, New York), pp. 331-340.

Elliott, L.L. (**1962**). "Backward and forward masking of probe tones of different frequencies," J.Acoust.Soc.Am. **34**, 1116-1117.

Florentine, M., Buus, S., Scharf, B., and Zwicker, E. (**1980**). "Frequency selectivity in normally-hearing and hearing-impaired observers," J.Speech Hear.Res. **23**, 646-669.

Houtgast, T. (**1974**). "Auditory analysis of vowel-like sounds," Acustica, **31**, 320-324.

Lacerda, F., and Moreira, H.O. (**1982**). "How does the peripheral auditory system represent formant transitions? A psychophysical approach," in *The Representation of Speech in the Peripheral Auditory System*, edited by R. Carlson and B. Granstrom (Elsevier Biomedical Press, Amsterdam), pp. 89-94.

Miller, M.I., and Sachs, M.B. (**1983**). "Representation of stop consonants in the discharge patterns of auditory-nerve fibers," J.Acoust.Soc.Am. **74**, 502-517.

Moore, B.C.J., and Glasberg, B.R. (**1983**). "Masking patterns for synthetic vowels in simultaneous and forward masking," J.Acoust.Soc.Am. 73, 906-917.

Moore, B.C.J., and O'Loughlin, B.J. (**1986**). "The use of nonsimultaneous masking to measure frequency selectivity and suppression," in *Frequency Selectivity in Hearing*, edited by B.C.J. Moore (Academic Press Inc., London), pp. 179-250.

Pick, G.F., Evans, E.F., and Wilson, J.P. (**1977**). "Frequency resolution in patients with hearing loss of cochlear origin," in *Psychophysics and Physiology of Hearing*, edited by E.F. Evans and J.P. Wilson (Academic Press, New York).

Sidwell, A., and Summerfield, Q. (**1985**). "The effect of enhanced spectral contrast on the internal representation of vowel-shaped noise," J.Acoust. Soc.Am. **78**, 495-506.

Sidwell, A., and Summerfield, Q. (**1986**). "The auditory representation of symmetrical CVC syllables," Speech Communications **5**, 283-297.

Spiegel, M.F. (**1987**). "Speech masking. I. Simultaneous and nonsimultaneous masking within stop /d/ and flap /r/ closures," J.Acoust.Soc.Am. **82**, 1492-1502.

Stelmachowicz, P.G., Jesteadt, W., Gorga, M.P., and Mott, J. (**1985**). "Speech perception ability and psychophysical tuning curves in hearing-impaired listeners," J.Acoust.Soc.Am. **77**, 620-627.

Tyler, R.S. (**1986**). "Frequency resolution in hearing-impaired listeners," in *Frequency Selectivity in Hearing*, edited by B.C.J. Moore (Academic Press, London), pp. 309-371

Tyler, R.S. (**1988**). The psychophysical representation of speech in the peripheral auditory system. J.Phonetics, in press.

Tyler, R.S., and Lindblom, B. (**1982**). "Preliminary study of simultaneous-masking and pulsation-threshold patterns of vowels," J.Acoust.Soc.Am. **71**, 220-224.

Comments

Moore:

There is a problem in using a narrowband noise masker in forward masking, since the subject may lack an effective cue to distinguish the signal from the masker (e.g. Moore and Glasberg, 1985). This problem mainly occurs when the signal frequency is close to the centre frequency of the masker. Thus, the forward-masking pattern obtained with such a masker does not give a direct indication of the internal representation of the masker; the pattern may show a peak simply because the signal is "confused" with the masker when its frequency is close to that of the masker, but is not "confused" with the masker when their center frequencies are sufficiently different. I am also concerned about your assumption that the forward-masking pattern is determined primarily by the last 10-15 ms of the masker. Since the amount of forward masking increases with masker duration up to at least 200 ms, the preceding portions of the masker must play some role. If the portion of the masker 30-40 ms before the signal is closer in frequency to the signal than the portion immediately before the signal, then the earlier part of the masker might well contribute substantially to the masking observed.

Moore, B.C.J. and Glasberg, B.R. (1985). "The danger of using narrow-band noise maskers to measure 'suppresion'," J.Acoust.Soc.Am. 77, 2137-2141.

Reply by Tyler:

The problem you describe occurs when there is a perceptual similarity between the masker and signal. With a tonal signal the problem is greatest for a narrowband noise masker and is minimal for a broadband masker.

The masker used in the present study is unlike any for which you have demonstrated a cueing effect, because in the present study the spectrum is changing over time. "Cueing" effects with these stimuli will have to be addressed experimentally. I can say that for me, the format-transition masker was perceptually very distinct from the tonal signal.

I believe that the forward-masking patterns reflect activity produced by the previous 40-50 ms of the masker, and possibly longer. However I do not agree that the experiments where masker duration is increased are the most relevant here. The study that I cited (Elliot, 1962) varied the interstimulus interval between the masker offset and signal onset. I think this study is more relevant and my recollection is that it suggests that maskers that are within 10-15 ms of the signal will have the largest effect. When the masker and signal are seperated by more than 60 ms, the amount of masking is limited. I would be very surprised if masker components 200 ms earlier than the signal contributed significantly in the present experiment.

Effects of selective outer hair cell lesions on the frequency selectivity of the auditory system

David W. Smith[1], David B. Moody, and William C. Stebbins

Kresge Hearing Research Institute, University of Michigan Medical School, Ann Arbor, Michigan, USA

Introduction

Current notions of outer hair cell (OHC) function suggest a key role in determining both the frequency selectivity and sensitivity of the auditory system (cf., Khanna, 1984). Studies of OHCs in isolation have shed much light on the physiological basis for the process of frequency selectivity, yet these data tell us very little about the role of these processes in the behavior of hearing. While a direct dependence has long been assumed, there have been few demonstrations of the relationship between these physiological mechanisms and hearing, per se.

Dallos *et al.* (1977) measured both individual auditory neuron physiological tuning curves (FTCs) and psychophysical tuning curves (PTCs) in chinchillas with selective OHC loss following kanamycin treatment. Post-drug analyses of hearing from regions with selective damage to OHCs showed broadly tuned FTCs with selective loss of tip tuning. However, the associated PTCs were elevated by approximately 40 dB, yet retained sharp tuning. Dallos and colleagues have suggested that one possible explanation for the differences seen in the behavioral and physiological data is that tuning undergoes additional sharpening beyond the level of the VIIIth nerve.

A similar finding was reported by Nienhuys and Clark (1979), who compared critical bands in cats before and after systemic treatment with kanamycin. Critical bands measured at frequencies corresponding to regions of selective OHC loss were normal. Broadening of critical bands was only realized when OHC loss was accompanied by an IHC loss of greater than 40 percent. Nienhuys and Clark's data agree well with those of Dallos *et al.* (1977) and they, too, conclude that normal frequency selectivity is mediated by IHCs alone.

The behavioral data of Dallos *et al.* (1977) and Nienhuys and Clark (1979), however, are at odds with the physiological data showing losses in frequency

---

[1]Present address: Department of Otolaryngology, University of Toronto, Toronto, Ontario, Canada.

selectivity with loss of normal OHC function (c.f., Liberman and Dodds, 1984). Moreover, they do not agree with the human psychophysical data which show deterioration in frequency resolution associated with hearing losses of cochlear origin (Jesteadt, 1980; Wightman *et al.*, 1977).

The data to be reported here are from recent studies that help define the role of the OHC in determining the frequency selectivity of the auditory system. These studies take advantage of the unique reactivity of the aminoglycoside antibiotic dihydrostreptomycin (DHSM) in the patas monkey (Stebbins, Moody, Hawkins and Norat, 1987). In the patas monkey, DHSM produces a progressive loss of OHCs over large regions of the organ of Corti while leaving the IHCs relatively unaffected. The psychophysical tuning curve, the behavioral analog of the physiological tuning curve, was used as the index of frequency selectivity. Since the PTC is an indicator of normal cochlear function, describing both sensitivity and selectivity characteristics of the filter process, changes in these measures in response to controlled pathology can tell us much about the role of the damaged receptors in normal auditory processing.

Methods

The following experiments were performed in order to ascertain the effects of alterations of OHC function on a behavioral measure of auditory sensitivity and frequency selectivity. Complete descriptions of these techniques can be found in the literature (Smith, Moody, Stebbins and Norat, 1987). Briefly, steady and pulsed-tone thresholds were measured at half-octaves from 63 Hz to 40 kHz. Psychophysical tuning curves were also measured at frequencies of 500 Hz, 2, 4, and 8 kHz at the probe tone level of 10 dB SL. Tuning curves at 2, 4, and 8 kHz were also measured at probe-tone levels of 30 and 60 dB SL. Following collection of stable baseline data, the animals received dihydrostreptomycin-sulfate at 20 mg/kg/day until a hearing loss was evident at 16 kHz, whereupon treatments were discontinued. Post-drug threshold and PTC measurements were continued until the data showed no further changes for 30 days. The animals were then sacrificed and ears taken for histological examination.

Results

While the extent and time course of the hearing loss and range of affected frequencies varied from subject to subject, the systematic changes seen in PTCs measured from regions of OHC loss are in agreement for all subjects and all frequencies where a shift in threshold was evident.

Of the four subjects in these studies, two showed very slow progressive hearing losses with similar patterns of receptor lesions (M-155 and M-157); the third (M-156) showed a very rapid loss of sensitivity, although the extent of cochlear damage was similar to M-155 and M-157; and the fourth (M-154) required substantially longer drug treatment to produce an initial loss of sensitivity, and subsequently experienced a significantly greater loss of both outer and inner hair cells. All four animals showed identical systematic changes in tuning function. To illustrate the main findings, data from only one of these subjects will be discussed in detail.

A potential confounding factor in using the PTC to analyze functional changes in pathological cochleae is the dependence of PTC shape upon the absolute level at which measurements are taken (Nelson and Freyman, 1984; Smith, Moody, and Stebbins, 1987). Tuning curves broaden as the absolute level of the signal is increased. Since a loss of OHCs is associated with a 40-60 dB increase in threshold, post-drug measurement levels will necessarily be higher than those prior to drug administration. To serve as comparisons, therefore, tuning curves measured at levels of 30 and 60 dB SL are also presented to help differentiate the effects of signal level from the effects of the pathological changes.

Figure 1 presents the final audiogram (lower panel) and cytocochleogram (upper panel), plotted as percent remaining hair cells as a function of distance

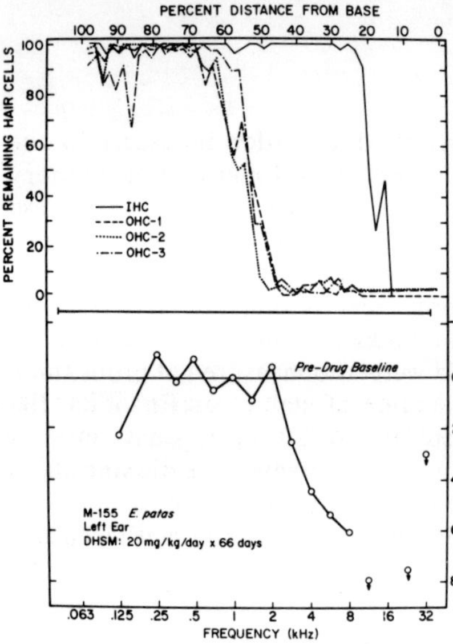

Figure 1. Cytocochleogram (upper panel) for M-155, plotted as percent remaining hair cells as a function of distance along the basilar membrane from the base. Corresponding final audiogram (lower panel) is given as steady-tone threshold shift as a function of frequency. Actual length of basilar membrane, 22.59 mm.

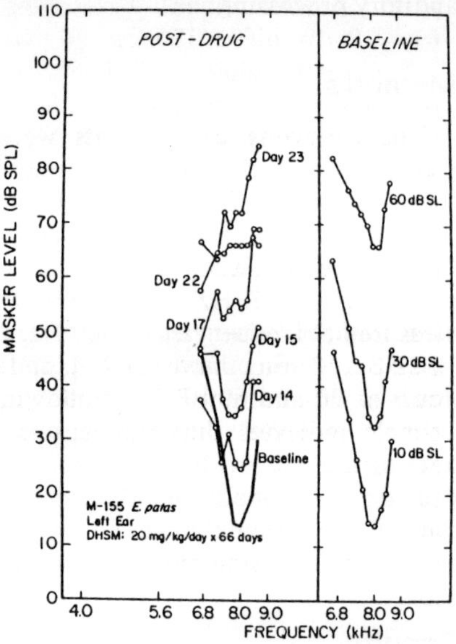

Figure 2. Systematic progression of changes in 8 kHz PTC for M-155 measured on various days post-drug (left panel). Normal PTCs measured at 10, 30, and 60 dB SL (right panel).

along the basilar membrane from the base, for subject M-155. Histologic evaluation of the organ of Corti for this subject showed an absence of IHCs in the basal-most 15% of the cochlea with a sharp transition to nearly complete retention of IHCs throughout the remaining apical 80% of the basilar membrane. Light microscopic evaluation of remaining IHCs revealed normal-appearing cells in which stereocilia were present and of normal shape and arrangement, the cell body was of normal shape and size, and there was no evidence of vacuolization within the cell. The OHCs were absent from the basal half of the cochlea with a transition to nearly normal populations in the apical 50% of the organ of Corti. The result of this pattern of hair cell loss was a region with normal IHCs and devoid of OHCs over approximately one-third of the basilar membrane.

As can be seen in the lower panel of Figure 1, threshold shifts were tonotopically related to regions of hair cell loss. Losses of 20 to 60 dB were evident at frequencies between 2.8 and 8 kHz, corresponding to the regions of selective OHC loss. Increases in threshold above 8 kHz were so large as to preclude measurement. Thresholds were normal at 2 kHz and below, except for a 20-dB shift at 125 Hz.

Progressive changes in 8 kHz tuning curves from M-155, as a function of time post drug, can be seen in the left panel of Figure 2. The initial changes in tuning-curve shape were reliably seen as two distinct phenomena. The first was observed as an elevation and shift of the characteristic frequency (CF) toward lower frequencies. Elevations of the PTC tip of up to 50 dB were associated with either no change, or a hypersensitivity, in the low-frequency tail. For example, at days 14, 15, and 17, the tuning curve tip was elevated by more than 40 dB, yet the low-frequency tail at 6.8 kHz was either at, or was less than, baseline values. By days 22 and 23, the plot was elevated by nearly 60 dB and resembled a low-pass filter. Comparisons of pathological tuning curves with normal PTCs recorded in the same subject at similar SPLs (right panel) indicates that the lack of tuning in post-drug PTCs cannot be accounted for on the basis of increases in measurement level. Changes in tuning brought on by increases in SPLs were a decrease in tip-to-tail depth and a broadening of the filter function. In contrast, PTCs underwent a complete detuning and transition from bandpass to low-pass function with a loss of OHCs.

Figure 3 presents the progressive changes in 4 kHz PTCs for M-155. Data averaged across days 36-39 showed a 30-dB loss of sensitivity and a shift of CF toward lower frequencies, while a hypersensitivity was present in the low-frequency tail. At day 40, the PTC tip was elevated by over 40 dB and yet little effect was seen in the low-frequency tail. By day 41, with a 50-dB increase in tip threshold, an elevation of the low-frequency tail was apparent. Since masking functions were not measured at SPLs of greater than 110 dB, the magnitude of the threshold shifts prevented assessment of high-frequency tail function above 4.4 kHz. However, extrapolation from the 4.2 kHz masker at 85 dB SPL, to these higher levels at 4.4 kHz, yields a low-pass filter function. Again, comparisons of normal PTCs at 10, 30, and 60 dB SL

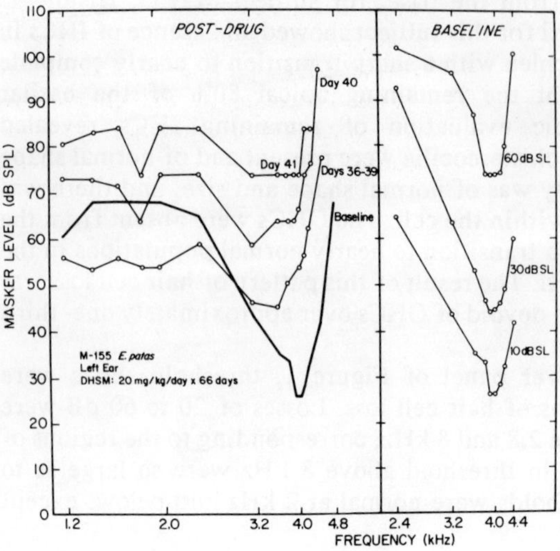

Figure 3. Systematic changes in 4 kHz PTC for M-155 measured on various days post-drug (left panel). Normal PTCs for same subject at 10, 30, and 60 dB SL (right panel).

(right panel) and pathological tuning curves at roughly equivalent SPLs failed to explain these changes on the basis of increases in test signal levels. Even at the highest test level of 60 dB SL, the normal PTCs retained sharp bandpass function. However, this property was rapidly lost with increases in threshold associated with loss of OHC function.

Discussion

For purposes of simplifying discussion of the role of various processes upon psychophysical frequency selectivity, the general phenomena evident in the data from the four subjects have been incorporated into idealized PTCs presented in Figure 4. Changes associated with OHC loss are depicted in the left panel. For purposes of comparison, similar idealized data are presented in the right panel for changes in PTC shape associated with changes in absolute measurement levels. Subsequent discussions will refer to this figure.

When comparisons are made of normal PTCs taken at high signal levels (right panel), with pathological PTCs taken at roughly equivalent SPLs (left panel), it becomes immediately obvious that the changes in PTCs following OHC loss cannot be accounted for on the basis of increased measurement levels. Following systemic drug treatment, tuning curves undergo a rapid increase in threshold and nearly complete detuning in response to OHC loss. In the present study, this transition from low-threshold sharply-tuned PTC to high-threshold low-pass filter can only be explained as a change in the tuning mechanism brought on by loss of OHC function.

In these studies, increases in threshold were invariably followed by a rapid and nearly complete loss of psychophysical tuning. The rate of increase in threshold varied across frequency and length of time post-drug, but could be

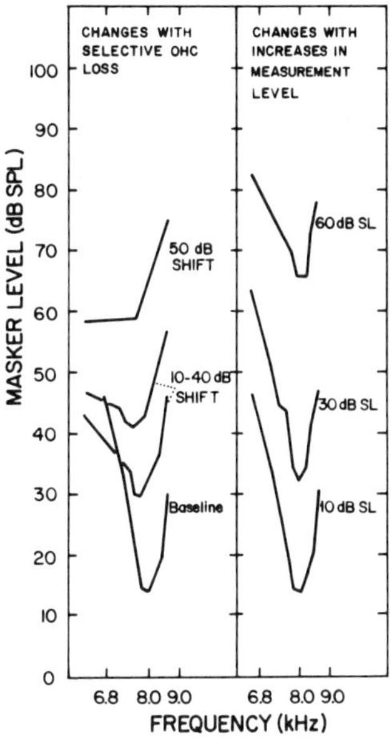

Figure 4. Idealized PTCs for changes associated with selective loss of OHCs (left panel). Idealized PTCs for changes associated with increases in measurement level (right panel).

as rapid as 10-20 dB/day. The pattern of change in tuning was systematic and entirely dependent upon threshold and is, therefore, presumably a function of orderly alterations in the processing mechanism.

As seen in the idealized PTCs presented in the left panel of Figure 4, with increases of up to 40 dB, there was a selective elevation and broadening of the tip region in the PTC response. The CF was also shifted toward lower frequencies. The slope of the high-frequency tail remained relatively constant, yet was elevated in a more or less linear fashion with increases in threshold at CF. Following threshold shifts of greater than 50 dB, the tip response was completely absent and the filter took on low-pass characteristics. As can be seen from comparisons of the cytocochleograms and corresponding final audiograms, threshold shifts to both steady and pulsed tones were on the order of 40-60 dB at frequencies corresponding to regions completely lacking OHCs. This suggests that the final transition of the PTC to low-pass filter function concomitant with threshold shifts of greater than 40-50 dB is a result of complete removal of OHC influence. The orderly covariation of threshold and tuning implies a common origin for both processes at the level of the OHC.

The results of these studies are in both qualitative and quantitative agreement with the data from previous physiological studies, indicating the dependence of the sensitivity and sharply tuned response of the FTC on normal OHC function. Temporary or permanent inhibition or alteration of outer hair cell activity results in a filter lacking a sharply-tuned tip. In the extreme, these anomalous filter functions resemble low-pass filters. It is likely that this residual low-pass tuning seen following complete degeneration of OHCs in both the behavioral and physiological responses reflects the passive mechanical interactions of the basilar membrane and surrounding fluids. Because of the remarkable similarity of FTCs and PTCs in both normal and pathological ears, it is suggested that those processes which determine the tuning of the auditory system as a whole are peripheral phenomena.

The psychophysical data presented here corroborate suggestions of Evans (1975), Evans and Wilson (1973), and Khanna (1984), that the observed physiological filter function is a composite of two interacting processes, the first being a low-pass filter process dependent upon the passive mechanical properties of the basilar membrane and dynamics of the surrounding fluids. This mechanical system is relatively immune to trauma. The second process, the so-called "second filter", is a sharply tuned response near the high-frequency cutoff of the first filter. This active process reflects the function of the OHC subsystem which is demonstrably physiologically labile.

PTC low-frequency tail response to selective lesions of OHC

The data also indicate that moderate increases in threshold at CF produce a hypersensitivity in the response of the low-frequency tail of the PTC. This increase in sensitivity, which always accompanies a hyposensitivity of the tip response, is similar to that recently observed by Liberman and Dodds (1984) in single-unit FTCs arising from identified IHCs innervating areas of selective OHC damage or loss. Zwislocki (1984) suggests that a disruption in the normal shearing motion between the tectorial and basilar membranes, caused by depletion of OHCs, explains this finding. Since these same processes form the basis for psychophysical frequency selectivity, he suggests this same hypersensitivity should be obtainable in psychophysical tuning curves. These data, showing an increase in sensitivity at the low-frequency tail accompanying increases in threshold of 10-40 dB, indicating initial selective insult to OHCs, probably represent this same phenomena.

Acknowledgements

We would like to thank Dr. Richard Altschuler and the Otopathology Laboratory at Kresge Hearing Research Institute for their skilled histological preparations. We also wish to thank Charlotte Lieser for her assistance in the preparation of this manuscript. Research funded by NIH grant #NS-05785 and a Horace H. Rackham Graduate School Dissertation Grant to DWS. This manuscript was prepared while DWS was an NINCDS Institutional Post-Doctoral Fellow at Boys Town National Institute.

References

Dallos, P., Ryan, A., Harris, D., McGee, T. and Ozdamer, O. (1977). "Cochlear frequency selectivity in the presence of hair-cell damage," in *Psychophysics and Physiology of Hearing*, edited by E.F. Evans and J.P. Wilson (Academic Press, New York), pp. 249-258.

Evans, E.F. (**1975**). "The sharpening of cochlear frequency selectivity in the normal and abnormal cochlea," Audiology **14**, 197-201.

Evans, E.F. and Wilson, J.P. (**1973**). "The frequency selectivity of the cochlea," in *Basic Mechanisms of Hearing*, edited by A.R. Moller (Academic Press, New York), pp. 519-551.

Jesteadt, W. (**1980**). "Frequency analysis in normal and hearing-impaired listeners," Ann.Otol.Rhinol.Laryngol. **89**, 88-95.

Khanna, S.M. (**1984**). "Inner ear function based on the mechanical tuning of the hair cells," in *Hearing Science: Recent Advances* edited by C.I. Berlin (College Hill Press, San Diego), pp. 213-239.

Liberman, M.C. and Dodds, L.W. (**1984**). "Single-neuron labeling and chronic cochlear pathology. III: Stereocilia damage and alteration of threshold tuning curves," Hearing Res. **16**, 55-74.

Nelson, D.A. and Freyman, R.L. (**1984**). "Broadened forward-masked tuning curves from intense masking tones: Delay-time and probe-level manipulations," J.Acoust.Soc.Am. **75**, 1570-1577.

Nienhuys, T.G.W. and Clark, G.M. (**1979**). "Critical bands following the selective destruction of cochlear inner and outer hair cells," Acta Otolaryngol. **88**, 350-358.

Smith, D.W., Moody, D.B. and Stebbins, W.C. (**1987**). "Effects of changes in absolute signal level on psychophysical tuning curves in quiet and noise in patas monkeys," J.Acoust.Soc.Am. **82**, 63-68.

Smith, D.W., Moody, D.B., Stebbins, W.C. and Norat, M.A. (**1987**). "Effects of outer hair cell loss on the frequency selectivity of the patas monkey auditory system," Hearing Res. **29**, 125-138.

Stebbins, W.C., Moody, D.B., Hawkins, J.E. jr., and Norat, M. (**1986**). "The species-specific nature of the ototoxicity of dihydrostreptomycin in the patas monkey," J.Neurotoxicol. **8**, 33-44.

Wightman, F.L., McGee, T. and Kramer, M. (**1977**). "Factors influencing frequency selectivity in normal and hearing-impaired listeners," in *Psychophysics and Physiology of Hearing* edited by E.F. Evans and J.P. Wilson (Academic Press, New York), pp. 295-306.

Zwislocki, J.J. (**1984**). "How OHC lesions can lead to neural cochlear hypersensitivity," Acta Otolaryngol. **97**, 529-534.

Comments

Evans:

Did you examine the afferents to the apparently intact inner hair cells? C.M. Hackeny and D. Furness (unpublished data) in our group have demonstrated swollen afferent terminals on IHC's in guinea pigs poisoned with Kanamycin, using the same regime (400 mg/kg/day × 8 days) that Harrison and I used to show determination in cochlear nerve fibre frequency selectivity related to apparently selective OHC loss (Evans and Harrison, 1976). It is not, of course, clear how this could affect frequency selectivity, but we may need to be cautious.

Evans, E.F. & Harrison, R.V. (1976). "Correlation between outer hair cell damage and deterioration of cochlear nerve tuning properties in the guinea pig." J. Physiol. 256, 43-44P.

Reply by Smith et al.:

I agree with your suggestion of caution. Any model of selective OHC loss must show that the IHC and, for that matter, the remainder of the ear remains otherwise normal. We have looked quite carefully at the remaining IHC's and they appear morphologically normal in every respect. However, we have not examined the afferent terminals in any detail. As you point out, given current conceptions of IHC function, it is unclear how these swellings might have any effect on selectivity.

One piece of our data might have some relevance, though. One of our animals (M-154) required a substantially longer drug treatment to produce an initial shift in threshold and, consequently, produced an approximate 50% loss of IHC's throughout most of the organ of Corti. Yet, when compared to the other three subjects with all IHCs present, there were no differences in either day to day systematic changes in tuning or in final post-drug selectivity measurements, i.e. the behavioural tuning correlated with presence/absence of OHC. The ability of the residual tuning to "survive" a loss of 50% of IHC's suggests to us that the IHC's **alone** contribute very little or nothing to the tuning process. This, of course, is consistent with the physiological data and with most current modelling efforts.

Another point is that since DHSM was obviously circulated throughout the entire cochlea, yet we showed post-drug was unaffected at low frequencies, i.e. 500 H_3 and 2 KH_3 PTCs for M-155 overlay baseline functions. Had DHSM produced some non-specific pathology, in afferouts they should have been apparent there.

Abnormal two-sound interactions in hydropic cochleas of the guinea pig

Y. Cazals and K. Horner

Laboratoire d'Audiologie expérimentale, Inserm unité 229, Université Bordeaux II, Hôpital Pellegrin, 33076 Bordeaux, France.

Introduction

Endolymphatic hydrops is a peculiar anatomo-pathology which has been observed in human temporal bones of patients who presented various diseases such as meningitis, syphilis, otosclerosis but was seen most often associated with Ménière's disease (Hallpike and Cairns, 1938; Schucknecht and Gulya, 1983; Paparella, 1984). An experimental hydrops can be induced in various mammals by the surgical blockage of the endolymphatic duct (Kimura and Schucknecht, 1965). This technique has been used quite often to perform anatomical studies but much less often to study physiological alterations. In recent electrophysiological experiments on the guinea pig we have shown a progressive and fluctuating threshold elevation closely resembling the typical evolution of Ménière's disease (Horner and Cazals, 1987). Indeed in a first period of about three months, thresholds at the low and middle frequencies, below 8 kHz, fluctuate by up to 25 dB within a few days and losses at the very high frequencies also develop (Fig.1); then in the following months losses occur at all frequencies and the audiogram becomes flat at 50-60 dB SPL and deteriorates progressively. We also observed that at the period of selective threshold elevation at low and middle frequencies eighth nerve compound responses at threshold for these frequencies can show abrupt latency decreases bringing them as short as those for the high frequencies (see Fig. 1) thus suggesting that they could originate from the base of the cochlea (Horner and Cazals, 1987). It was the aim of this study to investigate whether these abrupt modifications in temporal cochlear excitation were associated with altered tonotopic excitation.

An altered tonotopic cochlear excitation has been speculated at least fourty years ago (de Maré, 1948) to occur in pathological ears and still remains a matter of debate on perceptive anomalies (Thornton and Abbas, 1980; Turner *et al.*, 1983; Burns and Turner, 1986) and to our knowledge there is no physiological evidence to settle the matter. Experimental hydrops is one of the rare ways of obtaining an animal model of selective low and middle frequency loss (see also Aran and Cazals, 1978) and appeared particularly

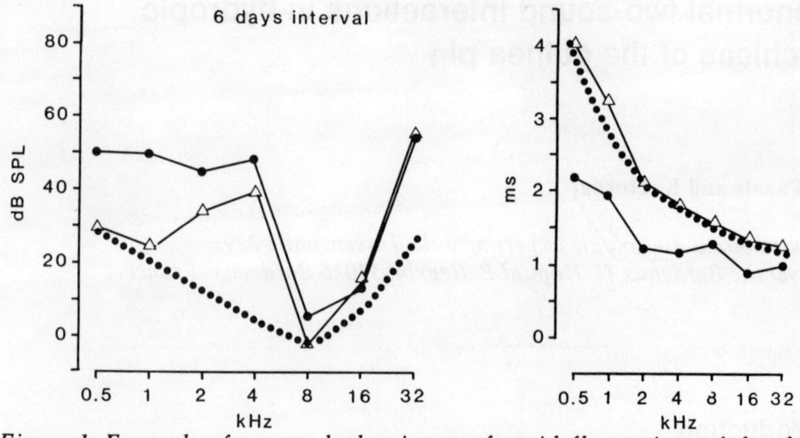

Figure 1. Examples from one hydropic ear of rapid fluctuations of threshold (left) and of latencies at threshold (right) obtained one day (open triangles) and 6 days later (black circles) in comparison with reference curves from control ears (dotted lines).

interesting for physiological investigations of altered tonotopy. In this perspective experiments on patterns of simultaneous masking with high-pass noise and pure tones were performed on hydropic ears of guinea pigs presenting the various audiograms and latency modifications occuring during the development of hydrops.

High-pass masking

The basic principle and the use of the high-pass masking technique were first experimentally illustrated on 8th nerve compound action potential by Teas *et al.* (1962) and its validity and limitations to frequencies above about 1-2 kHz were shown on single fibers responses by Evans and Elberling (1982). Since the objective in this study was to mask frequencies above about 6 kHz the technique appeared quite appropriate.

Guinea pigs were chronically implanted with an electrode on the round window and some weeks later operated for hydrops induction. Then over several months their compound action potential audiograms were regularly measured together with the associated response latencies using tone pips of 2 ms rise/fall time. At various times post-operation animals presenting the typical CAP audiogram and latency patterns as indicated above were tested. A high-pass masking noise with a frequency cut-off set at 6.4 kHz was presented continuously at various intensity levels and the CAP audiograms were measured.

Data obtained from control ears and from different pathological ears are presented in Fig.2. When the audiogram showed a sensitivity loss at low and middle frequencies and normal latencies at threshold (upper right quadrant)

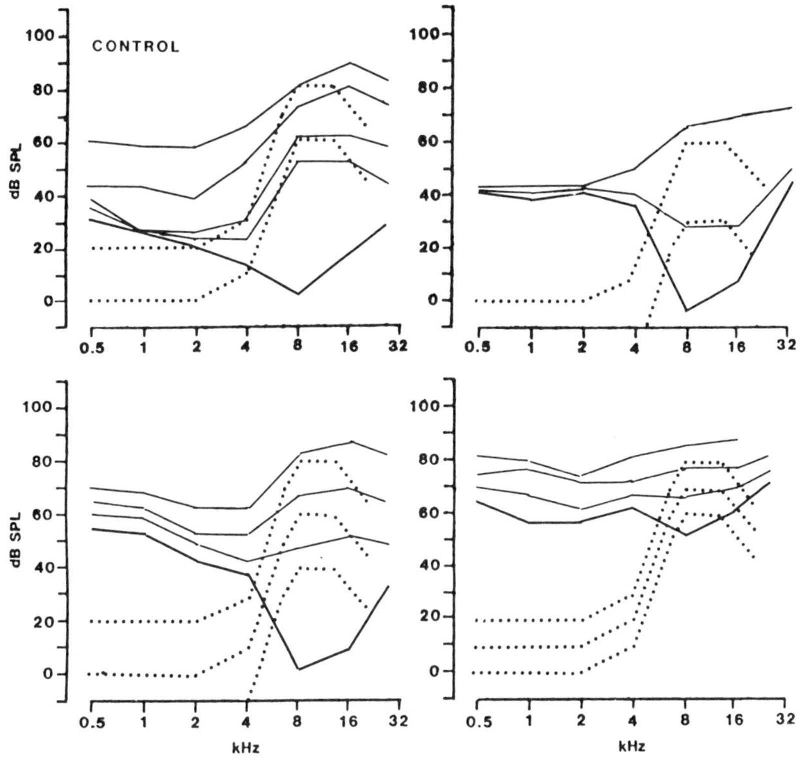

Figure 2. Audiograms obtained under continuous masking with high-pass noise (spectrum shown in dotted lines) at different intensities for a control (upper left) and three hydropic ears presenting various threshold curves (continuous lines at the bottom of each graph).

the high-pass noise increased thresholds at high frequencies without affecting frequencies below 4 kHz. When the latencies were short (lower left quadrant) the high-pass noise affected thresholds at all frequencies. When the audiogram was flat, and latencies short (lower right quadrant), the high-pass noise also affected threshold at all frequencies. However in control animals (upper left quadrant) when the noise was set at the same high levels (i.e. above 60 dB SPL in 30 Hz band) so that the 8 kHz threshold was elevated above 60 dB SPL, thresholds at the lower frequencies were also elevated. The observations on pathological ears appear therefore normal which prevents any clear-cut conclusion as to the tonotopic source of these low and middle frequency responses.

Tuning and interaction curves

It was then reasoned that if a low-mid frequency stimulates the base of the cochlea it should, when presented simultaneously with a high frequency pip, produce some masking on the response evoked by the latter. Or inversely a high frequency tone should produce some masking on responses to low or middle frequency pips. Since partial masking could be expected the evoked response to a tone pip alone was first recorded from which was then subtracted the response to the same tone pip with the simultaneous presentation of a continuous masking tone. Experiments on control animals showed that such waveform subtractions allowed the detection of derived CAP as small as about 15 microvolts and permitted to draw what we call interaction curves. In the same conditions we also measured the classical tuning curves corresponding to total masking (Dallos and Cheatham, 1976).

Data obtained from control and pathological ears are presented in Fig.3. Examples from a control ear of tuning curves for total masking and interaction curves are shown (upper row of Fig.3) for various stimuli at different levels high enough to compare directly with pathological ears. The tuning curves are quite similar to those reported previously (Dallos and Cheatham, 1976; Cazals *et al.*, 1982). The family of interaction curves for tone pips at about 60 dB SPL showed some broad frequency selectivity with thresholds of interactions close to absolute thresholds. In line with the aim of this study it should be noted in particular that for normal ears in the response to a 2 kHz tone pip at 60 dB SPL interactions can be detected with pure tones of 4 and 8 kHz at threshold i.e. at 10 or 0 dB SPL.

Results from hydropic ears showed that tuning for total masking was not significantly modified: for several ears showing the various types of audiogram, tuning curves were quite similar to those obtained, at the same level in dB SPL, in control ears. As concerns interaction curves, when thresholds at the high frequencies were normal or near normal but latencies at threshold for the low or middle frequencies were short (middle row of Fig. 3), in the response to a 8-kHz pip close to its threshold (10 dB SPL) interaction was detected with a 4-kHz and 2-kHz pure tones at 55 and 60 dB SPL. However, in the response to a 2-kHz pip or a 4-kHz pip slightly above threshold, i.e. about 60 dB SPL, no interaction was detected with an 8 kHz pure tone until its intensity was raised to about 60 dB SPL. When the audiogram was slightly elevated at 8 kHz the interaction level of a pure tone at 8 kHz with the low frequency pips decreased. These results indicate that some interactions are considerably reduced in hydropic ears since tone pips of 2 or 4 kHz do not appear to excite the base of the cochlea to the same extent as in normal ears. When the audiogram was flat with all thresholds above 60 dB SPL (lower row of Fig.3), tuning and interaction curves were found to differ considerably between different ears.

The absence of interaction in the response to a 2-kHz pip of an 8-kHz pure tone seems to be in contradiction with the existence of an interaction of a 2-kHz pure tone in the response to an 8-kHz pip. The difference between the

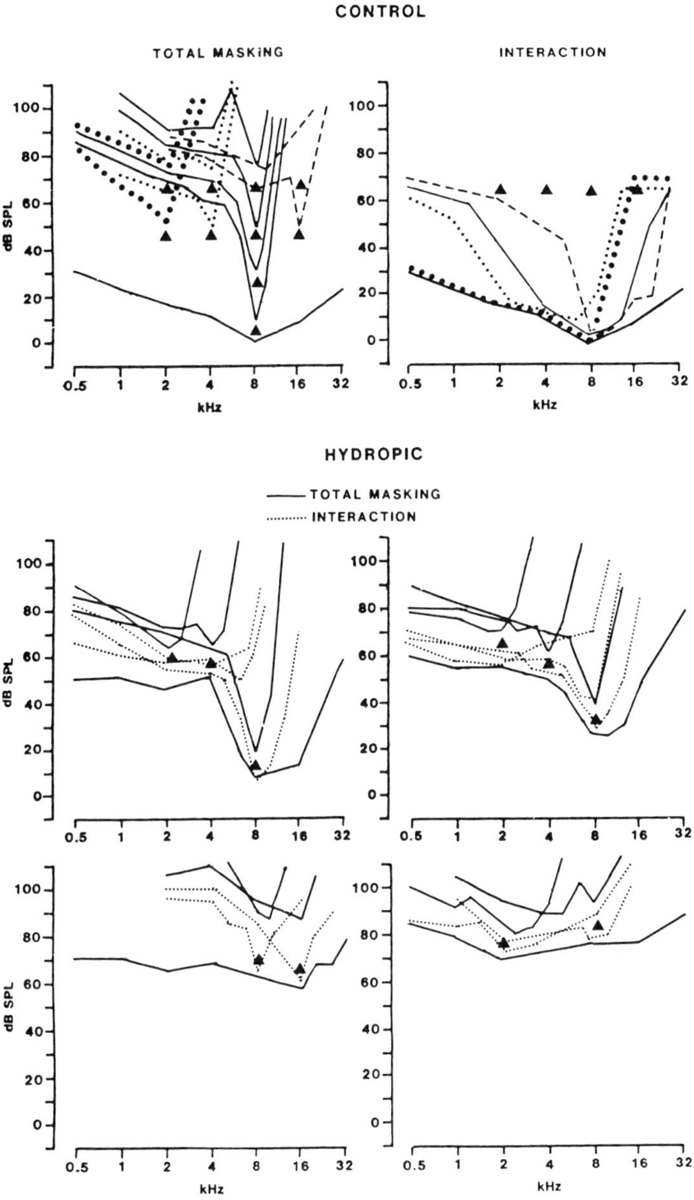

Figure 3. Tuning curves for total masking and interaction curves for a control and four hydropic ears. presenting different audiograms (continuous line at the bottom of each graph).

two conditions being only the duration of stimuli, and assuming that the 8 kHz stimulus just above threshold stimulates only a limited basal part of the cochlea, the observed difference certainly reflects differences in cochlear excitation of the base between the steady state and the impulse stimulation at 2 kHz.

Pure tone masked audiograms

Abnormal spread of masking has often been reported for pathological ears (see Tyler, 1986 for a review). In this study tuning curves showed some abnormal broadening only when the audiogram was flat. We therefore checked further for abnormal spread of masking by investigating the masking patterns of pure tones at different times during the evolution of hearing sensitivity loss in hydropic ears. The results obtained are shown in Fig.4. In

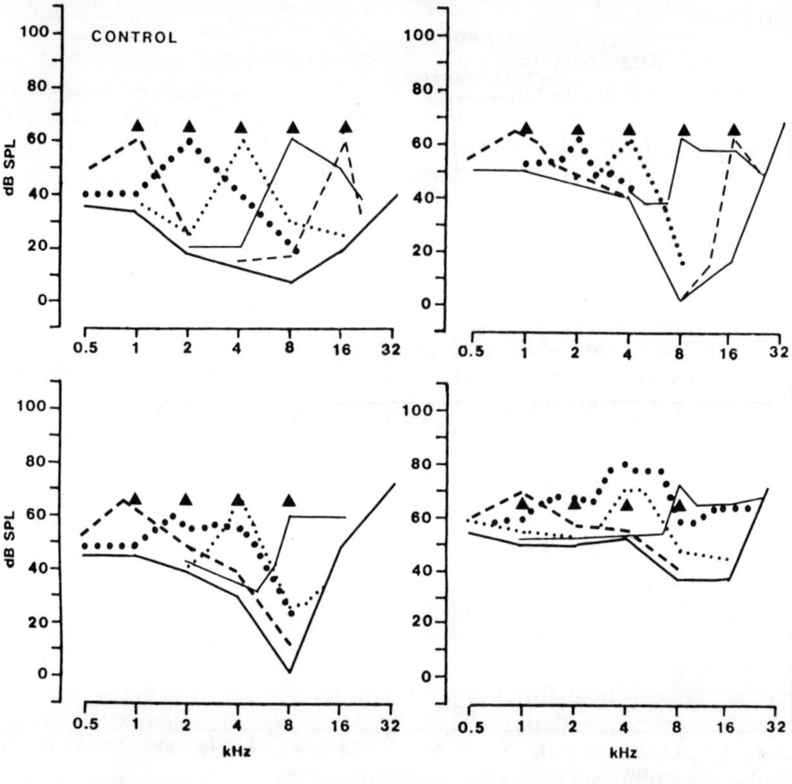

Figure 4. Masking curves of pure tones in a control and three hydropic ears with various audiograms (continuous line at the bottom of each graph).

control ears pure tone masking patterns always showed a clear peak at the frequency of the masker (upper left quadrant) but the broadness of the peak varied considerably between different animals. In hydropic ears it can be seen that when thresholds at the low and middle frequencies are elevated (upper right and lower left quadrants) the masking patterns are quite similar to those observed in control ears. Results presented in the lower left quadrant show some spread of masking toward the high frequencies in particular for the 2 kHz tone but similar masking patterns could also be observed in some control ears. When thresholds started to be elevated at all frequencies (lower right quadrant) an abnormal masking for the 2 kHz tone affecting more the thresholds around 4 kHz was found whereas no obvious anomaly was observed for other frequencies. In a later stage when the audiogram was flat with all thresholds at 60 dB SPL or more the masking patterns for all tones appeared very broad.

Discussion

The overall data from this study do not support the hypothesis of an abnormal tonotopic excitation of the base of the cochlea by the low or middle frequencies when the sensitivity loss affects exclusively frequencies below about 8 kHz. Indeed they indicate the contrary that the low and middle frequencies when presented as impulse stimuli do not excite the base of the cochlea to the same extent as they do in normal ears. The abnormal interactions described in the present study could be a consequence of the presence of hydrops throughout the cochlea including the base (Kimura, 1967) which does not affect absolute thresholds for the high frequencies. The difference in response of the base between the steady state and the impulse stimuli revealed in this study give grounds for our interpretation of some clinical results from our laboratory. Indeed it was shown that glycerol administration to Ménière's patients, presumably reducing temporarily the hydrops, could result in changes of basal responses to tone bursts of low but not of high frequencies (Dauman *et al.*, 1986).

Assuming that the low frequency responses do arise from their tonotopic location, then the atrophy of the short and middle stereocilia of the outer hair cells which is primarily seen in the upper cochlear turns (Horner *et al.*, 1988), probably underlies the abnormal fluctuant, short latency responses. The data of the present study are in agreement with psychoacoustic investigations of altered tonotopic excitation in various cases of low frequency hearing loss which showed less disturbance than could be predicted (Turner *et al.*, 1983). The reduced interactions for brief stimuli in early stages of hydrops together with the later spread of masking, could be at the origin of some distortions in auditory perception known to occur in Ménière's disease (Hood, 1983). In particular the alterations of the 2 kHz region may be more specifically related to deficiencies in speech perception (Lindeman, 1971).

In conclusion we hypothetise that in hydropic ears the swelling of scala media alters the cochlear mechanics for low and middle frequencies at all cochlear turns, whereas changes of hair cells tufts are responsible for tonotopically related deficiencies.

Acknowledgements

The authors gratefully acknowledge the financial support of the Fondation de France and EPR Aquitaine.

References

Aran, J-M. and Cazals, Y. (**1978**) "Electrocochleography : animal experiments," in *Evoked electrical activity in the auditory nervous system*, edited by R.F. Naunton and C. Fernandez, (Academic, New York), pp 239-257.

Burns, E.M. and Turner C. (**1986**) "Pure-tone pitch anomalies. II. Pitch-intensity effects and diplacusis in impaired ears," J.Acoust.Soc.Am. 79, 1530-1540.

Cazals, Y. Aran, J-M. and Erre J-P. (**1982**) "Frequency sensitivity and selectivity of acoustically evoked potentials after complete cochlear hair cell destruction," Brain Res. **231**, 197-203.

Dallos, P. and Cheatham M.A. (**1976**) "Compound action potential (AP) tuning curves," J.Acoust.Soc.Am. **59**, 591-597.

Dauman, R., Aran, J-M. and Portmann, M. (**1986**) "Summating potential and water balance in ménière's disease," Ann.Otol.Rhinol.Laryngol., **95**, 389-395.

de Marè, G. (**1948**). "Investigations into the functions of the auditory apparatus in perception deafness," Acta Oto-laryngol. Suppl. **74**, 107-116.

Evans, E.F. and Elberling C. (**1982**) "Location-specific components of the gross cochlear action potential," Int.Audiol. **21**, 204-227.

Hallpike, C. and Cairns, H. (**1938**) "Observations on the pathology of Ménière's syndrome," J.Laryngol.Otol. **63**, 625-655.

Hood, J.D. (**1983**) "Audiology," in *Ménière's disease: a comprehensive appraisal*, edited by W.J.Oosterveld (John Wiley and sons) pp 35-53.

Horner, K.C. and Cazals, Y. (**1987**) "Rapidly fluctuating thresholds at the onset of experimentally induced hydrops in the guinea pig," Hearing Res. **26**, 319-326.

Horner, K.C., Guilhaume, A. and Cazals, Y. (**1988**) "Atrophy of middle and short stereocilia on outer hair cells of guinea pigs's cochleas with experimental hydrops." Hearing Res. **32**, 41-48.

Kimura, R.S. (**1967**) "Experimental blockage of the endolymphatic duct and sac and it's effect on the inner ear of the guinea pig. A study on endolymphatic hydrops." Ann.Otol.Rhinol.Laryngol. **76**, 665-687.

Kimura, R.S. and Schucknecht H.F. (**1965**) "Membranous hydrops of the inner ear of the guinea pig after obliteration of the endolymphatic sac," Pract.Otorhinolaryngol. **27**, 343-354.

Lindeman H.E. (**1971**) "Relations between audiological findings and complaints by persons suffering from noise-induced hearing loss," Am. Ind.Hyg.Assoc. **32**, 447.

Paparella, M.M. (**1984**) "Pathology of Meniere's disease," Ann.Otol.Rhinol. Laryngol. Suppl. **112**, 31-35.

Schucknecht, H.F. and Gulya, A.J. (**1983**) "Endolymphatic hydrops an overview and classification," Ann.Otol.Rhinol.Laryngol. **92**, 1-20.

Teas, D., Eldredge, D. and Davis H. (**1962**) "Cochlear responses to acoustic transients : an interpretation of whole nerve action potentials," J.Acoust. Soc.Am. **34**, 1438-1459.

Thornton, A.R and Abbas, P.J. (**1980**) "Low frequency hearing loss: perception of filtered speech, psychophysical tuning curves, and masking," J.Acoust.Soc.Am. **67**, 638-643.

Turner, C., Burns, E.M. and Nelson, D.A. (**1983**) "Pure tone pitch perception and low-frequency hearing loss," J.Acoust.Soc.Am. **73**, 966-975.

Tyler, R.S. (**1986**) "Frequency resolution in hearing impaired listeners," in *Frequency selectivity in hearing*, editor B.C.J. Moore (Academic, London) pp 309-171.

Permuted title index